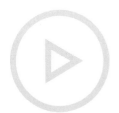

IMPORTANT:

HERE IS YOUR REGISTRATION CODE TO ACCESS
YOUR PREMIUM McGRAW-HILL ONLINE RESOURCES.

MCGRAW-HILL
ONLINE RESOURCES

For key premium online resources you need THIS CODE to gain access. Once the code is entered, you will be able to use the Web resources for the length of your course.

If your course is using **WebCT** or **Blackboard**, you'll be able to use this code to access the McGraw-Hill content within your instructor's online course.

Access is provided if you have purchased a new book. If the registration code is missing from this book, the registration screen on our Website, and within your WebCT or Blackboard course, will tell you how to obtain your new code.

Registering for McGraw-Hill Online Resources

TO gain access to your McGraw-Hill web resources simply follow the steps below:

1. USE YOUR WEB BROWSER TO GO TO: http://www.mhhe.com/medicalassisting,2/e
2. CLICK ON **FIRST TIME USER**.
3. ENTER THE REGISTRATION CODE* PRINTED ON THE TEAR-OFF BOOKMARK ON THE RIGHT.
4. AFTER YOU HAVE ENTERED YOUR REGISTRATION CODE, CLICK **REGISTER**.
5. FOLLOW THE INSTRUCTIONS TO SET-UP YOUR PERSONAL UserID AND PASSWORD.
6. WRITE YOUR UserID AND PASSWORD DOWN FOR FUTURE REFERENCE. KEEP IT IN A SAFE PLACE.

TO GAIN ACCESS to the McGraw-Hill content in your instructor's **WebCT** or **Blackboard** course simply log in to the course with the UserID and Password provided by your instructor. Enter the registration code exactly as it appears in the box to the right when prompted by the system. You will only need to use the code the first time you click on McGraw-Hill content.

Thank you, and welcome to your McGraw-Hill online Resources!

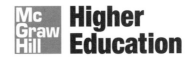

REGISTRATION CODE

Registration code no longer necessary.

Mc Graw Hill **Higher Education**

* YOUR REGISTRATION CODE CAN BE USED ONLY ONCE TO ESTABLISH ACCESS. IT IS NOT TRANSFERABLE.
ISBN-13: 978-0-07-297145-3
ISBN-10: 0-07-297145-2 T/A Medical Assisting, 2/e

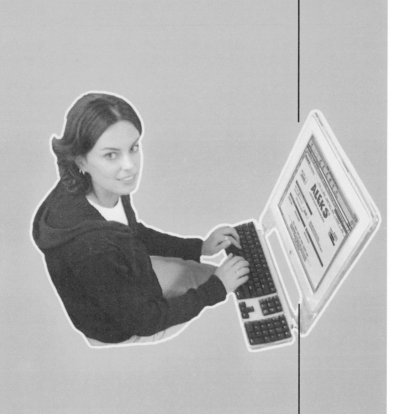

SECOND EDITION

ADMINISTRATIVE PROCEDURES

for Medical Assisting

Barbara Ramutkowski, RN, BSN
Pima Medical Institute
Tucson, Arizona

Kathryn A. Booth, RN, MS
Total Care Programming and Wildwood Medical Clinic
Henrico, North Carolina

Donna Jeanne Pugh, RN, BSN
Florida Metropolitan University
Jacksonville, Florida

Sharion K. Thompson, BS, AAB, RMA, CPT
Sanford Brown Institute
Middleburg Heights, Ohio

Leesa G. Whicker, BA, CMA
Central Piedmont Community College
Charlotte, North Carolina

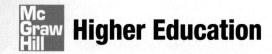

Boston   Burr Ridge, IL   Dubuque, IA   Madison, WI   New York   San Francisco   St. Louis
Bangkok   Bogotá   Caracas   Kuala Lumpur   Lisbon   London   Madrid   Mexico City
Milan   Montreal   New Delhi   Santiago   Seoul   Singapore   Sydney   Taipei   Toronto

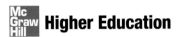

Higher Education

ADMINISTRATIVE PROCEDURES FOR MEDICAL ASSISTING, SECOND EDITION

Published by McGraw-Hill, a business unit of The McGraw-Hill Companies, Inc., 1221 Avenue of the Americas, New York, NY 10020. Copyright © 2005, 1999 by The McGraw-Hill Companies, Inc. All rights reserved. No part of this publication may be reproduced or distributed in any form or by any means, or stored in a database or retrieval system, without the prior written consent of The McGraw-Hill Companies, Inc., including, but not limited to, in any network or other electronic storage or transmission, or broadcast for distance learning.

Some ancillaries, including electronic and print components, may not be available to customers outside the United States.

This book is printed on M-real paper.
Printed in China

6 7 8 9 0 CTP/CTP 0 9 8 7
ISBN-13: 978-0-07-294785-4
ISBN-10: 0-07-294785-3
Part of
ISBN-13: 978-0-07-297450-8
ISBN-10: 0-07-297450-8

Publisher: *David Culverwell*
Senior Sponsoring Editor: *Roxan Kinsey*
Developmental Editor: *Patricia Forrest*
Editorial Coordinator: *Connie Kuhl*
Outside Developmental Services: *Julie Scardiglia*
Senior Marketing Manager: *James F. Connely*
Senior Project Manager: *Sheila M. Frank*
Senior Production Supervisor: *Laura Fuller*
Media Project Manager: *Sandra M. Schnee*
Media Technology Producer: *Janna Martin*
Designer: *Laurie B. Janssen*
Cover Designer: *Studio Montage*
Lead Photo Research Coordinator: *Carrie K. Burger*
Supplement Producer: *Brenda A. Ernzen*
Compositor: *Interactive Composition Corporation*
Typeface: *10/12 Slimbach*
Printer:*CTPS*

Cover photo credits: Front (left to right); Total Care Programming, Inc., Total Care Programming, Inc., Photodisc V18 Health & Medicine, © Ed Bock/CORBIS, © Royalty-Free/CORBIS, PhotoDisc: V40 Health & Medicine 2, Total Care Programming, Inc. Back (left to right); Total Care Programming, Inc., Photodisc, V21, Time and Technology, Photodisc: VL08 Emergency Room, © Royalty-Free/CORBIS, Total Care Programming, Inc., © JFPI Studios, Inc./CORBIS, Total Care Programming, Inc.

Library of Congress Cataloging-in-Publication Data

Administrative procedures for medical assisting/Barbara Ramutkowski . . . [et al.] — 2nd ed.
  p. cm.
 Includes index.
 ISBN 0-07-294785-3
 1. Medical assistants. 2. Prickett-Ramutkowski, Barbara.

 R728.8.A28   2005
 610.73'72069—dc22   2004045908
                                      CIP

WARNING NOTICE: The clinical procedures, medicines, dosages, and other matters described in this publication are based upon research of current literature and consultation with knowledgeable persons in the field. The procedures and matters described in this text reflect currently accepted clinical practice. However, this information cannot and should not be relied upon as necessarily applicable to a given individual's case. Accordingly, each person must be separately diagnosed to discern the patient's unique circumstances. Likewise, the manufacturer's package insert for current drug product information should be consulted before administering any drug. Publisher disclaims all liability for any inaccuracies, omissions, misuse, or misunderstanding of the information contained in this publication. Publisher cautions that this publication is not intended as a substitute for the professional judgment of trained medical personnel.

www.mhhe.com

Brief Contents

PART ONE

Introduction to Medical Assisting   2

SECTION 1
Foundations and Principles   4

Chapter 1   The Profession of Medical Assisting   5
Chapter 2   Types of Medical Practice   21
Chapter 3   Legal and Ethical Issues in Medical Practice, Including HIPAA   37
Chapter 4   Communication With Patients, Families, and Coworkers   59

PART TWO

Administrative Medical Assisting   80

SECTION 1
Office Work   82

Chapter 5   Using and Maintaining Office Equipment   83
Chapter 6   Using Computers in the Office   100
Chapter 7   Managing Correspondence and Mail   119
Chapter 8   Managing Office Supplies   140
Chapter 9   Maintaining Patient Records   156
Chapter 10   Managing the Office Medical Records   176

SECTION 2
Interacting With Patients   195

Chapter 11   Telephone Techniques   196
Chapter 12   Scheduling Appointments and Maintaining the Physician's Schedule   210

Chapter 13   Patient Reception Area   226
Chapter 14   Patient Education   240

SECTION 3
Financial Responsibilities   255

Chapter 15   Processing Health-Care Claims   256
Chapter 16   Medical Coding   278
Chapter 17   Patient Billing and Collections   293
Chapter 18   Accounting for the Medical Office   312

APPENDIXES

Appendix I   Medical Assistant Role Delineation Chart   345
Appendix II   Prefixes and Suffixes Commonly Used in Medical Terms   347
Appendix III   Latin and Greek Equivalents Commonly Used in Medical Terms   349
Appendix IV   Abbreviations Commonly Used in Medical Notations   350
Appendix V   Symbols Commonly Used in Medical Notations   352
Appendix VI   Professional Organizations and Agencies   353

Glossary   355

Index   365

Contents

PART ONE

Introduction to Medical Assisting 2

SECTION 1

Foundations and Principles 4

Chapter 1 The Profession of Medical Assisting 5

Growth of the Medical Assisting Profession 7

Medical Assistant Credentials 8

Membership in a Medical Assisting Association 9

Training Programs and Other Learning Opportunities 10

Career Opportunities/Unit Secretary 13

Daily Duties of Medical Assistants 14

Tips for the Office/Recycling in the Medical Office, Hospital, Laboratory, or Clinic 15

Personal Qualifications of Medical Assistants 15

On-the-Job Rights of the Medical Assistant 18

The AAMA Role Delineation Study 18

Chapter 2 Types of Medical Practice 21

Medical Specialties 22

Working With Other Allied Health Professionals 25

Career Opportunities/Medical Office Administrator 27

Specialty Career Options 31

Professional Associations 34

Chapter 3 Legal and Ethical Issues in Medical Practice, Including HIPAA 37

Medical Law and Ethics 38

OSHA Regulations 44

Quality Control and Assurance 48

Code of Ethics 49

HIPAA 50

Confidentiality Issues and Mandatory Disclosure 55

Caution: Handle With Care/Notifying Those at Risk for Sexually Transmitted Disease 55

Chapter 4 Communication With Patients, Families, and Coworkers 59

Communicating With Patients and Families 60

The Communication Circle 61

Understanding Human Behavior and How It Relates to the Provider-Patient Relationship 62

Types of Communication 63

Improving Your Communication Skills 64

Communicating in Special Circumstances 67

PROCEDURE 4-1 Communicating With the Anxious Patient 69

Caution: Handle With Care/Multicultural Attitudes About Modern Medicine 70

Communicating With Coworkers 73

Managing Stress 74

Preventing Burnout 75

The Policy and Procedures Manual 76

PART TWO

Administrative Medical Assisting 80

SECTION 1

Office Work 82

Chapter 5 Using and Maintaining Office Equipment 83

Office Communication Equipment 84

Tips for the Office/Routing Calls Through an Automated Menu 86

Office Automation Equipment 89

PROCEDURE 5-1 How to Use a Postage Meter 91

PROCEDURE 5-2 How to Use a Dictation-Transcription Machine 92

Purchasing Decisions 95

Maintaining Office Equipment 96

Chapter 6   Using Computers in the Office   100

The Computer Revolution   101
A Brief History of the Computer   102
Types of Computers   102
Components of the Computer   103
Diseases and Disorders/Carpal Tunnel Syndrome   104
Using Computer Software   107
PROCEDURE 6-1   Creating a Form Letter   108
Tips for the Office/Saving Time and Money Online   109
Selecting Computer Equipment   112
Security in the Computerized Office   114
Computer System Care and Maintenance   115
Career Opportunities/Dental Office Administrator   116
Computers of the Future   117

Chapter 7   Managing Correspondence and Mail   119

Correspondence and Professionalism   120
Choosing Correspondence Supplies   120
Written Correspondence   122
Effective Writing   125
Editing and Proofreading   125
Preparing Outgoing Mail   130
PROCEDURE 7-1   Creating a Letter   132
Mailing Equipment and Supplies   134
U.S. Postal Service Delivery   134
Other Delivery Services   136
PROCEDURE 7-2   Sorting and Opening Mail   136
Processing Incoming Mail   137
Tips for the Office/How to Spot Urgent Incoming Mail   137

Chapter 8   Managing Office Supplies   140

Organizing Medical Office Supplies   141
Taking Inventory of Medical Office Supplies   144
PROCEDURE 8-1   Step-by-Step Overview of Inventory Procedures   145
Ordering Supplies   147
Tips for the Office/Ordering by Telephone or Fax or Online   150

Chapter 9   Maintaining Patient Records   156

Importance of Patient Records   158
Contents of Patient Charts   159
Initiating and Maintaining Patient Records   163
Tips for the Office/Talking With the Older Patient   164
The Six Cs of Charting   164
Types of Medical Records   165

Appearance, Timeliness, and Accuracy of Records   167
Medical Transcription   169
Career Opportunities/Medical Transcriptionist   170
Correcting and Updating Patient Records   171
PROCEDURE 9-1   Correcting Medical Records   172
PROCEDURE 9-2   Updating Medical Records   172
Release of Records   173

Chapter 10   Managing the Office Medical Records   176

The Importance of Records Management   177
Filing Equipment   177
Filing Supplies   179
Filing Systems   180
PROCEDURE 10-1   Creating a Filing System for Patient Records   183
PROCEDURE 10-2   Setting Up an Office Tickler File   184
The Filing Process   184
Tips for the Office/Evaluating Your Office Filing System   187
File Storage   187
PROCEDURE 10-3   Developing a Records Retention Program   190
Career Opportunities/Medical Record Technologist   191

SECTION 2
Interacting With Patients   195

Chapter 11   Telephone Techniques   196

Using the Telephone Effectively   197
Communication Skills   197
Managing Incoming Calls   198
Tips for the Office/Screening Incoming Calls   199
Types of Incoming Calls   200
Using Proper Telephone Etiquette   202
PROCEDURE 11-1   Handling Emergency Calls   203
Taking Messages   205
PROCEDURE 11-2   Retrieving Messages From an Answering Service   206
Telephone Answering Systems   206
Placing Outgoing Calls   206
Telephone Triage   207
Telecommunications   208
Facsimile (Fax) Machines   208

Chapter 12   Scheduling Appointments and Maintaining the Physician's Schedule   210

The Appointment Book   211
Appointment Scheduling Systems   214

PROCEDURE 12-1 Creating a Cluster Schedule 217

Arranging Appointments 218

Special Scheduling Situations 219

Tips for the Office/Scheduling Emergency
Appointments 219

Scheduling Outside Appointments 221

PROCEDURE 12-2 Scheduling and Confirming
Surgery at a Hospital 221

Maintaining the Physician's Schedule 222

Chapter 13 Patient Reception Area 226

First Impressions 227

The Importance of Cleanliness 230

Caution: Handle With Care/Maintaining Cleanliness
Standards in the Reception Area 231

The Physical Components 232

Keeping Patients Occupied and Informed 233

Tips for the Office/Tailoring Office Magazines to
Patient Interests 234

Patients With Special Needs 235

PROCEDURE 13-1 Creating a Pediatric
Playroom 236

PROCEDURE 13-2 Creating a Reception Area
Accessible to Differently Abled Patients 237

Chapter 14 Patient Education 240

The Educated Patient 241

Types of Patient Education 242

PROCEDURE 14-1 Developing a Patient
Education Plan 242

Promoting Good Health Through Education 243

The Patient Information Packet 245

Educating Patients With Special Needs 247

Educating the Patient/Instructing Patients With
Hearing Impairments 248

Patient Education Prior to Surgery 249

PROCEDURE 14-2 Informing the Patient of
Guidelines for Surgery 250

Additional Educational Resources 252

Career Opportunities/Occupational Therapy
Assistant 252

SECTION 3
Financial Responsibilities 255

Chapter 15 Processing Health-Care
Claims 256

Basic Insurance Terminology 257

Types of Health Plans 258

The Claims Process: An Overview 262

Fee Schedules and Charges 266

Preparing and Transmitting Health-Care Claims 269

PROCEDURE 15-1 Completing the CMS-1500
Claim Form 273

Tips for the Office/Data Elements for HIPAA
Electronic Claims 275

Chapter 16 Medical Coding 278

Diagnosis Codes: The ICD-9-CM 279

PROCEDURE 16-1 Locating an ICD-9-CM
Code 282

Procedure Codes: The CPT 283

HCPCS 286

PROCEDURE 16-2 Locating a CPT Code 287

Avoiding Fraud: Coding Compliance 287

Career Opportunities/Medical Coder, Physician
Practice 289

Chapter 17 Patient Billing and
Collections 293

Basic Accounting 294

Standard Payment Procedures 294

Standard Billing Procedures 298

PROCEDURE 17-1 How to Bill With
the Superbill 301

Standard Collection Procedures 301

Tips for the Office/Choosing a Collection Agency 306

Credit Arrangements 306

Career Opportunities/Coding, Billing, and Insurance
Specialist 309

Common Collection Problems 310

Chapter 18 Accounting for the Medical
Office 312

The Business Side of a Medical Practice 313

Bookkeeping Systems 314

PROCEDURE 18-1 Organizing the Practice's
Bookkeeping System 319

Banking for the Medical Office 321

PROCEDURE 18-2 Making a Bank Deposit 324

PROCEDURE 18-3 Reconciling a Bank
Statement 326

Tips for the Office/Telephone Banking 327

Managing Accounts Payable 328

Managing Disbursements 328

PROCEDURE 18-4 Setting Up the Accounts Payable
System 329

Handling Payroll 331

Tips for the Office/Handling Payroll Through
Electronic Banking 335

Calculating and Filing Taxes 335

PROCEDURE 18-5 Generating Payroll 337

Managing Contracts 339

APPENDIXES

Appendix I   Medical Assistant Role Delineation Chart   345

Appendix II   Prefixes and Suffixes Commonly Used in Medical Terms   347

Appendix III   Latin and Greek Equivalents Commonly Used in Medical Terms   349

Appendix IV   Abbreviations Commonly Used in Medical Notations   350

Appendix V   Symbols Commonly Used in Medical Notations   352

Appendix VI   Professional Organizations and Agencies   353

Glossary   355

Index   365

Procedures

PROCEDURE 4-1   Communicating With the Anxious Patient   69

PROCEDURE 5-1   How to Use a Postage Meter   91

PROCEDURE 5-2   How to Use a Dictation-Transcription Machine   92

PROCEDURE 6-1   Creating a Form Letter   108

PROCEDURE 7-1   Creating a Letter   132

PROCEDURE 7-2   Sorting and Opening Mail   136

PROCEDURE 8-1   Step-by-Step Overview of Inventory Procedures   145

PROCEDURE 9-1   Correcting Medical Records   172

PROCEDURE 9-2   Updating Medical Records   172

PROCEDURE 10-1   Creating a Filing System for Patient Records   183

PROCEDURE 10-2   Setting Up an Office Tickler File   184

PROCEDURE 10-3   Developing a Records Retention Program   190

PROCEDURE 11-1   Handling Emergency Calls   203

PROCEDURE 11-2   Retrieving Messages From an Answering Service   206

PROCEDURE 12-1   Creating a Cluster Schedule   217

PROCEDURE 12-2   Scheduling and Confirming Surgery at a Hospital   221

PROCEDURE 13-1   Creating a Pediatric Playroom   236

PROCEDURE 13-2   Creating a Waiting Room Accessible to Differently Abled Patients   237

PROCEDURE 14-1   Developing a Patient Education Plan   242

PROCEDURE 14-2   Informing the Patient of Guidelines for Surgery   250

PROCEDURE 15-1   Completing the CMS-1500 Claim Form   273

PROCEDURE 16-1   Locating an ICD-9-CM Code   282

PROCEDURE 16-2   Locating a CPT Code   287

PROCEDURE 17-1   How to Bill With the Superbill   301

PROCEDURE 18-1   Organizing the Practice's Bookkeeping System   319

PROCEDURE 18-2   Making a Bank Deposit   324

PROCEDURE 18-3   Reconciling a Bank Statement   326

PROCEDURE 18-4   Setting Up the Accounts Payable System   329

PROCEDURE 18-5   Generating Payroll   337

Preface

Administrative Procedures for Medical Assisting, 2nd Edition, acquaints the student with all aspects of the administrative skills of the medical assisting profession. From the general to the specific, it covers key concepts, skills, and tasks that should be familiar to the medical assistant. The book speaks directly to the student, with chapter introductions, case studies, procedures, and chapter summaries written to engage the student's attention and build a sense of positive anticipation about joining the profession of medical assisting.

When referring to patients in the third person, we have alternated between passages that describe a male patient and passages that describe a female patient. Thus, the patient will be referred to as "he" half the time and as "she" half the time. The same convention is used to refer to the physician. The medical assistant is consistently addressed as "you."

Patient Education

Throughout the book we provide the medical assistant with the information needed to educate patients so that patients can participate fully in their health care. Whenever tasks involving interaction with patients are described, the focus is on the patient's needs and on the role of the medical assistant in making the patient an active participant in her own care. Several chapters are primarily or exclusively devoted to interaction with patients—such as Chapter 4, on communicating with patients, and Chapter 13, on planning and maintaining the patient reception area.

There is a particular focus on patient education. It is always desirable for patients to be as knowledgeable as possible about their health. Patients who do not understand what is expected of them may become confused, frightened, angry, and uncooperative; educated patients are better able to understand why compliance is important. Chapter 14 is devoted entirely to patient education. Elsewhere throughout the book, information that focuses on patient education is provided.

We have also made a consistent effort to discuss patients with special needs. Several chapters in Part II, Administrative Medical Assisting, contain special sections of text devoted to the particular concerns of certain patient groups. These groups include the following:

- **Pregnant women.** Pregnancy has profound effects on every aspect of health, all of which must be taken into account when working with pregnant patients. Where appropriate, we have addressed special concerns for pregnant patients.

- **Elderly patients.** Special care is often required with elderly patients. The body undergoes many changes with age, and patients may have difficulty adjusting to their changing physical needs. The special needs of elderly patients are highlighted in Chapter 13, Patient Reception Area, and a "Tips for the Office" feature in Chapter 9, Maintaining Patient Records, discusses talking with the older patient.

- **Children.** The special needs of children are complex, because not only their bodies but also their minds and social situations are very different from those of adults. Dealing with children usually means dealing with their parents as well, and medical assistants must hone their communication skills to meet the needs of both patient and parent when working with children. One chapter that focuses on children is Chapter 13, which includes a special text section and a procedure for designing a patient reception area to accommodate children.

- **Patients with disabilities.** Many different diseases and disabilities require extra effort or consideration on the part of the medical assistant. Patients in wheelchairs and patients with diabetes, hemophilia, or visual or hearing impairments all require specific accommodations. For example, Chapter 13 deals with such patients; it includes a section that discusses the Americans With Disabilities Act and one about the Older Americans Act of 1965 and the implications of both laws for providing comfort and safety in the office setting.

- **Patients from other cultures.** Communicating with patients from other cultures, especially when language barriers are involved, poses a special challenge for the medical assistant. In addition, patients from other cultures may have attitudes about medicine or about social interaction that differ sharply from those of the medical assistant's culture. Chapter 4 is one chapter that deals in depth with patients from other cultures. It contains a text section and a Caution: Handle With Care feature about different cultures' attitudes toward medicine.

Because safety is a primary concern for both the patient and the medical assistant, we have emphasized this aspect of medical assisting work.

Areas of Competence

A key feature of *Administrative Procedures* that will enhance its usefulness to both students and instructors is its reference to the areas of competence defined in the 2003 AAMA (American Association of Medical Assistants) Role Delineation Study. The study, which replaces the 1990 DACUM (*Developing A CurriculUM*) analysis, provides a comprehensive list of duties and skills that medical assistants must master at the entry level. The Committee on Accreditation of Allied Health Education Personnel (CAAHEP) requires that all medical assistants be proficient in the 71 entry-level areas of competence when they begin medical assisting work. The opening page of each chapter provides a list of the areas of competence that the chapter covers, and the complete Medical Assistant Role Delineation Chart is provided as an appendix. (A correlation chart also appears in the *Instructor's Resource Binder.*) The chapter-by-chapter listing of areas of competence allows instructors to identify skills that have been covered in the course and helps students find the chapters that cover specific skills and duties.

We have been careful to ensure that the text provides ample coverage of topics used to construct the AMT (Association of Medical Technologists) Registered Medical Assistant (RMA) Exam. A correlation chart appears in the *Instructor's Resource Binder.*

Organization of the Text

Administrative Procedures for Medical Assisting, 2nd Edition, is divided into two parts. Part I provides a basic explanation of the role of the medical assistant in a medical practice, such as an overview of the profession, different types of medical practices, legal and ethical issues—including important information on HIPAA (Health Information Portability and Accountability Act) regulations—and communication with patients, their families, and coworkers. Part II explores the administrative duties of the medical assistant, including basic office work, patient interaction, and the financial responsibilities of a medical practice.

The ordering of chapters within each part allows the student and the instructor to build a knowledge base starting with the fundamentals and working toward an understanding of highly specialized tasks. Part 2 introduces the basics of working with office equipment before covering the details of maintaining patient records, scheduling appointments, and processing insurance.

Chapters are also grouped into sections when their subjects relate to a broader topic or area of skills. Each section is set apart and includes the list of chapters within that section.

Each chapter opens with a page of material that includes the chapter outline and objectives, a list of key terms, and the areas of competence covered in the chapter. The main text of each chapter begins with an overview of chapter content and includes a case study for students to consider as they read the chapter. The main text of each chapter is organized into topics that move from the general to the specific. Color photographs, anatomic and technical drawings, tables, charts, and text features help educate the student about various aspects of medical assisting. The text features, set off in boxes within the text, include the following:

- **Case Studies** are provided at the beginning of all chapters. They represent situations similar to those that the medical assistant may encounter in daily practice. Students are encouraged to consider the case study as they read each chapter. Case Study Questions in the end-of-chapter review check students' understanding and application of chapter content.

- **Procedures** give step-by-step instructions on how to perform the specific administrative tasks a medical assistant will be required to perform. A list of the procedures, which follows the Table of Contents, details the procedures found in each chapter, the AAMA competency number associated with each specific procedure, and if information related to that procedure is included on the student CD.

- **"Tips for the Office"** features provide guidelines on keeping the administration of the medical office running smoothly and efficiently.

- **"Educating the Patient"** focuses on ways to instruct patients about caring for themselves outside the medical office.

- **"Diseases and Disorders"** features give detailed information on specific medical conditions, including how to recognize, prevent, and treat them.

- **"Caution: Handle With Care"** boxes cover the precautions to be taken in certain situations or when performing certain tasks.

- **"Career Opportunities"** provide the student with information on various specialized medical professions or duties related to the medical assistant's role within the healthcare team.

Each chapter closes with a summary of the chapter material, focusing on the role of the medical assistant. The summary is followed by an end-of-chapter review that consists of the following elements:

- Case Study Questions
- Discussion Questions
- Critical Thinking Questions
- Application Activities
- Internet Activities

These questions and activities allow students to practice specific skills.

The book also includes a glossary and several appendices for use as reference tools. The Glossary lists all the words presented as key terms in each chapter, along with a pronunciation guide and the definition of each term. The appendices include the Medical Assistant Role Delineation Chart, commonly used prefixes and suffixes, Latin and Greek terms, abbreviations and symbols used in medical terminology, and a comprehensive list of professional organizations and agencies.

The Student CD-ROM provides a comprehensive learning program that is correlated to each chapter of the text and reinforces competencies required to become a medical assistant. Short video clips and pictures introduce skills and case studies for application. In addition, numerous interactive exercises and applications are provided for every chapter in the text. The Student CD, included with each student textbook, provides the following menu choices:

- Administrative Practice
- Clinical Practice
- Anatomy and Physiology Review
- Games
  - Spin the Wheel
  - Key Term Concentration
- Interactive Review
- Audio Glossary
- Progress Report
- Online Learning Center

Ancillaries

The *Student Workbook* provides an opportunity for the student to review the material and skills presented in the textbook. On a chapter-by-chapter basis, it provides:

- Vocabulary review exercises, which test knowledge of key terms in the chapter
- Content review exercises, which test the student's knowledge of key concepts in the chapter
- Critical thinking exercises, which test the student's understanding of key concepts in the chapter
- Application exercises, which test mastery of specific skills
- Case studies, which apply the chapter material to real-life situations or problems
- Competency checklists for the procedures in the text

The *Instructor's Resource Binder* provides the instructor with materials to help organize lessons and classroom interactions. It includes:

- A complete lesson plan for each chapter, including an introduction to the lesson, teaching strategies, alternate teaching strategies, case studies, assessment, chapter close, resources, and an answer key to the student textbook
- Procedure competency checklists, reproduced from the *Student Workbook*
- An answer key to the *Student Workbook*
- Charts that show the location in the student textbook, the *Student Workbook,* and the *Instructor's Resource*

Binder, of material that correlates with the 2003 AAMA Role Delineation Study Areas of Competence, the SCANS Competencies, the National Health Care Skill Standards, and the AMT Registered Medical Assistant (RMA) Certification Exam Topics

- Power Point Presentations on the IPC CD-ROM

The Instructor Resource CD-ROM provides easy-to-use resources for class preparation. The Instructor Resource CD-ROM includes the following:

- Exam*View*® Pro Test Generator with answer rationales and correlations to AAMA competencies
- PowerPoint® Presentations
- Correlations to AAMA and AMT Standards
- Course syllabi

Together, the Student Edition, the *Student Workbook,* and the *Instructor's Resource Binder* form a complete teaching and learning package. The *Administrative Procedures for Medical Assisting* course will prepare students to enter the medical assisting field with all the knowledge and skills needed to be a useful resource to patients, a valued asset to employers, and a credit to the medical assisting profession.

Acknowledgments

The publisher and authors would like to thank the reviewers and contributors for their assistance in shaping this revision. We appreciate their suggestions, insights, and commitment to providing information that is relevant and valuable to medical assisting students.

In addition, many people and organizations provided invaluable assistance in the process of illustrating the highly technical and detailed topics covered in the text. Their contributions helped ensure the accuracy, timeliness, and authenticity of the illustrations in the book.

We would like to thank the following organizations for providing source materials and technical advice: the American Association of Medical Assistants, Chicago, Illinois; Becton Dickinson Microbiology Systems, Sparks, Maryland; Becton Dickinson VACUTAINER Systems, Franklin Lakes, New Jersey; Bibbero Systems, Petaluma, California; Burdick, Schaumberg, Illinois; the Corel Corporation, Ottawa, Ontario, Canada; Hamilton Media, Hamilton, New Jersey; Nassau Ear, Nose, and Throat, Princeton, New Jersey; Princeton Allergy and Asthma Associates, Princeton, New Jersey; Richmond International, Boca Raton, Florida; Winfield Medical, San Diego, California.

We would like to express our appreciation to the following New Jersey physicians and medical facilities for allowing us to photograph a variety of procedures and procedural settings at their facilities: the Eric B. Chandler Medical Center, New Brunswick; Helene Fuld School of Nursing of New Jersey, Trenton; Mercer Medical Center, Trenton; Mercer County Vocational-Technical Health

CHAPTER 7

Managing Correspondence and Mail

AREAS OF COMPETENCE

2003 Role Delineation Study

ADMINISTRATIVE

Administrative Procedures
- Perform basic administrative medical assisting functions

GENERAL

Communication Skills
- Recognize and respond effectively to verbal, nonverbal, and written communications
- Utilize electronic technology to receive, organize, prioritize, and transmit information

KEY TERMS

annotate
clarity
concise
courtesy title
dateline
editing
enclosure
full-block letter style
identification line
key
letterhead
modified-block letter style
proofreading
salutation
simplified letter style
template

CHAPTER OUTLINE

- Correspondence and Professionalism
- Choosing Correspondence Supplies
- Written Correspondence
- Effective Writing
- Editing and Proofreading
- Preparing Outgoing Mail
- Mailing Equipment and Supplies
- U.S. Postal Service Delivery
- Other Delivery Services
- Processing Incoming Mail

OBJECTIVES

After completing Chapter 7, you will be able to:

7.1 List the supplies necessary for creating and mailing professional-looking correspondence.
7.2 Identify the types of correspondence used in medical office communications.
7.3 Describe the parts of a letter and the different letter and punctuation styles.
7.4 Compose a business letter.
7.5 Explain the tasks involved in editing and proofreading.
7.6 Describe the process of handling incoming and outgoing mail.
7.7 Compare and contrast the services provided by the U.S. Postal Service and other delivery services.

Chapter openers include chapter outlines, objectives, key terms, and the competencies covered in each chapter.

Specific administrative or clinical tasks are illustrated in a step-by-step format in the Procedures boxes.

Patient instruction on self care outside the medical office is the focus in the Educating the Patient boxes.

Introduction

Medical assisting is one of the fastest-growing occupations in allied health care today. Health care is changing at a rapid rate, from advanced technology to implementing cost-effective medicine while maintaining quality patient care. The medical assistant is the perfect complement to this changing industry. Employers are looking for health care professionals who are "generalists." A generalist is someone who is trained in all departments in the facility in which they are employed. Medical assistants who graduate from an accredited institution will gain the skills that enable them to multitask. A multitasking professional is someone who is able to work in the administrative areas, the clinical areas, and the financial areas. Employers are seeking credentialed health care professionals who are dedicated to the profession and the patient.

This chapter will introduce the professional standards that are required in medical assisting.

CASE STUDY

Medical assistants are considered generalists in most medical environments. The following scenarios describe how the medical assistant functions as a generalist or multiskilled professional. As you review the scenarios, make note of the many duties the medical assistant performs.

Scenario 1 Kim is 28 years old. She has been working as a medical assistant for 6 years. She is currently working in a family practice office with two doctors, two other medical assistants, and a medical records clerk. Her role is primarily administrative; she is mainly responsible for phone reception and patient check-in and check-out.

A 29-year-old female patient calls complaining of lower back pain. As Kim listens to the patient describe her condition, she determines the severity of the patient's discomfort and schedules an appointment. When the patient arrives at the office, Kim greets her and collects the necessary demographic and insurance information, and escorts her to an exam room on the way out. The patient is instructed to see Kim on the way out and gives the patient a prescription. Kim collects the payment and files the...

PROCEDURE 9.1

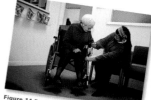

Correcting Medical Records

Objective: To follow standard procedures for correcting a medical record

Materials: Patient file, other pertinent documents that contain the information to be used in making corrections (for example, transcribed notes, telephone notes, physician's comments, correspondence), good ballpoint pen

Method

1. Always make the correction in a way that does not suggest any intention to deceive, cover up, alter, or add information to conceal a lack of proper medical care.
2. When deleting information, never block it out, never use correction fluid to cover it up, and never in any other way erase or obliterate the original wording. Draw a line through the original information so that it is still legible. Write the correct information above or below it or in the margin. The

location on the chart for the new information should be clear. You may need to attach another sheet of paper or another document with the correction on it. Note in the record "See attached document A" or similar wording to indicate where the corrected information can be found.

4. Place a note near the correction stating why it was made (for example, "error, wrong date; error, interrupted by phone call.") This indication can be a brief note in the margin or an attachment to the record. As a general rule of thumb, do not make any changes without noting the reason for them.
5. Enter the date and time, and initial the correction.
6. If possible, have another staff member or the physician witness and initial the correction to the record when you make it.

Figure 14-5. When instructing elderly patients, remember that each patient is an individual with unique needs.

Patients With Mental Impairments

Patients with impaired mental functions include those with **dementia**, Alzheimer's disease, mental retardation, drug addictions, and emotional problems. These patients can be challenging to deal with because communication may be difficult. Tact and empathy are important. A key to dealing with these patients is to speak at their level of understanding. Again, you must try to meet patients' needs without talking down to them.

Patients With Hearing Impairments

Patients with hearing impairments may have conditions ranging from mild impairment to total hearing loss. It is a common mistake to treat these patients as though they have mental impairments. Although you may have difficulty communicating with these patients, remember that their inability to hear has nothing to do with their level of intelligence. The Educating the Patient section provides techniques for educating patients who have hearing impairments.

Patients With Visual Impairments

As with hearing impairment, the level of visual impairment can vary significantly from patient to patient. Determining the severity of a patient's condition allows you to tailor your instruction to the patient's needs.

instructions are an essential aspect of patient care. Patients can refer to the instructions as necessary or can ask a relative to do so.

- Adjust procedures as needed. When demonstrating a procedure to elderly patients, keep in mind any physical limitations they may have, and adjust the procedure accordingly. Make sure patients understand the instructions by asking them to perform the procedure for you.

Educating the Patient

Instructing Patients With Hearing Impairments

Educating patients who have hearing impairments need not be difficult if you pay a little extra attention in the following areas.

- Try to eliminate all background noise. Talk in a quiet room, if possible.
- Make sure the room is well lit.
- Face the patient, and make sure the patient can see your mouth. Having the patient watch your mouth movements can help him understand what you are saying.
- Speak loudly and clearly, but do not shout.
- Use visual aids as necessary.
- Tell patients to let you know right away if they cannot hear you or do not catch something you have said. Even patients who do not have hearing impairments often appear to understand what a medical professional is saying rather than admit they are confused. It is a good idea to ask patients to repeat information to you to check their understanding. Also, periodically ask if they

would like you to go over any particular part of the explanation or instructions again.

An additional point to keep in mind when dealing with patients who have hearing impairments is that loss of hearing can cause them to withdraw and feel isolated. Being empathic and patient greatly enhances the educational process.

Elderly Patients With Hearing Loss

Most people experience a gradual loss of hearing as they get older. In addition to the preceding suggestions, try to talk in a lower pitch whenever possible. As people get older, they often have more trouble understanding higher tones.

Patients Who Wear Hearing Aids

When talking to a patient who wears a hearing aid, it is best to speak at a normal level. Many hearing aids make a normal voice louder but filter out loud noises. If you raise your voice, the hearing aid may filter it out. Consequently, the patient may hear only broken speech.

248   CHAPTER 14

Handle With Care boxes cover precautions to be taken when performing certain tasks.

Career Opportunities boxes provide information on professions and duties related to medical assisting.

Diseases and Disorders boxes detail medical conditions and how to recognize, prevent, and treat them.

A summary of the chapter material and an end-of-chapter review close out each chapter.

CAUTION Handle With Care

Multicultural Attitudes About Modern Medicine

Patients' cultural backgrounds have a great effect on their attitudes toward health and illness. Patients from different cultural backgrounds often have beliefs about the causes of illness, what symptoms mean, and what to expect from health-care professionals that are different from those of modern medicine. Understanding some of these perceptions, behaviors, and expectations will help you communicate effectively with patients of different cultures.

Beliefs About Causes of Illness

Some cultures have beliefs about the causes of illness that differ sharply from accepted notions in the mainstream culture. As an example, many cultures believe that some illnesses are caused by hot or cold forces in the body. Some believe that winds and drafts cause illness or that illness can be caused by blood that is too thick or too thin. Others believe that having bad feelings toward others can create ill health.

Because of such beliefs, it may be hard to obtain information from patients about possible reasons for their medical problems. It may also be hard for some patients to realize the importance of taking medication to treat certain illnesses. In this case, you may have to be very persuasive and firm when giving the instructions for medication usage. It may be necessary to involve other [...] suading the patient [...]

express pain very emotionally because their culture may feel that suppressing pain is harmful. In contrast, people from other cultures may not admit that they are in pain, thinking that acknowledging pain is a sign of weakness. People of all cultures may be more likely to report physical symptoms of illness than they are to report psychologic symptoms of illness. Be aware of nonverbal indications of pain or other symptoms.

Treatment Expectations

Patients from other cultures may be totally unaccustomed to some of the practices of modern medicine. Patients of certain ethnic or cultural groups often consult other types of healers before seeing a doctor. They are likely to have different expectations of treatment from each.

Patients from other cultures may be wary of certain treatments because these treatments are so different from what they are accustomed to, especially true of some of the medical [...] interventions considered to [...] as laser surgery [...]

Career Opportunities

Dental Office Administrator

To gain medical assistant credentials, you must fulfill the requirements of either the American Association of Medical Assistants (for a Certified Medical Assistant) or the American Medical Technologists (for a Registered Medical Assistant). After obtaining your medical assistant certification or registration, you may wish to acquire additional skills in specialty areas through course work or on-the-job training. Although this course work or training may not lead to an additional certification or degree, it will enable you to expand your role in the medical office and advance your career as the demand for skilled health professionals increases.

Skills and Duties

A dental office administrator carries out clerical and administrative duties for a dentist or a dental group. His duties may vary with the size of the practice. In a large practice he may oversee the clerical staff, including [...] reception desk, maintaining records, [...] services. [...] administrator mostly [...]

6. Supervision. In a large dental practice, the administrator trains and oversees clerical staff and secretaries.

Workplace Settings

Dental office administrators may work in a private practice, a group practice, or a dental clinic.

Education

Dental office administrators often learn the dental and medical terminology they need on the job. They may acquire secretarial training by taking courses, either in a business/vocational school or in a junior or community college. A high school diploma is usually required. Further education may be necessary in a practice where the administrator must supervise other staff members.

Where to Go for More Information

American Academy of Dental Practice Administrators
1063 Whippoorwill Lane
Palatine, IL 60067
(312) 934-4404

Diseases and Disorders

Carpal Tunnel Syndrome

As the number of computers used in the home and workplace has escalated in recent years, the number of cases of carpal tunnel syndrome has also risen dramatically. Carpal tunnel syndrome is a hand disorder that is often associated with computer use. The term for this condition comes from the name for a canal (the carpal tunnel) located in the wrist. Several tendons pass through this tunnel, allowing the hand to open and close.

Carpal tunnel syndrome results from repetitive motion, such as keyboarding, for hours at a time. This motion may cause swelling to develop around the tendons and carpal tunnel. The swelling compresses the nerve. The people most likely to develop carpal tunnel syndrome are workers whose jobs require them to perform repetitive hand and finger motions.

Symptoms

The symptoms associated with carpal tunnel syndrome include the following:

- Tingling or burning in the hands or fingers
- Weakness or numbness in the hands or fingers
- Hands that go to sleep frequently
- Difficulty opening or closing the hands
- Pain that stems from the wrist and travels up the arm

Tips for Prevention

If you use a keyboard for extended periods, you should practice proper techniques to prevent carpal tunnel syndrome.

- While seated, hold your arms relaxed at your sides, and check to make sure that your keyboard is positioned slightly higher than your elbows. As you input, keep your elbows at your sides, and relax your shoulders (see Figure 6-2).
- Use only your fingers to press keys, and do not use more pressure than necessary. Use a wrist rest, and keep your wrists relaxed and straight.

- When you need to strike difficult-to-reach keys, move your whole hand rather than stretching your fingers. When you need to press two keys at the same time, such as "Control" and "F1," use two hands.
- Try to break up long periods of keyboard work with other tasks that do not require computer use.

Tips for Relieving Symptoms

If you have symptoms of carpal tunnel syndrome, try these suggestions for relief.

- Elevate your arms
- Wear a splint on the hand and forearm
- Discuss your symptoms with a physician, who may prescribe medication

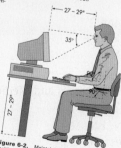

Figure 6-2. Maintaining proper posture and hand positions helps to avoid strain or injury of the back, eyes, neck, or wrist when keyboarding.

---

simply slide your finger across the touch pad. To click on an item, you push a button similar to that on a mouse or trackball, or you tap your finger on the touch pad.

Modem. This term *modem* is a shortened form of the words *modulator-demodulator.* A modem is used to transfer information from one computer to another over telephone

lines. Because modems allow information to be transferred both to and from a computer, they are considered input/output devices. The speed at which a modem transfers data is called the baud rate. Although the current standard modem speed is 28,800 baud, modem speeds are continually being improved. Modems are essential for any medical office that needs to transfer files electronically, as when submitting insurance claim forms.

REVIEW

CHAPTER 18

CASE STUDY QUESTIONS

Now that you have completed this chapter, review the case study at the beginning of the chapter and answer the following question:

1. What should Ben do to properly record the payment?

Discussion Questions

1. Name three things that are required in a single-entry accounting system.
2. What are the three terms that are used in the double-entry accounting system?
3. Why is the reconciliation of the bank statement so important?
4. Why is a petty cash fund useful?
5. When creating a payroll information sheet, name what it should contain.

Critical Thinking Questions

1. Why is it important for an employer to have an Employer Identification Number?
2. Discuss the importance of having separate accounts for employee deductions.

3. Name some of the banking tasks of the medical practice.
4. Name some of the requirements of the Fair Labor Standards Act.

Application Activities

1. Record the following disbursements made on September 9, 2004, in a disbursements journal:
   - Check no. 1234, payee—Tom Jones (electrician), check amount—$125
   - Check no. 1235, payee—Postmaster (postage), check amount—$32
   - Check no. 1236, payee—Gateway Property Management (rent), check amount—$900
2. Simulate an office petty cash account, using your own personal expenses. Determine a starting amount, and use it for 2 weeks to buy small items. For each purchase, obtain a receipt, or write a petty cash voucher. Record each withdrawal you make from the petty cash account using a petty cash record. At least once during the 2-week period, write a check to replenish the account.
3. Prepare your personal federal income tax return, using information from the Wage and Tax Statement (Form W-2) and the Employee's Withholding Allowance Certificate (Form W-4) provided by your employer.

Occupations Center, Trenton; Plainfield Health Center, Plainfield; Princeton Allergy and Asthma Associates, Princeton; the Princeton Medical Group, Princeton; Robert Wood Johnson University Hospital, New Brunswick; Robert Wood Johnson University Hospital at Hamilton, Hamilton; St. Francis Medical Center, Trenton; St. Peter's Medical Center, New Brunswick; Dr. Edward von der Schmidt, neurosurgeon, Princeton; Wound Care Center/Curative Network, New Brunswick.

We would also like to thank the following facilities and educational institutions for graciously allowing us to photograph procedures and other technical aspects related to the profession of medical assisting: Total Care Programming Inc., Henrico, North Carolina; Wildwood Medical Clinic, Henrico, North Carolina; Central Piedmont Community College, Charlotte, North Carolina; and Roanoke Rapids Clinic, Roanoke Rapids, Virginia.

Reviewers

Every area of the text was reviewed by practitioners and educators in the field. Their insights helped shape the direction of the book.

Kaye Acton, CMA
  Alamance Community College
  Graham, NC

Jannie R. Adams, PhD, RN, MS-HSA, BSN
  Clayton College and State University,
  School of Technology
  Morrow, GA

Cathy Kelley Arney, CMA, MLT (ASCP), AS
  National College of Business and Technology
  Bluefield, VA

Joseph Balabat, MD
  Dean of Academics
  Sanford Brown Institute

Marsha Benedict, CMA-A, MS, CPC
  Baker College of Flint
  Flint, MI

Michelle Buchman
  Springfield College
  Springfield, MO

Patricia Celani, CMA
  ICM School of Business and Medical Careers
  Pittsburgh, PA

Theresa Cyr, RN, BN, MS
  Heald Business College
  Honolulu, HI

Barbara Desch
  San Joaquin Valley College
  Visalia, CA

Herbert J. Feitelberg, BA, DPM
  King's College
  Charlotte, NC

Geri L. Finn
  Remington College, Dallas Campus
  Garland, TX

Kimberly L. Gibson, RN, DOE
  Sanford Brown Institute
  Middleburg Heights, OH

Barbara G. Gillespie, MS
  San Diego & Grossmont Community College Districts
  El Cajon, CA

Cindy Gordon, MBA, CMA
  Baker College
  Muskegon, MI

Mary Harmon
  MedTech College
  Indianapolis, IN

Glenda H. Hatcher, BSN
  Southwest Georgia Technical College
  Thomasville, GA

Helen J. Hauser, RN, MSHA, RMA
  Phoenix College
  Phoenix, AZ

Christine E. Hetrick
  Cittone Institute
  Mt. Laurel, NJ

Beulah A. Hofmann, RN, MSN, CMA
  Ivy Tech State College
  Terre Haute, IN

Karen Jackson
  Education America
  Garland, TX

Latashia Y. D. Jones, LPN
  CAPPS College, Montgomery Campus
  Montgomery, AL

Donna D. Kyle-Brown, PhD, RMA
  CAPPS College, Mobile Campus
  Mobile, AL

Sharon McCaughrin
  Ross Learning
  Southfield, MI

Tanya Mercer, BS, RMA
  Kaplan Higher Education Corporation
  Roswell, GA

T. Michelle Moore-Roberts
  CAPPS College, Montgomery Campus
  Montgomery, AL

Linda Oprean
  Applied Career Training
  Manassas, VA

Julie Orloff, RMA, CMA, CPT, CPC
  Ultrasound Diagnostic School
  Miami, FL

Delores W. Orum, RMA
  CAPPS College
  Montgomery, AL

Katrina L. Poston, MA, RHE
Applied Career Training
Arlington, VA

Manuel Ramirez, MD
Texas School of Business
Friendswood, TX

Beatrice Salada, BAS, CMA
Davenport University
Lansing, MI

Melanie G. Sheffield, LPN
Capps Medical Institute
Pensacola, FL

Kristi Sopp, RMA
MTI College
Sacramento, CA

Carmen Stevens
Remington College, Fort Worth Campus
Fort Worth, TX

Deborah Sulkowski, BS, CMA
Pittsburgh Technical Institute
Oakdale, PA

Fred Valdes, MD
City College
Ft. Lauderdale, FL

Janice Vermiglio-Smith, RN, MS, PhD
Central Arizona College
Apache Junction, AZ

Erich M. Weldon, MICP, NREMT-P
Apollo College
Portland, Oregon

Terri D. Wyman, CMRS, CMS
Ultrasound Diagnostic School
Springfield, MA

Previous Edition Reviewers

Janet Aaberg, MS
San Diego Community Colleges
San Diego, CA

Jeri Adler, BA, AA, CMA, CMT
Lane Community College
Eugene, OR

Sr. Patricia Carter, BSN, MS
Stautzenberger College
Findlay, OH

Gwendolyn J. Coleman, RN
Weakley County Vocatonal Center
Dresden, TN

Lisa Cook, RMA, CMA
Eton Technical Institute
Port Orchard, WA

Barbara Dahl, CMA
Whatcom Community College
Bellingham, WA

Joyce Deutsch, RN, CPC-H, CMA
Indiana Business College
Evansville, IN

Suzanne Ezzo, RN, AST, BS, LVT
Sawyer School
Pittsburgh, PA

Tracie Fuqua, AAS, CMA
Wallace State College
Hanceville, AL

Jeanette Girkin, EdD, CMA
Tulsa Junior College
Tulsa, OK

Glenn Grady, MEd, BSMT (ASCP), CMA
Miller-Motte Business College
Wilmington, NC

Christine E. Hollander, CMA, BS
Denver Institute of Technology
Denver, CO

Sue A. Hunt, MA, RN, CMA
Middlesex Community College
Bedford/Lowell, MA

Gwynne Mangiore
Missouri College For Doctors' Assistants
St. Louis, MO

Diane Morlock, CMA
Stautzenberger College
Toledo, OH

Deborah Newton, BS, MA, EMT-I, CMA
Montana State University, College of Technology
Great Falls, MT

Virginia Opitz, RN, BSN, MS, CRRN
North Western Business College
Chicago, IL

Tom Palko, MEd, MCS, MT (ASCP)
Arkansas Tech University
Russellville, AR

Hilda Palko, BS, MT (ASCP), CMA
Russellville, AR

Savatore M. Passanese, AS, BA, MS, PhD
Niagara County Community College
Sanborn, NY

Debra Rosch, CMA
Minnesota School of Business
Brooklyn Center, MN

Jay Shahed, BS, PhD
Robert Morris College
Chicago, IL

Connie W. Stack, BSAH, MLT (ASCP), CMA
Anson Community College
Polkton, NC

Patricia A. Stang, CMA, CPT
Medix School
Baltimore, MD

Geraldine M. Todaro, CMA, CLPLb
    Stark State College of Technology
    Canton, OH
Kimberly C. Wilson, MT (AMT), CMA
    Spencerian College
    Louisville, KY
Chris Kientzle, CMA-C, RMA
    Sanford Brown College
    Hazelwood, MO
Clare Lewandowski, BS, MA, PhD
    Columbus State Community College
    Columbus, OH
Joan Winters, BS, MS, DLM (ASCP), MT (ASCP)
    Wayne Community College
    Goldsboro, NC

Contributors

Kaye Acton, CMA
    Alamance Community College
    Graham, North Carolina
Jannie R. Adams, PhD, RN, MS-HSA, BSN
    Clayton College and State University, School
    of Technology
    Morrow, Georgia
Cathy Kelley Arney, CMA, MLT (ASCP), AS
    National College of Business and Technology
    Bluefield, Virginia
Russell E. Battiata
    National School of Technology
    Miami, Florida

Marti A. Burton, RN, BS
    Canadian Valley Technology Center
    El Reno, Oklahoma
Ann Coleman
    Society of Nuclear Medicine
    Reston, Virginia
Barbara G. Gillespie, MS
    San Diego and Grossmont Community
    College Districts
    El Cajon, California
Regina Hoffman, PhD
    Midlands Technical College
    Columbia, South Carolina
Donna D. Kyle-Brown, PhD, RMA
    CAPPS College, Mobile Campus
    Mobile, Alabama
Cynthia Newby, CPC
    Chestnut Hill Enterprises
Melanie G. Sheffield, LPN
    Capps Medical Institute
    Pensacola, Florida
Cynthia T. Vincent, MMS, PA-C
    Wildwood Medical Clinic
    Henrico, North Carolina
Terri D. Wyman, CMRS, CMS
    Ultrasound Diagnostic School
    Springfield, Massachusetts

ADMINISTRATIVE PROCEDURES
for Medical Assisting

PART One

Introduction to Medical Assisting

"The medical assisting profession is filled with challenges and rewards every day. Everything is important when you are assisting a patient. You should get to know your patient, and his family, if possible, in order to understand the patient's specific needs. This is especially true with an elderly patient. Treat your patient like a family member. Be considerate and concerned, and always maintain a pleasant attitude.

"It is also essential to know your physician well, and how he or she likes to work. Let the physician know all the information the patient has shared with you, to help him or her make a better diagnosis. Keep informed about what the physician has recommended for treatment. The patient will have questions along the way. It's good medicine to be able to give him solid information about his condition and reinforce the doctor's orders when necessary. A skilled physician and an organized, cooperative, receptive medical assistant promote and maintain exceptional patient care."

Sue Haines
Medical Assistant, Princeton, New Jersey

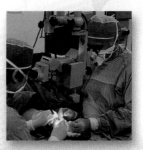

SECTION ONE
Foundations and Principles

Chapter 1   The Profession of Medical Assisting

Chapter 2   Types of Medical Practice

Chapter 3   Legal and Ethical Issues in Medical Practice,
             Including HIPAA

Chapter 4   Communication With Patients, Families, and Coworkers

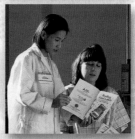

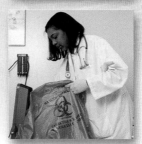

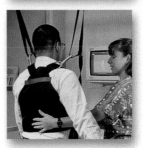

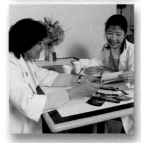

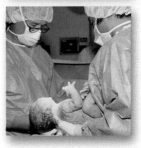

SECTION 1

FOUNDATIONS AND PRINCIPLES

CHAPTER 1

The Profession of Medical Assisting

CHAPTER 2

Types of Medical Practice

CHAPTER 3

Legal and Ethical Issues in Medical Practice, Including HIPAA

CHAPTER 4

Communication With Patients, Families, and Coworkers

The Profession of Medical Assisting

AREAS OF COMPETENCE

2003 Role Delineation Study

GENERAL

Professionalism
- Display a professional manner and image
- Demonstrate initiative and responsibility
- Prioritize and perform multiple tasks
- Promote the CMA credential
- Enhance skills through continuing education

Communication Skills
- Recognize and respond effectively to verbal, nonverbal, and written communications

Legal Concepts
- Perform within legal and ethical boundaries
- Recognize professional credentialing criteria

KEY TERMS

accreditation

American Association of Medical Assistants (AAMA)

Certified Medical Assistant (CMA)

CLIA (Clinical Laboratory Improvement Amendments)

contaminated

cross-training

externship

HIPAA (Health Insurance Portability and Accountability Act)

managed care organization (MCO)

OSHA (Occupational Safety and Health Act)

portfolio

practitioner

Registered Medical Assistant (RMA)

résumé

CHAPTER OUTLINE

- Growth of the Medical Assisting Profession
- Medical Assistant Credentials
- Membership in a Medical Assisting Association
- Training Programs and Other Learning Opportunities
- Daily Duties of Medical Assistants
- Personal Qualifications of Medical Assistants
- On the Job
- The AAMA Role Delineation Study

OBJECTIVES

After completing Chapter 1, you will be able to:

1.1 Describe the job responsibilities of a medical assistant
1.2 Discuss the professional training of a medical assistant
1.3 Identify the personal characteristics a medical assistant needs
1.4 Define multiskilled health professional
1.5 Explain the importance of continuing education for a medical assistant
1.6 Describe the process and benefits of certification and registration
1.7 List the benefits of becoming a member of a professional association

Introduction

Medical assisting is one of the fastest-growing occupations in allied health care today. Health care is changing at a rapid rate, from advanced technology to implementing cost-effective medicine while maintaining quality patient care. The medical assistant is the perfect complement to this changing industry. Employers are looking for health care professionals who are "generalists." A generalist is someone who is trained in all departments in the facility in which they are employed. Medical assistants who graduate from an accredited institution will gain the skills that enable them to multitask. A multitasking professional is someone who is able to work in the administrative areas, the clinical areas, and the financial areas. Employers are seeking credentialed health care professionals who are dedicated to the profession and the patient.

This chapter will introduce the professional standards that are required in medical assisting.

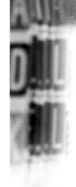

CASE STUDY

Medical assistants are considered generalists in most medical environments. The following scenarios describe how the medical assistant functions as a generalist or multiskilled professional. As you review the scenarios, make note of the many duties the medical assistant performs.

Scenario 1 Kim is 28 years old. She has been working as a medical assistant for 6 years. She is currently working in a family practice office with two doctors, two other medical assistants, and a medical records clerk. Her role is primarily administrative; she is mainly responsible for phone reception and patient check-in and check-out.

A 29-year-old female patient calls complaining of lower back pain. As Kim listens to the patient describe her condition, she determines the severity of the patient's discomfort and schedules a same-day appointment. When the patient arrives at the office, Kim greets her at the front desk, verifies her address and insurance information, and escorts her to an exam room. After the physician completes the exam, the patient is instructed to see Kim on the way out. Kim reviews the patient's prescriptions and schedules a diagnostic test and laboratory work for the patient at another facility. Kim then collects the patient co-pay and gives the patient a receipt. After the patient leaves, Kim prepares the insurance forms for reimbursement and files the patient's chart.

Scenario 2 David is 38 years old. He has been working as a medical assistant for 13 years. He currently works as a clinical medical assistant in an urgent care center that specializes in occupational medicine and basic emergency medicine. He is flexible and works a combination of days, afternoons, and weekends. He normally works with two doctors, two nurses, and four other medical assistants during his shift. The center's patients usually arrive on a walk-in basis.

A 40-year-old man signs in with the receptionist. She helps the patient complete the necessary forms for the medical chart. After the chart is completed, she places the chart at the clinical station. David reviews the medical chart and makes note that the patient, a truck driver, is here for an occupational physical. He obtains the protocol from the trucking company file and verifies the testing requested by the company. He then escorts the patient to an exam room and interviews the patient regarding his medical history. He explains all the testing that will be completed and escorts the patient to the laboratory. David collects a urine drug screen, following precise directions, and collects a blood specimen. David then performs an auditory and visual screening and escorts the patient back to the exam room. The patient is given a gown with instructions on how to put it on. After a few minutes, David obtains an EKG on the patient. The patient is now ready for the physical part of the exam, which is performed by the doctor. David verifies the information again and gives the chart to the doctor. After the doctor is finished with the exam, David returns to the patient, explains how the physical is reported to his employer, and escorts him to the x-ray technician for a chest x-ray. After the patient leaves, David completes the paperwork, submits the laboratory work to an outside reference lab, and submits the x-ray to be read by a radiologist.

As you read this chapter, consider the following questions:

1. How are the two jobs different?
2. How are the two jobs the same?
3. How do these two medical assistants function as multiskilled health-care professionals?

Growth of the Medical Assisting Profession

As a medical assistant you will be an allied health professional trained to work in a variety of health-care settings: medical offices, clinics, and ambulatory care facilities. Your role, with varied and challenging administrative and clinical duties, will be integral to creating a health-care facility that operates smoothly and provides a patient-centered approach to quality health care. Your specific responsibilities will likely depend on the location and size of the facility as well as its medical specialties.

Medical assisting is now one of the fastest-growing occupations. As the health services industry expands, the U.S. Department of Labor predicts that medical assisting will grow at a much faster rate than the average rate for all occupations through the year 2010. The growth in the number of physicians' group practices and other health-care practices that use support personnel will in turn continue to drive up demand for medical assistants.

According to the U.S. Department of Labor Bureau of Statistics, in the year 2000, medical assistants held approximately 329,000 jobs. Of these, 60% were in physicians' offices, and approximately 15% were in hospitals, including outpatient and inpatient facilities. The rest were in nursing homes and the offices of other health **practitioners** (those who practice a profession), such as chiropractors, optometrists, and podiatrists. Some medical assistants worked in other health-care facilities.

Modern health insurance, Medicare, and Medicaid now make medical care available to more people, and the number of physicians is increasing. Thus, more medical assistants will be needed to run these physicians' offices.

The following factors will also increase job opportunities for medical assistants: growth of outpatient clinics and health maintenance organizations (HMOs), and the population increase. Specifically, greater numbers of older people now require a relatively higher level of medical care. Today, the elderly are the fastest-growing segment of the U.S. population. Statistics show that the entire population will grow 22% from 2000 to 2005, but that those aged 65 and older will increase to 78.5%. The older population has unique needs and problems.

History of the Medical Assisting Profession

With the emergence of formal training programs for medical assistants and the continuous changes in health care today, the role of the medical assistant has become dynamic and wide ranging. These changes have raised the expectations for medical assistants. The knowledge base of the modern medical assistant includes:

- administrative and clinical skills
- patient insurance product knowledge (specific to the workers' geographical locations)

- compliance, especially of OSHA and HIPAA guidelines
- exceptional customer service
- practice management
- current patient treatments and education

The medical assisting profession today requires a commitment to self-directed, lifelong learning. Health care is changing rapidly because of new technology, new health-care delivery systems, and new approaches to facilitating cost-efficient, high-quality health care. A medical assistant who can adapt to change and is continually learning will be in high demand.

Creating the American Association of Medical Assistants

The seed of the idea for a national association of medical assistants—to be called the **American Association of Medical Assistants (AAMA)**—was planted at the 1955 annual state convention of the Kansas Medical Assistants Society. The next year, at an American Medical Association (AMA) meeting, the AAMA was officially created. In 1978 the U.S. Department of Health, Education, and Welfare declared medical assisting an allied health profession. In the early 1970s the American Medical Technologists (which has been a national certifying body for laboratory personnel since 1939) began a program to register medical assistants at accredited schools. You will read more about the benefits of joining one of these organizations later in the chapter. Figure 1-1 shows the pins worn by medical assistants who are certified by the AAMA and by those registered by the American Medical Technologists.

The AAMA's Purpose. The AAMA works to raise standards of medical assisting to a more professional level. It is the only professional association devoted exclusively to the medical assisting profession. Its creator and first

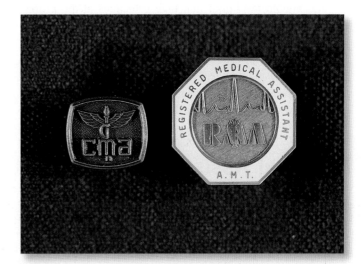

Figure 1-1. The pin on the left is worn by members of the American Association of Medical Assistants. The pin on the right is worn by medical assistants registered by the American Medical Technologists.

president, Maxine Williams, had extensive experience in orchestrating medical assisting projects for the Kansas Medical Assistants Society. She also served as cochair of the planning committee that formed the AAMA.

The AAMA Creed.   To maintain the professional standards of the medical assisting profession, the AAMA has developed the following creed, which is reprinted here with the permission of the organization:

> *I believe in the principles and purposes of the profession of medical assisting.*
> *I endeavor to be more effective.*
> *I aspire to render greater service.*
> *I protect the confidence entrusted to me.*
> *I am dedicated to the care and well-being of all people.*
> *I am loyal to my physician-employer.*
> *I am true to the ethics of my profession.*
> *I am strengthened by compassion, courage, and faith.*

AAMA Code of Ethics.   The AAMA has also established a code of ethics, which is reprinted here with the permission of the organization:

> The Code of Ethics of AAMA shall set forth principles of ethical and moral conduct as they relate to the medical profession and the particular practice of Medical Assisting.
>
> Members of AAMA dedicated to the conscientious pursuit of their profession, and thus desiring to merit the high regard of the entire medical profession and the respect of the general public which they serve, do pledge themselves to strive always to:

A. render service with full respect for the dignity of humanity

B. respect confidential information obtained through employment unless legally authorized or required by responsible performance of duty to divulge such information

C. uphold the honor and high principles of the profession and accept its disciplines

D. seek to continually improve the knowledge and skills of medical assistants for the benefit of patients and professional colleagues

E. participate in additional service activities aimed toward improving the health and well-being of the community

Medical Assistant Credentials

According to Donald A. Balasa, JD, MBA, AAMA executive director and staff legal counsel, "voluntary credentialing . . . is usually national in its scope and most often sponsored by a nongovernmental, private-sector entity" (Balasa, 1994). Employers today prefer or even insist that their medical assistants have credentialing within their discipline. Understanding why employers are aggressively

recruiting credentialed medical assistants is of utmost importance for medical assisting educators as well as all medical assistants. Listed here are some explanations as to why credentialing is becoming so important for a medical assistant's entry into and advancement within the allied health force.

Malpractice

The United States continues to be one of the most litigious nations in the civilized world. Disputes that used to be settled by discussion and mediation are now being referred to attorneys and ending up in courts of law. Lawsuit mania is particularly acute in the world of health care. Employers of allied health professionals have correctly concluded that having credentialed personnel or staff will lessen the likelihood of a successful legal challenge to the quality of work of employees.

Managed Care Organizations

Managed care is a growing trend in today's health-care industry. The cost limitations imposed by **managed care organizations (MCOs)** are causing mergers and buyouts throughout the nation. Small physician practices are being consolidated or merged into larger providers of health care, and the resulting economies of scale can make the delivery of health care more cost-effective. Human resource directors of MCOs place great importance in professional credentials for their employees and therefore are more likely to establish certification or registry as a mandatory professional designation for medical assistants.

State and Federal Regulations

Certain provisions of the **OSHA (Occupational Safety and Health Act)** and the **CLIA (Clinical Laboratory Improvement Amendments)** are making mandatory credentialing for medical assistants a logical step in the hiring process. Presently, OSHA and CLIA do not require that medical assistants be credentialed, but there are various components of these statutes and their regulations that can be met by demonstrating that medical assistants in a clinical setting are certified.

CMA Certification

The **Certified Medical Assistant (CMA)** credential is awarded by the Certifying Board of the AAMA. The AAMA's certification examination evaluates mastery of medical assisting competencies based on the 2003 Role Delineation Study, discussed later in this chapter. The National Board of Medical Examiners (NBME) also provides technical assistance in developing the tests.

CMAs must recertify the CMA credential every 5 years. This mandate requires you to learn about new medical developments through education courses or participation in an examination. Hundreds of continuing education courses are sponsored by local, state, and national AAMA groups. The AAMA also offers self-study courses through its Continuing Education Department. As described in the AAMA's publication *Certified Medical Assistants: Health-Care's Most Versatile Professionals,* the advantages of CMA certification include respect and recognition from peers in the medical assisting profession.

As of June 1998, only applicants of medical assisting programs accredited by the Commission on Accreditation of Allied Health Education Programs (CAAHEP) and the Accrediting Bureau of Health Education Schools (ABHES) are eligible to take the certification examination. The examination is administered nationwide every January and June at more than 100 test sites. The AAMA offers the *Candidate's Guide to the Certification Examination* to help applicants prepare for the examination. This guide explains the test format and test-taking strategies. It also includes a sample examination with answers and information about study references.

RMA Registration

The **Registered Medical Assistant (RMA)** credential is given by the American Medical Technologists (AMT), an organization founded in 1939. RMA credentialing by the AMT ensures that you have taken and passed the AMT certification examination for the Registered Medical Assistant. RMA is a generic term used by the American Registry of Medical Assistants since 1950 and by the AMT since 1984.

The AMT sets forth certain educational and experiential requirements to earn the RMA credential. These include:

- Graduation from an accredited high school or acceptable equivalent.
- Graduation from a medical assistant program or institution accredited by the Accrediting Bureau of Health Education Schools (ABHES), from a medical assistant program accredited by a regional accrediting commission, or from a formal medical services training program of the U.S. Armed Forces. Alternatively, the applicant can have been employed in the profession of medical assisting for a minimum of 5 years, not more than 2 of which may have been as an instructor in a postsecondary medical assistant program.
- Passing the AMT examination for RMA certification.

Major Areas of the RMA/CMA Examinations

The RMA and CMA qualifying examinations are rigorous. Participation in an accredited program, however, will help you learn what you need to know. The examinations cover several distinct areas of knowledge. These include:

- General medical knowledge, including terminology, anatomy, physiology, behavioral science, medical law, and ethics

- Administrative knowledge, including medical records management, collections, insurance processing, and the **Health Insurance Portability and Accountability Act (HIPAA)**
- Clinical knowledge, including examination room techniques, medication preparation and administration, pharmacology, and specimen collection

Membership in a Medical Assisting Association

Professional associations set high standards for quality and performance in a profession. They define the tasks and functions of an occupation. In addition, they provide members with the opportunity to communicate and network with one another. They also present their goals to the profession and to the general public. Becoming a member of a professional association helps you achieve career goals and further the profession of medical assisting.

Professional Support for CMAs

When you become a member of the AAMA, you will have a large support group of active medical assistants. Membership benefits include:

- Professional publications, such as *The CMA*
- A large variety of educational opportunities, such as chapter-sponsored seminars and workshops about the latest administrative, clinical, and management topics (Figure 1-2)

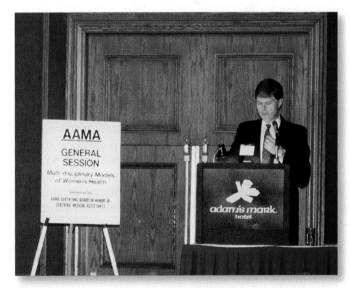

Figure 1-2. Local and state chapters of the AAMA and AMT frequently sponsor seminars and workshops on administrative, clinical, or management topics. In this picture, Donald A. Balasa, executive director and staff legal counsel for the AAMA, addresses a group at the annual AAMA national convention.

- Group insurance
- Legal counsel
- Local, state, and national activities that include professional networking and multiple continuing education opportunities

Professional Support for RMAs

The AMT offers many benefits for RMAs. These include:

- Professional publications
- Membership in the AMT Institute for Education
- Group insurance programs—liability, health, and life
- State chapter activities
- Legal representation in health legislative matters
- Annual meetings and educational seminars
- Student membership

Training Programs and Other Learning Opportunities

Formal programs in medical assisting are offered in a variety of educational settings. They include vocational-technical high schools, postsecondary vocational schools, community and junior colleges, and 4-year colleges and universities. Vocational school programs usually last 1 or 2 years and award a certificate or diploma. Community and junior college programs are usually 2-year associate degree programs.

Accreditation

Accreditation is the process by which programs are officially authorized. Two agencies recognized by the U.S. Department of Education accredit programs in medical assisting: CAAHEP and ABHES.

Accredited programs must cover the following topics: anatomy and physiology; medical terminology; medical law and ethics; psychology; oral and written communications; laboratory, clinical, and administrative procedures; typing; transcription; record keeping; accounting; and insurance processing. High school students may prepare for these courses by studying mathematics, health, biology, typing, office skills, bookkeeping, and computers. You may obtain current information about accreditation standards for medical assisting programs from the AAMA.

Medical assisting programs must also include an externship. An **externship** is practical work experience for a specified time frame in physicians' offices, hospitals, or other health-care facilities.

Additionally, the AAMA lists its minimum standards for accredited programs (called essentials). This list of essentials ensures that all personnel—administrators and faculty—are qualified to perform their jobs.

The AAMA requires that administrative personnel exhibit leadership and management skills. They must also be able to fully perform the functions identified in documented job descriptions. Faculty members must develop and evaluate lesson plans, assess student progress toward the program's objectives, and be knowledgeable regarding course content. They must be qualified through work experience and be able to effectively direct and evaluate student learning and laboratory experiences.

The AAMA also has accreditation requirements for financial and physical resources. Each program's financial resources must meet its obligations to students. Schools must also have adequate physical resources—classrooms, laboratories, clinical and administrative facilities, and equipment and supplies.

The Benefits of Certification/Registration

Certification or registration is not required to practice as a medical assistant. You may practice with a high school diploma or equivalent. Your career options will be greater, however, if you graduate from an accredited school and you become certified or registered.

Graduation from an accredited program helps your career in three ways. First, it shows that you have completed a program that meets nationally accepted standards. Second, it provides recognition of your education by professional peers. Third, it makes you eligible for registration or certification (Heyman, 1993).

A solid medical assisting program provides the following:

- Facilities and equipment that are up to date
- Student to instructor ratio of 20:1
- Job placement services
- A cooperative education program and opportunities for continuing education

Externships

In an externship you will obtain work experience while completing a medical assisting program. You will practice skills learned in the classroom in an actual medical office environment.

Externship Requirements. Externships are mandatory in accredited schools. Each program has its own externship requirements. Familiarize yourself with the program requirements as soon as possible. You may be able to obtain an externship site of your choice either at a practice already affiliated with the school or at a practice you find on your own.

The externship is offered in cooperative medical offices or hospitals for a predetermined period (several weeks to several months). Another experienced medical assistant, nurse manager, or licensed nurse practitioner in the externship office often becomes your mentor. This mentor advises and supervises you during the externship.

Externship Duties. Your duties will be planned to meet your program's requirements for real-world work experience. Approach the externship with a positive attitude. Accept any guidance, constructive criticism, or praise as a learning experience.

Obtaining a Reference. Your externship also offers you the opportunity to acquire a good reference. A reference is usually written by your supervisor, who will describe your performance, strengths, and skills. You may use this reference later with prospective employers. Because you may be required to provide a list of references when applying for future jobs, ask your externship mentor to prepare a letter of reference for your **portfolio** (a collection of your résumé, reference letters, and other documents of interest, such as awards for volunteer service in a health-related field). Send a thank-you note to your supervisor for allowing you to do an externship and for writing you a reference.

Volunteer Programs

Volunteering is a rewarding experience. Before you even begin a medical assisting program, you can gain experience in a health-care profession through volunteer work. As a volunteer, you will get hands-on training and learn what it is like to assist patients who are ill, disabled, or frightened.

You may volunteer as an aide in a hospital, clinic, nursing home, or doctor's office or as a typist or filing clerk in a medical office or medical record room. Some visiting nurse associations and hospices (homelike medical settings that provide medical care and emotional support to terminally ill patients and their families) also offer volunteer opportunities. These experiences may help you decide if you want to pursue a career as a medical assistant.

The American Red Cross also offers volunteer opportunities for the student medical assistant. The Red Cross needs volunteers for its disaster relief programs locally, statewide, nationally, and abroad.

As part of a disaster relief team at the site of a hurricane, tornado, storm, flood, earthquake, or fire, volunteers learn first-aid and emergency triage skills. Red Cross volunteers gain valuable work experience that may help them obtain a job.

Because volunteers are not paid, it is usually easy to find work opportunities. Just because you are not paid for volunteer work, however, does not mean the experience is not useful for meeting your career goals.

Include information about any volunteer work on your **résumé**—a typewritten document that summarizes your employment and educational history. Be sure to note specific duties, responsibilities, and skills developed during the volunteer experience (Figure 1-3).

Multiskill Training

Today many hospitals and health-care practices are embracing the idea of a multiskilled health-care professional (MSHP). An MSHP is a cross-trained team member who is able to handle many different duties.

The AAMA includes the word *multiskill* in its definition of the profession of medical assisting:

> Medical assisting is a multiskilled allied health profession whose practitioners work primarily in ambulatory settings, such as medical offices and clinics. Medical assistants function as members of the healthcare delivery team and perform administrative and clinical procedures. (AAMA, 1991)

An MSHP may be trained to perform certain clinical procedures. She is not, however, trained to make judgments or interpretations concerning a patient's diagnosis or treatment, as a physician would.

Reducing Health-Care Costs. As a result of health-care reform and downsizing (a reduction in the number of staff members) to control the rising cost of health care, medical practices are eager to reduce personnel costs by hiring multiskilled health professionals. These individuals, who perform the functions of two or more people, are the most cost-efficient employees.

Expanding Your Career Opportunities. Career opportunities are vast if you are self-motivated and willing to learn new skills. If you continue to learn about new administrative and clinical techniques and procedures, you will be an important part of the health-care team.

As you read this book, look for a boxed feature titled Career Opportunities. This feature highlights additional skills medical assistants can learn and integrate into their jobs to make themselves more marketable as multiskilled health professionals. Following are several examples of positions that are sometimes combined with a medical assistant position:

- Office manager
- Medical laboratory technician
- ECG technician
- Medical transcriptionist 80-100 wpm
- Medical biller
- Hospital admissions coordinator
- A professional who performs physical exams for applicants to insurance companies
- An administrative assistant at insurance companies (particularly in managed care companies), hospitals, and clinics

If you are multiskilled, you will have an advantage when job hunting. Prospective employers are eager to hire multiskilled medical assistants and may create positions for them.

ALICIA HOLT
114 Herald Avenue
Winston, MO 43840
660-555-1212

POSITION: Full-time medical assistant

EDUCATION:

June 1996–June 1998   Associate Degree in Science, Mayerville Community College
                        Will take the medical assisting certification examination
                        after graduation

September 1991–June 1995   Winston Central High School

WORK EXPERIENCE:

May 1998–June 1998   Medical assistant extern
                        Dr. J. D. Perez, pediatrician,
                        Mayerville Pediatrics, Mayerville, MO

September 1994–present General office clerk
                        Cunningham Medical Supply Company, Winston, MO

June 1994–September 1994   Waitress
                        Bonelli's Italian Restaurant, Winston, MO

VOLUNTEER EXPERIENCE:

May 1995–present   Recreational aide
                        Watson House for Autistic Children, Mayerville, MO

June 1993–present   Receptionist and information clerk
                        Riverside General Hospital, Atherton, MO

SPECIAL SKILLS:

                        Typing 55 wpm
                        WordPerfect and Excel
                        Medical Transcription
                        CPR (certified)
                        First Aid (certified)

                        References available upon request.

Figure 1-3. This medical assistant's résumé includes information about her volunteer work.

Unit Secretary

To gain medical assistant credentials, you must fulfill the requirements of either the American Association of Medical Assistants (for a Certified Medical Assistant) or the American Medical Technologists (for a Registered Medical Assistant). After obtaining your medical assistant certification or registration, you may wish to acquire additional skills in specialty areas through course work or on-the-job training. Although this course work or training may not lead to an additional certification or degree, it will enable you to expand your role in the medical office and advance your career as the demand for skilled health professionals increases.

Skills and Duties

Unit secretaries work in nursing stations or units in a hospital. They keep the nursing station functioning smoothly and free the nursing staff to focus on patient care. A unit secretary usually reports to a head nurse or a unit manager.

The unit secretary has four main areas of responsibility.

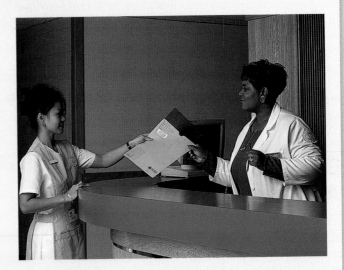

1. *Reception.* The unit secretary greets patients and gives them directions. She welcomes visitors and directs them to the rooms of the patients they wish to visit.

2. *Communication.* The unit secretary answers the phone and responds to pages. She addresses patient requests received over the intercom system, such as a request for a nurse or a doctor to come to the patient's room. The unit secretary also delivers mail and messages to patients. Unit secretaries with a command of medical terminology may be involved in coordinating the scheduling of medical personnel for the unit.

3. *Clerical duties.* The unit secretary updates records in patients' charts, transcribes physicians' orders, adds x-rays and laboratory reports to patients' charts, and processes the necessary paperwork for admissions, discharges, transfers, and deaths. In addition, she provides patient information, such as charts and schedules, to doctors and other hospital staff. The unit secretary also schedules patients' visits to other medical units in the hospital, such as laboratories. She keeps track of supply inventories for the unit, places orders for supplies and equipment as needed, and schedules necessary maintenance and repair services.

4. *Safety.* In some hospitals the unit secretary may be responsible for checking each room in the unit to make sure that all equipment—such as lamps, televisions, radios, and furniture—is in good working order. Other safety-related duties include keeping work areas free from clutter and making emergency code calls when necessary.

Workplace Settings

Most unit secretaries work at a nursing station or in a unit or ward in a hospital, but some find work in nursing homes. In some locations the work is divided differently than in a hospital. For example, a clinic might employ one person to handle scheduling and telephone reception and another staff member to greet patients and collect check-in information. Thus the clerical duties of the unit secretary might be separate from those of the receptionist.

Education

Unit secretaries need a high school diploma, and they receive their training on the job, although courses are available that provide valuable background. Sometimes a person who volunteers as a unit secretary in a hospital may be promoted to a paid position.

Where to Go for More Information

American Hospital Association
One North Franklin, Suite 2706
Chicago, IL 60606
(312) 422-3000

National Health Council
1730 M Street, NW, Suite 500
Washington, DC 20036
(202) 785-3910

You can gain multiskill training by showing initiative and a willingness to learn every aspect of the medical facility in which you are working. When you begin working within a medical facility, establish goals regarding your career path and discuss them with your immediate supervisor. Indicate that you would like to become **cross-trained** in every aspect of the medical facility. Begin your mastery of the department that you are currently working in and branch out to other departments once you master the skills needed for your current position. This will demonstrate a commitment to your profession as well as a strong work ethic. Cross-training is a valuable marketing tool to include on your résumé.

Daily Duties of Medical Assistants

As a medical assistant you will be the physician's "right arm." Duties include maintaining an efficient office, preparing and maintaining medical records, assisting the physician during examinations, and keeping examining rooms in order. You may also handle the payroll for the office staff (or supervise a payroll service), obtain equipment and supplies, and serve as the link between the physician and representatives of pharmaceutical and medical supply companies. In small practices you will usually handle all duties. In larger practices you may specialize in a particular duty.

Administrative Duties

Your administrative duties may include:

- Greeting patients
- Handling correspondence
- Scheduling appointments
- Answering telephones
- Creating and maintaining patient medical records
- Handling billing, bookkeeping, and insurance processing
- Performing medical transcription
- Arranging for hospital admissions
- Scheduling teleconferences for doctors at different locations to discuss cases
- Supervising personnel
- Developing and conducting public outreach programs to market the physician's professional services
- Negotiating leases of equipment and supply contracts
- Creating a recycling program for the practice (Tips for the Office gives more information on this topic.)
- Serving as liaison between the physician and other individuals, such as pharmaceutical sales representatives and lawyers
- Performing as a HIPAA compliance officer

Clinical Duties

Your clinical duties may vary according to state law. They may include:

- Assisting the doctor during examination
- Asepsis and infection control
- Performing diagnostic tests
- Giving injections, where allowed
- Performing electrocardiograms (ECGs)
- Drawing blood for testing
- Disposing of **contaminated** (soiled, or stained) supplies
- Explaining treatment procedures to patients
- Performing first aid and cardiopulmonary resuscitation (CPR)
- Patient education
- Preparing patients for examinations
- Preparing and administering medications as directed by the physician, and following state laws for invasive procedures
- Facilitating treatment for patients from diverse cultural backgrounds and for patients with hearing or vision impairments, or physical or mental disabilities
- Recording vital signs and medical histories
- Removing sutures or changing dressings on wounds
- Sterilizing medical instruments

Other clinical duties may include instructing patients about medication and special diets, authorizing drug refills as directed, and calling pharmacies to order prescriptions. You may also assist with minor surgery or teach patients about special procedures before laboratory tests, surgery, x-rays, or ECGs.

Laboratory Duties

Your laboratory duties may include:

- Performing tests, such as a urine pregnancy test, on the premises
- Collecting, preparing, and transmitting laboratory specimens
- Teaching patients to collect specific specimens properly
- Arranging laboratory services
- Meeting safety standards and fire protection mandates
- Performing as an OSHA compliance officer

Specialization

You may also choose to specialize in a specific area of health care. For example, podiatric medical assistants make castings of feet, expose and develop x-rays, and assist podiatrists in surgery. Ophthalmic medical assistants help ophthalmologists (doctors who provide eye care) by administering diagnostic tests, measuring and

Tips for the Office

Recycling in the Medical Office, Hospital, Laboratory, or Clinic

You may easily incorporate recycling procedures into the daily routine of a medical office, hospital, laboratory, or clinic. Medical facilities generate a tremendous amount of recyclable paper material. Recycling may be required by state law. Purchase paper products that can be recycled, or those made of postconsumer recycled materials, and take care in disposing of them (Roseen, 1991).

Some states levy large fines for noncompliance with recycling regulations. It is thus important to have a well-organized office recycling program. There are two essential aspects of recycling: disposal and purchasing. To create a complete recycling program, ensure that materials are disposed of properly and that purchased products have been made from recycled materials.

You may easily call the town's recycling center for guidelines for packaging recycled materials and for a pickup schedule. The recycling center may also provide containers for recyclable materials. You must fulfill all town and state legal recycling requirements.

Most paper products that do not have a glossy coating (like some fax paper) are recyclable. Each recycling center will provide a list of paper materials that can and cannot be recycled.

You must also research disposal techniques for biohazardous materials and follow regulations listed in the office policy manual and OSHA guidelines. These materials cannot be recycled and must be disposed of properly. They must not be mixed with recyclable waste. You will follow the office policy manual and OSHA guidelines for hazardous medical wastes—including blood products, gloves, cotton swabs, body fluids, and sharps (needles or instruments that puncture the skin). These materials must be disposed of following standard guidelines and in a specially designed protective container.

You must keep recycling issues in mind at all times. Always choose products made from recycled materials—including paper (computer paper and letterhead), printer cartridges, pencils, and many other products.

---

recording vision, testing the functioning of eyes and eye muscles, and performing other duties. (Medical specialties and medical assistant specialties are fully discussed in Chapter 2.)

Personal Qualifications of Medical Assistants

There are several personal qualifications that you must have to be an effective and productive medical assistant. You must enjoy working with all types of people, possess good critical thinking skills, and be able to pay attention to detail. Empathy, willingness to learn, flexibility, self-motivation, professionalism, integrity, and sound judgment are other important traits. Additionally, you must have a neat, professional appearance, possess good communication skills, and know how to remain calm in a crisis.

Critical Thinking Skills

You will develop critical thinking skills over time, as you apply knowledge about and experience with human nature, medicine, and office administration to new situations. Critical thinking skills include quickly evaluating circumstances, solving problems, and taking action.

Critical thinking skills are used every day. One example is prioritizing your work—deciding which are the most important tasks of the day and which are less important. On a day where everything seems to be "top priority," you must use your professional judgment, knowledge of office policies, and experience with physicians and coworkers to determine what should get done first, second, third, and so on.

You must use critical thinking skills to assess how to react to emergency situations. If you see a patient suddenly pass out in the physician's waiting room, you must quickly see that the patient receives first aid, notify a physician, and alert the patient's family.

Attention to Detail

The profession of medical assisting requires attention to detail. You must check every detail when administering drugs, processing bills and insurance forms, and completing patient charts.

The need for attention to detail is illustrated in the common request to call a patient's pharmacy to order a prescription. You must accurately relay information from the doctor's prescription to the pharmacist. You must ask the pharmacist to read back the information to ensure that he has heard it correctly. Then you must document, in the chart, what has been ordered and when.

Empathy

Empathy is the ability to "put yourself in someone else's shoes" and to identify with and understand another person's feelings. Patients who are ill, frustrated, or frightened appreciate empathic medical personnel.

Many patients require empathy during a medical crisis. For example, a patient with the flu may describe how coughing has prevented him from getting a full night's sleep. You may display empathy by saying, "I know how the flu can disrupt sleep. I just got over it last week myself. It's important to rest in bed, though, even if you can't always sleep."

Willingness to Learn

You must always display a willingness to learn. You will gain new skills more easily and become better acquainted with the administrative and clinical topics and issues related to the practice in which you work if you are willing to learn. Keep an open mind, listen carefully to the professionals with whom you work, observe procedures carefully, listen actively to others, and do your own homework to learn more about medical topics so you can apply new information to your daily activities. For example, if you work in a pediatric practice, you might take a continuing education class on child development at a local community college, at a YWCA, or in a workshop offered by a professional association such as the AAMA or AMT (Figure 1-4).

Flexibility

You will encounter new people and situations every day. An attitude of flexibility will allow you to adapt and to handle them with professionalism.

An example of the need for flexibility occurs when a physician's schedule changes to include evening and weekend hours. The staff may also be asked to change schedules. You must make it a priority to be flexible and to meet the employer's needs.

Self-Motivation

You must be self-motivated and willing to offer assistance with work that needs to be done, even if it is not your assigned job. For example, if you think of a more efficient way to organize patient check-in, discuss it with your supervisor. She may agree and be willing to give your idea a try. If a coworker is on vacation, offer to pitch in and work extra time to keep the office running smoothly.

Professionalism

You should exhibit courtesy, conscientiousness, and a generally businesslike manner at all times on the job. It is important to act professionally with coworkers, patients,

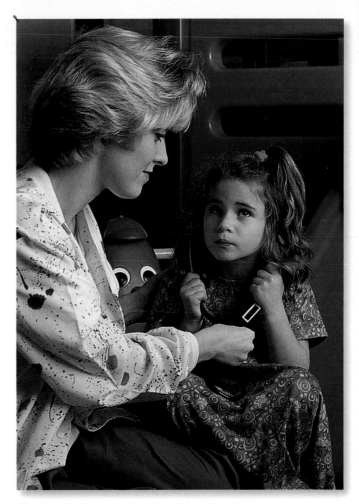

Figure 1-4. A medical assistant who works part-time in a pediatric practice might volunteer one day a week at a preschool to learn more about working with children.

doctors, and others in the work setting. You are an agent of your employer—you represent the doctor or doctors in the practice.

One example of professional behavior includes treating all patients with dignity and kindness. Another is making sure that you have completed and documented all your daily duties before leaving work at the end of each day.

You can start acting like a professional even while you are in the classroom studying to become a medical assistant. Presenting a neat appearance, showing courtesy and respect for peers and instructors, having a good attendance record, and arriving on time to class are all important elements that contribute to professionalism in school and in the workplace.

Neat Appearance

A medical professional always strives to maintain a neat appearance in the workplace. Personal cleanliness is an important part of maintaining a neat appearance. Your appearance is your first impression to your patients, coworkers, and the physicians you work with. Medical facilities and staff are considered "conservative" work environments. Your appearance should reflect a conservative style. Listed here are a few professional guidelines to follow in the medical environment:

- Your uniforms should be clean, pressed crisply, and in good repair. Your uniform should fit your body type and should not be ill-fitting.
- Your shoes should be comfortable, white, clean, and in good condition. Laces should be white and clean. Avoid athletic-looking shoes. Polish your shoes on a daily basis. Only leather shoes that are not open are permitted in a patient treatment area.
- Choose a hairstyle that is flattering and conservative. Hair should be clean and pulled back from your face and off your collar if long. Natural colors for hair are the only acceptable color in a medical environment.
- Your nails should be a short working length, no more than ¼ inch. Nail polish should be pale or clear. A French manicure is acceptable. Acrylic nails should be avoided. Many medical facilities are banning acrylic nails.
- Avoid heavy perfumes and colognes. Many patients and coworkers could be allergic to perfume and cologne.
- Jewelry should be kept to a minimum and in good taste. No more than one ring should be worn. Rings may tear through latex gloves. Ears can be pierced with one hole, and small earrings are appropriate. Any earrings that dangle can be torn off by a patient, such as pediatric patients. Males should not wear earrings in the medical environment.
- Tattoos should never be in a location where they can be seen by a patient.
- Body piercing and tongue piercing is not acceptable in a medical environment. Patients may view this as a visual threat and question your level of competence. Many physicians will rule you out on the first interview if a body piercing (other than ears) is present.
- Bath or shower daily and use an antiperspirant.
- Brush your teeth at least twice daily and schedule regular dental visits to maintain oral health and hygiene.
- Schedule regular checkups with your personal physician.
- Get plenty of rest and eat a well-balanced diet.
- If you are not required to wear a uniform, choose clothing that is conservative and business-appropriate. Avoid fad fashions. Wear low-heeled or flat, polished shoes and a lab coat if working with patients.

Some activities may make it difficult to maintain a neat appearance—replacing the toner in the copy machine, for example, or filling the developing solution in the x-ray machine. Always store a spare uniform or business outfit at your workplace.

Attitude

Your attitude will leave an impression of the type of person you are. In the medical environment, many people depend on you, including coworkers and patients. Your attitude can make or break your career. Professionals always project a positive, caring attitude. They respond to criticism as a learning experience. They take direction from authority without question. They function as a vital member of a medical team. A negative attitude will not be acceptable in a team-oriented medical environment. Many people do not know they have a negative attitude. Ask yourself these questions, and determine if you need to make improvements on your attitude before you begin your new career.

- Do I have repeated conflict with friends or family?
- Have I had a conflict at work that has resulted in voluntary or involuntary termination?
- Do I have conflict with authority figures, such as my instructors?
- Do people make comments about my attitude?

In the workplace environment, professional medical assistants are pleasant, smiling, and conducting themselves in a businesslike and professional manner.

Integrity and Honesty

People with integrity hold themselves to high standards. Everything they do, every task they complete, is performed with a goal of excellence. Individuals with integrity take extreme pride in everything they do. The characteristics of integrity are honesty, dependability, and reliability. Integrity and honesty are key in providing superior customer service to your patients. You must follow through on everything you say you are going to do. For example, if you tell a patient that you are going to return their call regarding a medication, you must call the patient at the time you indicated. Professionals with integrity are honest with the staff and physicians they work with. If you make an error, be honest about it. In order to have integrity, you must be dependable and reliable. Your office staff and physician must be able to trust you and the decisions you make.

Diplomacy

Diplomacy is the ability to communicate with patients, coworkers, managers, and physicians in a manner that is not offensive and that both expresses and inspires cooperation. Communicating with diplomacy is communicating with tact. Medical assistants are often exposed to situations that they may not agree with. A professional has the ability to look at both sides of a situation and to deal with it with courtesy and professionalism.

Proper Judgment

You should demonstrate proper judgment in every task. Before making an important decision, you must carefully evaluate each possible outcome.

An example of a situation that requires proper judgment is assessing when an exception should be made in a doctor's schedule of patients. Suppose the next patient on the schedule is in the waiting room. She is having a routine checkup. An unscheduled patient comes in with chest pains. You use proper judgment and allow the patient with chest pains to see the doctor first.

Communication Skills

Effective communication involves careful listening, observing, speaking, and writing. Communication even involves good manners—being polite, tactful, and respectful. You must use good communication skills during every patient discussion and in every interaction you have with physicians, other staff members, and other professionals with whom your practice does business. (Communication skills are discussed in Chapter 4.)

Remaining Calm in a Crisis

There is always the potential for a crisis or emergency in the health-care field. During a crisis you must remain calm and be prepared to handle any situation.

An example of the need for calm and effective action occurs when a patient appears to suffer a stroke while sitting in the waiting room of a busy medical office. You must quickly direct your peers to alert the doctor and remove the other patients from the room while you begin emergency first-aid measures.

On the Job
Rights of the Medical Assistant

You have the right to be free from any kind of discrimination in the workplace and during the hiring process. These rights are set forth under Title VII of the 1964 Civil Rights Act.

Title VII. The main prohibitions of the civil rights statute are as follows:

> It shall be unlawful employment practice for an employer to fail or refuse to hire or to discharge any individual, or otherwise to discriminate against any individual with respect to his or her compensation, terms, conditions, or privileges of employment, because of such individual's race, color, religion, sex, or national origin, or to limit, segregate, or classify employees or applicants for employment in any way which would deprive or tend to deprive any individual of employment opportunities or

otherwise adversely affect his or her status as an employee, because of such individual's race, color, religion, sex, or national origin. (Lindgren and Taub, 1993)

This law also protects workers from receiving lower pay than the opposite sex for the same work and from denial of a promotion opportunity because of gender.

Sexual Harassment. Title VII also addresses and defines sexual harassment:

> Unwelcome sexual advances, requests for sexual favors, and other verbal or physical conduct of a sexual nature . . . when submission to such conduct is made either explicitly or implicitly a term or condition of an individual's employment, submission to or rejection of such conduct by an individual is used as the basis for employment decisions affecting such individual, or such conduct has the purpose or effect of unreasonably interfering with an individual's work performance or creating an intimidating, hostile, or offensive working environment. (Lindgren and Taub, 1993)

Sexual harassment occurs in a variety of circumstances, and anyone may be sexually harassed. A man or a woman may be the victim or the harasser, and the victim does not have to be of the opposite sex. The victim may be the person being directly harassed or even a coworker who overhears the harassment. The victim has the responsibility to let the harasser know that the conduct is offensive. The victim should also report any instance of sexual harassment to a supervisor or personnel department.

The AAMA Role Delineation Study

In 1996 the AAMA formed a committee whose goal was to revise and update its standards for the accreditation of programs that teach medical assisting. The committee's findings were published in 1997 as the "AAMA Role Delineation Study: Occupational Analysis of the Medical Assisting Profession." The study included a new Role Delineation Chart that outlines the areas of competence you must master as an entry-level medical assistant. The Role Delineation Chart was further updated in 2003.

Areas of Competence

The Medical Assistant Role Delineation Chart, shown in Appendix I, provides the basis for medical assisting education and evaluation. Mastery of the areas of competence listed in this chart is required for all students in accredited medical assisting programs. The chart shows three general areas of competence: administrative, clinical, and general, or trandisciplinary. Each of these three areas is divided into two or more narrower areas, for a total of ten specific areas of competence. Within each area, a bulleted list of statements describes the medical assistant's role.

Uses of the Role Delineation Chart

According to the AAMA, the Role Delineation Chart may be used to:

- Describe the field of medical assisting to other health-care professionals
- Identify entry-level areas of competence for medical assistants
- Help practitioners assess their own current competence in the field
- Aid in the development of continuing education programs
- Prepare appropriate types of materials for home study

Summary

There are many kinds of on-the-job training, training programs, and careers for medical assistants. As you make the decision to become a medical assistant, you must evaluate your skills and the type of position you would like to obtain. An important goal will be to obtain a real-life view of the medical assistant's daily administrative, clinical, and laboratory duties. These skills and duties are outlined under the areas of competence listed in the AAMA Role Delineation Chart.

You must also research how to obtain on-the-job training or choose a training program that will adequately teach you those skills, how to conduct a job search, and whether or not to become a certified or registered medical assistant, and take advantage of the benefits of membership in medical assisting organizations such as the AAMA.

Additionally, you must be aware that the medical assisting profession will continue to change. You will need to stay abreast of changes in technology, procedures, and local, state, and federal regulations governing the way you perform daily duties.

REVIEW

CHAPTER 1

CASE STUDY *QUESTIONS*

Now that you have completed this chapter, review the case study at the beginning of the chapter and answer the following questions:

1. How are the two jobs different?
2. How are the two jobs the same?
3. How do these two medical assistants function as multiskilled health-care professionals?

Discussion Questions

1. Why are more employers recruiting credentialed medical assistants?
2. Name two of the most important personal qualities required of a medical assistant and explain why each is important for success.
3. What is the purpose of the AAMA Role Delineation Chart?
4. Discuss ways to gain real-world work experience in the field of medical assisting.

Critical Thinking Questions

1. Describe an effective medical assistant, and explain two ways a new medical assistant may learn to be an efficient and effective employee.
2. How will the "aging boom" affect health care and the profession of medical assisting in the future?
3. What is a self-directed, lifelong learner? How can a medical assistant achieve this goal?
4. Why is it important to stay current on changes in technology and health care?

Application Activities

1. With a partner, pick one of the following two situations. Without showing your partner, write a description of how you would display the personal attribute stated at the end of the scenario. After you and your partner have written your descriptions, compare them with each other.

   Patient Situation

   Patient says: "I have such a horrible headache. I've been feeling tired lately too."

   Attribute You Wish to Display

   Empathy

   Patient Situation

   Doctor: "I'm really backed up on paperwork. Could you come in an hour early tomorrow morning to help me organize it? You will be paid for the overtime."

   Attribute You Wish to Display

   Flexibility

2. List several challenging but realistic short-term and long-term goals for a medical assistant.
3. A. Think of all the personal qualifications you possess. List those that will help you as a medical assistant.
   B. List all of the personal qualifications you need to develop or improve in order to work successfully in the career of medical assisting.
   C. Describe the actions you will take to acquire the personal qualifications to become a multiskilled medical assistant.

Types of Medical Practice

AREAS OF COMPETENCE

2003 Role Delineation Study

GENERAL

Professionalism
- Work as a member of the health-care team
- Promote the CMA credential
- Enhance skills through continuing education

Legal Concepts
- Perform within legal and ethical boundaries
- Recognize professional credentialing criteria

CHAPTER OUTLINE

- Medical Specialties
- Working With Other Allied Health Professionals
- Specialty Career Options
- Professional Associations

OBJECTIVES

After completing Chapter 2, you will be able to:

2.1 Describe medical specialties and specialists.

2.2 Explain the purpose of the American Board of Medical Specialties.

2.3 Describe the duties of several types of allied health professionals with whom medical assistants may work.

2.4 Name professional associations that may help advance a medical assistant's career.

KEY TERMS

acupuncturist
allergist
anesthetist
cardiologist
chiropractor
dermatologist
doctor of osteopathy
endocrinologist
family practitioner
gastroenterologist
gerontologist
gynecologist
internist
massage therapist
nephrologist
neurologist
oncologist
orthopedist
osteopathic manipulative medicine (OMM)
otorhinolaryngologist
pathologist
pediatrician
physiatrist
physician assistant (PA)
plastic surgeon
primary care physician
radiologist
surgeon
triage
urologist

Introduction

Medical assistants are an integral part of a health-care delivery team. It is important to recognize the many different physician specialists and allied health professions. Medical assistants are often asked to call and process insurance referrals to different specialties and diagnostic departments. Therefore, a working knowledge of the different specialties and allied health professionals demonstrates professionalism and competence.

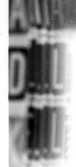

CASE STUDY

Susan has worked as a medical assistant for 12 years. She is considering furthering her educational background in a different allied health profession. She has a strong interest in nursing and in the laboratory.

As you read this chapter, consider the following questions:

1. What are Susan's career options in nursing? How much further education would she need in order to become a nurse?
2. What are Susan's career options in a laboratory setting? How much further education would she need in order to work in a laboratory?

Medical Specialties

Since the beginning of the twentieth century, some physicians have specialized in particular areas of study. There are now approximately 22 major medical specialties. Within each specialty are several subspecialties. For example, cardiology is a major specialty; pediatric cardiology is a subspecialty. As advances in the diagnosis and treatment of diseases and disorders unfold, the demand for specialized care increases and more medical specialties emerge.

If you graduate from an accredited medical assisting program, you will be well equipped to work with a physician specialist. If you work in the office of a physician specialist, you must continue to learn all the new skills that apply to that specialty. First, however, it is helpful to understand the education and licensing process any medical doctor must undergo to become a board-certified physician.

Physician Education and Licensure

The educational requirements for physicians are rigorous and take several years to complete. To earn the title MD (doctor of medicine), thereby qualifying as a licensed physician, a student must complete a bachelor's degree with a concentration typically in the sciences. Then she must attend a medical school accredited by the Liaison Committee on Medical Education (LCME). Upon completing medical school, she is awarded the degree of MD, but this is not the end of her medical training. She must also pass the U.S. Medical Licensing Examination (USMLE). This examination, commonly known as medical boards, has three parts. Part 1 is usually taken after the second year of medical school, part 2 during the fourth year of medical school, and part 3 during the first or second year of postgraduate medical training.

After medical school an MD begins a residency—a period of practical training in a hospital. The first year of residency is known as an internship. Once it is completed an MD can become certified by the National Board of Medical Examiners (NBME). After completing her internship

and passing her medical boards, the MD becomes certified as an NBME Diplomate. If she wishes to specialize in a particular branch of medicine, she must complete an additional 2 to 6 years of residency. She also will apply to the American Board of Medical Specialties (ABMS) to take an examination in her specialty area. After passing the examination, she will be board-certified in her area of specialization. For example, a physician who specializes in pediatrics would receive certification from the American Board of Pediatrics.

The ABMS is an organization of many different medical specialty boards. Its primary purpose is to maintain and improve the quality of medical care and to certify doctors in various specialties. This organization helps the member boards develop professional and educational standards for physician specialists.

Family Practice

Family practitioners (sometimes called general practitioners) are MDs who are generalists and treat all types and ages of patients. They do not specialize in a particular branch of medicine. Many patients seek medical care from a family practitioner and may never have visited a medical specialist. Family practitioners are called **primary care physicians** by insurance companies. The term refers to individual doctors who oversee patients' long-term health care. Some people, however, have internists as their primary care physicians.

A family practitioner sends a patient to a specialist when she has a specific condition or disease that requires advanced care. For example, a family practitioner refers a patient with a lump in her breast to an **oncologist,** a specialist who treats tumors, or to a general surgeon. Either of these doctors may order a mammogram or perform a needle biopsy of the lump to determine if it is malignant.

If you work in a general practice, you will encounter patients with many different conditions and illnesses. As in any medical setting, you must become knowledgeable about preventing the transmission of viruses. This important topic is discussed in several parts of this book.

If you work for a general practitioner, you will often be responsible for arranging patient appointments with specialists. It is important, therefore, for you to know about the duties of each medical specialist. One or more of these specialties may interest you, and you may decide to seek a position as a medical assistant for a physician in that specialty.

Allergy

Allergists diagnose and treat physical reactions to substances, including mold, dust, fur, and pollen from plants or flowers. An individual with allergies is hypersensitive to substances like drugs, chemicals, or elements in nature. An allergic reaction may be minor, such as a rash; serious, such as asthma; or life-threatening, such as swelling of the airways or nasal passages.

Anesthesiology

Anesthetists use medications that cause patients to lose sensation or feeling during surgery. These health-care practitioners administer anesthetics before and during surgery. They also educate patients regarding the anesthetic that will be used and its possible postoperative effects. An anesthesiologist is an MD. A certified registered nurse anesthetist (CRNA) is a registered nurse who has completed an additional program of study recognized by the American Association of Nurse Anesthetists.

Cardiology

Cardiologists diagnose and treat cardiovascular diseases (diseases of the heart and blood vessels). Cardiologists also read electrocardiograms (ECGs) for hospital laboratories. They educate patients about the positive role healthy diet and regular exercise play in preventing and controlling heart disease.

Dermatology

Dermatologists diagnose and treat diseases of the skin, hair, and nails. Their patients have conditions ranging from warts and acne to skin cancer. Dermatologists treat boils, skin injuries, and infections. They remove growths—such as moles, cysts, and birthmarks—and they treat scars and perform hair transplants.

Doctor of Osteopathy

Doctors of osteopathy, who hold the title of DO, practice a "whole-person" approach to health care. DOs feel that patients are more than just a sum of their body parts, and they treat the patient as a whole person instead of concentrating on specific symptoms. Osteopathic physicians understand how all the body's systems are interconnected and how each one affects the other. They focus special attention on the musculoskeletal system, which reflects and influences the condition of all other body systems.

One key concept that DOs believe is that structure influences function. If a problem exists in one part of the body, it may affect the function in both that area and other areas. DOs focus on the body's ability to heal itself, and they actively engage patients in the healing process. By using **osteopathic manipulative medicine (OMM)** techniques, DOs can help restore motion to these areas of the body, thus improving function and often restoring health.

Emergency Medicine

Physicians who specialize in emergency medicine work in hospital emergency rooms. They diagnose and treat patients with conditions resulting from an unexpected medical crisis or accident. Common emergencies include trauma, such as gunshot wounds or serious injuries from car accidents; other injuries, such as severe cuts; and sudden illness, such as alcohol or food poisoning.

Endocrinology

Endocrinologists diagnose and treat disorders of the endocrine system. This system regulates many body functions by circulating hormones that are secreted by glands throughout the body. An example of a disorder treated by an endocrinologist is hyperthyroidism, an abnormality of the thyroid gland. Symptoms include weight loss, shakiness, and weakness.

Gastroenterology

Gastroenterologists diagnose and treat disorders of the gastrointestinal tract. These disorders include problems related to the functioning of the stomach, intestines, and associated organs.

Gerontology

Gerontologists study the aging process. Geriatrics is the branch of medicine that deals with the diagnosis and treatment of problems and diseases of the older adult. A specialist in geriatrics may also be called a geriatrician. As the population of older adults continues to increase, there will be greater need for physicians who specialize in diagnosing and treating diseases of the elderly.

Gynecology

Gynecology is the branch of medicine that is concerned with diseases of the female genital tract. **Gynecologists** perform routine physical care and examination of the female reproductive system. Many gynecologists are also obstetricians.

Internal Medicine

Internists specialize in diagnosing and treating problems related to the internal organs. The internal medicine subspecialties include cardiology, critical care medicine, diagnostic laboratory immunology, endocrinology and metabolism, gastroenterology, geriatrics, hematology, infectious diseases, medical oncology, nephrology, pulmonary disease, and rheumatology. Internists must be certified as specialists in these areas.

Nephrology

Nephrologists study, diagnose, and manage diseases of the kidney. They may work in either a clinic or hospital setting. A medical assistant working with a nephrologist may assist in the operation of a dialysis unit for the treatment of patients with kidney disease. In a rural setting a medical assistant might help a doctor operate a mobile dialysis unit that can be taken to the patient's home or to a medical practice that does not have this technology.

Neurology

Neurology is the branch of medical science that deals with the nervous system. **Neurologists** diagnose and treat disorders and diseases of the nervous system, such as strokes. The nervous system is made up of the brain, spinal cord, and nerves that receive, interpret, and transmit messages throughout the body.

Nuclear Medicine

Nuclear medicine is a fast-growing specialty related to radiology. Both fields use radiation to diagnose and treat disease, but radiology beams radiation through the body from an outside source, whereas nuclear medicine introduces a small amount of a radioactive substance into the body and forms an image by detecting radiation as it leaves the body. The radiation that patients are exposed to is comparable to that of a diagnostic x-ray. Radiology reveals interior anatomy whereas nuclear medicine reveals organ function and structure. Noninvasive, painless nuclear medicine procedures are used to identify heart disease, assess organ function, and diagnose and treat cancer.

Obstetrics

Obstetrics involves the study of pregnancy, labor, delivery, and the period following labor called postpartum (Figure 2-1). This field is often combined with gynecology. A

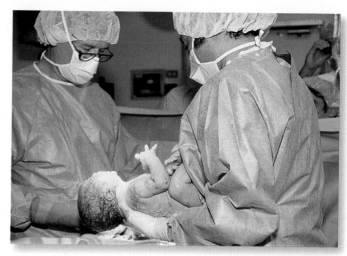

Figure 2-1. Obstetricians who are part of a private practice are usually connected with a specific hospital where they help their patients through labor and delivery.

physician who practices both specialties is referred to as an obstetrician/gynecologist, or OB/GYN.

Oncology

Oncologists, as stated earlier in the chapter, identify tumors, determine if they are benign or malignant, and treat patients with cancer. Treatment may involve chemotherapy, which is the administration of drugs to destroy cancer cells. Treatment may also involve radiation therapy, which kills cancer cells through the use of x-rays. Oncologists treat both adults and children.

Ophthalmology

An ophthalmologist diagnoses and treats diseases and disorders of the eye. This physician specialist examines patients' eyes for poor vision or disease. Other responsibilities include prescribing corrective lenses or medication, performing surgery, and providing follow-up care after surgery. (Ophthalmologists are sometimes confused with optometrists, but the latter are not MDs. Optometrists, however, perform eye exams to determine the general health of the eye and to prescribe corrective eyeglasses or contact lenses.)

Orthopedics

Orthopedics is a branch of surgery that works to maintain function of the musculoskeletal system and its associated structures. An **orthopedist** diagnoses and treats diseases and disorders of the muscles and bones. Some orthopedists concentrate on treating sports-related injuries, either exclusively for professional athletes or for nonprofessionals of all ages. They are called sports medicine specialists.

Otorhinolaryngology

Otorhinolaryngology involves the study of the ear, nose, and throat. An **otorhinolaryngologist** diagnoses and treats diseases of these body structures. This physician specialist is also referred to as an ear, nose, and throat (ENT) specialist.

Pathology

Pathology is the study of disease. It provides the scientific foundation for all medical practice. The **pathologist** studies the changes a disease produces in the cells, fluids, and processes of the entire body (sometimes by performing autopsies, examinations of the bodies of the deceased) to advance the clinical practice of medicine.

There are two basic types of pathologists. Governments and police departments use forensic pathologists to determine facts about unexplained or violent deaths. Anatomic pathologists often work at hospitals in a research capacity, and they may read biopsies (samplings of cells that could be malignant).

Pediatrics

Pediatrics is concerned with the development and care of children and the diseases of childhood. A **pediatrician** diagnoses and treats childhood diseases and teaches parents skills to keep their children healthy.

Physical Medicine

Physical medicine specialists **(physiatrists)** diagnose and treat diseases and disorders with physical therapy. Physical medicine specialists' patients include both adults and children.

Plastic Surgery

A **plastic surgeon** performs the reconstruction, correction, or improvement of body structures. Patients may be accident victims or disfigured due to disease or abnormal development. Plastic surgery involves facial reconstruction, face-lifts, and skin grafting. Plastic surgery is also used to repair problems like cleft lip and cleft palate.

Radiology

Radiology is the branch of medical science that uses x-rays and radioactive substances to diagnose and treat disease. **Radiologists** specialize in taking and reading x-rays.

Surgery

Surgeons use their hands and medical instruments to diagnose and correct deformities and treat external and

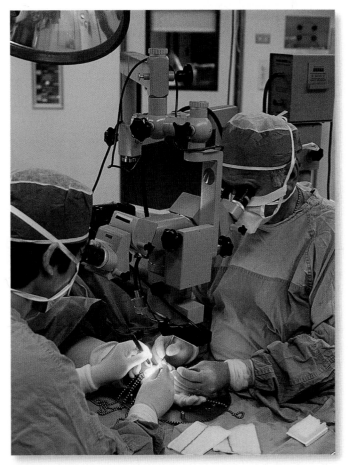

Figure 2-2. Most surgeons specialize in a particular type of surgery, such as heart surgery or hand surgery.

internal injuries or disease (Figure 2-2). They work with many different specialists to surgically treat a broad range of disorders. General surgeons may, for example, perform operations as diverse as breast lumpectomy and repair of a pacemaker. There are also subspecialties of surgery, such as neurosurgery, vascular surgery, and orthopedic surgery.

Urology

A **urologist** diagnoses and treats diseases of the kidney, bladder, and urinary system. A urologist's patients include infants, children, and adults of all ages.

Working With Other Allied Health Professionals

You will always work as a member of a health-care team. That health-care team will include doctors, nurses, specialists, and the patients themselves. You must know the duties of the other allied health professionals in your workplace. Even if you do not work with other allied health professionals in the office, you may contact them through correspondence or by telephone. Understanding the duties of other health-care team members will help make you a more effective medical assistant.

Acupuncturist

Acupuncturists treat people with pain or discomfort by inserting thin, hollow needles under the skin. The points used for insertion are selected to balance the flow of *qi,* or life energy, in the body. The theory of acupuncture relates to Chinese beliefs about how the body works. Qi is composed of two opposite forces called yin and yang. If the flow of qi is unbalanced, insufficient, or interrupted, then emotional, spiritual, mental, and physical problems will result. The acupuncturist works to balance these two forces in perfect harmony. Although there are variations in types of acupuncture—Chinese, Korean, and Japanese—all practitioners will focus on many pulse points along different meridians, the channels through which qi flows.

Chiropractor

Chiropractors treat people who are ill or in pain without using drugs or surgery. They primarily use manual treatments, although they may also employ physical therapy treatments, exercise programs, nutritional advice, and lifestyle modification to help correct the problem causing the pain. The manual treatments, called adjustments, realign the vertebrae in the spine and restore the function of spinal nerves. Chiropractors use diagnostic testing such as x-rays, muscle testing, and posture analysis to determine the location of spinal misalignments, also called *subluxations.* They then develop a treatment plan based on these findings. The treatment plan generally requires several adjustments per week for several weeks or months. Because the treatment does not involve drugs or surgery, the body needs time for healing and correction to occur.

Electroencephalographic Technologist

Electroencephalography (EEG) is the study and recording of the electrical activity of the brain. It is used to diagnose diseases and irregularities of the brain. The EEG technologist (sometimes called a technician) attaches electrodes to the patient's scalp and connects them to a recording instrument. The machine then provides a written record of the electrical activity of the patient's brain. EEG technologists work in hospital EEG laboratories, clinics, and physicians' offices.

Electrocardiograph Technician

The electrocardiograph (ECG) technician is a trained professional who operates an electrocardiograph machine, as pictured in Figure 2-3. An ECG records the electrical

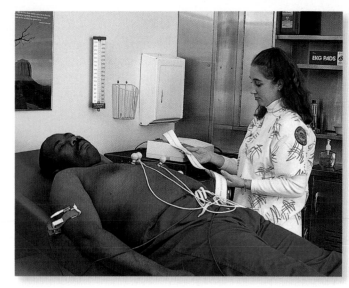

Figure 2-3. The electrocardiograph (ECG) technician is responsible for operating an electrocardiograph machine, which detects heart abnormalities and monitors patients with cardiac problems.

impulses reaching the heart muscles. Physicians and cardiologists use the readings from this machine to detect heart abnormalities and to monitor patients with known cardiac problems. Electrocardiograph technicians work in hospitals.

Massage Therapist

Massage therapists use pressure, kneading, stroking, vibration, and tapping to promote muscle and full-body relaxation as well as to increase circulation and lymph flow. Increasing circulation helps remove blood and waste products from injured tissues and brings fresh blood and nutrients to the areas to speed healing. Massage is one of the oldest methods of promoting healing and is used to treat strains, bruises, muscle soreness or tightness, lower-back pain, and dislocations. It can also relieve muscle spasm, restore motion and function to a body part, and decrease edema.

Medical Records Technologist

There are two types of medical records technologists: the Registered Records Administrator (RRA) and the Accredited Records Technician (ART). These technologists are responsible for organizing, analyzing, and evaluating medical records. Other responsibilities include compiling administrative and health statistics, coding symptoms, and inputting and retrieving computerized health data. These positions involve typing medical reports, preparing statistical reports on patient treatments, and supervising clerical personnel in the medical records department. Accredited records technicians and registered records

Medical Office Administrator

To gain medical assistant credentials, you must fulfill the requirements of either the American Association of Medical Assistants (for a Certified Medical Assistant) or the American Medical Technologists (for a Registered Medical Assistant). After obtaining your medical assistant certification, you may wish to acquire additional skills in specialty areas through course work or on-the-job training. Although this course work or training may not lead to an additional certification or degree, it will enable you to expand your role in the medical office and advance your career as the demand for skilled health professionals increases.

Skills and Duties

A medical office administrator manages the practice of a single physician (solo practice) or of a group practice. His duties are determined, in part, by the size of the practice. If the practice is large, he may have more managerial duties. If it is small, he may act as the receptionist, secretary, and records clerk. (Occasionally, in a solo practice, the practice nurse performs many or all of these functions.) Large group practices with 10 to 15 physicians may have one medical office administrator, while larger group practices with 40 to 50 physicians (such as managed care organizations) may have a highly trained practice administrator who oversees and coordinates the work of several assistant administrators.

The medical office administrator's reception duties begin with greeting and welcoming new patients. He may provide a medical history form for patients and answer any questions they may have. The administrator must have a knowledge of medical terminology in order to answer patients' questions.

This health-care professional coordinates the practice's records and filing. For example, he ensures that x-rays and test results are attached to the appropriate records and that insurance information is up to date. The medical office administrator may also schedule appointments for patients as well as referrals with other specialists. He may also keep track of the medical and nursing staff schedule. Sometimes the administrator is the person who calls patients ahead of time to confirm their appointments.

In a solo or small practice, the medical office administrator may perform general secretarial tasks, such as handling the mail and answering the telephone. He must have strong computer and word processing skills as well as shorthand, typing, and bookkeeping skills. In a large practice the administrator may train and oversee clerical staff and secretaries.

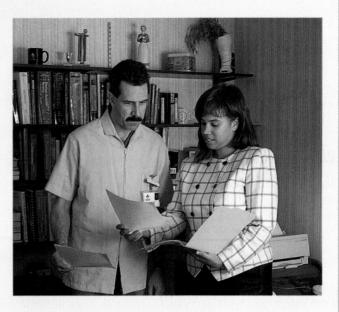

He may also interview and evaluate applicants for clerical jobs.

Workplace Settings

Medical office administrators may work in solo practices, group practices, or medical clinics. Specialized health-care facilities, such as nursing homes, may also employ medical office administrators.

Education

Although medical office administrators may learn the medical terminology they need on the job, they usually acquire their secretarial and clerical background through course work, either in a business/vocational school or in a junior or community college. The educational requirements for a medical office administrator vary with the size of the practice and the extent of the administrator's responsibilities. Upper-level positions require a graduate degree.

Where to Go for More Information

American Academy of Medical Administrators
30555 Southfield Road, Suite 150
Southfield, MI 48076
(313) 540-4310

Medical Group Management Association
104 Inverness Terrace East
Englewood Cliffs, CA 80112
(313) 799-1111

National Association of Medical Staff Services
P.O. Box 23590
Knoxville, TN 37933-1590
(615) 531-3571

administrators work in hospitals, nursing homes, health maintenance organizations, physicians' offices, and government agencies.

Medical Secretary

A medical secretary assists medical, professional, and technical personnel by performing secretarial and clerical support. These functions include taking dictation and typing as well as composing and preparing letters on a word processor. Other functions include maintaining medical and administrative files. A medical secretary may work in a hospital, nursing home, physician's office, or clinic.

Medical Technology

Medical technology is an umbrella term that refers to the development and design of clinical laboratory tests (such as diagnostic tests), procedures, and equipment. Two types of allied health professionals who work in medical technology are the medical technologist and the medical laboratory technician.

Medical Technologist. Medical technologists perform laboratory tests and procedures with clinical laboratory equipment. They examine specimens of human body tissues and fluids, analyze blood factors, and culture bacteria to identify disease-causing organisms. They also supervise and train technicians and laboratory aides. Medical technologists have 4-year degrees and may specialize in areas such as blood banking, microbiology, and chemistry. These technologists are employed in clinics, hospitals, private practices, colleges, pharmaceutical companies, government, research, and industry.

Medical Laboratory Technician. Medical laboratory technicians (MLTs) have 1- to 2-year degrees and are responsible for clinical tests performed under the supervision of a physician or medical technologist. They perform tests in the areas of hematology, serology, blood banking, urinalysis, microbiology, and clinical chemistry. Medical laboratory technicians work in hospital laboratories, commercial laboratories, medical clinics, and physicians' offices.

Medical Transcriptionist

Medical transcriptionists translate a physician's dictation about patient treatments into comprehensive, typed records. Attorneys, insurance companies, and medical specialists need accurate medical records. Medical transcriptionists work in doctors' offices, hospitals, clinics, laboratories, and radiology departments and for medical transcription services and insurance companies. Medical assistants often have medical transcription duties.

Mental Health Technician

A mental health technician, sometimes called a psychiatric aide or counselor, works in a variety of health-care settings with emotionally disturbed and mentally retarded patients. This health professional assists the psychiatric team by observing behavior and providing information to help in the planning of therapy. The mental health technician also participates in supervising group therapy and counseling sessions. This technician may work in a psychiatric clinic, specialized nursing home, psychiatric unit of a hospital, or community health center. Other places of employment include crisis centers and shelters. Training varies widely, from on-the-job training to advanced degrees, depending on job responsibilities and medical setting.

Nuclear Medicine Technologist

A nuclear medicine technologist performs tests to oversee quality control, to prepare and administer radioactive drugs, and to operate radiation detection instruments. This allied health professional is also responsible for correctly positioning the patient, performing imaging procedures, and preparing the information for use by a physician. A nuclear medicine technologist may work in a hospital, public health institution, or physician's office or—with appropriate clinical experience—in a teaching position at a college or university. There are 2- and 4-year training programs. The registration examination is administered by the American Registry of Radiologic Technologists.

Occupational Therapist

An occupational therapist works with patients who have physical injuries or illnesses, psychologic or developmental problems, or problems associated with the aging process. This health professional helps patients attain maximum physical and mental health by using educational, vocational, and rehabilitation therapies and activities. The occupational therapist may work in a hospital, clinic, extended care facility, rehabilitation hospital, or government or community agency. To become an occupational therapist, you need a 4-year degree, followed by a 9- to 12-month internship at an accredited hospital. Then you must pass the national board examination, in order to earn the title of OTR—registered occupational therapist.

Pharmacist

Pharmacists are professionals who have studied the science of drugs and who dispense medication and health supplies to the public. Pharmacists know the chemical and physical qualities of drugs and are knowledgeable about the companies that manufacture drugs.

Pharmacists inform the public about the effects of prescription and nonprescription (over-the-counter) medications. Pharmacists are employed in hospitals, clinics, and nursing homes. They may also work for government agencies, pharmaceutical companies, privately owned pharmacies, or chain store pharmacies. Some pharmacists own their own stores.

There are three levels of pharmacists, each with different training requirements. A pharmacy technician (CPhT) can typically receive on-the-job training. Formal training, although not required by most states, includes certificate programs and 2-year college programs offering associate degrees in science. Voluntary certification is by examination. A registered pharmacist (RPh) requires 5 years of college training with a bachelor's degree in science. Pharmacists must be registered by the state and must pass a state board examination. A doctor of pharmacy (PharmD) requires 6 to 7 years of college training, which may be followed by a residency in a hospital setting.

Phlebotomist

Phlebotomists are allied health professionals trained to draw blood for diagnostic laboratory testing. They work in medical clinics, laboratories, and hospitals. Although medical assistants are also trained to draw blood for standard types of tests, phlebotomists are trained at a more advanced level to be able to draw blood under difficult circumstances or in special situations. For example, if a blood sample is needed for a potassium-level test, it must be drawn in a particular manner that only phlebotomists are trained to do. In most states phlebotomists must be certified by the National Phlebotomy Association or registered by the American Society of Clinical Pathologists.

Physical Therapist

A physical therapist (PT) plans and uses physical therapy programs for medically referred patients. The PT helps these patients to restore function, relieve pain, and prevent disability following disease, injury, or loss of body parts. A physical therapist uses various treatment methods, which include therapy with electricity, heat, cold, ultrasound, massage, and exercise. The physical therapist also helps patients accept their disabilities. A physical therapist may work in a hospital, outpatient clinic, rehabilitation center, home-care agency, nursing home, voluntary health agency, private practice, or sports medicine center. A physical therapist must have a bachelor's degree in physical therapy and must pass a state board examination.

Physician Assistant

A **physician assistant (PA)** is a health-care provider who practices medicine under the supervision of a physician. Physician assistants are licensed by the state in which they practice. PAs are trained in medicine with a curriculum similar in content but shorter in duration than medical school. Most physician assistants are nationally certified and hold the title PA-C. National certification is maintained through cycles of examinations and continuing medical education.

The scope of the physician assistant's practice corresponds to the supervising physician's practice. Duties may include taking patient histories, performing physical examinations, ordering and interpreting laboratory tests, performing procedures, assisting in surgery, diagnosing medical conditions, and developing and carrying out treatment plans. Physician assistants can prescribe medication in most states. PAs work in a wide variety of health-care settings, including hospitals, clinics, private physician offices, schools, prisons, and governmental agencies. They also serve as faculty in physician assistant programs. Medical assistants may work with physician assistants, particularly in outpatient settings.

Radiographer

A radiographer (x-ray technician) is one of the most common positions for individuals whose education is in radiologic technology. The radiographer assists a radiologist in taking x-ray films. These films are used to diagnose broken bones, tumors, ulcers, and disease. A radiographer usually works in the radiology department of a hospital. The x-ray technician may, however, use mobile x-ray equipment in a patient's room or in the operating room. A radiographer may be employed in a hospital, laboratory, clinic, physician's office, government agency, or industry.

Registered Dietitian

Registered dietitians help patients and their families make healthful food choices that provide balanced, adequate nutrition (Figure 2-4). Dietitians are sometimes called nutritionists. Dietitians may assist food-service directors at health-care facilities and prepare and serve food to groups. They may also participate in food research and teach nutrition classes. Dietitians work in community health agencies, hospitals, clinics, private practices, and managed care settings. They may also teach at colleges and universities, and they serve as consultants to organizations and individuals.

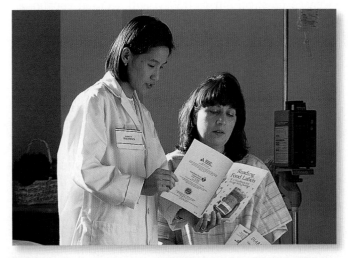

Figure 2-4. Registered dietitians work closely with patients who need to modify their food choices for better health.

Radiologic Technologist

A radiologic technologist is a health-care professional who has studied the theory and practice of the technical aspects of the use of x-rays and radioactive materials in the diagnosis and treatment of disease. A radiologic technologist may specialize in radiography, radiation therapy, or nuclear medicine. Radiologic technologists generally work in hospitals; some work in medical laboratories, medical practices, and clinics.

Respiratory Therapist

A respiratory therapist evaluates, treats, and cares for persons with respiratory problems. The respiratory therapist works under the supervision of a physician and performs therapeutic procedures based on observation of the patient. Using respiratory equipment, the therapist treats patients with asthma, emphysema, pneumonia, and bronchitis. The respiratory therapist plays an active role in newborn, pediatric, and adult intensive care units. The therapist may work in a hospital, nursing home, physician's office, or commercial company that provides emergency oxygen equipment and services to home-care patients.

Nursing Aide/Assistant

Nursing aides assist in the direct care of patients under the supervision of the nursing staff. Typical functions include making beds, bathing patients, taking vital signs, serving meals, and transporting patients to and from treatment areas. Nursing assistants are often employed in psychiatric and acute care hospitals, nursing homes, and home health agencies. On-the-job training can range from 1 week to 3 months.

Practical/Vocational Nurse

Licensed practical nurses (LPNs) and licensed vocational nurses (LVNs) provide nursing care to the sick. Both terms refer to the same type of nurse. Duties involve taking and recording patient temperatures, blood pressure, pulse, and respiration rates. They also include administering some medications under supervision, dressing wounds, and applying compresses. LPNs and LVNs are not allowed, however, to perform certain other duties, such as some intravenous (IV) procedures or the administration of certain medications.

Practical/vocational nurses assist registered nurses and physicians by observing patients and reporting changes in their conditions. LPNs/LVNs work in hospitals, nursing homes, clinics, and physicians' offices and in industrial medicine. To meet the needs of the growing aging population in this country, employment opportunities for LPNs and LVNs in long-term care settings have increased.

LPNs/LVNs must graduate from an accredited school of practical (vocational) nursing (usually a 1-year program).

They are also required to take a state board examination for licensure as LPNs/LVNs.

Associate Degree Nurse

Associate degrees in nursing (ADNs) are offered at many junior colleges and community colleges and at some universities. These programs combine liberal arts education and nursing education. The length of the ADN program is typically 2 years. ADNs are also considered RNs if they pass the state boards.

Diploma Graduate Nurse

Diploma programs are usually 3-year programs designed as cooperative programs between a community college and a participating hospital. The programs combine course work and clinical experience in the hospital.

Baccalaureate Nurse

A baccalaureate degree refers to a 4-year college or university program. Graduates of a 4-year nursing program are awarded a bachelor of science in nursing (BSN) degree. The curriculum includes courses in liberal arts, general education, and nursing courses. Graduates are prepared to function as nurse generalists and in positions that go beyond the role of hospital staff nurses. BSNs are also considered RNs if they pass the state boards.

Registered Nurse

A nurse who graduates from a nursing program and passes the state board examination for licensure is considered an RN, indicating formal, legal recognition by the state. The RN is a professional who is responsible for planning, giving, and supervising the bedside nursing care of patients. An RN may work in an administrative capacity, assist in daily operations, oversee programs in hospital or institutional settings, or plan community health services.

Registered nurses work in a variety of settings. These settings include hospitals, nursing homes, public health agencies, industry, physicians' offices, government agencies, and educational settings. Some RNs continue their education to earn master's or doctoral degrees.

Nurse Practitioner

A nurse practitioner (NP) is an RN who functions in an expanded nursing role. The NP usually works in an ambulatory patient care setting alongside physicians. An NP may work in an independent nurse practitioner practice with no physicians. An independent nurse practitioner takes health histories, performs physical examinations, conducts screening tests, and educates patients and families about disease prevention.

An NP who works in a physician's practice may perform some duties that a physician would, such as administering

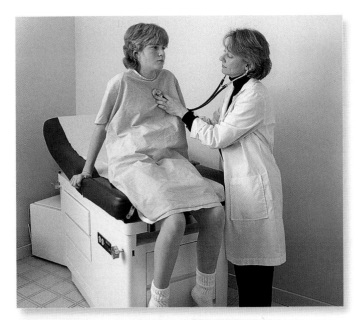

Figure 2-5. Many nurse practitioners work in physicians' offices and are trained to perform routine examinations.

physical examinations and treating common illnesses and injuries (Figure 2-5). For example, in an OB/GYN practice the NP can perform a standard annual gynecologic examination, including taking a Pap smear or a culture to test for yeast infection. The nurse practitioner emphasizes preventive health care.

The NP must be an RN with at least a master's degree in nursing and must complete 4 to 12 months of an apprenticeship or formal training. With specific formal training the student may become a pediatric nurse practitioner, an obstetric nurse practitioner (midwife), or a psychiatric nurse practitioner. The nurse practitioner works with medical assistants.

Specialty Career Options

The various medical specialties can open up many career possibilities for medical assistants. Deciding to specialize may become one of your career goals five or more years from now. Remember that you may need additional training or education for some of these positions. Your hard work will be rewarded, however, as you gain additional job responsibilities.

Choosing an area in which to specialize involves research and careful thought. Local and medical college libraries can supply a great deal of information about the areas in which you may specialize. State employment agencies or schools can help you make career choices.

It is also helpful to check the help-wanted section in local newspapers for information about jobs in specialized areas. Many newspapers separate health-care career opportunities into easy-to-find boxed sections. You may also directly contact companies you would like to work for. Ask about job opportunities, and find out what skills and training the employer requires.

Anesthetist's Assistant

Anesthetist's assistants provide anesthetic care under an anesthetist's direction. Hospitals and high-technology surgical centers frequently employ anesthetist's assistants. These assistants gather patient data and assist in evaluation of patients' physical and mental status. They also record planned surgical procedures, assist with patient monitoring, draw blood samples, perform blood gas analyses, and conduct pulmonary function tests.

Certified Laboratory Assistant

Certified laboratory assistants perform routine procedures in bacteriology, chemistry, hematology, parasitology, serology, and urinalysis. Laboratory assistants work under the supervision of a medical technologist or hospital anatomic pathologist. They work in laboratories at hospitals, clinics, and physicians' offices and in independent laboratories. One-year training programs are offered by hospitals, vocational schools, and community colleges.

Dental Assistant

A dental assistant can practice without formal education or training. In this case, on-the-job training is provided. A dental assistant performs many administrative and laboratory functions that are similar to the duties of a medical assistant. For example, a dental assistant may serve as chair-side assistant, provide instruction in oral hygiene, and prepare and sterilize instruments. To perform expanded clinical and chair-side functions such as those of a hygienist, a dental assistant must have at least 1 year of training in theory and clinical application. This formal education also requires work experience in a dental office.

Dental assistants often work in a private practice. They also work in clinics, dental schools, and local health agencies. Insurance companies hire dental assistants to process dental claims.

Emergency Medical Technician/Paramedic

An emergency medical technician (EMT), sometimes called a paramedic, works under the direction of a physician through a radio communication network. This health professional assesses and manages medical emergencies that occur away from hospitals or other medical settings, such as in private homes, schools, offices, or public areas. An EMT is trained to **triage** patients (to assess the urgency and type of condition presented as well as the immediate medical needs) and to initiate the appropriate treatment for a variety of medical emergencies. While transporting patients to the medical facility, an EMT records, documents, and radios the patient's condition to the physician, describing how the injury occurred. An EMT may work for an ambulance service, fire department, police department, hospital emergency department, private industry, or voluntary care service. Training requirements vary by state but typically require a high school diploma and driver's license, 100 hours of classroom training, and an average of 6 months of practical training on an ambulance squad or in a hospital emergency room.

Occupational Therapist Assistant

Occupational therapist assistants work under the supervision of an occupational therapist. They help individuals with mental or physical disabilities reach their highest level of functioning through the teaching of fine motor skills, trades (occupations), and the arts. Duties include preparing materials for activities, maintaining tools and equipment, and documenting the patient's progress. Occupational therapist assistants must earn a 2-year degree (OTA).

Ophthalmic Assistant

An ophthalmic assistant aids ophthalmologists with the routine functions of the practice. This health professional performs simple vision testing, takes medical histories, administers eyedrops, and changes dressings. There are three levels in this category of allied health professional (from most senior to least senior): ophthalmic technologist, ophthalmic technician, and ophthalmic assistant. Duties are determined by the supervising ophthalmologist. No states currently require certification for these positions.

Pathologist's Assistant

Pathologist's assistants work under the supervision of a pathologist. Pathologist's assistants sometimes work with forensic pathologists—professionals who study the human body and diseases for legal purposes, in cooperation with government or police investigations. They may prepare frozen sections of dissected body tissue. Assistants working for anatomic pathologists (professionals who study the human body and diseases in a research capacity) may maintain supplies, instruments, and chemicals for the anatomic pathology laboratory. Pathologist's assistants perform laboratory work about 75% of the workday. Assistants also perform a variety of administrative duties. They work in community hospitals, university medical centers, and private laboratories.

Pediatric Medical Assistant

A pediatric medical assistant assists the pediatrician in administrative and clinical duties (Figure 2-6). These duties include obtaining medical histories and preparing patients for examination. Other duties include performing routine

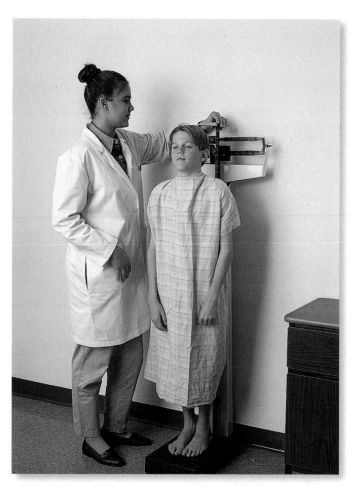

Figure 2-6. If you enjoy working with children, you might consider working as a pediatric medical assistant.

tests, sterilizing supplies and equipment, typing, filing, and clerical work. This health professional also educates patients and their parents or guardians about follow-up care and maintains patients' records. A pediatric medical assistant should be able to communicate well with children. Other helpful skills include patience and organizational skills. Pediatric medical assistants work with pediatricians in private practice, hospitals, and clinics.

Pharmacy Technician

Pharmacy technicians perform specific routine tasks related to record keeping and preparing and dispensing drugs. Duties include preparing medications for administration and making sure patients receive the correct medication. Pharmacy technicians usually work in hospitals or similar facilities under the supervision of a nurse, pharmacist, or other health-care professional. In a commercial pharmacy they work under the pharmacist's supervision. Opportunities are also available with pharmaceutical firms and wholesale pharmaceutical distributors.

Training can be on the job or through certificate programs and 2-year college programs (associate degree).

treatment to patients who have cancer. He may also be responsible for maintaining radiation treatment equipment. The technologist shares responsibility with the radiologist for the accuracy of treatment records. A radiation therapy technologist may work in a hospital, laboratory, clinic, physician's office, or government agency. Training requires a high school diploma and graduation from a 2- or 4-year program in radiography.

Respiratory Therapy Technician

Respiratory therapy technicians work under the supervision of a physician and a respiratory therapist. Respiratory therapists perform procedures such as artificial ventilation. They also clean, sterilize, and maintain the respiratory equipment and document the patient's therapy in the medical record. Respiratory therapy technicians work in hospitals, nursing homes, physicians' offices, and commercial companies that provide emergency oxygen equipment and therapeutic home care.

Speech/Language Pathologist

A speech/language pathologist treats communication disorders, such as stuttering, and associated disorders, such as hearing impairment. This health professional evaluates, diagnoses, and counsels patients who have these problems. A speech/language pathologist may work in a school, hospital, research setting, or private practice or may teach at a college or university.

Speech/language pathologists usually have a master's degree in speech/language pathology or audiology. Certification and licensing requirements vary by state, usually depending on the work setting (public school, private practice, clinic, and so on).

Surgeon's Assistant

A surgeon's assistant provides patient services under the direction, supervision, and responsibility of a licensed surgeon. This health professional's tasks include obtaining a patient's history and physical data. She then discusses the data with a physician or surgeon to determine what procedures to use to treat the problem. A surgeon's assistant may also assist in performing diagnostic and therapeutic procedures. She must be calm and have good judgment in the high-pressure environment of the operating room. Surgeon's assistants work primarily in hospitals.

Surgeon's assistants are considered a subcategory of physician assistant. Training programs are usually affiliated with 2- and 4-year colleges and with university schools of medicine and allied health. These programs include practical work in the surgery unit of an affiliated hospital.

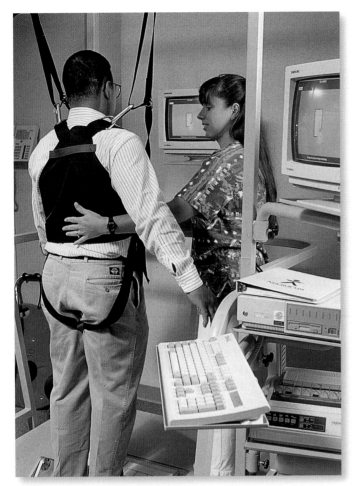

Figure 2-7. Physical therapy assistants provide guidance and support to patients who are recovering from a physical injury or from surgery on a limb or joint.

National certification is voluntary by examination and earns the title CPhT (certified pharmacy technician).

Physical Therapy Assistant

A physical therapy assistant (PTA) works under the direction of a physical therapist to assist with patient treatment. The assistant follows the patient care program created by the physical therapist and physician. This health professional performs tests and treatment procedures, assembles or sets up equipment for therapy sessions, and observes and documents patient behavior and progress (Figure 2-7). A physical therapy assistant may practice in a hospital, nursing home, rehabilitation center, or community or government agency.

Radiation Therapy Technologist

A radiation therapy technologist assists the radiologist. He may, for example, assist with administering radiation

Professional Associations

Membership in a professional association enables you to become involved in the issues and activities relevant to your field and presents opportunities for continuing education. It is a good idea to become informed about such associations, even those, such as the American Medical Association, that are open to physicians only. The physician you work for may ask you to obtain information about the group's activities and meetings. Table 2-1 summarizes professional associations related to the field of medicine and medical assisting.

American Association of Medical Assistants

The American Association of Medical Assistants (AAMA), as described in Chapter 1, was created to serve the interests

TABLE 2-1	Professional Medical Organizations	
Professional Organization	**Membership Requirements**	**Advantages of Membership**
American Association of Medical Assistants (AAMA)	Interested individuals and those who practice medical assisting may join the AAMA.	Offers flexible continuing education programs; publishes bimonthly *The Professional Medical Assistant;* offers legal counsel, professional recognition, various member discounts
American Association for Medical Transcription (AAMT)	Interested individuals and those who practice medical transcription may join the AAMT.	Educates and develops medical transcriptionists as medical language specialists; offers advice and support for self-employed medical transcriptionists
American College of Physicians (ACP)	Physicians and medical students may join.	Provides education and information resources to the field of internal medicine and its subspecialties
American Hospital Association (AHA)	Institutional health-care providers and other individuals may join.	Provides consultant referral service and access to health-care information resources
American Medical Association (AMA)	Physicians and medical students may join.	Provides large information source; publishes *Journal of the American Medical Association (JAMA);* offers AMA/Net
American Medical Technologists (AMT)	Medical assistants, medical technologists, medical laboratory technicians, dental assistants, and phlebotomy technicians may join.	Offers national certification as Registered Medical Assistant (RMA); offers certification to other health-care professionals, publications, state chapter activities, continuing education programs
American Pharmaceutical Association (APhA)	Pharmaceutical professionals and physicians may join.	Helps members improve skills; active in pharmacy policy development, networking, publishing, research, public education
American Society of Clinical Pathologists (ASCP)	Any professional involved in laboratory medicine or pathology may join.	Resource for improving the quality of pathology and laboratory medicine; offers educational programs and materials; certifies technologists and technicians
American Society of Phlebotomy Technicians (ASPT)	Interested individuals and those who practice phlebotomy may join.	Offers national certification as a phlebotomy technician and continuous education programs

of medical assistants and to further the medical assisting profession. The AAMA offers self-paced continuing education classes; workshops and seminars at the local, state, and national levels; and job networking opportunities. Other benefits include legal counsel, group health insurance, professional recognition, and member discounts.

American Association for Medical Transcription

The American Association for Medical Transcription (AAMT) is the professional organization for the advancement of medical transcription. The AAMT also educates medical transcriptionists as medical language specialists. The AAMT offers advice and support to the many medical transcriptionists who are self-employed.

American College of Physicians

Founded in 1915, the American College of Physicians (ACP) is the largest medical specialty organization in the world. It is the only society of internists dedicated to providing education and information resources to the entire field of internal medicine and its subspecialties.

American Hospital Association

The American Hospital Association (AHA) is the nation's largest network of institutional health-care providers. These providers represent every type of hospital: rural and city hospitals, specialty and acute care facilities, free-standing hospitals, academic medical centers, and health systems and networks. The AHA works to support and promote the interests of hospitals and health-care organizations across the country. Organizations as well as individual professionals may join the AHA. Membership benefits include use of the AHA consultant referral service, accessed, for example, by hospitals that need experts in areas not addressed by in-house personnel. Members also have access to AHA's health-care information resources, including teleconferencing and AHA database services.

American Medical Association

The American Medical Association (AMA) was founded in 1847. Its members include 300,000 physicians from every medical specialty. The AMA promotes science and the art of medicine and works to improve public health. The AMA is the world's largest publisher of scientific and medical information and publishes ten monthly medical specialty journals. The AMA also accredits medical programs in the United States and Canada.

The AMA provides an online service called AMA/Net for physicians and medical assistants, offering up-to-date information about current medical topics. To use the AMA/Net, the medical office must have a computer, telephone, and modem.

American Medical Technologists

American Medical Technologists (AMT) was established in 1939 as a not-for-profit organization. The AMT offers national certification as a Registered Medical Assistant (RMA) to medical assisting practitioners. It also offers certification to medical technologists, medical laboratory technicians, dental assistants, and phlebotomy technicians. Membership benefits include continuing education classes, workshops and seminars, and job networking opportunities.

American Pharmaceutical Association

The American Pharmaceutical Association (APhA), the national professional society of pharmacists, was founded in 1852. The APhA represents the interests of pharmaceutical professionals, and it strives to help individual members improve their skills. The APhA works to advance the field of pharmacy and the safety of patients. The APhA is active in pharmacy policy development, networking, publishing, research, and public education.

Summary

There are many medical settings in which you can serve as a medical assistant. Some settings will be in specialized branches of medicine. It is important to gain an understanding of the major areas of medicine, as well as the various subspecialties, in order to choose and plan for the type of setting in which you would like to work.

Learning about various allied health professionals—such as pharmacists, nurse practitioners, and medical transcriptionists—will help you interact with others on the job. Learning about specialty career options—such as physical therapy assistants, certified laboratory assistants, and ophthalmic assistants—can give you ideas about integrating new skills into your job as a multiskilled health professional.

Joining a professional organization will enable you to stay informed about issues and activities in the medical assisting field and the specialty or subspecialty in which you work. Professional organizations also provide other benefits to members, such as group health insurance; job networking opportunities; state or chapter meetings, seminars, workshops, and guest presentations; and member discounts. Membership in a professional organization helps you be recognized as a professional. Therefore, it is an important addition to your résumé.

REVIEW

CHAPTER 2

CASE STUDY QUESTIONS

Now that you have completed this chapter, review the case study at the beginning of the chapter and answer the following questions:

1. What are Susan's career options in nursing? How much further education would she need in order to become a nurse?
2. What are Susan's career options in a laboratory setting? How much further education would she need in order to work in a laboratory?

Discussion Questions

1. Why is geriatrics a growing medical specialty?
2. How might learning about specialty career options help motivate medical assistants in their careers?
3. How do professional organizations help medical assistants perform their job duties?

Critical Thinking Questions

1. How might a medical assistant's experience working with a medical specialist differ from her experience working with a general practitioner, in terms of learning about medicine?
2. If you worked for an obstetrician or OB/GYN, how might you use your spare time to learn more about the specialty and do your job better?
3. Why might a medical assistant be interested in joining a professional association such as the American Hospital Association?

Application Activities

1. Interview a medical assistant, such as a physical therapy assistant, who has chosen a specialty career option. What additional education or training did she need to obtain the position? What are her administrative and clinical duties? What does she like about her job? What does she find most challenging? How did she come to choose the specialty? Report your findings to the class.
2. Create a job-hunting plan for a medical assistant interested in learning about job opportunities in a specialty medical assisting career. Your plan should consist of at least four different ways for the medical assistant to look for jobs.
3. Pick three medical specialties, and identify the skills required for a medical assistant in each specialty.

Legal and Ethical Issues in Medical Practice, Including HIPAA

AREAS OF COMPETENCE

2003 Role Delineation Study

CLINICAL

Fundamental Principles

- Apply principles of aseptic technique and infection control
- Comply with quality assurance practices

Patient Care

- Coordinate patient care information with other health-care providers

GENERAL

Legal Concepts

- Perform within legal and ethical boundaries
- Prepare and maintain medical records
- Document accurately
- Follow employer's established policies dealing with the health-care contract
- Implement and maintain federal and state health-care legislation and regulations
- Comply with established risk management and safety procedures
- Recognize professional credentialing criteria

KEY TERMS

abandonment
agent
arbitration
assault
authorization
battery
bioethics
breach of contract
civil law
contract
crime
criminal law
defamation
disclosure
durable power of attorney
electronic transaction record
ethics
expressed contract
felony
fraud
implied contract
law
law of agency
liable
living will
malpractice claim
misdemeanor
moral values
negligence
Notice of Privacy Practices (NPP)
Privacy Rule
protected health information (PHI)
Security Rule
subpoena
tort
treatment, payment, and operations (TPO)
uniform donor card
use
void

CHAPTER OUTLINE

- Medical Law and Ethics
- OSHA Regulations
- Quality Control and Assurance
- Code of Ethics
- HIPAA
- Confidentiality Issues and Mandatory Disclosure

OBJECTIVES

After completing Chapter 3, you will be able to:

3.1 Define ethics, bioethics, and law.

3.2 Discuss the measures a medical practice must take to avoid malpractice claims.

3.3 Describe OSHA requirements for a medical office.

3.4 Describe procedures for handling an incident of exposure to hazardous materials.

3.5 Compare and contrast quality control and quality assurance procedures.

3.6 Explain how to protect patient confidentiality.

3.7 Discuss the impact that HIPAA regulations have in the medical office.

Introduction

Medical law plays an important role in medical facility procedures and the way we care for patients. We live in a litigious society, where patients, relatives, and others are inclined to sue health-care practitioners, health-care facilities, manufacturers of medical equipment and products, and others when medical outcomes are not acceptable. It is important for a medical professional to understand medical law, ethics, and protected health information as it pertains to HIPAA. There are two main reasons for medical professionals to study law and ethics: The first is to help you function at the highest professional level by providing competent, compassionate health care to patients, and the second is to help you avoid legal problems that can threaten your ability to earn a living.

A knowledge of medical law and ethics can help you gain perspective in the following three areas:

1. *The rights, responsibilities, and concerns of health-care consumers.* Not only do health-care professionals need to be concerned about how law and ethics impact their respective professions, they must also understand how legal and ethical issues affect patients. As medical technology advances and the use of computers increases, patients want to know more about their options and rights as well as more about the responsibilities of health-care practitioners. Patients want to know who and how their information is used and the options they have regarding health-care treatments. Patients have come to expect favorable outcomes from medical treatment, and when these expectations are not met, lawsuits may result.

2. *The legal and ethical issues facing society, patients, and health-care professionals as the world changes.* Every day new technologies emerge with solutions to biological and medical issues. These solutions often involve social issues, and we are faced with decisions, for example, regarding reproductive rights, fetal stem cell research, and confidentiality with sensitive medical records.

3. *The impact of rising costs on the laws and ethics of health-care delivery.* Rising costs, both of health-care insurance and of medical treatment in general, can lead to questions concerning access to health-care services and the allocation of medical treatment. For example, should everyone, regardless of age or lifestyle, have the same access to scarce medical commodities such as transplant organs or highly expensive drugs?

In today's society, medical treatment and decisions surrounding health care have become complex. It is therefore important to be knowledgeable and aware of the issues and the laws that govern patient care.

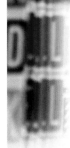

CASE STUDY

A medical assistant is very busy on a Monday morning. She has drawn blood on a patient that she has known for years and has been very comfortable chatting with this patient. The patient is checking out at the front desk in the reception area, and she notices that he forgot his prescription for Dilantin, a medication for seizure control. She rushes up to the front area and, as he is opening the door, says to him, "Mr. Doe, you forgot your prescription for Dilantin."

As you read this chapter, consider the following questions:

1. Does the medical assistant's comment represent a breach of confidentiality?
2. Has any HIPAA rule been violated? If so, which one?

Medical Law and Ethics

In order to understand medical law and ethics, it is helpful to understand the differences between laws and ethics. A **law** is defined as a rule of conduct or action prescribed or formally recognized as binding or enforced by a controlling authority. Governments enact laws to keep society running smoothly and to control behavior that could threaten public safety. **Ethics** is considered a standard of behavior and a concept of right and wrong beyond what the legal consideration is in any given situation. **Moral values** serve as a basis for ethical conduct. Moral values are formed through the influence of the family, culture, and society.

Classifications of Law

There are two types of law that pertain to health-care practitioners: criminal law and civil law.

Criminal Law. A **crime** is an offense against the state committed or omitted in violation of a public law. **Criminal law** involves crimes against the state. When a state or federal criminal law is violated, the government brings criminal charges against the alleged offender, for example, *Ohio v. John Doe.* State criminal laws prohibit such crimes as murder, arson, rape, and burglary. A criminal act may be classified as a felony or misdemeanor. A **felony** is a crime punishable by death or by imprisonment in a state or federal prison for more than one year. Some examples of a felony include abuse (child, elder, or domestic violence), manslaughter, fraud, attempted murder, and practicing medicine without a license.

Misdemeanors are less serious crimes than felonies. They are punishable by fines or by imprisonment in a facility other than a prison for one year or less. Some examples of misdemeanors are thefts under a certain dollar amount, attempted burglary, and disturbing the peace.

Civil Law. **Civil law** involves crimes against the person. Under civil law, a person can sue another person, a business, or the government. Court judgments in civil cases often require the payment of a sum of money to the injured party. Civil law includes a general category of law known as torts. A **tort** is broadly defined as a civil wrong committed against a person or property that causes physical injury or damage to someone's property or that deprives someone of his or her personal liberty and freedom. Torts may be intentional (willful) or unintentional (accidental).

Intentional Torts. When one person intentionally harms another, the law allows the injured party to seek a remedy in a civil suit. The injured party can be financially compensated for any harm done by the person guilty of committing the tort. If the conduct is judged to be malicious, punitive damages may also be awarded. Examples of intentional torts include the following:

- Assault. **Assault** is the open threat of bodily harm to another, or acting in such as way as to put another in the "reasonable apprehension of bodily harm."
- Battery. **Battery** is an action that causes bodily harm to another. It is broadly defined as any bodily contact made without permission, In health-care delivery, battery may be charged for any unauthorized touching of a patient, including such actions as suturing a wound, administering an injection, or performing a physical examination.

- Defamation of character. Damaging a person's reputation by making public statements that are both false and malicious is considered **defamation** of character. Defamation of character can take the form of slander and libel. Slander is speaking damaging words intended to negatively influence others against an individual in a manner that jeopardizes his or her reputation or means of livelihood.
- False imprisonment. False imprisonment is the intentional, unlawful restraint or confinement of one person by another. Preventing a patient from leaving the facility might be seen as false imprisonment.
- Fraud. **Fraud** consists of deceitful practices in depriving or attempting to deprive another of his or her rights. Health-care practitioners might be accused of fraud for promising patients "miracle cures" or for accepting fees from patients while using mystical or spiritual powers to heal.
- Invasion of privacy. Invasion of privacy is the interference with a person's right to be left alone. Entering an exam room without knocking can be considered an invasion of privacy. The improper use of or a breach of confidentiality of medical records may be seen as an invasion of privacy.

Unintentional Torts. The most common torts within the health-care delivery system are those committed unintentionally. Unintentional torts are acts that are not intended to cause harm but are committed unreasonably or with a disregard for the consequences. In legal terms, such acts constitute negligence. **Negligence** is charged when a health-care practitioner fails to exercise ordinary care and the patient is injured. The accused may have performed an act or failed to perform an act that a reasonable person would or would not have performed. Under the principles of negligence, civil liability exists only in cases in which the act is judicially determined to be wrongful. Health-care practitioners, for example, are not necessarily liable for a poor-quality outcome in delivering health care. Practitioners become liable only when their conduct is determined to be malpractice, the negligent delivery of professional services.

Contracts

A **contract** is a voluntary agreement between two parties in which specific promises are made for a consideration. The elements of a contract are important to health-care practitioners because health-care delivery takes place under various types of contracts. To be legally binding, four elements must be present in a contract:

1. Agreement—One party makes an offer and another party accepts it. Certain conditions pertain to the offer:
   - It can relate to the present or the future.
   - It must be communicated.
   - It must be made in good faith and not under duress or as a joke.

- It must be clear enough to be understood by both parties.
- It must define what both parties will do if the offer is accepted.

For example, a physician offers a service to the public by obtaining a license to practice medicine and opening for business. Patients accept the physician's offer by scheduling appointments, submitting to physical examinations, and allowing the physician to prescribe or perform medical treatment. The contract is complete when the physician's fee is paid.

2. Consideration—Something of value is bargained for as part of the agreement. The physician's consideration is providing service; the patient's consideration is payment of the physician's fee.

3. Legal subject matter—Contracts are not valid and enforceable in court unless they are for legal services or purposes. For example, a contract entered into by a patient to pay for services of a physician in private practice would be **void** (not legally enforceable) if the physician was not licensed to practice medicine. **Breach of contract** may be charged if either party fails to comply with the terms of a legally valid contract.

4. Contractual capacity—Parties who enter into the agreement must be capable of fully understanding all its terms and conditions. For example, a mentally incompetent individual or a person under the influence of drugs or alcohol cannot enter into a contract.

Types of Contracts. The two main types of contracts are expressed contracts and implied contracts. An **expressed contract** is clearly stated in written or spoken words. A payment contract is an example of an expressed contract. **Implied contracts** are those in which the acceptance or conduct of the parties, rather than expressed words, creates the contract. A patient who rolls up a sleeve and offers an arm for an injection is creating an implied contract.

Malpractice

Malpractice claims are lawsuits by a patient against a physician for errors in diagnosis or treatment. Negligence cases are those in which a person believes that a medical professional did not perform an essential action or performed an improper one, thus harming the patient.

Following are some examples of malpractice:

- Postoperative complications. For example, a patient starts to show signs of internal bleeding in the recovery room. The incision is reopened, and it is discovered that the surgeon did not complete closure of all the severed capillaries at the operation site.
- *Res ipsa loquitur.* This Latin term, which means "The thing speaks for itself," refers to a case in which the doctor's fault is completely obvious. For example, if a lung cancer patient has to have the right lung removed

and the surgeon instead removes the left lung, the patient will most likely sue the surgeon for malpractice. Another example is a case in which a surgeon accidentally leaves a surgical instrument inside the patient.

Following are examples of negligence:

- Abandonment. A health-care professional who stops care without providing an equally qualified substitute can be charged with **abandonment.** For example, a labor and delivery nurse is helping a woman in labor. The nurse's shift ends, but all the other nurses are busy and her replacement is late for work. Leaving the woman would constitute abandonment.
- Delayed treatment. A patient shows symptoms of some illness or disorder, but the doctor decides, for whatever reason, to delay treatment. If the patient later learns of the doctor's decision to wait, the patient may believe he has a negligence case.

Negligence cases are sometimes classified using the following three legal terms.

1. *Malfeasance* refers to an unlawful act or misconduct.
2. *Misfeasance* refers to a lawful act that is done incorrectly.
3. *Nonfeasance* refers to failure to perform an act that is one's required duty or that is required by law.

The Four Ds of Negligence. The American Medical Association (AMA) lists the following four Ds of negligence:

1. Duty. Patients must show that a physician-patient relationship existed in which the physician owed the patient a duty.
2. Derelict. Patients must show that the physician failed to comply with the standards of the profession. For example, a gynecologist has routinely taken Pap smears of a patient and then, for whatever reason, does not do so. If the patient then shows evidence of cervical cancer, the physician could be said to have been derelict.
3. Direct cause. Patients must show that any damages were a direct cause of a physician's breach of duty. For example, if a patient fell on the sidewalk and damaged her cast, she could not prove that the cast was damaged because it was incorrectly or poorly applied by her physician. It would be clear that the damage to the cast resulted from the fall. If, however, the patient's leg healed incorrectly because of the way the cast had been applied, she might have a case.
4. Damages. Patients must prove that they suffered injury.

To go forward with a malpractice suit, a patient must be prepared to prove all four Ds of negligence.

Malpractice and Civil Law. Malpractice lawsuits are part of civil law. Civil law is concerned with individuals' private rights (as opposed to criminal offenses against public law). Under civil law, a breach of some obligation that causes harm or injury to someone is known as a tort. A tort can be intentional or unintentional. Both negligence and breach of contract are considered torts. Breach of contract is the failure to adhere to a contract's terms. The implied physician-patient contract includes requirements like maintaining patient confidentiality. (Remember that an implied contract is one that is not created by specific, written words, but rather is defined by the conduct of the parties. Usually the parties involved have some special relationship.)

Settling Malpractice Suits.

Malpractice suits often require a trial in a court of law. Sometimes, however, they are settled through arbitration. **Arbitration** is a process in which the opposing sides choose a person or persons outside the court system, often with special knowledge in the field, to hear and decide the dispute. (Your local or state medical society has information about your state's policy on arbitration.) If injury, failure to provide reasonable care, or abandonment of the patient is proved to have occurred, the doctor must pay damages (a financial award) to the injured party.

If the doctor you work with becomes involved in a lawsuit, you should be familiar with subpoenas. A **subpoena** is a written court order addressed to a specific person, requiring that person's presence in court on a specific date at a specific time. If you were directly involved in the patient case that precipitated the lawsuit, you might be subpoenaed. Another important term to know is *subpoena duces tecum,* which is a court order to produce documents. If you are in charge of patient records at the practice, you may be required to locate, assemble, photocopy, and arrange for delivery of patient records for this purpose.

Law of Agency.

According to the **law of agency,** an employee is considered to be acting as a doctor's **agent** (on the doctor's behalf) while performing professional tasks. The Latin term *respondeat superior,* or "Let the master answer," is sometimes used to refer to this relationship. For example, the employee's word is as binding as if it were the doctor's (so you should never, for example, promise a patient a cure). Therefore, the doctor is responsible, or **liable,** for the negligence of employees. A negligent employee, however, may also be sued directly, because individuals are legally responsible for their own actions. Therefore, a patient can sue both the doctor and the involved employee for negligence. The employer, or the employer's insurance company, can also sue the employee.

The American Association of Medical Assistants (AAMA) recommends that you purchase your own malpractice insurance and have a personal attorney. Most likely, in a case of negligence the doctor would be sued (because you as an employee are acting on the doctor's behalf), and you are usually covered by the doctor's malpractice insurance. Even if you are young and think you do not have many assets, you should still obtain your own insurance.

Courtroom Conduct.

Most health-care practitioners will never have to appear in court. If you should be asked to appear, the following suggestions may prove helpful:

- Attend court proceedings as required. Failure to appear in court could result in either charges of contempt of court or the case being forfeited.
- Do not be late for scheduled hearings.
- Bring required documents to court and present them only when requested to do so.
- Before testifying, refresh your memory concerning all the facts observed about the matter in question, such as dates, times, words spoken, and circumstances.
- Speak slowly, clearly, and professionally. Do not use medical terms. Do not lose your temper or attempt to be humorous.
- Answer all questions in a straightforward manner, even if the answers appear to help the opposing side.
- Answer only the question asked, no more and no less.
- Appear well groomed, and dress in clean, conservative clothing.

How Effective Communication Can Help Prevent Lawsuits.

Patients who see the medical office as a friendly place are generally less likely to sue. Physicians, medical assistants, and other medical office staff who have pleasant personalities and are competent in their jobs will have less risk of being sued. Medical assistants can help by:

- Developing good listening skills and nonverbal communication techniques so that patients feel the time spent with them is not rushed
- Setting aside a certain time during the day for returning patients' phone calls
- Checking to be sure that all patients or their authorized representatives sign informed consent forms before they undergo medical or surgical procedures
- Avoiding statements that could be construed as an admission of fault on the part of the physician or other medical staff
- Using tact, good judgment, and professional ability in handling patients
- Refraining from making overly optimistic statements about a patient's recovery or prognosis
- Advising patients when their physicians intend to be gone
- Making every effort to reach an understanding about fees with the patient before treatment so that billing does not become a point of contention

Terminating Care of a Patient

A physician may wish to terminate care of a patient. Terminating care is sometimes called withdrawing from a case. Following are some typical reasons a physician may choose to withdraw from a case:

- The patient refuses to follow the physician's instructions.
- The patient's family members complain incessantly to or about the physician.
- A personality conflict develops between the physician and patient that cannot be reasonably resolved.
- The patient insists on having pain medication refilled beyond what the physician considers medically necessary.
- The patient habitually does not pay or fails to make satisfactory arrangements to pay for medical services. A physician may stop treatment of such a patient and end the physician-patient relationship only if adequate notice is given to the patient.
- The patient fails to keep scheduled appointments. To protect the physician from charges of abandonment, all missed appointments should be noted in the patient's chart.

A physician who terminates care of a patient must do so in a formal, legal manner, following these four steps.

1. Write a letter to the patient, expressing the reason for withdrawing from the case and recommending that the patient seek medical care from another physician as soon as possible. Figure 3-1 shows an example of a letter of termination.

2. Send the letter by certified mail with a return receipt requested.
3. Place a copy of the letter (and the return receipt, when received) in the patient's medical record.
4. Summarize in the patient record the physician's reason for terminating care and the actions taken to inform the patient.

Standard of Care

You are expected to fulfill the standards of the medical assisting profession for applying legal concepts to practice. According to the AAMA, medical assistants should uphold legal concepts in the following ways:

- Maintain confidentiality
- Practice within the scope of training and capabilities
- Prepare and maintain medical records
- Document accurately
- Use appropriate guidelines when releasing information
- Follow employer's established policies dealing with the health-care contract
- Follow legal guidelines and maintain awareness of health-care legislation and regulations
- Maintain and dispose of regulated substances in compliance with government guidelines

---

LETTER OF WITHDRAWAL FROM CASE

Dear Mr._____:

I find it necessary to inform you that I am withdrawing from further professional attendance upon you for the reason that you have persisted in refusing to follow my medical advice and treatment. Since your condition requires medical attention, I suggest that you place yourself under the care of another physician without delay. If you so desire, I shall be available to attend you for a reasonable time after you have received this letter, but in no event for more than five days.

This should give you ample time to select a physician of your choice from the many competent practitioners in this city. With your approval, I will make available to this physician your case history and information regarding the diagnosis and treatment which you have received from me.

Very truly yours,

_____, MD

Figure 3-1. Physicians are required to inform patients in writing if they wish to withdraw from a case.
Source: Medicolegal Forms With Legal Analysis, American Medical Association, © 1991.

- Follow established risk-management and safety procedures
- Recognize professional credentialing criteria
- Help develop and maintain personnel, policy, and procedure manuals

Often laws dictate what medical assistants may or may not do. For instance, in some states it is illegal for medical assistants to draw blood. No states consider it legal for medical assistants to diagnose a condition, prescribe a treatment, or let a patient believe that a medical assistant is a nurse or any other type of caregiver. In addition to what is stated by law, you and the physician must establish the procedures that are appropriate for you to perform.

Administrative Duties and the Law

Many of a medical assistant's administrative duties are related to legal requirements. Paperwork for insurance billing, patient consent forms for surgical procedures, and correspondence (such as a physician's letter of withdrawal from a case) must be handled correctly to meet legal standards. Documentation, such as making appropriate and accurate entries in a patient's medical record, is legally important. You may also maintain the physician's appointment book. This book is considered a legal document. It can prove, for instance, that the physician, if unable to see a patient, arranged for the patient to be seen by another physician in the same practice. In other words, the physician provided a qualified substitute as required by law.

You may also be responsible for handling certain state reporting requirements. Items that must be reported include births; certain diseases such as acquired immunodeficiency syndrome (AIDS) and other sexually transmitted diseases; drug abuse; suspected child abuse or abuse of the elderly; injuries caused by violence, such as knife and gunshot wounds; and deaths. Reports are sent to various state departments, depending on the content of the report. For example, suspected child abuse cases are reported to the state department of social services. Addressing these state requirements is called the physician's public duty.

Phone calls must be handled with an awareness of legal issues. For example, if the physician asks you to contact a patient by phone and you call the patient at work, you should not identify yourself or the physician by name to someone else without the patient's permission. You can say, for example, "Please tell Mrs. Arnot that her doctor's office is calling." If you do not take this precaution, the physician can be sued for invasion of privacy. You must abide by similar guidelines if you are responsible for making follow-up calls to a patient after a surgical procedure.

Documentation

Patient records are often used as evidence in professional medical liability cases, and improper documentation can contribute to or cause a case to be lost. Physicians should keep records that clearly show what treatment was performed and when it was done. It is important that physicians be able to demonstrate that nothing was neglected and that the care given fully met the standards demanded by law. One cliché to remember is "If it is not written down, then it was not done." Pay attention to spelling in charts and keep a medical dictionary handy if you are not sure of a spelling. Today's health-care environment requires complete documentation of actions taken and actions not taken. Medical staff members should pay particular attention to the following situations.

Referrals. Make sure the patient understands whether the referring physician's staff will make the appointment and notify the patient, or whether the patient must call to set up the appointment. Document in the chart that the patient was referred and the time and date of the appointment, and follow up with the specialist to verify that the appointment was scheduled and kept. Note whether reports of the consultation were received in your office, and document any further care of the patient from the referring physician.

Missed Appointments. At the end of the day, a designated person in the medical office should gather all patient charts of those who missed or canceled appointments without rescheduling. Charts should be dated, stamped, and documented "No Call/No Show" or "Canceled/No Reschedule." The treating physician should review these records and note whether follow-up is indicated.

Dismissals. To avoid charges of abandonment, the physician must formally withdraw from a case. Be sure that a letter of withdrawal or dismissal has been filed in the patient's records. All mailing confirmations should be filed in the record, such as the return receipt from certified mail.

All Other Patient Contact. Patient records should include reports of all tests, procedures, and medications prescribed, including prescription refills. Make sure all necessary informed consent papers have been signed and filed in the chart. Make entries into the chart of all telephone conversations with the patient. Correct documentation requires the initials or signature of the person making the notation on the patient's chart as well as the date and time.

Controlled Substances and the Law

You must also follow the correct procedures for the safekeeping and disposal of controlled substances, such as narcotics, in the medical office. It is important to know the right dosages and potential complications of these drugs, as well as prescription refill rules, in order to understand and interpret the directions of the physician in a legally responsible manner. Prescription pads must be kept secure so that they do not fall into the wrong hands.

Communication and the Law

Communication with the patient and disclosure of information are sensitive legal areas. You are not allowed to decide what information should be given to the patient or by whom. You can, however, provide support and show respect for the patient as a person. In cases involving sexually transmitted diseases (STDs), for example, clear, nonjudgmental communication is of the utmost importance. Sensitivity is also required in dealing with special issues such as illiteracy. For example, a patient may not want to admit being unable to read written instructions. In general, your role in maintaining smooth communication between the patient and the medical office is to help prevent misunderstandings that could lead to legal confrontations.

Legal Documents and the Patient

You need to be aware of two legal documents that are typically completed by a patient prior to major surgery or hospitalization: the living will and the uniform donor card. Traditionally, these documents were completed outside the medical office or in the hospital. The current trend, however, is for medical practice personnel, including medical assistants, to assist patients in developing these important documents.

Living Wills. A **living will,** sometimes called an advance directive, is a legal document addressed to the patient's family and health-care providers. The living will states what type of treatment the patient wishes or does not wish to receive if she becomes terminally ill, unconscious, or permanently comatose (sometimes referred to as being in a persistent vegetative state). For example, a living will typically states whether a patient wishes to be put on life-sustaining equipment should she become permanently comatose. Some living wills contain DNR (do not resuscitate) orders. These orders mean the patient does not wish medical personnel to try to resuscitate her should the heart stop beating. Living wills are a means of helping families of terminally ill patients deal with the inevitable outcome of the illness and may help limit unnecessary medical costs.

The living will is signed when the patient is mentally and physically competent to do so. It must also be signed by two witnesses. Medical practices can help patients develop a living will, sometimes in conjunction with organizations that make available preprinted living will forms. The Partnership for Caring (based in Washington, D.C.) is one such organization.

Patients who have living wills are asked to name, in a document called a **durable power of attorney,** someone who will make decisions regarding medical care on their behalf, if they are unable to do so. Often, a durable power of attorney for health care form is completed in conjunction with a living will.

The Uniform Donor Card. In 1968 the Uniform Anatomical Gift Act was passed, setting forth guidelines for all states to follow in complying with a person's wish to make a gift of one or more organs (or the whole body) upon death. An anatomical gift is typically designated for medical research, organ transplants, or placement in a tissue bank. The **uniform donor card** is a legal document that states one's wish to make such a gift. People often carry the uniform donor card in their wallets. Many medical practices offer the service of helping their patients obtain and complete a uniform donor card.

Confidentiality Issues

The physician is legally obligated to keep patient information confidential. Therefore, you must be sure that all patient information is discussed with the patient privately and shared with the staff only when appropriate. For example, the billing department will have to see patient records to code diagnoses and bill appropriately. Also, a staff member who has to make an appointment for a patient to get a herpes test at an outside location will need the patient record to do so.

You must avoid discussing cases with anyone outside the office, even if the patient's name is not mentioned. Only the patient can waive this confidentiality right. All patients' records must be kept out of sight of other patients or visitors as well as night staff, such as janitorial service employees. Confidentiality also is required in the handling of test results.

OSHA Regulations

The Occupational Safety and Health Administration (OSHA), a division of the U.S. Department of Labor, has created federal laws to protect health-care workers from health hazards on the job. Medical personnel may accidentally contract a dangerous or even fatal disease by coming into contact with a virus a patient is carrying. Medical assistants may also be exposed to toxic substances in the office. OSHA regulations describe the precautions a medical office must take with clothing, housekeeping, record keeping, and training to minimize the risk of disease or injury.

Some of the most important OSHA regulations are those for controlling workers' exposure to infectious disease. These regulations are set forth in the Occupational Safety and Health Administration Bloodborne Pathogens Protection Standard of 1991. A pathogen is any microorganism that causes disease. Microorganisms are microscopic living bodies, such as viruses or bacteria, that may be present in a patient's blood or other body fluids (saliva or semen).

Of particular concern to medical workers are the human immunodeficiency virus (HIV), which causes AIDS, and the hepatitis B virus (HBV). AIDS damages the body's immune system and thus its ability to fight disease. AIDS is always fatal. HBV is a highly contagious disease that is potentially fatal. It causes inflammation of the liver and may cause liver failure. Every year, about 8700 health-care workers become HBV-infected at work, and about 200 die from the disease.

OSHA requires that medical professionals in medical practices follow what are called Universal Precautions. They were developed by the Centers for Disease Control and Prevention (CDC) to prevent medical professionals from exposing themselves and others to blood-borne pathogens. Exposure can occur, for example, through skin that has been broken from a needle puncture or other wound and through mucous membranes, such as those in the nose and throat. If these areas come into contact with a patient's (or coworker's) blood or body fluids, a virus could be transferred from one person to another.

Hospitals are required to follow what are called Standard Precautions, also developed by the CDC. Standard Precautions combine Universal Precautions with body substance isolation guidelines.

Protective Gear

The more exposure that is involved, the more protective clothing you need to wear (Figure 3-2). Procedures that usually involve exposure to blood, other body fluids, or broken skin require gloves. There are several kinds of gloves for different situations.

- Disposable gloves are worn only once and then discarded. Do not use a pair that has been torn or damaged.
- Utility gloves are stronger and may be decontaminated. They are used for housecleaning tasks.
- Examination gloves are used for procedures that do not require a sterile environment.
- Sterile gloves are used for sterile procedures such as minor surgery.

Appropriate masks, goggles, or face shields must be used for procedures in which a worker's eyes, nose, or mouth may be exposed. These are procedures that may involve spraying or splashes—for example, examining blood. If potentially infected substances might get onto a worker's clothing, the worker must wear a protective laboratory coat, gown, or apron. Fluid-resistant material is recommended by OSHA.

The law requires that the physician/employer provide all necessary protective clothing to the employee free of charge. The employer also pays for cleaning, maintaining, and replacing the protective items.

Decontamination

After a procedure, you must decontaminate all exposed work surfaces with a 10% bleach solution or with a germ-killing solution containing glutoraldohydes approved by the Environmental Protection Agency (EPA). Replace protective coverings on equipment and surfaces if they have been exposed. Regularly decontaminate receptacles such as bins, pails, and cans as part of routine housekeeping procedures. Never pick up broken glass with your hands. Use tongs, even when wearing gloves, so that the sharp glass does not cut the gloves and expose the skin.

Dispose of any potentially infectious waste materials in special "biohazard bags," which are leakproof and labeled with the biohazard symbol (Figure 3-3). Wastes that fall into this category include blood products, body fluids, human tissues, and vaccines; table paper, linen, towels, and gauze with body fluids on them; and gloves, diapers, sanitary napkins, and cotton swabs. Disposal of sharp instruments ("sharps") is discussed in the next section.

Sharp Equipment

Disposable sharp equipment that has been used must not be bent, broken, recapped, or otherwise tampered with, so as to prevent possible exposure to medical workers. It should be placed in a leakproof, puncture-resistant, color-coded, and appropriately labeled container. Reusable sharp equipment must be placed as soon as possible into a puncture-resistant container and taken to a reprocessing area.

Both disposable and reusable instruments are sterilized in their appropriate containers. Sterilizing is usually accomplished by means of an autoclave, a machine that uses pressurized steam. Sterilization of disposable instruments is usually handled by an outside waste management company.

Exposure Incidents

You must give special attention to what to do in case of an exposure incident. This may happen when a medical worker accidentally sticks herself with a used needle. These "puncture exposure incidents" are the most common kind of exposure.

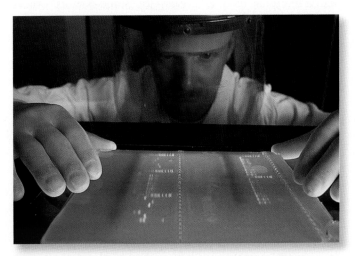

Figure 3-2. Researchers must wear full protective gear in a laboratory that studies infectious diseases. Regulations for such gear are set by OSHA.

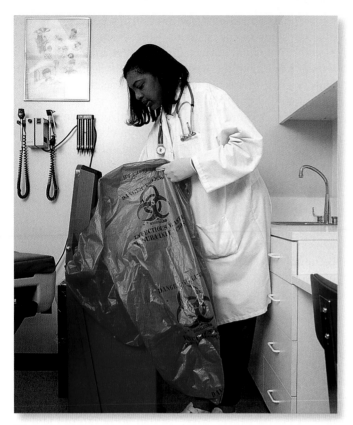

Figure 3-3. The medical assistant may be responsible for disposing of wastes such as gloves, table paper, and gauze with body fluids on them in containers that display the biohazard symbol.

When an exposure incident occurs, the physician/employer must be notified immediately. Quick and proper treatment can help prevent the development of HBV. Timely action can also prevent exposing other people to any infection the worker may have acquired. Reporting the incident to the physician/employer also may encourage him to revise the office's safety procedures in some way to help prevent the same type of incident from happening again.

Postexposure Procedures

OSHA requires specific postexposure evaluation and follow-up procedures. If an exposure incident occurs, the employer must offer the exposed employee a free medical evaluation by a health-care provider of the employer's choice. The employer must refer the employee to a licensed health-care provider who will counsel the employee about what happened and how to prevent the spread of any potential infection. The health-care provider will also take a blood sample and prescribe the appropriate treatment. The employee has the right to refuse both the medical evaluation and the treatment.

When a medical worker starts a job, the physician/employer is required to offer the worker, at no cost, the opportunity to have an HBV vaccination within 10 days.

An employee who refuses vaccination must sign a waiver. The employee can change his mind at any time and decide to have the vaccination. If an employee who declined the HBV vaccination is exposed to a patient who is HBV-positive or who is being tested for HBV, it is recommended that the employee be tested for HBV and receive the vaccination if necessary. (The employee may decline to be tested, however.) If the patient is being tested for HBV, the employee is legally required to be informed of the test results. (This is true for HIV as well, and the employee still has the right to refuse testing.) The employee may agree to give blood but not be tested. The blood sample must be kept on hand for 90 days in case the worker later develops symptoms of HBV or HIV infection and then decides to be tested.

The health-care provider that performs the postexposure evaluation must give the employer a written report stating whether HBV vaccination was recommended and received. The report must also state that the employee, if tested, was informed of the blood test results. Any information beyond this must be kept confidential.

If you plan to do an externship in a medical office, the physician does not have to provide you with the HBV vaccine. She may, however, deny you the opportunity to do the externship if you have not received the vaccination elsewhere. Many accredited medical assisting programs offer the vaccine to their students.

Laundry

OSHA has regulations for handling potentially infectious laundry. Hospitals have their own laundry facilities because these facilities are cost-effective. Some larger clinics also have their own laundry facilities. Most doctors' offices, however, send laundry out. Laundry must be bagged and labeled. Any wet laundry to be transported should be packed so that it does not leak. The laundry service the medical office uses should abide by all OSHA regulations. Laundry workers must wear gloves and handle contaminated materials as little as possible. Some doctors' offices use only disposable items, such as paper robes, and do not need laundry service.

Hazardous Materials

You may encounter hazardous equipment and toxic substances in the office. These hazards include vaccines, disinfectants, and laser equipment.

OSHA's Occupational Health and Safety Act of 1970 sets minimum requirements for workplace safety. It also requires employers to keep an inventory of all hazardous materials used in the workplace. Containers of hazardous substances must be labeled in a specific way, listing any potentially harmful ingredients. The employer must post Material Safety Data Sheets (MSDS) about these substances. These sheets specify whether the substance is cancer-causing, list other possible risks, and state OSHA's requirements for controlling exposure. All employees are entitled to be informed about hazardous substances in the workplace and to be trained in how to use them safely.

Training Requirements

Training requirements are part of OSHA's hazardous substance regulations. Every employee who may be exposed to hazardous or infectious substances on the job must be given free information and training during working hours at least once a year. Training must also be held when a new chemical or piece of medical equipment is introduced into the office or when a procedure changes. Training must cover the following topics:

- How to obtain a copy of the OSHA regulations and an explanation of them
- The causes and symptoms of blood-borne diseases
- How blood-borne pathogens are transmitted
- The facility's Exposure Control Plan and how to obtain a copy
- What tasks might result in exposure
- The use and limitations of all the precautions
- All aspects of personal protective equipment
- All aspects of HBV vaccination
- Emergency procedures
- Postexposure procedures
- Warning labels, signs, and color coding

Beyond this federal law, state training requirements vary. The states of Washington and Florida require medical assistants to take a short course specifically covering HIV laws and precautions. Your instructor will familiarize you with your state's policy. OSHA has its own training institute, supports various other training resources, and develops training videotapes and tests for trainees. In some doctors' offices, the laboratory supervisor conducts training for the office staff. Anyone who has gone through a training session can then train others.

General Regulations

General work area laws restrict eating, drinking, smoking, applying cosmetics or lip balm, and handling contact lenses in the work area. These laws also forbid storing food or drinks in refrigerators that are used to store blood or other potentially infectious material. Refrigerators must have working thermometers to ensure proper cooling temperature (see Figure 3-4).

There are also required procedures for various specific on-the-job injuries. For instance, for eye injuries such as burns and chemical splashes, OSHA requires flushing the eye(s) for 15 minutes with a constant water flow.

Documentation

Lastly, OSHA's record-keeping and documentation requirements are intended to protect the legal rights and

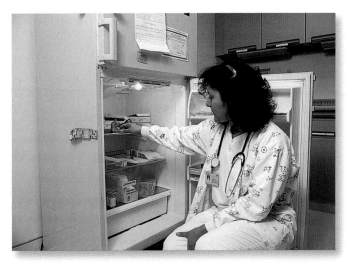

Figure 3-4. OSHA laws require blood or other potentially infectious material to be stored separately from food and drinks. Refrigerators storing such material should have working thermometers to ensure proper cooling temperature.

safety of everyone in the medical office. The office must have a written Exposure Control Plan describing all precautions against exposure to hazards and blood-borne pathogens and specifying what to do if exposure occurs. Employee medical and exposure records must be kept on file during employment and 30 years afterward. If an employer retires or closes the practice, the employee records are forwarded to the director of OSHA. Also, a log of occupational injuries and illnesses, OSHA Form 200, must be kept for 5 years. The employer must also keep on file for 3 years records documenting an employee's training: dates, topics covered, and names and qualifications of the trainers.

OSHA Inspections

In response to a complaint, or sometimes at random, OSHA may send a compliance officer to inspect a medical office. In 1995 approximately 29,000 inspections were performed. The penalties for not complying with regulations vary according to the severity of the offense. For example, if an inspector finds that the medical assistants have not worn gloves for 2 months because the employer did not make them available, that would entail a severe penalty. If four assistants were wearing gloves but one had forgotten to put them on, there would be a lesser penalty. There are reductions for complying on the spot—perhaps no penalty will be charged. In a serious case, the office could be charged up to $10,000 per broken regulation, multiplied by the number of employees. The penalties are paid directly to OSHA, but the money goes into the federal treasury. If a serious violation occurs in a physicians' office laboratory, the laboratory's payments from Medicare may be suspended.

Quality Control and Assurance

A medical office often has a physicians' office laboratory to perform different types of clinical tests, depending on the physician's specialty and state laws. The Clinical Laboratory Improvement Amendments of 1988 (CLIA '88) lists the regulations for laboratory testing. Physicians must display a certificate from CLIA confirming that their office complies with CLIA regulations. These regulations set standards for the quality of work performed in a laboratory and the accuracy of test results. Congress passed these laws after publicity about deaths caused by errors in the test used to diagnose cancer of the uterus.

According to CLIA '88, there are three categories of laboratory tests: waived tests, moderate-complexity tests, and high-complexity tests. Waived tests, the simplest kind, require the least amount of judgment and pose an insignificant risk to the patient in the event of an error. The laboratory applies for a certificate of waiver from the U.S. Department of Health and Human Services, which grants permission to perform any test on the list of waived tests and to bill it to Medicare or Medicaid. Tests that patients can do at home with kits approved by the department's Food and Drug Administration (FDA), such as the blood glucose test, also fall under this heading.

Most tests are in the moderate-complexity category. Cholesterol testing and checking for the presence or absence of sperm are examples. CLIA lists all waived and moderate-complexity tests and considers all other tests to be of high complexity.

Under CLIA '88, medical assistants are always allowed to perform waived tests. These tests are listed in Figure 3-5. Medical assistants can also perform moderate-complexity tests as long as the physician can ensure that the assistant is appropriately trained and experienced according to federal guidelines. Some state laws may be stricter than the federal laws, so the medical office should check with the state health department to see if there are any local rules about what kinds of tests medical assistants may perform. As you advance in your career, you will most likely be trained to do more and more types of tests, receiving training either by senior staff members or through outside programs.

Elements of the Quality Assurance Program

CLIA '88 also requires every medical office to have a quality assurance (QA) program. This program must include a quality control (QC) program specifically for the laboratory. The goal is to track and improve the quality of all aspects of the medical practice—including patient care, laboratory procedures, record keeping, employee evaluations, finances, legal responsibilities, public image, staff morale, insurance issues, and patient education. Documentation is

Waived Tests

- Dipstick or tablet reagent urinalysis (nonautomated) for the following: bilirubin, glucose, hemoglobin, ketone, leukocytes, nitrite, pH, protein, specific gravity, and urobilinogen
- Fecal occult blood
- Ovulation tests—visual color tests for human luteinizing hormone
- Urine pregnancy tests—visual color comparison determination
- Erythrocyte sedimentation rate—nonautomated
- Hemoglobin—(nonautomated) by copper sulfate
- Blood glucose—by glucose monitoring devices cleared by FDA specifically for home use
- Spun microhematocrit
- Hemoglobin—(automated) by single analyte instruments with self-contained or component features to perform specimen-reagent interaction, providing direct measurement and readout

Figure 3-5. Under CLIA '88, medical assistants are always allowed to perform waived tests.

required by QA regulations, to provide evidence that QA procedures are in place in the office. This documentation becomes extremely important if there is an inspection or a legal dispute.

Any QA program must include the following elements:

- Written policies on the standards of patient care and professional behavior
- A QC program
- Training and continuing education programs
- An instrument maintenance program
- Documentation requirements
- Evaluation methods

Software programs are available to help medical offices develop a QA program and procedures manual.

The Laboratory Program

The laboratory QC program must cover testing concerns such as patient preparation procedures, collection of the specimen (blood, urine, or tissue), labeling, preservation and transportation, test methods, inconsistent results, use and maintenance of equipment, personnel training, complaints and investigations, and corrective actions. The accuracy of the tests, and the instruments and chemicals that are used, must be monitored through QC procedures and documented.

Code of Ethics

Medical ethics is a vital part of medical practice, and following an ethical code is an important part of your job. Ethics deals with general principles of right and wrong, as opposed to requirements of law. A professional is expected to act in ways that reflect society's ideas of right and wrong, even if such behavior is not enforced by law. Often, however, the law is based on ethical considerations.

Bioethics: Social Issues

Bioethics deals with issues that arise related to medical advances. Here are three examples of bioethical issues.

1. A treatment for Parkinson's disease was developed that uses fetal tissue. Some women, upon learning about this treatment, might get pregnant just to have an abortion and sell the fetal tissue. Is this ethical?

2. If a couple cannot have a baby because of a medical condition of the mother, using a surrogate mother is an option some couples choose. The surrogate mother is artificially inseminated with the sperm of the husband and carries the baby to term. The couple then raises the child. Ethically speaking, who is the real mother, the woman who bears the child or the woman who raises the child? If the surrogate mother wants to keep the baby after it is born, does she have a right to do so?

3. When a liver transplant is needed by both a famous patient who has had a history of alcohol abuse and a woman who is a recipient of public assistance, what criteria are considered when determining who receives the organ? Who makes the decision? Ethically, treating physicians should not make the decision of allocating limited medical resources. Decisions regarding the allocation of limited medical resources should consider only the likelihood of benefit, the urgency of need, and the amount of resources required for successful treatment. Nonmedical criteria, such as ability to pay, age, social worth, perceived obstacles to treatment, patient's contribution to illness, or the past use of resources should not be considered.

Practicing appropriate professional ethics has a positive impact on your reputation and the success of your employer's business. Many medical organizations, therefore, have created guidelines for the acceptable and preferred manners and behaviors, or etiquette, of medical assistants and physicians.

The principles of medical ethics have developed over time. The Hippocratic oath, in which medical students pledge to practice medicine ethically, was developed in ancient Greece. It is still used today and is one of the original bases of modern medical ethics. Hippocrates, the fourth-century-B.C. Greek physician commonly called the "father of medicine," is traditionally considered the author of this oath, but its authorship is actually unknown.

Among the promises of the Hippocratic oath are to use the form of treatment believed to be best for the patient, to refrain from harmful actions, and to keep a patient's private information confidential.

The AMA defines ethical behavior for doctors in *Code of Medical Ethics: Current Opinions with Annotations* (Chicago: American Medical Association, 1996). Medical assistants as well as doctors need to be aware of these principles.

> A physician shall be dedicated to providing competent medical service with compassion and respect for human dignity.

This concept means that medical professionals will respect all aspects of the patient as a person, including intellect and emotions. The doctor must decide what treatment would result in the best, most dignified quality of life for the patient, and the doctor must respect a patient's choice to forgo treatment.

> A physician shall deal honestly with patients and colleagues and strive to expose those physicians deficient in character or competence or who engage in fraud or deception.

Medical professionals, including medical assistants, should respect colleagues, but they must also respect and protect the profession and public welfare enough to report colleagues who are breaking the law, acting unethically, or unable to perform competently. Dilemmas may arise where one suspects, but is not able to prove, for instance, that a coworker has a substance abuse problem or another problem that is affecting performance. Ignoring such a situation in medical practice could cost someone's life as well as lead to lawsuits.

In terms of billing, a doctor should bill only for direct services, not for indirect ones, such as referrals. The doctor also should not bill for services that do not really pertain to the practice of medicine, such as dispensing drugs.

It is also unethical for the doctor to influence the patient about where to fill prescriptions or obtain other medical services when the doctor has a personal financial interest in any of the choices.

> A physician shall respect the law and also recognize a responsibility to seek changes in requirements that are contrary to the patient's best interests.

Several legal or employer requirements have come under scrutiny as being contrary to a patient's best interests. Among them are discharging patients from the hospital after a certain time limit for certain procedures, which may be too soon for many patients. Insurance company payment policies have sometimes been criticized as unfair. So have health maintenance organization (HMO) financial policies that may conflict with a doctor's preference in treatment.

CODE OF ETHICS

The Code of Ethics of the AAMA shall set forth principles of ethical and moral conduct as they relate to the medical profession and the particular practice of medical assisting.

Members of the AAMA dedicated to the conscientious pursuit of their profession, and thus desiring to merit the high regard of the entire medical profession and the respect of the general public which they serve, do pledge themselves to strive always to:

A. render service with full respect for the dignity of humanity;

B. respect confidential information obtained through employment unless legally authorized or required by responsible performance of duty to divulge such information;

C. uphold the honor and high principles of the profession and accept its disciplines;

D. seek to continually improve the knowledge and skills of medical assistants for the benefit of patients and professional colleagues;

E. participate in additional service activities aimed toward improving the health and wellbeing of the community;

Figure 3-6. The AAMA's Code of Ethics sets the ethical standard for the profession of medical assisting. (Reprinted with permission of the American Association of Medical Assistants.)

A physician shall respect the rights of patients, of colleagues, and of other health professionals and shall safeguard patient confidences within the constraints of law.

A document called the Patient's Bill of Rights, established by the American Hospital Association in 1973 and revised in 1992, lists ethical principles protecting the patient. Some states have even passed this code of ethics into law. Among a patient's rights are the right to information about alternative treatments, the right to refuse to participate in research projects, and the right to privacy.

A physician shall continue to study; apply and advance scientific knowledge; make relevant information available to patients, colleagues, and the public; obtain consultation; and use the talents of other health professionals when indicated.

Keeping up with the latest advancements in medicine is crucial for providing high-quality, ethical care. Most states require doctors to accumulate "continuing education units" to maintain a license to practice. These units are earned by means of educational activities such as courses and scientific meetings. The AAMA requires medical assistants to renew their certification every 5 years, by either accumulating continuing education credits through the AAMA or retaking the certification examination.

A physician shall, in the provision of appropriate patient care, except in emergencies, be free to choose whom to serve, with whom to associate, and the environment in which to provide medical services.

Ethically, doctors can set their hours, decide what kind of medicine to practice and where, decide whom to accept as a patient, and take time off as long as a qualified substitute performs their duties. Doctors may decline to accept new patients because of a full workload. In an emergency, however, a doctor may be ethically obligated to care for a patient, even if the patient is not of the doctor's choosing. The doctor should not abandon that patient until another physician is available.

A physician shall recognize a responsibility to participate in activities contributing to an improved community. This ethical obligation holds true for the allied health professions as well.

In addition to knowing the physician's codes of ethics, medical assistants should follow the AAMA's Code of Ethics, which appears in Figure 3-6 and in Chapter 1.

HIPAA

Today, health care is considered a trillion-dollar industry, growing rapidly with technology and employing millions of health-care workers in numerous fields. The U.S. Department of Labor recognizes 400 different job titles in the health-care industry.

On August 21, 1996, the U.S. Congress passed the Health Insurance Portability and Accountability Act (HIPAA). The primary goals of the act are to improve the portability and continuity of health-care coverage in group and individual markets; to combat waste, fraud, and abuse in health-care insurance and health-care delivery; to promote the use of medical savings accounts; to improve access to long-term care services and coverage; and to simplify the administration of health insurance.

The purposes of the act are to:

- Improve the efficiency and effectiveness of health-care delivery by creating a national framework for health privacy protection that builds on efforts by states, health systems, and individual organizations and individuals

- Protect and enhance the rights of patients by providing them access to their health information and controlling the inappropriate use or disclosure of that information
- Improve the quality of health care by restoring trust in the health-care system among consumers, health-care professionals, and the multitude of organizations and individuals committed to the delivery of care

HIPAA is divided into two main sections of law: Title I, which addresses health-care portability, and Title II, which covers the prevention of health-care fraud and abuse, administrative simplification, and medical liability reform.

Title I: Health-Care Portability

The issue of portability deals with protecting health-care coverage for employees who change jobs, allowing them to carry their existing plans with them to new jobs. HIPAA provides the following protections for employees and their families:

- Increases workers' ability to get health-care coverage when starting a new job
- Reduces workers' probability of losing existing health-care coverage.
- Helps workers maintain continuous health-care coverage when changing jobs.
- Helps workers purchase health insurance on their own if they lose coverage under an employer's group plan and have no other health-care coverage available.

The specific protections of this title include the following:

- Limits the use of exclusions for preexisting conditions
- Prohibits group plans from discriminating by denying coverage or charging extra for coverage based on an individual's or a family member's past or present poor health.
- Guarantees certain small employers, as well as certain individuals who lose job-related coverage, the right to purchase health insurance.
- Guarantees, in most cases, that employers or individuals who purchase health insurance can renew the coverage regardless of any health conditions of individuals covered under the insurance policy.

Title II: Prevention of Health-Care Fraud and Abuse, Administrative Simplification, and Medical Liability Reform

HIPAA Privacy Rule. The HIPAA Standards for Privacy of Individually Identifiable Health Information provide the first comprehensive federal protection for the privacy of health information. The **Privacy Rule** is designed to provide strong privacy protections that do not interfere with patient access to health care or the quality of health-care delivery. This act creates, for the first time, national standards to protect individuals' medical records and other personal health information. The privacy rule is intended to:

- Give patients more control over their health information
- Set boundaries on the use and release of health-care records
- Establish appropriate safeguards that health-care providers and others must achieve to protect the privacy of health information
- Hold violators accountable, with civil and criminal penalties that can be imposed if they violate patients' privacy rights
- Strike a balance when public responsibility supports disclosure of some forms of data—for example, to protect public health

Before the HIPAA Privacy Rule, the personal information that moves across hospitals and doctors' offices, insurers or third-party payers, and state lines fell under a patchwork of federal and state laws. This information could be distributed—without either notice or authorization—for reasons that had nothing to do with a patient's medical treatment or health-care reimbursement. For example, unless otherwise forbidden by state or local law, without the Privacy Rule, patient information held by a health plan could, without the patient's permission, be passed on to a lender who could then deny the patient's application for a home mortgage or a credit card or could be given to an employer who could use it in personnel decisions.

Individually identifiable health information includes:

- Name
- Address
- Phone numbers
- Fax number
- Dates (birth, death, admission, discharge, etc.)
- Social Security number
- E-mail address
- Medical record numbers
- Health plan beneficiary numbers
- Account numbers
- Certificate or license numbers
- Vehicle identifiers and serial numbers, including license plate numbers
- Device identifiers and serial numbers
- Web Universal Resource Locators (URLs)
- Internet Protocol (IP) address numbers

The core of the HIPAA Privacy Rule is the protection, use, and disclosure of **protected health information (PHI).** Protected health information means individually identifiable health information that is transmitted or maintained by electronic or other media, such as computer storage devices. The Privacy Rule protects all PHI held or transmitted by a covered entity, which includes health-care providers, health plans, and health-care clearing-houses. Other covered entities include employers, life insurers, schools or universities, and public health authorities. Protected health information can come in any form or media, such as electronic, paper, or oral, including verbal communications among staff members, patients, and other providers. *Use* and *disclosure* are the two fundamental concepts in the HIPAA Privacy Rule. It is important to understand the differences between these terms.

Use. **Use** refers to performing any of the following actions to individually identifiable health information by employees or other members of an organization's workforce:

- Sharing
- Employing
- Applying
- Utilizing
- Examining
- Analyzing

Information is used when it moves within an organization.

Disclosure. **Disclosure** occurs when the entity holding the information performs any of the following actions so that the information is outside the entity:

- Releasing
- Transferring
- Providing access to
- Divulging in any manner

Information is disclosed when it is transmitted between or among organizations.

Under HIPAA, *use* limits the sharing of information within a covered entity, while *disclosure* restricts the sharing of information outside the entity holding the information.
The Privacy Rule covers the following PHI:

- The past, present, or future physical or mental health or condition of an individual
- Health care that is provided to an individual
- Billing or payments made for health care provided

Information that is not individually identifiable or unable to be tied to the identity of a particular patient is not subject to the Privacy Rule.

Managing and Storing Patient Information. Medical facilities have undergone many changes to the way they manage and store patient information. The Privacy Rule compliance was enforced in April of 2003. Many facilities contracted consultants that specialized in HIPAA and became certified in HIPAA compliance. For the health-care provider, the Privacy Rule requires activities such as:

- Notifying patients of their privacy rights and how their information is used

- Adopting and implementing privacy procedures for its practice, hospital, or plan
- Training employees so that they understand the privacy procedures
- Designating an individual to be responsible for seeing that the privacy procedures are adopted and followed
- Securing patient records containing individually identifiable health information so that they are not readily available to those who do not need them

Under HIPAA, patients have an increased awareness of their health information privacy rights, which includes the following:

- The right to access, copy, and inspect their health-care information
- The right to request an amendment to their health-care information
- The right to obtain an accounting of certain disclosures of their health-care information
- The right to alternate means of receiving communications from providers
- The right to complain about alleged violations of the regulations and the provider's own information policies

Sharing Patient Information. When sharing patient information, HIPAA will allow the provider to use health-care information for **treatment, payment, and operations (TPO).**

- Treatment—Providers are allowed to share information in order to provide care to patients
- Payment—Providers are allowed to share information in order to receive payment for the treatment provided
- Operations—Providers are allowed to share information to conduct normal business activities, such as quality improvement

If the use of patient information does not fall under TPO, then written authorization must be obtained *before* sharing information with anyone.
Patient information may be disclosed without authorization to the following parties or in the following situations:

- Medical researchers
- Emergencies
- Funeral directors/coroners
- Disaster relief services
- Law enforcement
- Correctional institutions
- Abuse and neglect
- Organ and tissue donation centers
- Work-related conditions that may affect employee health
- Judicial/administrative proceedings at the patient's request or as directed by a subpoena or court order

When using or disclosing PHI, a provider must make reasonable efforts to limit the use or disclosure to the minimum amount of PHI necessary to accomplish the intended purpose. Providing only the minimum necessary information means taking reasonable safeguards to protect an individual's health information from incidental disclosure. State laws may impose more stringent requirements regarding the protection of patient information. Health-care providers and staff should only have access to information they need to fulfill their assigned duties. The minimum necessary standard does not apply to disclosures, including oral disclosures, among health-care providers for treatment purposes. For example, a physician is not required to apply the minimum necessary standard when discussing a patient's medical chart information with a specialist at another hospital.

Patient Notification. Since the effective date of the HIPAA Privacy Rule, medical facilities have made major changes in how they inform patients of their HIPAA compliance. You may have noticed, as a patient yourself, the forms and information packets that are now provided by your health-care providers. The first step in informing patients of HIPAA compliance is the communication of patient rights. These rights are communicated through a document called **Notice of Privacy Practices (NPP)**. A notice must:

- Be written in plain, simple language.
- Include a header that reads: "This Notice describes how medical information about you may be used and disclosed and how you can get access to this information. Please review carefully."
- Describe the covered entity's uses and disclosures of PHI.
- Describe an individual's rights under the Privacy Rule.
- Describe the covered entity's duties.
- Describe how to register complaints concerning suspected privacy violations.
- Specify a point of contract.
- Specify an effective date.
- State that the entity reserves to right to change its privacy practices.

The second step in patient notification is to implement a document that explains the policy of the medical facility on obtaining **authorization** for the use and disclosure of patient information for purposes other than TPO. The authorization form must be written in plain language. Some of the core elements of an authorization form include:

- Specific and meaningful descriptions of the authorized information
- Persons authorized to use or disclose protected health information
- Purpose of the requested information
- Statement of the patient's right to revoke the authorization
- Signature and date of the patient

Security Measures. Health-care facilities can undertake a number of measures in order to help reduce a breach of confidentiality, including for information that is either stored or delivered electronically (i.e., stored in computers or computer networks, or delivered via computer networks or the Internet).

HIPAA Security Rule. In February 2003, the final regulations were issued regarding the administrative, physical, and technical safeguards to protect the confidentiality, integrity, and availability of health information covered by HIPAA. The **Security Rule** specifies how patient information is protected on computer networks, the Internet, disks, and other storage media and extranets. The rapidly increasing use of computers in health care today has created new dangers for breaches of confidentiality. The Security Rule mandates that:

- A security officer must be assigned the responsibility for the medical facility's security
- All staff, including management, receives security awareness training
- Medical facilities must implement audit controls to record and examine staff who have logged into information systems that contain PHI
- Organizations limit physical access to medical facilities that contain electronic PHI
- Organizations must conduct risk analyses to determine information security risks and vulnerabilities
- Organizations must establish policies and procedures that allow access to electronic PHI on a need-to-know basis

Computers are not the only concern regarding security of the workplace. The facility layout can propose a possible violation if not designed correctly. All facilities must take measures to reduce the identity of patient information. Some examples of facility design that can help reduce a breach of confidentiality include the security of patient charts, the reception area, the clinical station, and faxes sent and received.

Chart Security. Patient charts can be kept confidential by following these rules:

- Charts that contain a patient's name or other identifiers cannot be in view at the front reception area or nurse's station. Some offices have placed charts in plain jackets to prevent information from being seen.
- Charts must be stored out of the view of a public area, so that they cannot be seen by unauthorized individuals.
- Charts should be placed on the filing shelves without the patient name showing.
- Charts should be locked when not in use. Many facilities have purchased filing equipment that can be locked and unlocked without limiting the availability of patient information.

- Every staff member who uses patient information must be logged and a confidentiality statement signed. Signatures of staff should be on file with the office.

Reception Area Security. The following steps can be taken to secure the reception area:

- Log off or turn your monitor off when leaving your terminal or computer.
- The computer must be placed in an area where other patients cannot see the screen.
- Many facilities are purchasing flat screen monitors to prevent visibility to the screen.
- The sign-in sheet must be monitored and not left out in patient view. The names of patients must be blacked out so the next patient cannot read the names. It is best to put another system in place and to eliminate the sign-in sheet.
- Many offices are reviewing the reception area with regard to phone conversations. Some offices are creating call centers away from the reception/waiting area.

Medical Assistant Clinical Station Security. Medical assistants should follow these guidelines to protect PHI at the clinical station:

- Log off or turn your monitor off when leaving your terminal or computer.
- When placing charts in exam room racks or in shelves, the name of the patient or other identifiers must be concealed from other patients.
- HIPAA does not have a regulation about calling patients' names in the reception area, but to increase privacy in your facility, you may suggest a numbering system to identify patients.
- When discussing a patient with another staff member or with the physician, make sure your voice is lowered and that all doors to the exam rooms are closed. Avoid discussing patient conditions in heavy traffic areas.
- When discussing a condition with a patient, make sure that you are in a private room or area where no one can hear you.
- Avoid discussing patients in lunchrooms, hallways, or any place in a medical facility where someone can overhear you.

Fax Security. A lot of information is exchanged over the fax machine in a medical office. The fax machine is a vital link among physicians, hospitals, insurance companies, and other medical staff members. Private health information can be exchanged via faxes sent to covered entities. Here are some recommendations to help safeguard information exchanged via fax machines:

- Fax cover page: State clearly on the fax cover sheet that confidential and protected health information is included. Further state that the information included is to be protected and must not be shared or disclosed without the appropriate authorizations from the patient.
- Location of the fax machine: Keep the fax machine in an area that is not accessible by individuals who are not authorized to view PHI.
- Faxes with protected health information: Faxes that your office receives with PHI must be stored promptly in a protected, secure area.
- Fax number: Always confirm the accuracy of fax numbers to minimize the possibility of faxes being sent to the wrong person. Call people to tell them the fax is being sent.
- Confirmation: Program the fax machine to print a confirmation for all faxes sent, and staple the confirmation sheet to each document sent.
- Training: Train all staff members to understand the importance of safeguarding PHI sent or received via fax.

Violations and Penalties. Every staff member is responsible for adhering to HIPAA privacy and security regulations to ensure that PHI is secure and confidential. Anyone who uses or shares patient information is ethically obligated to comply with HIPAA. If PHI is abused or confidentiality is breached, the medical facility can incur substantial penalties or even the incarceration of staff. Violations of HIPAA law can result in both civil and criminal penalties.

Civil Penalties. Civil penalties for HIPAA privacy violations can be up to $100 for each offense, with an annual cap of $25,000 for repeated violations of the same requirement.

Criminal Penalties. Criminal penalties for the knowing, wrongful misuse of individually identifiable health information can result in the following penalties:

- For the knowing misuse of individually identifiable health information: up to $50,000 and/or one year in prison.
- For misuse under false pretenses: up to $100,000 and/or 5 years in prison.
- For offenses to sell for profit or malicious harm: up to $250,000 and/or 10 years in prison.

Administrative Simplification. The main key to the set of rules established for HIPAA administrative simplification is standardizing patient information throughout the health-care system with a set of transaction standards and code sets. The codes and formats used for the exchange of medical data are referred to as **electronic transaction records.** Regulated transaction information is given a transaction set identifier. For example, a health-care professional claim would be given an identifier of ASC X12N 837. This is a standard transaction code given to any facility that submits a health-care claim to an insurance company.

Standardized code sets are used for encoding data elements. The following books are used for the standardized code sets for all health-care facilities:

- *ICD-9-CM*, Volumes 1 and 2. This book is used to identify diseases and conditions.
- *CPT 4*. This book is used to identify physician services or procedures.
- *HCPCS*. This book is used to identify health-related services that are not physician or hospital services and procedures, such as radiology or hearing and vision services.

Confidentiality Issues and Mandatory Disclosure

Related to law, ethics, and quality care is the issue of when the medical assistant can disclose information and when it must be kept confidential. The incidents that doctors are legally required to report to the state were outlined earlier in the chapter. A doctor can be charged with criminal action for not following state and federal laws.

Ethics and professional judgment are always important. Consider the question of whether to contact the partners of a patient who has a sexually transmitted disease and whether to keep the patient's name from those people. The law says that the physician must instruct patients on how to notify possibly affected third parties and give them referrals to get the proper assistance. If the patient refuses to inform involved outside parties, then the doctor's office may offer to notify current and former partners. The Caution: Handle With Care section addresses this issue.

In general, the patient's ethical right to confidentiality and privacy is protected by law. Only the patient can waive the right to confidentiality. A physician cannot publicize a patient case in journal articles or invite other health professionals to observe a case without the patient's written consent. Most states also prohibit a doctor from testifying in court about a patient without the patient's approval. When a patient sues a physician, however, the patient automatically gives up the right to confidentiality.

In terms of rights to the patient's chart, the physician owns the chart, but the patient owns the information. The patient has a right to a copy of the chart for a reasonable fee. (It is illegal for the patient to be denied a copy of his chart if he is unable to pay the fee.)

Following are six principles for preventing improper release of information from the medical office.

1. When in doubt about whether to release information, it is better not to release it.
2. It is the patient's, not the doctor's, right to keep patient information confidential. If the patient wants to disclose the information, it is unethical for the physician not to do so.
3. All patients should be treated with the same degree of confidentiality, whatever the health-care professional's personal opinion of the patient might be.
4. You should be aware of all applicable laws and of the regulations of agencies such as public health departments.
5. When it is necessary to break confidentiality and when there is a conflict between ethics and confidentiality, discuss it with the patient. If the law does not dictate what to do in the situation, the attending physician should make the judgment based on the urgency of the situation and any danger that might be posed to the patient or others.
6. Get written approval from the patient before releasing information. For common situations, the patient should sign a standard release-of-records form.

CAUTION *Handle With Care*

Notifying Those at Risk for Sexually Transmitted Disease

Few things are more difficult for a patient with a sexually transmitted disease (STD) than telling current and former partners about the diagnosis. In fact, some patients elect not to do so. When patients refuse to alert their partners, the medical office can offer to make those contacts. Often that responsibility lies with the medical assistant.

You are most likely to encounter such a situation if you are a medical assistant working in a family practice, an obstetrics/gynecology practice, or a clinic. Becoming familiar with all facets of the situation—from ensuring patient confidentiality to handling potentially difficult confrontations—will help you best serve the patient.

The first step is to get the appropriate information from the patient who has contracted the STD. Because the patient may be sensitive about revealing former and current partners, help him feel more comfortable. First, spend some time talking about the STD. How much does the patient know about it? Educate him about implications, including the probable short- and long-term effects of the disease. Explain how the STD

continued ⟶

Notifying Those at Risk for Sexually Transmitted Disease *(continued)*

is transmitted. Alert the patient as to precautions to take so he will not continue to transmit the disease to others. Help the patient understand why it is important for people who may have contracted the disease from him to be told they may have it.

Then, offer to contact the patient's former and current partners. Fully explain each step in the notification process, assuring the patient that his name will not be revealed under any circumstances. Answer any questions and address any concerns about the notification process. If the patient is still reluctant to provide information, give him some time to think about it away from the office, and follow up periodically with a phone call.

Once the patient agrees to reveal names, write down the names and other information, preferably phone numbers. To make sure you have correct information, read it back to the patient, spelling each person's name in turn and reciting the phone number or address. Write down the phonetic pronunciations of any difficult names. Tell the patient when you will make the notifications.

You now are ready to contact these individuals. Professionals who work with STD patients recommend guidelines for contacting current and former partners to alert them about potential exposure to an STD. Note that these guidelines are applicable only to STDs other than AIDS.

Determine how you will contact each individual: in writing, in person, or by phone.

1. If you use U.S. mail, mark the outside of the addressed envelope "Personal." On a note inside, simply ask the person to call you at the medical office. Do not put the topic of the call in writing.

2. If you make the contact in person, ask where you can talk privately. Even if the person appears to be alone, others may still be able to overhear the conversation.

3. If you use the phone, identify yourself and your office, and ask for the specific individual. Do not reveal the nature of your call to anyone but that person. If pressed, tell the person who answers the phone that you are calling regarding a personal matter.

Once on the phone or alone with the person, confirm that you are talking to the correct person. Mention that you wish to talk about a highly personal matter, and ask if it is a good time to continue the discussion. If not, arrange for a more appropriate time.

Inform the individual that she has come in contact with someone who has a sexually transmitted disease. Recommend that the person visit a doctor's office or clinic to be tested for the disease.

Be prepared for a variety of reactions, from surprise to anger. Respond calmly and coolly. Expect to respond to questions and statements such as:

- Who gave you my name?
- Do I have the disease?
- Am I really at risk? I haven't had intercourse recently (or) I've only had intercourse with my spouse.
- I feel fine. I just went to my doctor recently.

Let the person know that you cannot reveal the name of the partner because the information is strictly confidential. Assure the person that you will not reveal her name to anyone either.

Explain that exposure to the disease does not mean a person has contracted it. Encourage the person to get tested to know for sure.

Tell the person that she is still at risk, even if she hasn't had intercourse recently or has had it only with a spouse. Let the person know that someone with whom she came in close contact at some point has contracted the disease.

Even if the person says, "I feel fine," she may still have the disease. Again, stress the importance of getting tested.

Provide your name and phone number for contact about further questions. Recommend local offices and clinics for testing, and provide phone numbers. If the person will come to your office, offer to make the appointment.

Finally, document the results of your call. Log in the original patient's file the date that you completed notification. Include any pertinent details about the notification. Alert the patient when all people on the list have been notified.

The AMA has several standard forms for authorization of disclosure and includes disclosure clauses in many other forms. For example, the consent-to-surgery form includes a clause about consenting to picture taking and observation during the surgery. When using a standard form, cross out anything that does not apply in that particular situation. Medical practices often develop their own customized forms.

Summary

You must carefully follow all state, federal, and individual practice rules and laws while performing your daily duties. You must also follow the AAMA Code of Ethics for medical assistants. It is an important part of your duties to help the doctor avoid malpractice claims—lawsuits by the patient against the physician for errors in diagnosis or treatment.

To perform effectively as a medical assistant, you must maintain an office that follows all OSHA regulations for safety, hazardous equipment, and toxic substances. The office also must meet QC and QA guidelines for all tests, specimens, and treatments. It is your responsibility to follow HIPAA guidelines, to ensure patient privacy and confidentiality of patient records, to fully document patient treatment, and to maintain patient records in an orderly and readily accessible fashion.

REVIEW

CHAPTER 3

CASE STUDY *QUESTIONS*

Now that you have completed this chapter, review the case study at the beginning of the chapter and answer the following questions:

1. Does the medical assistant's comment represent a breach of confidentiality?
2. Has any HIPAA rule been violated? If so, which one?

Discussion Questions

1. How does the law of agency make it possible for a patient to sue both the medical assistant and the physician for an act of negligence committed by the medical assistant?
2. Under HIPAA, what rights do patients have regarding confidentiality and ownership of their medical records? When does a patient give up the right to confidentiality?
3. Are health-care professionals legally liable for all unsatisfactory outcomes?
4. What are two scenarios that would void a contract between physician and patient?

Critical Thinking Questions

1. What is an example of a bioethical issue? Give two opposing views of the issue.
2. What are two different situations that could turn into a malpractice or abandonment suit if committed by physicians or their medical staff members?
3. Describe implied consent and two ways that a patient can accept treatment by implied consent.

Application Activities

1. Research a controversial topic from the following list:
   Euthanasia
   Surrogacy
   Abortion
   Fetal stem cell research
   Cloning
   Emergency contraceptive (morning-after pill)

   Write a three-page report that presents both the pro side and the con side of the issue. Write a closing paragraph that gives your personal opinion and views and how you have been conditioned in that belief, for example, social, cultural, and religious beliefs.
2. Choose teams of four people, and stage debates on the controversial topics listed in question 1. Research your topics thoroughly and present arguments on both sides. Your purpose is to state facts and persuade your audience to your beliefs.

   Rules for the debate:
   - Participants must be courteous and professional
   - Presentations must be factual
   - Opening arguments are four minutes for each side
   - Each side presents, and then for three minutes each side is allowed to counter any fact
   - Closing arguments are five minutes for each side
   - Have the class vote on which side was more persuasive.
3. In a medical law textbook or journal, research a malpractice case. Prepare a 10-minute presentation for the class in which you summarize both sides of the case (patient and caregiver). Include when and where the case took place. Explain how the case was settled and whether the settlement took place in a court of law or through arbitration. Close with your opinion about whether the case was settled fairly.
4. Research a piece of legislation on a health-care issue or practice, either a bill passed in the last 5 years or a bill currently being considered in Washington. What impact has this bill had or might this bill have on the medical assisting profession? Summarize your findings in a one- to two-page report.

CHAPTER 4

Communication With Patients, Families, and Coworkers

AREAS OF COMPETENCE

2003 Role Delineation Study

GENERAL

Professionalism
- Display a professional manner and image
- Demonstrate initiative and responsibility
- Work as a member of the health-care team
- Adapt to change
- Treat all patients with compassion and empathy
- Promote the practice through positive public relations

Communication Skills
- Recognize and respect cultural diversity
- Adapt communications to an individual's ability to understand
- Recognize and respond effectively to verbal, nonverbal, and written communications
- Serve as liaison

Legal Concepts
- Perform within legal and ethical boundaries
- Document accurately

KEY TERMS

- active listening
- aggressive
- assertive
- body language
- burnout
- closed posture
- conflict
- empathy
- feedback
- hierarchy
- homeostasis
- hospice
- interpersonal skills
- open posture
- passive listening
- personal space
- rapport

CHAPTER OUTLINE

- Communicating With Patients and Families
- The Communication Circle
- Understanding Human Behavior and How It Relates to the Provider-Patient Relationship
- Types of Communication
- Improving Your Communication Skills
- Communicating in Special Circumstances
- Communicating With Coworkers
- Managing Stress
- Preventing Burnout
- The Policy and Procedures Manual

OBJECTIVES

After completing Chapter 4, you will be able to:

4.1 Identify elements of the communication circle.
4.2 Give examples of positive and negative communication.

4.3 List ways to improve listening and interpersonal skills.

4.4 Explain the difference between assertiveness and aggressiveness.

4.5 Give examples of effective communication strategies with patients in special circumstances.

4.6 Discuss ways to establish positive communication with coworkers and superiors.

4.7 Explain how stress relates to communication and identify strategies to reduce stress.

4.8 Describe how the office policy and procedures manual is used as a communication tool in the medical office.

Introduction

The ability to recognize human behaviors and the ability to communicate effectively are vital to a medical assistant and the pursuit for success. This chapter has taken a psychological approach to understanding human behavior and the challenges that influence therapeutic communication in a health-care setting. Patients will often have more interaction with the medical assistant than with any other health-care practitioner in the facility. It is important that patients develop a good rapport and feel confident in the care they are receiving from your office. The medical assistant sets the tone for the communication cycle and must be aware of all the obstacles that can affect human communication. As a medical assistant, you are often exposed to all kinds of patients. You will see patients from different cultures, socioeconomic backgrounds, educational levels, ages, and lifestyles. You must be able to communicate with each patient with professionalism and diplomacy.

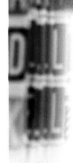

CASE STUDY

Mary is 23 years old and has been a medical assistant for 6 months. She is currently working in a walk-in clinic in a large urban city. She has interviewed three patients this morning. One patient is a homeless transient male who appears to have some type of mental incapacity; the second is a teenage girl who suspects she might be pregnant; and the third is a well-dressed professional male who complains of a sore throat.

As you read this chapter, consider how you would answer the following questions relative to each of the patients:

1. How will Mary adapt her communication style to communicate with each patient?
2. What types of communication roadblocks will she encounter with each one?
3. What types of communication techniques will she use for each patient?

Communicating With Patients and Families

Think about the last time you had a doctor's appointment. How well did the staff and physicians communicate with you? Were you greeted cordially and pleasantly invited to take a seat, or did someone thrust a clipboard at you and say "Fill this out"? If you had a long wait in the waiting room or examination room, did someone come in to explain the delay? Did you become frustrated and angry because nobody told you what was happening?

As a medical assistant, you are a key communicator between the office and patients and families. The way you greet patients, explain procedures, ask and answer questions, and attend to the individual needs of patients forms your communication style. Your interaction with the patient sets the tone for the office visit and can significantly influence how comfortable the patient feels in your practice. Developing strong communication skills in the medical office is just as important as mastering administrative and clinical tasks.

Customer service is the most important part of communication to families and patients. Your mastery of clinical and administrative skills is only a portion of your skills; customer service and communication skills are the other 70%.

A definition of customer service includes the following two points:

1. The patient comes first
2. Patient needs are satisfied

In today's health-care environment, patients are consumers and are more educated than ever before. Patients have more options in choosing a physician or a health-care facility. Patients who feel that they were not given exceptional customer service will choose another physician or facility to meet their needs. Another reason a facility must strive for exceptional customer service is that a medical facility grows rapidly from referral business. A medical facility that acquires a reputation for having an "unfriendly" staff will feel the negative impact from that reputation.

Listed here are some examples of customer service in the physician's office:

- Using proper telephone techniques
- Writing or responding to telephone messages
- Explaining procedures to patients
- Expediting insurance referral requests
- Assisting in billing issues
- Answering questions or finding answers to patient questions
- Ensuring that patients are comfortable in your office
- Creating a warm and reassuring environment

From a business perspective, exceptional customer service is vital to a medical facility's success. Any business that does not provide exceptional customer service will not grow and thrive in today's business economy.

The Communication Circle

As you interact with patients and their families, you will be responsible for giving information and ensuring that the patient understands what you, the doctor, and other members of the staff have communicated. You will also be responsible for receiving information from the patient. For example, patients will describe their symptoms. They may also discuss their feelings or ask questions about a treatment or procedure. The giving and receiving of information forms the communication circle.

Elements of the Communication Circle

The communication circle involves three elements: a message, a source, and a receiver. Messages are usually verbal or written. (As you will see later in the chapter, some messages are nonverbal.) The source sends the message, and the receiver receives it. The communication circle is formed as the source sends a message to the receiver and the receiver responds (Figure 4-1).

Consider this example, in which Simone, a medical assistant who works in a physical therapy office, is speaking with Mrs. Sommer, a patient who is having therapy for a back injury. Watch the communication circle at work.

| Simone: | The physical therapist says you're making great progress and that you can start on some simple back exercises at home. |

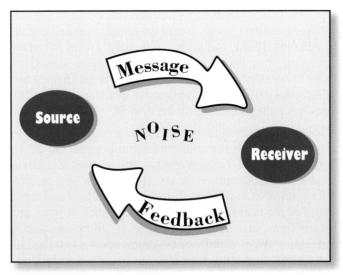

Figure 4-1. The process of communication involves an exchange of messages through verbal and nonverbal means.

	I'd like to go over them with you. Then I'll give you a sheet that illustrates the exercises. How does that sound to you?
Mrs. Sommer:	I'm a little nervous about doing exercises. I still have some pain when I bend over.
Simone:	I understand. It's important, though, to start using those muscles again. Why don't you show me exactly where it hurts. Then we can go over proper body mechanics, such as bending down to pick something up and getting in and out of chairs, the car, and bed. Then we'll just start with one or two of the exercises and save the rest for next time, when you're feeling more ready.
Mrs. Sommer:	Yes, I only feel up to doing a little bit today.

The medical assistant (the source) gives a verbal message (about back exercises) to the patient (the receiver). The patient responds by drawing attention to her pain and uneasiness about certain movements. The patient's response is also a message to the medical assistant, who responds in turn. The giving and receiving of information continues within the communication circle until the exchange is finished.

Feedback. Another word for response is **feedback**, which is verbal or nonverbal evidence that the receiver got and understood the message. When you communicate information to a patient or ask a patient a question, always look for feedback. For example, if you calculate a pregnant patient's due date and tell her she's 12 weeks pregnant, look for a response. If she responds, "Oh, good, that means I'm out of danger of having a miscarriage," you would respond that whereas most miscarriages occur in the first 12 weeks, some risk of miscarriage remains throughout the pregnancy. If she responds, "I thought I was 14 weeks pregnant," you would need to clarify how you worked out your calculation and compare it with hers, to uncover any discrepancy. Good communication in the medical office requires patient feedback at every step.

Noise. Anything that distorts the message in any way or interferes with the communication process can be referred to as noise. Noise refers not only to sounds, such as a siren or jackhammer on the street below the medical office suite. It also refers to room temperature and other types of physical comfort or discomfort, such as pain, and to emotions, such as fear or sadness. If patients are feeling uncomfortable in a chilly or hot room, upset about their illness, or in great pain, they may not pay close attention to what you are saying. Conversely, if you are feeling upset about a personal problem outside work or if you are unwell or preoccupied with all the things you have on your to-do list, you may not communicate well.

As you deal with each patient, try to screen out or eliminate both literal and figurative noise. For example, before you start a conversation with a patient in an examination room, you might ask, "Are you too chilly or too hot? Is the temperature in here comfortable for you?" If there is construction going on outside the building, see if there is a less noisy inner room or office that you might be able to use. If a patient seems nervous or upset, address those feelings before you launch into a factual discussion.

If you are feeling stressed or out of sorts, that feeling constitutes a type of noise. Try to take a "breather" between patients or a break from desk work—walk downstairs, get some fresh air, stretch your legs. Feeling dehydrated or hungry affects your communication efforts too. Limit your caffeine and sugar intake. Drink plenty of water and juice throughout the day. Eat a good lunch and healthful snacks. Leave your personal problems at home.

Humanizing the Communication Process in the Medical Office

As highly structured managed care organizations and technological advances rapidly change the face of health care, many patients feel that health care is becoming impersonal. Every time you communicate with patients, you can counteract this perception by playing a humanistic role in the health-care process. Being humanistic means that you work to help patients feel attended to and respected as individuals, not just as descriptions on a chart. Good communication supports this patient-centered approach.

Make a point of developing and using strong communication skills to show patients that you, the doctors, and other staff members care about them and their feelings. Taking care to treat patients as people helps humanize the communication process in the medical office.

Understanding Human Behavior and How It Relates to the Provider-Patient Relationship

Understanding human behavior is important when you are communicating with patients. Medical assistants are exposed to many different personality types in addition to different illnesses. When you understand why a person is behaving in a certain way, you can adjust your communication style to adapt to that person. Abraham Maslow, a well-known human behaviorist, developed a model of human behavior known as the **hierarchy** (i.e., a classification) of needs. This hierarchy states that human beings are motivated by unsatisfied needs and that certain lower needs have to be satisfied before higher needs, like self-actualization, are met. Maslow felt that people are basically trustworthy, self-protecting, and self-governing and that humans tend toward growth and love. He believed that humans are not violent by nature, but are violent only when their needs are not being met.

Deficiency Needs

According to Maslow, there are general types of needs—physiological, safety, love, and esteem—that must be satisfied before a person can act unselfishly. He called these needs *deficiency needs.*

Physiological Needs. Physiological needs are humans' very basic needs, such as air, water, food, sleep, and sex. When these needs are not satisfied, we may feel sickness, irritation, pain, and discomfort. These feelings motivate us to alleviate them as soon as possible to establish **homeostasis** (that is, a state of balance or equilibrium). Once those feelings are alleviated, we may think about other things.

Safety Needs. People have the need and desire for establishing stability and consistency. These basic needs are security, shelter, and existing in a safe environment.

Love Needs. Humans have a desire to belong to groups: clubs, work groups, religious groups, family, and so on. We need to feel loved and accepted by others. Humans are like pack animals—we place great importance in belonging to society.

Esteem Needs. Humans like to feel that they are important and have worthiness to society. There are two types of self-esteem. The first results from competence or mastery of a task, such as completing an educational program. The second is the attention and recognition that comes from others.

Self-Actualization

The need for self-actualization is "the desire to become more and more what one is, to become everything that one is capable of becoming." To reach this level, a person utilizes many tools to maximize potential, such as education. Successful people have reached this level on the hierarchy ladder.

When working and communicating with patients, remember this hierarchy of human needs and observe what need a patient is deficient in. For example, if an elderly patient has recently lost her husband, she may feel lonely and deficient in the love need. You may see homeless patients who are deficient in their physiological and safety needs. You may have a young girl as a patient who is overweight and has low self-esteem. On the other hand, you may have a high-level executive as a patient who has reached self-actualization. Each of these scenarios would require a communication style adjustment in order for you to effectively communicate with these patients.

Types of Communication

Communication can be positive or negative. It can also be verbal, nonverbal, or written. To help ensure effective communication with patients, familiarize yourself with these different types of communication. (Written communication is discussed in Chapter 7.)

Positive Communication

In the medical office, communication that promotes patients' comfort and well-being is essential. Treating patients brusquely or rudely is unacceptable in the health-care setting. It is your responsibility—not the patient's—to set the stage for positive communication.

When information—even bad news—is communicated with some positive aspect, patients are more likely to listen attentively and respond positively themselves. For example, you might explain to a patient who is about to get an injection, "This will sting, but only for a couple of seconds. When we're through, you're free to go." You would not just say, "This is going to hurt."

Other examples of positive communication are:

- Being friendly, warm, and attentive ("It's good to see you again, Mrs. Armstrong. I know you're on your lunch hour, so let's get started right away.")
- Verbalizing concern for patients ("Are you comfortable?" "I understand it hurts when I do this; I'll be gentle." "This paperwork won't take long at all.")
- Encouraging patients to ask questions ("I hope I've explained the procedure well. Do you have any questions, or are there any parts you would like to go over again?")
- Asking patients to repeat your instructions to make sure they understand
- Looking directly at patients when you speak to them
- Smiling (naturally, not in a forced way)

- Speaking slowly and clearly
- Listening carefully

Negative Communication

Most people do not purposely try to communicate negatively. Some people, however, may not realize that their communication style has a negative impact on others. Look for and ask for feedback to help you curb negative communication habits. Ask yourself, "Do the physicians and my other coworkers seem glad to speak with me? Are they open and responsive to me?" "Do patients seem at ease with me, or are they very quiet, turned off, or distant?" (Note that some patients may respond this way because of the way they feel, not because of the way you are communicating with them.) Here are some examples of negative communication:

- Mumbling
- Speaking brusquely or sharply
- Avoiding eye contact
- Interrupting patients as they are speaking
- Rushing through explanations or instructions
- Treating patients impersonally
- Making patients feel they are taking up too much of your time or asking too many questions
- Forgetting common courtesies, such as saying please and thank you
- Showing boredom

A good way to avoid negative communication is to open your eyes and ears to others in service-oriented workplace settings. The next time you buy something at a store, call a company for information over the phone, or eat out at a restaurant, take note of the way the staff treats you. Do they answer your questions courteously? Do they give you the information you ask for? Do they make you feel welcome? What specifically makes their communication style positive or negative? Remember, you can always improve your communication skills.

Body Language

Verbal communication refers to communication that is spoken. Nonverbal communication is also known as **body language.** Body language includes facial expressions, eye contact, posture, touch, and attention to personal space. In many instances, people's body language conveys their true feelings, even when their words may say otherwise. A patient might say "I'm OK about that," but if she is sitting with her arms folded tightly across her chest and avoids looking at you, she may not mean what she says.

Facial Expression. Your face is the most expressive part of your body. You can often tell whether someone has understood your message simply by his facial expression. For example, when you are explaining a procedure to a patient, look at his expression. Does it seem puzzled? Is his brow wrinkled? Does he look surprised? Facial expressions can give you clues about how to tailor your communication efforts. They also serve as a form of feedback.

Eye Contact.   Eye contact is an important part of positive communication. Look directly at patients when speaking to them. Looking away or down communicates that you are not interested in the person or that you are avoiding her for some reason.

There may be cultural differences in the ways patients react to eye contact. In some cultures, for example, it is common to avoid eye contact out of respect for someone who is considered a superior. Thus, children may be taught not to look adults in the eye.

Posture.   The way you hold or move your head, arms, hands, and the rest of your body can project strong nonverbal messages. During communication, posture can usually be described as open or closed.

Open Posture.   A feeling of receptiveness and friendliness can be conveyed with an **open posture**. In this position, your arms lie comfortably at your sides or in your lap. You face the other person, and you may lean forward in your chair. This demonstrates that you are listening and are interested in what the other person has to say. Open posture is a form of positive communication.

Closed Posture.   A **closed posture** conveys the opposite, a feeling of not being totally receptive to what is being said. It can also signal that someone is angry or upset. A person in a closed posture may hold his arms rigidly or fold them across his chest. He may lean back in his chair, away from the other person. He may turn away to avoid eye contact. Slouching is a kind of closed posture that can convey fatigue or lack of caring. Watch for patients with closed postures that may indicate tension or pain. Avoid closed postures yourself—they have a negative effect on your communication efforts.

Touch.   Touch is a powerful form of nonverbal communication. A touch on the arm or a hug can be a means of saying hello, sharing condolences, or expressing congratulations. Family background, culture, age, and gender all influence people's perception of touch. Some people may welcome a touch or think nothing of it. Others may view touching as an invasion of their privacy. In general, in the medical setting, a touch on the shoulder, forearm, or back of the hand to express interest or concern is acceptable.

Personal Space.   When communicating with others, it is important to be aware of the concept of personal space. **Personal space** is an area that surrounds an individual. By not intruding on patients' personal space, you show respect for their feelings of privacy.

In most social situations, it is common for people to stand 4 to 12 ft away from each other. For personal conversation, you would typically stand between 1½ and 4 ft away from a person. Some patients may feel uncomfortable—and may become anxious—when you stand or sit close to them. Others prefer the reassurance of having people close to

them when they speak. Watch patients carefully. If they lean back when you lean forward or if they fold their arms or turn their head away, you may be invading their personal space. If they lean or step toward you, they may be seeking to close up the personal space.

Improving Your Communication Skills

Sharpening your communication skills should be an ongoing effort and will help you become a more effective communicator. Good communication skills can enhance the quality of your interaction with patients and coworkers alike. Among the skills involved in communication are listening skills, interpersonal skills, therapeutic communication skills, and assertiveness skills.

Listening Skills

Listening involves both hearing and interpreting a message. Listening requires you to pay close attention not only to what is being said but also to nonverbal cues, such as those communicated through body language.

Listening can be passive or active. **Passive listening** is simply hearing what someone has to say without the need for a reply. An example is listening to a news program on the radio; the communication is mainly one-way. **Active listening** involves two-way communication. You are actively involved in the process, offering feedback or asking questions. Active listening takes place, for example, when you interview a patient for her medical history. Active listening is an essential skill in the medical office.

There are several ways to improve your listening skills:

- Prepare to listen. Position yourself at the same level (sitting, standing) as the person who is speaking, and assume an open posture (Figure 4-2).
- Relax and listen attentively. Do not simply pretend to listen to what is being said.
- Maintain eye contact.
- Maintain appropriate personal space.
- Think before you respond.
- Provide feedback. Restate the speaker's message in your own words to show that you understand.
- If you do not understand something that was said, ask the person to repeat it.

Interpersonal Skills

When you interact with people, you use **interpersonal skills.** When you make a patient feel at ease by being warm and friendly, you are demonstrating good interpersonal skills. In addition to warmth and friendliness, valuable interpersonal skills include empathy, respect, genuineness, openness, and consideration and sensitivity.

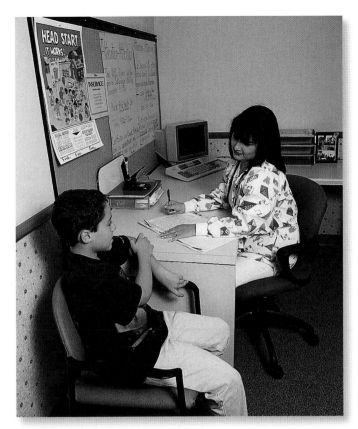

Figure 4-2. Active listening requires two-way communication and positive body language.

Warmth and Friendliness. A friendly but professional approach, a pleasant greeting, and a smile get you off to a good start when communicating with patients. When your approach is sincere, patients will be more relaxed and open.

Empathy. The process of identifying with someone else's feelings is **empathy.** When you are empathetic, you are sensitive to the other person's feelings and problems. For example, if a patient is experiencing a migraine headache and you have never had one, you can still let her know you are trying to imagine, or relate to, her situation. In other words, you can acknowledge the severity of her pain and show support and care. You must, however, always remain objective in your interaction with patients.

Respect. Showing respect can mean using a title of courtesy such as "Mr." or "Mrs." when communicating with patients. It can also mean acknowledging a patient's wishes or choices without passing judgment.

Genuineness. Being genuine in your interactions with patients means that you refrain from "putting on an act" or just going through the motions of your job. Patients like to know that their health-care providers are real people. In a medical setting, being genuine means caring for each patient on an individual basis, giving patients the full attention they deserve, and showing respect for them. Being genuine in your communication with patients encourages them to place trust in you and in what you say.

Openness. Openness means being willing to listen to and consider others' viewpoints and concerns and being receptive to their needs. An open individual is accepting of others and not biased for or against them.

Consideration and Sensitivity. You should always try to show consideration toward patients and act in a thoughtful, kind way. You must be sensitive to their individual concerns, fears, and needs.

Therapeutic Communication Skills

Therapeutic communication is the ability to communicate with a patient in terms that they can understand and, at the same time, feel at ease and comfortable in what you are saying. It is also the ability to communicate with other members of the health team in technical terms that are appropriate in a health-care setting. Therapeutic communication techniques are methodologies that can improve communication with patients.

Therapeutic communication involves the following communication skills:

- Being Silent. Silence allows the patient time to think without pressure.

- Accepting. This skill gives the patient an indication of reception. It shows that you have heard the patient and follow the patient's thought pattern. Some indicators of acceptance include nodding; saying "Yes," "I follow what you said," and other such phrases; and body language.

- Giving Recognition. Show patients that you are aware of them by stating their name in a greeting or by noticing positive changes. With this skill, you are recognizing the patient as a person or individual.

- Offering Self. Make yourself available to the needs of the patient.

- Giving a Broad Opening. Allow the patient to take the initiative in introducing the topic. Ask open-ended questions such as "Is there something you'd like to talk about?" or "Where would you like to begin?"

- Offering General Leads. Give the patient encouragement to continue by making comments such as "Go on" or "And then?"

- Making Observations. Make your perceptions known to the patient. Say things like "You appear tense today" or "Are you uncomfortable when you . . . ?" By calling patients' attention to what is happening to them, you encourage them to notice it for themselves so that they can describe it to you.

- Encouraging Communication. Ask patients to verbalize what they perceive. Make statements such as "Tell me when you feel anxious" or "What is happening?" Patients should feel free to describe their perceptions to you, and you must try to see things as they seem to the patients.

- Mirroring. Restate what the patient has said to demonstrate that you understand.

- Reflecting. Encourage patients to think through and answer their own questions. A reflecting dialogue may go like this:

  Patient: Do you think I should tell the doctor?

  Medical Assistant: Do you think you should?

  By reflecting patients' questions or statements back to them, you are helping patients feel that their opinions about their health are of value.

- Focusing. Focusing encourages the patient to stay on the topic.

- Exploring. Encourage patients to express themselves in more depth. Try to get as much detail as possible about a patent complaint, but avoid probing and prying if the patient does not wish to discuss it.

- Clarifying. Ask patients to explain themselves more clearly if they provide information that is vague or not meaningful.

- Summarizing. This skill involves organizing and summing up the important points of the discussion and gives the patient an awareness of the progress made toward greater understanding.

Ineffective Therapeutic Communication. In the previous section, the focus was on how to communicate effectively in a therapeutic environment. Oftentimes people think they are communicating thoroughly, but they are not. Here are some roadblocks that can interfere with your communication style:

- Reassuring. This type of communication indicates to the patient that there is no need for anxiety or worry. By doing this, you devalue the patient's feelings and give false hope if the outcome is not positive. The communication error here is a lack of understanding and empathy.

- Giving Approval. Giving approval is usually done by overtly approving of a patient's behavior. This may lead the patient to strive for praise rather than progress.

- Disapproving. Being disapproving is done by overtly disapproving of a patient's behavior. This implies that you have the right to pass judgment on the patient's thoughts and actions. Find an alternate attitude when dealing with patients. Adopting a moralistic attitude may take your attention away from the patient's needs and may direct it toward your own feelings.

- Agreeing/Disagreeing. Overtly agreeing or disagreeing with thoughts, perceptions, and ideas of patients is not an effective way to communicate. When you agree with patients, they will have the perception that they are right because you agree with them or because you share the same opinion. Opinions and conclusions should be the patient's, not yours. When disagreeing with patients, you become the opposition to them instead of their caregiver. Never place yourself in an argumentative situation regarding the opinions of a patient.

- Advising. If you tell the patient what you think should be done, you place yourself outside your scope of practice. You cannot advise patients.

- Probing. Probing is discussing a topic that the patient has no desire to discuss.

- Defending. Protecting yourself, the institution, and others from verbal attack are classified as defending. If you become defensive, the patient may feel the need to discontinue communication.

- Requesting an Explanation. This communication pattern involves asking patients to provide reasons for their behavior. Patients may not know why they behave in a certain manner. "Why" questions may have an intimidating effect on some patients.

- Minimizing Feelings. Never judge or make light of a patient's discomfort. It is important for you to perceive what is taking place from the patient's point of view, not your own.

- Making Stereotyped Comments. This type of communication involves using meaningless clichés when communicating with patients. An example of a stereotypical comment is "It's for your own good." These types of comments are given in an automatic, mechanical way as a substitute for a more reasonable and thoughtful explanation.

Defense Mechanisms. When working with patients, it is important to observe their communication behaviors. Patients will often develop *defense mechanisms,* which are unconscious, to protect themselves from anxiety, guilt, and shame.

Here are some common defense mechanisms that a patient may display when communicating with the doctor, medical assistant, or other health-care team members:

- Compensation: Overemphasizing a trait to make up for a perceived or actual failing

- Denial: An unconscious attempt to reject unacceptable feelings, needs, thoughts, wishes, or external reality factors

- Displacement: The unconscious transfer of unacceptable thoughts, feelings, or desires from the self to a more acceptable external substitute

- Dissociation: Disconnecting emotional significance from specific ideas or events

- Identification: Mimicking the behavior of another to cope with feelings of inadequacy

- Introjection: Adopting the unacceptable thoughts or feelings of others

- Projection: Projecting onto another person one's own feelings, as if they had originated in the other person

- Rationalization: Justifying unacceptable behavior, thoughts, and feelings into tolerable behaviors

- Regression: Unconsciously returning to more infantile behaviors or thoughts

- Repression: Putting unpleasant thoughts, feelings, or events out of one's mind

TABLE 4-1	A Comparison of Nonassertive, Assertive, Aggressive, and Nonassertive Aggressive Behavior			
	Nonassertive Behavior	**Assertive Behavior**	**Aggressive Behavior**	**Nonassertive Aggressive Behavior (NAG)**
Characteristics of the behavior	Emotionally dishonest, indirect, self-denying; allows others to choose for self; does not achieve desired goal	Emotionally honest, direct, self-enhancing, expressive; chooses for self; may achieve goal	Emotionally honest, direct, self-enhancing at the expense of another, expressive; chooses for others; may achieve goal at expense of others	Emotionally dishonest, indirect, self-denying; chooses for others; may achieve goal at expense of others
Your feelings	Hurt, anxious, possibly angry later	Confident, self-respecting	Righteous, superior, derogative at the time and possibly guilty later	Defiance, anger, self-denying; sometimes anxious, possibly guilty later
The other person's feelings toward you	Irritated, pity, lack of respect	Generally respected	Angry, resentful	Angry, resentful, irritated, disgusted
The other person's feelings about her/himself	Guilty of superior	Valued, respected	Hurt, embarrassed, defensive	Hurt, guilty or superior, humiliated

Adapted from Alberti, Robert E., and Emmons, Michael, *Your Perfect Right: A Guide to Assertive Behavior,* San Luis Obispo, California: Impact, 1970.

- Substitution: Unconsciously replacing an unreachable or unacceptable goal with another, more acceptable one

Assertiveness Skills

As a professional, you need to be **assertive,** that is, to be firm and to stand by your principles while still showing respect for others. Being assertive means trusting your instincts, feelings, and opinions (not in terms of diagnosing, which only the doctor can do, but in terms of basic communication with patients), and acting on them. For example, when you see that a patient looks uneasy, speak up. You might say, "You look concerned. How can I help you feel more comfortable?"

Being assertive is different from being aggressive. When people are **aggressive,** they try to impose their position on others or try to manipulate them. Aggressive people are bossy and can be quarrelsome. They do not appear to take into consideration others' feelings, needs, thoughts, ideas, and opinions before they act or speak.

To be assertive, you must be open, honest, and direct. Be aware of your body position: an open posture conveys the proper message. When you communicate, speak confidently and use "I" statements such as "I feel . . ." or "I think . . ." (Assertiveness is also discussed later in the chapter in the section on communicating with coworkers.)

Developing your assertiveness skills increases your sense of self-worth and your confidence as a professional. Being assertive will also help you prevent or resolve conflicts more peacefully and increase your leadership ability. People look up to and respect professionals who are assertive in the workplace. See Table 4-1 for a comparison of assertive, nonassertive, and aggressive behaviors.

Communicating in Special Circumstances

If you make an effort to develop good interpersonal skills, most patients will not be difficult to communicate with. You will, however, encounter patients in special circumstances, when they may be anxious or angry. These situations sometimes inhibit communication. Patients from different cultures may pose challenges to communication. Others may have some type of impairment or disability that makes communication difficult. Similarly, young patients, parents with children who are ill or injured, and patients with terminal illnesses may present communication difficulties. Learning about the special needs of these patients and polishing your own communication skills will help you become an effective communicator in any number of situations.

The Anxious Patient

It is common for patients to be anxious in a doctor's office or other health-care setting. This reaction is commonly known as the "white-coat syndrome." There can be many reasons for anxiety. A patient can become anxious because she is ill and does not know what is wrong with her—she may fear the worst. A patient may have recently been diagnosed with an illness that he knows nothing about, which may necessitate a severe lifestyle change. Fear of bad news or fear that some procedure is going to be painful can create anxiety. Anxiety can interfere with the communication process. For example, because of anxiety a patient may not listen well or pay attention to what you are saying.

Some patients—particularly children—may be unable to verbalize their feelings of fear and anxiety. Watch for signs of anxiety. They may include a tense appearance, increased blood pressure and rates of breathing and pulse, sweaty palms, reported problems with sleep or appetite, irritability, and agitation. Procedure 4-1 will help you communicate with patients who are anxious.

The Angry Patient

In a medical setting, anger may occur for many reasons. Anger may be a mask for fear about an illness or the outcome of surgery. Anger may come from a patient's feeling of being treated unfairly or without compassion. Anger may stem from a patient's resentment about being ill or injured. Anger may be a reaction to frustration, rejection, disappointment, feelings of loss of control or self-esteem, or invasion of privacy.

As a medical assistant, you will encounter angry patients and will need to help them express their anger constructively, for the sake of their health. At the same time, you must learn not to take expressions of anger personally; you may just be the unlucky target. A goal with angry patients is to help them refocus emotional energy toward solving the problem. Study the following steps in communicating with an angry patient.

1. Learn to recognize anger and its causes. Anger is easy to recognize in most people, but it can be subtle in others. Patients who speak in a tense tone, are stubborn, or appear to ignore your attempts at communication may be angry.

2. Remain calm and continue to demonstrate genuineness and respect. Communicate that you respect and care about the patient's feelings.

3. Focus on the patient's physical and medical needs.

4. Maintain adequate personal space. Place yourself on the same level as the patient. If the patient is standing, encourage him to sit down. Maintain an open posture to show that you are receptive to listening. Maintain eye contact, but avoid staring at the patient, which can make the person angrier.

5. Avoid the feeling that you need to defend yourself or to give reasons why the patient should not be angry. Instead, listen attentively and with an open mind to what the patient is saying. Most patients' anger will lessen if they know someone is really listening to them and showing an interest in their emotions and needs.

6. Encourage patients to be specific in describing the cause of their anger, their thoughts about it, and their feelings. Be empathic and acknowledge the patient's feelings and perceptions. Follow through with any promises you might make concerning correction of a problem, but avoid totally agreeing or disagreeing with the patient. State what you can and cannot do for the patient.

7. Present your point of view calmly and firmly to help the patient better understand the situation. If patients are receptive to your viewpoint, their perspective may change for the better.

8. Avoid a breakdown in communication. Allow the patient to voice anger. Trying to outtalk the patient or overexplain will only annoy and irritate him. You might also suggest that the patient spend a few moments alone to gather his thoughts or to cool off before continuing any type of communication.

9. If you feel threatened by a patient's anger or if it looks as if the patient's anger may become violent, leave the room and seek assistance from one of the physicians or other members of the office staff. Document any threats in the patient's chart.

Patients of Other Cultures

Our beliefs, attitudes, values, use of language, and views of the world are unique to us, but they are also shaped by our cultural background. In any health-care setting, you will most likely have contact with patients of diverse cultures and ethnic groups. Each culture and ethnic group has its own behaviors, traditions, and values. Rather than viewing these differences as barriers to communication, strive to understand and be tolerant of them.

Remember that these beliefs are neither superior nor inferior to your own. They are simply different. Never allow yourself to make value judgments or to stereotype a patient, a culture, or an ethnic group. Each patient is an individual in her own right.

Different Views and Perceptions. It is common for patients in many cultures to view health-care professionals as superior to themselves intellectually, socially, and economically. Patients from minority ethnic groups may feel that health-care professionals of the majority ethnic group cannot understand them or identify with them. In some cases, unfortunately, they may be right. The professional's attitude of superiority may stem from the feeling that because she knows more about medical issues than the patient does, she is somehow more important than the patient.

PROCEDURE 4.1

Communicating With the Anxious Patient

Objective: To use communication and interpersonal skills to calm an anxious patient

Materials: None

Method

1. Identify signs of anxiety in the patient.
2. Acknowledge the patient's anxiety. (Ignoring a patient's anxiety often makes it worse.)
3. Identify possible sources of anxiety, such as fear of a procedure or test result, along with supportive resources available to the patient, such as family members and friends. Understanding the source of anxiety in a patient and identifying the supportive resources available can help you communicate with the patient more effectively.
4. Do what you can to alleviate the patient's physical discomfort. For example, find a calm, quiet place for the patient to wait, a comfortable chair, a drink of water, or access to the bathroom (Figure 4-3).
5. Allow ample personal space for conversation. Note: You would normally allow a 1½- to 4-ft distance between yourself and the patient. Adjust this space as necessary.
6. Create a climate of warmth, acceptance, and trust.
   a. Recognize and control your own anxiety. Your air of calm can decrease the patient's anxiety.
   b. Provide reassurance by demonstrating genuine care, respect, and empathy.
   c. Act confidently and dependably, maintaining truthfulness and confidentiality at all times.
7. Using the appropriate communication skills, have the patient describe the experience that is causing anxiety, her thoughts about it, and her feelings. Proceeding in this order allows the patient to describe what is causing the anxiety and to clarify her thoughts and feelings about it.
   a. Maintain an open posture.
   b. Maintain eye contact, if culturally appropriate.
   c. Use active listening skills.
   d. Listen without interrupting.
8. Do not belittle the patient's thoughts and feelings. This can cause a breakdown in communication, increase anxiety, and make the patient feel isolated.
9. Be empathic to the patient's concerns.
10. Help the patient recognize and cope with the anxiety.
    a. Provide information to the patient. Patients are often fearful of the unknown. Helping them understand their disease or the procedure they are about to undergo will help decrease their anxiety.
    b. Suggest coping behaviors, such as deep breathing or other relaxation exercises.
11. Notify the doctor of the patient's concerns.

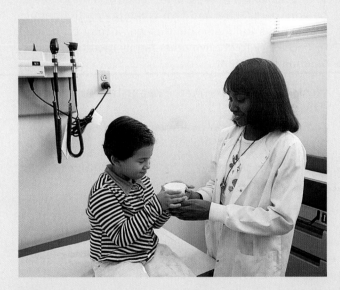

Figure 4-3. You can calm children's anxiety by spending time talking with them, playing a game, reading a story, or just offering a glass of water.

Do your best to treat patients of all cultures and ethnic groups with equal respect. Effective communication cannot take place unless you respect the patient's dignity and maintain the patient's sense of self-worth.

Maintaining an open mind will help you see and understand differences in cultural perceptions to which you must be sensitive. For example, patients may have different views of their role and the role of their families in the

Multicultural Attitudes About Modern Medicine

Patients' cultural backgrounds have a great effect on their attitudes toward health and illness. Patients from different cultural backgrounds often have beliefs about the causes of illness, what symptoms mean, and what to expect from health-care professionals that are different from those of modern medicine. Understanding some of these perceptions, behaviors, and expectations will help you communicate effectively with patients of different cultures.

Beliefs About Causes of Illness

Some cultures have beliefs about the causes of illness that differ sharply from accepted notions in the mainstream culture. As an example, many cultures believe that some illnesses are caused by hot or cold forces in the body. Some believe that winds and drafts cause illness or that illness can be caused by blood that is too thick or too thin. Others believe that having bad feelings toward others can create ill health.

Because of such beliefs, it may be hard to obtain information from patients about possible reasons for their medical problems. It may also be hard for some patients to realize the importance of taking medication to treat certain illnesses. In this case, you may have to be very persuasive and firm when giving the patient instructions for medication usage. It may be helpful or necessary to involve other family members in persuading the patient.

How Symptoms Are Presented and What They Mean

People from different cultures may differ in the way they perceive and report symptoms. Some may express pain very emotionally because their culture may feel that suppressing pain is harmful. In contrast, people from other cultures may not admit that they are in pain, thinking that acknowledging pain is a sign of weakness. People of all cultures may be more likely to report physical symptoms of illness than they are to report psychologic symptoms. Be aware of nonverbal indications of pain or other symptoms.

Treatment Expectations

Patients from other cultures may be totally unaccustomed to some of the practices of modern medicine. Patients of certain ethnic or cultural groups often consult other types of healers before seeing a doctor. They are likely to have different expectations of treatment from each.

Patients from other cultures may be wary of certain treatments because these treatments are so different from what they are accustomed to. This is especially true of some of the medical procedures and interventions considered to be state-of-the-art, such as laser surgery or diabetes management.

When dealing with patients of other cultures, keep in mind their perspectives on health care. Try to avoid generalizations and cultural stereotyping, however, because there can be a variation of attitudes within ethnic groups. Treat each patient as an individual, and you will be providing the best care possible.

---

health-care process. They may view the roles of men and women differently than you do. Patients may also have different views of the cause of their illness and how it should be treated. "Caution: Handle With Care" discusses different cultural views of health care.

The Language Barrier. Patients who cannot speak or understand English may have difficulty expressing their needs or feelings effectively. You may need to speak through an interpreter to gather and convey information or to discuss sensitive issues with a patient. Instead of using medical terms, which can be difficult to translate, try to say the same thing using basic, familiar words and simple phrases.

If the patient comes to the office often, take the time to learn some basic phrases in the patient's native language, such as "How are you feeling today?" and "Is there anything I can get you?" Even if the rest of your conversation must take place in English, your small efforts will be much appreciated.

The Patient With a Visual Impairment

When communicating with a patient who has a visual impairment, be aware of what you say and how you say it. Since people with visual impairments cannot usually rely on nonverbal clues, your tone of voice, inflection, and speech volume take on greater importance.

Following are some suggestions for communicating with a patient who has a visual impairment.

- Use large-print materials whenever possible.
- Make sure there is adequate lighting in all patient areas.
- Use a normal speaking voice.
- Talk directly and honestly. Explain instructions thoroughly.
- Do not talk down to the patient; preserve the patient's dignity.

The Patient With a Hearing Impairment

Hearing loss can range from mild to severe. How you communicate depends on the degree of impairment and on whether the patient has effective use of a hearing aid.

Following are some tips to help you communicate effectively with a hearing-impaired patient.

- Find a quiet area to talk, and try to minimize background noise.
- Position yourself close to and facing the patient. The patient will rely on visual clues such as the movement of your lips and mouth, your facial expression, and your body language (Figure 4-4).
- Speak slowly, so the patient can follow what you are saying.
- Remember that elderly patients lose the ability to hear high-pitched sounds first. Try speaking in lower tones.
- Speak in a clear, firm voice, but do not shout, especially if the patient wears a hearing aid.
- To verify understanding, ask questions that will encourage the patient to repeat what you said.
- Whenever possible, use written materials to reinforce verbal information.

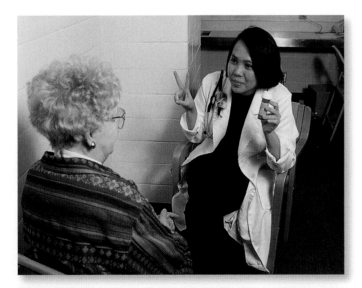

Figure 4-4. When communicating with a patient who has a hearing impairment, position yourself close to the patient and use gestures and effective body language.

The Patient Who Is Mentally or Emotionally Disturbed

There may be times when you will need to communicate with patients who are mentally or emotionally disturbed. When dealing with this type of patient, you need to determine what level of communication the patient can understand. Keep these suggestions in mind to improve communication.

- It is important to remain calm if the patient becomes agitated or confused.
- Avoid raising your voice or appearing impatient.
- If you do not understand, ask the patient to repeat what he said.

The Elderly Patient

Medical assistants now spend at least 50% of their time caring for older patients. Be aware of the vast differences in the capabilities of people of this age group. Do not stereotype all elderly patients as frail or confused. Most are not, and each patient deserves to be treated according to her own individual abilities.

Always treat elderly patients with respect. Regardless of their physical or mental state, elderly patients are adults. Do not talk down to them. Use the title "Mrs." or "Mr." to address older people unless they ask you to call them by their first name.

Denial or Confusion.   Some elderly patients deny that they are ill. For example, in a survey of elderly people, the majority of whom had at least one chronic condition, 85% reported that they were in good or excellent health (Bradley and Edinberg, 1990). Patients' perception of how they feel may be quite different from their actual state of health.

The reverse situation can also occur. Elderly patients may overreact to a problem and consider themselves sicker than they really are. They may become dependent, passive, or anxious. Elderly patients may also over- or underestimate their ability to perform certain tasks or to deal with certain limitations.

Elderly patients may be confused if they have some impairment in memory, judgment, or other mental abilities. Signs of confusion can occur with Alzheimer's disease, senility, depression, head injury, or misuse of medications or alcohol. Elderly patients may or may not be aware of their condition. They may have difficulty understanding instructions.

The following tips can help you communicate with elderly patients.

- Act as if you expect the patient to understand.
- Respond calmly to any confusion on the patient's part. Tell the truth. Use facts. Do not go along with misconceptions or make up explanations.
- Use simple questions and terms, but avoid using baby talk or speaking to the patient as if he were a child.

- Explain points slowly and clearly, using concrete terms rather than abstract expressions. Say, for example, "You may feel a pinprick and a sting when I put the needle in" instead of "You may feel some discomfort in your arm."
- Ask the patient to relax and speak slowly.
- If you do not understand the patient, simply say that you cannot understand her well and ask her to repeat what she said. Do not say you understand when in fact you do not. It is important not to belittle the patient. It is equally important to inform yourself about what could be very important information.

The Importance of Touch. Because they often live alone, many elderly patients experience a lack of physical touch. Using touch—offering to hold a patient's hand or placing an arm around his shoulder—communicates that you care about the patient's well-being.

Terminally Ill Patients

Terminally ill patients are often under extreme stress and can be a challenge to treat. It is important that health-care professionals respect the rights of terminal patients and treat them with dignity. It is also important that you communicate with the family and offer support and empathy as their loved one accepts her condition. You should also provide information on **hospice,** which is an area of medicine that works with terminally ill patients and their families. Hospice workers often go to the home of the terminally ill patient or work with patients in facilities. Hospice care is usually staffed with RNs who have specialized training in issues related to death and dying. They work with the family and patient in the beginning, assisting with medications, and they end by making arrangements with the funeral home and coroner.

Elisabeth Kübler-Ross, a world-renowned authority in the areas of death and dying, developed a model of behavior that patients will experience on learning their condition. This is called the Stages of Dying or Stages of Grief. This model is widely used today in work with terminally ill patients.

Kübler-Ross's Stages of Dying include five stages, which usually—but not always—progress in the following order:

1. Denial. Patients are in direct denial or periods of disbelief. This defense is generally temporary.
2. Anger. Patients may suddenly realize what is really happening and respond with anger. They can become difficult patients in this stage and display temper tantrums and fits of rage.
3. Bargaining. Patients attempt to make deals with physicians, clergy, and family members. Patients at this stage may become more cooperative and congenial.
4. Depression. The patient will begin to show signs of depression, such as withdrawal, lethargy, and sobbing.

The patient's body is beginning to deteriorate, and the patient may experience more pain and realize that relationships with family and friends will soon be gone.

5. Acceptance. Patients accept the fact that they are dying. They will begin arrangements for when they expire, making funeral or burial requests. The patient's family needs the most support at this stage.

Even though these stages have been generalized to dying, many experts have applied them to the grieving process as well.

The Young Patient

A doctor's office can be a frightening place for children. They often associate the doctor's office with getting a shot or being sick. Sometimes parents have misled their children about what to expect from a visit to the doctor. When dealing with children, it is better to recognize and accept their fear and anxiety than to dismiss these emotions. When children realize that you take their feelings seriously, they are more apt to be receptive to your requests and suggestions.

Explain any procedure, no matter how basic (such as testing a reflex with a reflex hammer), in very simple terms. Let the child examine the instrument.

Other suggestions include using praise ("You were very brave") and always being truthful. Do not tell children that a procedure will not hurt if it will, or you will lose their trust.

As children get older, you can use more detailed descriptions when explaining procedures. Remember that after the age of 7 or 8, children can tell if they are being talked down to or treated like babies. Encourage them to participate actively in their care, and direct any questions or instructions to them, when appropriate. You should also respect the adolescent's request not to have a parent present during private conversations.

Parents

Parents are naturally concerned about their children and are likely to be worried or anxious when a child is ill. Children often react to a situation based on how they see their parents react. Reassuring parents and keeping them calm can also help children relax.

The Patient With AIDS and the Patient Who Is HIV-Positive

Patients with acquired immunodeficiency syndrome (AIDS) and patients who have the human immunodeficiency virus (HIV), the virus that causes AIDS, have a grave illness to deal with. They also face a society that often stigmatizes them, saying they have only themselves to blame. These patients often feel guilty, angry, and depressed. Many literally hate themselves.

To communicate effectively with these patients, you need accurate information about the disease and the risks involved. Take the initiative to educate yourself about AIDS and HIV. Patients will have many questions. Part of your role as a good communicator will be to answer as many questions as you can. If a patient asks a question you cannot answer, tell the physician, so he can respond quickly.

Above all, remember that HIV is not transmitted through casual or common physical contact, such as brushing by a person in a crowded hall or shaking hands. It is transferred only through bodily fluids. Patients with AIDS and those who are HIV-positive need to know you are not afraid to be near them, to touch them, or to talk to them. Like any patient whose body is being ravaged by a serious illness, these patients need human contact (verbal and physical), and they need to be treated with dignity.

Patients' Families and Friends

Family members or friends sometimes accompany a patient to the office. These individuals can provide important emotional support to the patient. Always ask patients if they want a family member or friend to accompany them to the examination room, however. Do not just assume their preference. Acknowledge family members and friends, and communicate with them as you do with patients. They should be kept informed of the patient's progress, whenever possible, to avoid unnecessary anxiety on their part. You must always protect patient confidentiality, however. Too often, health-care workers think that it is acceptable to discuss patient cases in detail with family members, even without the consent of the patient.

Communicating With Coworkers

The quality of the communication you have with coworkers greatly influences the development of a positive or negative work climate and a team approach to patient care. In turn, the workplace atmosphere ultimately affects your communication with patients.

Positive Communication With Coworkers

In your interactions with coworkers, use the same skills and qualities that you use to communicate with patients. Have respect and empathy; be caring, thoughtful, and genuine; and use active listening skills. These skills will help you develop **rapport,** which is a harmonious, positive relationship, with your coworkers (Figure 4-5).

Following are some rules for communication in the medical office.

- Use proper channels of communication. For example, if you are having problems getting along with a coworker, try first to work it out with her. Do not go

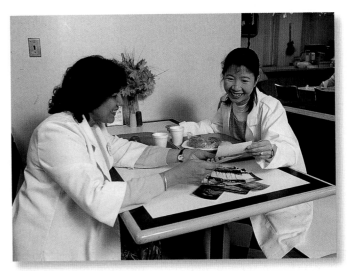

Figure 4-5. Rapport with coworkers is easy to build when you are open, friendly, and thoughtful.

over her head and complain to her supervisor. Your coworker may not have realized the effect of her behavior and may wish to correct it without involving her supervisor. If you go to the supervisor right away, working relationships can become even more strained.

- Have the proper attitude. You can avoid conflict and resolve most problems if you maintain a positive attitude. A friendly approach is much more effective than a hostile approach. Remember that many problems are simply the result of misinformation or lack of communication.

- Plan an appropriate time for communication. If you have something important to discuss, schedule a time to do so. For example, if you want to talk with the office manager about renewing the lease of a piece of office equipment, tell him you would like to discuss that topic and ask him to let you know a time that is convenient.

As an example of good communication with coworkers, consider this exchange between Mai Lee, a medical assistant, and Margot, a coworker in a pediatric practice. Note the way Mai Lee demonstrates assertiveness.

Mai Lee: I know you spent a lot of time choosing the new toys for the reception area. I love the wooden safari animal puzzles.

Margot: Thanks. I think the children really enjoy themselves now.

Mai Lee: I wanted to mention to you, though, that I'm concerned about the toy tea set with miniature cupcakes and sandwiches. Anything that's smaller than a golf ball is a choking hazard to infants and toddlers.

Margot: I don't think the little ones pay much attention to the tea set. It's mostly for older kids.

Mai Lee: Yes, but I'm still afraid that a baby could put one of those pieces in his mouth. What if we put up a little shelf in the play area that is low enough for kids 4 years old or more to reach but high enough to be out of reach of the babies. We could put the tea set on it in a clear plastic box and any other toys with small parts.

Margot: I see your point. Sounds like a good idea to me.

Mai Lee started with a statement that acknowledged the coworker's situation and feelings. Then she stated her own opinion. When her coworker disagreed, she repeated her concern, describing what might happen if the situation remained unchanged. Then she made a constructive suggestion for solving the problem without hurting the coworker's feelings. As you interact with coworkers, be sensitive to the timing of your conversations, the manner in which you present your ideas and thoughts, and your coworkers' feelings.

Communicating With Superiors

Positive or negative communication can affect the quality of your relationships with superiors. For example, problems arise when communication about job responsibilities is unclear or when you feel that one of your superiors does not trust or respect you, or vice versa.

Consider these suggestions when communicating with superiors.

- Keep superiors informed. If the office copier is not working properly, talk to your supervisor about it before a breakdown occurs that will hold everyone up. If several patients express the same types of complaint about the examination rooms, make sure the right people are told. If the doctor asks you to call a patient and you reach the patient, tell the doctor.

- Ask questions. If you are unsure about an administrative task or the meaning of a medical term, for example, do not hesitate to ask a superior. It is better to ask a question before acting than to make a mistake. It is also better to ask than to risk annoying someone because you carried out a task or wrote a term incorrectly. Asking questions of superiors means that you respect them professionally.

- Minimize interruptions. For example, before launching into a discussion, make sure the superior you are talking to has time to talk. Opening with "Can I interrupt you for a moment, or should I come back?" or "Do you have a minute to talk?" goes a long way toward establishing good communication. It is also better to go to your supervisor when you have several questions to ask rather than to interrupt her repeatedly.

- Show initiative. Any superior will greatly appreciate this quality. For example, if you think you can come up with a more efficient way to get the office newsletter written and distributed, write out a plan and show it to your supervisor. He is likely to welcome any ideas that improve office efficiency or patient satisfaction.

Dealing With Conflict

Conflict, or friction, in the workplace can result from opposition of opinions or ideas or even from a difference in personalities. Conflict can arise when the lines of communication break down or when a misunderstanding occurs. Conflict can also result from prejudices or preconceived notions about people or from lack of mutual respect or trust between a staff member and a superior. Whatever the cause, conflict is counterproductive to the efficiency of an office.

Following these suggestions can help prevent conflict in the office and improve communication among coworkers.

- Do not "feed into" other people's negative attitudes. For example, if a coworker is criticizing one of the doctors, change the subject.

- Try your best at all times to be personable and supportive of coworkers. For example, everyone has bad days. If a coworker is having a bad day, offer to pitch in and help or to run out and get her lunch if she is too busy to go out.

- Refrain from passing judgment on others or stereotyping them (women are bad at math, men don't know how to communicate, and so on). Coworkers should show respect for one another and try to be tolerant and nonjudgmental.

- Do not gossip. You are there to work. Act professionally at all times.

- Do not jump to conclusions. For example, if you get a memo about a change in your schedule that disturbs you, bring your concern to your supervisor. She may be able to be flexible on certain points. You do not know until you ask.

Managing Stress

Stress can be a barrier to communication. For example, if you are feeling very pressured at work, you might snap at a coworker or patient, or you might forget to give the physician an important message.

Professionals in the health-care field may experience high levels of stress in their daily work environment. Stress can result from a feeling of being under pressure, or it can be a reaction to anger, frustration, or a change in your routine. Stress can increase your blood pressure, speed up your breathing and heart rate, and cause muscle tension. To minimize stress—for the sake of your health as well as for good communication in the office—it is helpful to understand some basic information about stress.

Stress—Good or Bad?

A certain amount of stress is normal. A little bit of stress—the kind that makes you feel excited or challenged by the task at hand—can motivate you to get things done and push you toward a higher level of productivity. Ongoing

Potential Causes of Stress

- Death of a spouse or family member
- Divorce or separation
- Hospitalization (yours or a family member's) due to injury or illness
- Marriage or reconciliation from a separation
- Loss of a job or retirement
- Sexual problems
- Having a new baby
- Significant change in your financial status (for better or worse)
- Job change
- Children leaving or returning home
- Significant personal success, such as a promotion at work
- Moving or remodeling your home
- Problems at work, such as your boss's retiring, that may put your job at risk
- Substantial debt, such as a mortgage or overspending on credit cards

Figure 4-6. Be aware of the common causes of stress. Find stress-reducing techniques that work for you.

Tips for Reducing Stress

- Maintain a healthy balance in your life among work, family, and leisure activities.
- Exercise regularly.
- Eat balanced, nutritious meals and healthful snacks. Avoid foods high in caffeine, salt, sugar, and fat.
- Get enough sleep.
- Allow time for yourself, and plan time to relax.
- Rely on the support that family, friends, and coworkers have to offer. Don't be afraid to share your feelings.
- Try to be realistic about what you can and cannot do. Do not be afraid to admit that you cannot take on another responsibility.
- Try to set realistic goals for yourself.
- Remember that there are always choices, even when there appear to be none.
- Be organized. Good planning can help you manage your workload.
- Redirect excess energy constructively—clean your closet, work in the garden, do volunteer work, have friends over for dinner, exercise.
- Change some of the things you have control over.
- Keep yourself focused. Focus your full energy on one thing at a time, and finish one project before starting another.
- Identify sources of conflict, and try to resolve them.
- Learn and use relaxation techniques, such as deep breathing, meditation, or imagining yourself in a quiet, peaceful place. Choose what works for you.
- Maintain a healthy sense of humor. Laughter can help relieve stress. Joke with friends after work. Go see a funny movie.
- Try not to overreact. Ask yourself if a situation is really worth getting upset or worried about.
- Seek help from social or professional support groups, if necessary.

Figure 4-7. These tips will help you avoid and reduce stress in your professional and personal life.

stress, however, can be overwhelming and affect you physically. For example, it can lower your resistance to colds and increase your risk for developing heart disease, diabetes, high blood pressure, ulcers, allergies, asthma, colitis, cancer, and certain autoimmune diseases, which cause the body's immune system to attack normal tissue. Figure 4-6 shows the potential causes of stress.

Reducing Stress

Some stress at work is inevitable. An important goal is to learn how to manage or reduce stress. Take into account your strengths and limitations, and be realistic about how much you can handle at work and in your life outside work. Pushing yourself a certain amount can be motivating.

Pushing yourself too much is dangerous. Review Figure 4-7 for tips on reducing stress.

Preventing Burnout

Burnout is the end result of prolonged periods of stress without relief. Burnout is an energy-depleting condition that will affect your health and career. Certain personality types are more prone to burnout than others. If you are a highly driven, perfectionist-type person, you will be more susceptible to burnout. Experts often refer to such a person as a characteristic Type A personality. A more relaxed, calm, laid-back individual is considered a Type B person. Type B personalities are less prone to burnout but have the potential to suffer from it, especially if they work in health care.

According to some experts on stress, there are five stages that lead to burnout (Miller and Smith). The road to burnout follows this path:

1. The Honeymoon Phase. During the honeymoon phase, your job is wonderful. You have boundless energy and enthusiasm, and all things seem possible. You love the job and the job loves you. You believe it will satisfy all your needs and desires and solve all your problems. You are delighted with your job, your coworkers, and the organization.

2. The Awakening Phase. The honeymoon wanes and the awakening stage starts with the realization that your initial expectations were unrealistic. The job isn't working out the way you thought it would. It doesn't satisfy all your needs, your coworkers and the organization are less than perfect, and rewards and recognition are scarce.

   As disillusionment and disappointment grow, you become confused. Something is wrong, but you can't quite put your finger on it. Typically, you work harder to make your dreams come true. But working harder doesn't change anything and you become increasingly tired, bored, and frustrated. You question your competence and ability, and start losing your self-confidence.

3. Brownout Phase. As brownout begins, your early enthusiasm and energy give way to chronic fatigue and irritability. Your eating and sleeping patterns change, and you indulge in escapist behaviors such as partying, recreational drugs, alcoholism, and binge shopping. You become indecisive and your productivity drops. Your work deteriorates. Coworkers and superiors may comment on it.

   Unless interrupted, brownout slides into later stages. You become increasingly frustrated and angry and project the blame for your difficulties onto others. You are cynical, detached, and openly critical of the organization, superiors, and coworkers. You are beset with depression, anxiety, and physical illness.

4. Full-Scale Burnout Phase. Unless you wake up and interrupt the process or someone intervenes, brownout drifts remorselessly into full-scale burnout. Despair is the dominant feature of this final stage. It may take several months to get to this phase, but in most cases it takes three to four years. You experience an overwhelming sense of failure and a devastating loss of self-esteem and self-confidence. You become depressed and feel lonely and empty.

   Life seems pointless, and there is a paralyzing, "what's the use" pessimism about the future. You talk about "just quitting and getting away." You are exhausted physically and mentally. Physical and mental breakdowns are likely. Suicide, stroke, or heart attack is not unusual as you complete the final stage of what all started with such high hopes, energy, optimism, and enthusiasm.

5. The Phoenix Phenomenon. You can arise from the ashes of burnout (like a phoenix), but it takes time.

First, you need to rest and relax. Don't take work home. If you're like many people, the work won't get done and you'll only feel guilty for being "lazy."

Second, be realistic in your job expectations as well as your aspirations and goals. Whoever you're talking to about your feelings can help you, but be careful. Your readjusted aspirations and goals must be yours and not those of someone else. Trying to be and do what someone else wants you to be or do is a sure-fire recipe for continued frustration and burnout.

Third, create balance in your life. Invest more of yourself in family and other personal relationships, social activities, and hobbies. Spread yourself out so that your job doesn't have such an overpowering influence on your self-esteem and self-confidence.

The Policy and Procedures Manual

The policy and procedures manual is a key written communication tool in the medical office. No discussion of communication in the medical office would be complete without a description of this important document. The manual is used by permanent employees as well as by temporary employees who may be hired when others are ill or on vacation or when there is an unusually heavy workload. The manual covers all office policies and clinical procedures. It is usually developed as a joint effort by the physician (or physicians) and the staff (often the medical assistant).

Policies

Policies are rules or guidelines that dictate the day-to-day workings of an office. Although individual policies vary from office to office, most medical office manuals describe the following policy areas:

- Office purposes, objectives, and goals as set down by the physician(s)
- Rules and regulations
- Job descriptions and duties of staff personnel
- Office hours
- Dress code
- Insurance and other benefits
- Vacation, sick leave, and other time away from the office
- Salary and performance evaluations
- Maintenance of equipment and supplies
- Mailings
- Bookkeeping
- Scheduling of appointments and maintenance of patient records
- OSHA guidelines

The policy section of the manual also typically describes the chain of command for the office, or the person to whom each employee reports. This information is sometimes presented in chart form and called an organizational chart. For example, the receptionist, secretary, medical assistant, and billing person might report to the office manager. The office manager, in turn, might report directly to the physician or physicians. This chain of command varies from office to office, depending on the size and needs of the practice.

Procedures

Detailed instructions for specific procedures are covered in the procedures section of the manual. The areas discussed include clinical procedures and quality assurance programs.

Each clinical procedure should include instructions about the following:

- Purpose of the test, clinical application, and usefulness
- Specimen required and collection method; special patient preparation or restrictions
- Reagents, standards, controls, and media used; special supplies
- Instrumentation, including calibration and schedules
- Step-by-step directions
- Calculations
- Frequency and tolerance of controls; corrective action to be taken if tolerances are exceeded
- Expected values; values requiring special notification; interpretation of values

- Procedure notes (e.g., linearity or detection limits)
- Limitations of method (e.g., interfering substances and/or pitfalls and precautions)
- Method validation
- References
- Effective date and schedule for review
- Distribution

Developing a Manual

Although it is likely that your office will already have a manual, you may be involved in reorganizing, producing, or updating the manual. In any event, it is important to understand how a manual is developed.

Planning. To begin planning a manual, first determine a format, or how you will organize the information. The format depends on the office's needs and organization. Many offices prefer a loose-leaf notebook in which pages can easily be replaced when changes or updates are necessary. Figure 4-8 shows a sample page from a manual.

After determining a format, create an outline, organizing the topics and subtopics. Have it approved by the office manager and physician or physicians. In the procedures section, begin each procedure sheet on a new page. Include the following for each procedure page:

- The style to be used for each procedure, whether quantitative or qualitative

---

MILLSTONE MEDICAL ASSOCIATES

Policy and Procedures Manual

Procedure for Creating a Medical File for a New Patient

GOAL: To create a complete medical record for each new patient containing all necessary personal and medical information

PROCEDURE:
1. Establish that the patient is new to the doctor's office.
2. Ask the patient for all necessary insurance information. If the patient has an insurance card, make a photocopy of it for his file.
3. Ask the patient to fill out the patient information form. Keyboard the information onto a new patient information form, for legibility.
4. Review all information with the patient, to check for accuracy.
5. Label the new patient's folder, according to office procedure. Type either the patient's name (for an alphabetic file) or the correct number (for a numerical file).
6. If filing is done numerically, fill out a cross-reference form on the computer, along with a patient ID card to be stored in a secure location.
7. Add the patient's name to the necessary financial records, including the office ledger, whether on paper or on the computer.
8. After completing the folder label information, place the new patient information form inside the folder, along with any other personal or medical information that pertains to the patient.
9. On the outside of the patient's folder, clip a routing slip.

Figure 4-8. This page from a policy and procedures manual provides the office staff with information about creating a medical file for a new patient.

- The month and year the procedure was adopted
- The page number and total number of pages for that procedure
- A cover sheet for noting changes, additions, or corrections to the procedure, including whether the procedure replaces an earlier one
- The name of the writer and the name of the physician who approved the text of the procedure

Developing and Updating Material. Sources you may refer to for developing or updating the manual might include scientific or medical journals, manufacturer product literature, textbooks, standards publications, research and validation data, and written personal communications.

For more information on the design, development, and use of technical procedure manuals, contact the National Committee for Clinical Laboratory Standards (NCCLS) in Wayne, Pennsylvania.

Summary

As a medical assistant, you are a key communicator between the office and patients and families. The way you greet patients, the way you explain procedures, the manner in which you ask and answer questions, and your attentiveness to patients' individual needs combine to form your communication style. Effective communication skills—which include listening, interpersonal, and assertiveness skills—will help you improve your communication style. These skills will also enable you to develop good communication with patients under special circumstances. Patients with special needs include those who are anxious or angry, elderly, or from other cultures and those who have hearing or visual impairments.

Good communication skills also enable you to develop satisfying and professional working relationships with coworkers and superiors. Effective communication helps the office function smoothly, helps reduce conflicts and stress, and helps motivate individuals to achieve personal and professional goals.

An important communication document in the medical office is the policy and procedures manual. This manual covers all office policies and clinical procedures and is usually developed as a joint effort by the doctor (or doctors) and the staff (often the medical assistant).

CASE STUDY QUESTIONS

Now that you have completed this chapter, review the case study at the beginning of the chapter and answer the following questions:

1. How will Mary adapt her communication style to communicate with each patient?
2. What types of communication roadblocks will she encounter with each one?
3. What types of communication techniques will she use for each patient?

Discussion Questions

1. Discuss the difference between verbal and nonverbal communication. Give examples of each.
2. Name two interpersonal skills. Give an example of how you can demonstrate each skill.
3. Suggest some of the communication problems that can arise with patients from other cultures. How might you deal with these problems?
4. Discuss defense mechanisms and apply them to everyday communication with friends, family, and classmates.

Critical Thinking Questions

1. You are with a patient who is anxious about having her blood drawn. What specific steps would you take to address her anxiety, and what would you say to her at each step to prepare her for the procedure?
2. You would like to learn more about the financial aspect of the facility you are working in. Your office manager always appears to be busy, and you are uncomfortable approaching her with this idea. How would you communicate with her your willingness to learn another aspect of the office?
3. You notice that you have not been feeling well lately, and you suspect that it is job-related stress. What kinds of activities can you take part in to help reduce stress and prevent job burnout?

Application Activities

1. With a partner, practice your communication skills by assuming the roles of a medical assistant and a patient who is angry after having to wait for an hour in the office waiting room.
2. With a partner or group, take turns using body language to indicate a variety of emotions, and see if the others can correctly guess what message you are sending.
3. With a group of classmates, create an outline for an office policy and procedures manual. Identify sections that might need updating on an ongoing basis and why the updating might be necessary.
4. With a partner, take turns being blindfolded and communicate a list of activities each of you wants the other person to do. For example:
   - walk to the bathroom
   - purchase a candy bar out of the vending machine
   - find the light switch
   - turn on a computer

This activity will teach you how to communicate with someone who depends on you and allows the partner to feel what it is like to depend on someone.

PART Two

Administrative Medical Assisting

"In my 15 years as a medical assistant and transcriptionist in a large cardiology practice, I have gained invaluable experience that enhances the care of our patients. Cardiology patients require complex care. State-of-the-art equipment, pleasant office surroundings, and a well-educated, warm, and caring staff are key elements in helping patients feel at ease. As I work with patients, I do everything I can to help them feel comfortable in the office. Using reassuring words and good listening skills helps them overcome the anxieties they may have about their illness or a test they are about to have performed.

"Administrative duties are as important as clinical duties. For example, make sure the medical transcription work space is quiet and comfortable. Transcription requires intense concentration to ensure accuracy. Accuracy in all administrative tasks contributes to the success of each patient's treatment plan."

Kaye H. Listug
Medical Assistant, La Mesa, California

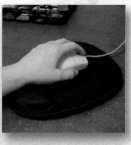

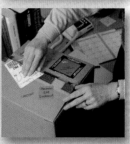

SECTION ONE
Office Work

Chapter 5 Using and Maintaining Office Equipment
Chapter 6 Using Computers in the Office
Chapter 7 Managing Correspondence and Mail
Chapter 8 Managing Office Supplies
Chapter 9 Maintaining Patient Records
Chapter 10 Managing the Office Medical Records

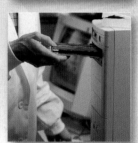

SECTION TWO
Interacting With Patients

Chapter 11 Telephone Techniques
Chapter 12 Scheduling Appointments and Maintaining the Physician's Schedule
Chapter 13 Patient Reception Area
Chapter 14 Patient Education

SECTION THREE
Financial Responsibilities

Chapter 15 Processing Health-Care Claims
Chapter 16 Medical Coding
Chapter 17 Patient Billing and Collections
Chapter 18 Accounting for the Medical Office

SECTION 1

OFFICE WORK

CHAPTER 5
Using and Maintaining Office Equipment

CHAPTER 6
Using Computers in the Office

CHAPTER 7
Managing Correspondence and Mail

CHAPTER 8
Managing Office Supplies

CHAPTER 9
Maintaining Patient Records

CHAPTER 10
Managing the Office Medical Records

Using and Maintaining Office Equipment

AREAS OF COMPETENCE

2003 Role Delineation Study

ADMINISTRATIVE

Administrative Procedures

- Perform basic administrative medical assisting functions

GENERAL

Operational Functions

- Perform inventory of office supplies and equipment
- Perform routine maintenance of administrative and clinical equipment

KEY TERMS

cover sheet

disclaimer

interactive pager

lease

maintenance contract

microfiche

microfilm

service contract

troubleshooting

voice mail

warranty

CHAPTER OUTLINE

- Office Communication Equipment
- Office Automation Equipment
- Purchasing Decisions
- Maintaining Office Equipment

OBJECTIVES

After completing Chapter 5, you will be able to:

5.1 Describe the types of office equipment used in a medical practice.

5.2 Explain how each piece of office equipment is used.

5.3 List the steps in making purchasing decisions for office equipment.

5.4 Compare and contrast leasing and buying.

5.5 Describe a warranty, a maintenance contract, and a service contract, and discuss the importance of each.

5.6 Identify when troubleshooting is appropriate and what actions may be taken.

5.7 List the information included in an equipment inventory.

Introduction

The medical office of today requires many different types of clerical equipment in order to function effectively and smoothly. The role of the medical assistant includes learning how to evaluate, purchase or lease, operate, and maintain this essential equipment.

Think how difficult it would be to communicate with others outside the office without the use of a communication system, which could include telephones, e-mail, beepers or pagers, answering machines, and fax machines. How limited would a medical practice become if the recording of the care given to a patient had to done *without* the use of a word processor, computer, or typewriter? What if all patient billing, bank deposits, and payroll management had to be done *without* the use of an adding machine or calculator? Without a shredder, each piece of confidential paper would have to be torn many times before discarding. Possibly the most difficult of all tasks would be the duplication of endless documents by hand because there is no copy machine!

In this chapter you will be learning about the use and maintenance of many important pieces of administrative medical office equipment. Additionally, you just might come away with a new appreciation of the importance they play in the function of the efficient medical practice.

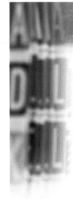

CASE STUDY

Meg is a CMA and is the first to arrive each morning at the busy medical practice where she works. As she unlocks the back door, she is thinking about the entry process. She knows she will set off an alarm as she enters and that she must go immediately to the security alarm box on the nearby wall and type in her security code number to turn off the system.

Meg walks to the front door and unlocks it. As she walks to her desk, she notices the fire extinguisher hanging on the wall. She makes a note to herself to call the maintenance company today to notify them that the expiration date on the extinguisher is this month. They will replace the old one with another extinguisher.

Meg next turns on all the lights. As she walks through the quiet front office, she sees three messages in the fax machine that have come in overnight. She picks them up and scans them quickly before she places them in the center of her desk.

She switches on the copy machines. On the top display is a four-digit number that indicates the number of copies each machine has made this month. Because it is the first of the month, she will call the leasing company today to report that number. Her office is billed based on how many copies are made each month.

Sitting at her desk, Meg turns off the telephone answering machine, which has been in operation throughout the night. There are four messages. As she listens, she makes careful notes before she discards each message and turns off the system. She knows that the phone will start ringing soon.

Meg turns on her computer and reviews all the tasks ahead of her today as a CMA in a busy medical practice. She has received e-mail from another doctor's office asking her to call about a new referral. Another e-mail is requesting medical records.

There is one more thing Meg must check before she settles in to her day's work. She makes her way to the break room and makes a big pot of coffee for all the staff. With a steaming coffee mug in hand, Meg walks back to her desk. Let the day begin!

As you read this chapter, consider the following questions:

1. What factors might go into the choice of an answering machine over the use of an answering service?
2. What backups for system failure might be important for the equipment in a medical office?
3. How could a misdialed phone number on the fax machine impact the life of a patient?
4. Why is routine maintenance of all office equipment important?

Office Communication Equipment

When you think of equipment for a medical office, you probably imagine x-ray machines, blood pressure monitors, and stethoscopes. You will, however, find many other kinds of equipment in a medical practice. Medical offices also use business communication equipment, which includes telephones, facsimile machines, computers, and photocopiers. One of your duties as a medical assistant may be to operate the medical office's communication equipment.

Just as medical equipment has evolved over the years, so has office equipment. The office communication equipment available years ago handled only the most basic tasks. Medical practices may have had a single telephone and a typewriter. If copies of patient records were required,

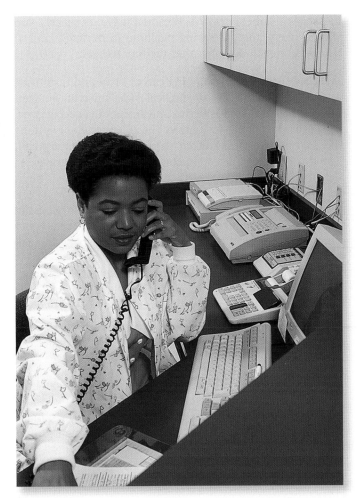

Figure 5-1. Most medical offices today rely on many up-to-date pieces of communication equipment.

medical assistants handwrote a duplicate set or used carbon paper to make additional copies.

Today technology allows almost instantaneous communication of information throughout the world. This instant communication can be critical for the fast-paced medical profession, where information often translates to the need for immediate treatment, sometimes in life-threatening situations. Communicating effectively within a medical office can be as vital as providing the correct treatment to patients—and often ensures that they receive such treatment (Figure 5-1).

Telephone Systems

Although the telephone is a common item in offices, it is one of the most important pieces of communication equipment in a medical practice. Not only is it the instrument patients use to communicate with the office, but it is also the primary means of communication with other doctors, hospitals, laboratories, and other businesses important to the practice.

Multiple Lines. Few practices can function with just one telephone line because if that line is in use, no other calls can come in or go out. Most medical offices have a telephone system that includes two or more telephones and several telephone lines. The six-button telephone is a popular choice in medical practices. This system has four lines for incoming or outgoing calls, an intercom line, and a button for putting a call on hold.

A telephone system can be set up so that incoming calls ring on all the telephones in the office. A more common setup in busy practices is to use a switchboard, a device that receives all calls. The receptionist then routes calls to the appropriate telephone extensions.

Patient Courtesy Phone. Some offices have a patient courtesy phone, which provides an outside local phone line strictly for the use of patients. Long-distance calls should be blocked from this phone. The addition of such a line leaves office lines free for business calls. This phone is located in the reception area. A patient courtesy phone provides a line of communication for patients to call for transportation or to contact work or family as needed. It is helpful to post a sign near the phone to indicate guidelines for its use. Calls are usually limited to two minutes.

Leaving a Message on an Answering Machine or Fax Machine. On occasion, it is also important to send a message to a patient's answering machine or fax machine. It is now required by law, including HIPAA, that you use these pieces of equipment correctly and confidentially. The goal in calling a patient's home is to speak directly to the patient or to leave a message with enough information to get the patient to call back. Be careful to avoid disclosing confidential patient information to anyone but the patient. Your primary concern is to guard the patient's private medical information. *Never* leave any information if you are unsure of the phone number dialed. Additionally, even if you know the number is correct, you cannot ensure that only the intended patient will receive the message. To guard the patient's privacy, *state only the following information:*

- The name of the individual for whom the message is intended
- The date and time of the call
- The name of your office or practice
- Your name as the contact person in the office
- The phone number of your office or practice
- The hours the office is open for a return call
- A request for a return call

Be especially careful of the hasty and indiscriminate use of fax machines. HIPAA law now states that the best format for the use of fax machines involves the use of a locked mailbox at the receiver's end of the transmission. Most in-home users, however, will not have this feature. It is always best to simply fax a request containing only the same information that was recommended for answering machines.

Automated Menu. Instead of using a switchboard, some medical practices route calls by means of an automated menu. Callers listen to the recorded menu and, in response, press a number on their telephone keypad. For example, the menu will say, "Press 2 to speak to Dr. Lowell." The caller presses 2, and the phone rings in Dr. Lowell's office. The Tips for the Office section provides more information on routing calls through an automated menu. If your office uses such a menu, make sure the voice prompts are clear and understandable.

Voice Mail. An automated menu is often used in conjunction with **voice mail,** which is an advanced form of answering machine. If a doctor is out of her office or taking another telephone call, the call is answered by voice mail, and the caller can leave a message. One of the benefits of a voice-mail system is that callers never receive a busy signal.

Answering Machine. Many offices use a telephone answering machine to answer calls after office hours, on weekends and holidays, and when the office is closed for any reason. A typical recorded message announces that the office is closed and states when it will reopen. The message must always indicate how the caller can reach the doctor or the answering service in an emergency.

An answering machine may be programmed simply to play a taped message from the office, or it may also record messages from callers. If callers can leave messages, you should check the answering machine to retrieve them at the start of each day and after the lunch break.

Answering Service. Instead of or in addition to an answering machine, most medical offices use an answering service. Unlike answering machines, answering services provide people to answer the telephone. They take messages and communicate them to the doctor on call. The doctor on call is responsible for handling emergencies that may occur when the office is closed, such as at night or on weekends or holidays.

Upon receiving a call from the answering service, the doctor calls the patient. For example, the doctor may recommend ways for the patient to alleviate her pain and ask her to come into the office the next morning.

Answering services can be used in two ways. The doctor's office may have an answering machine to record calls of a routine nature and give the number of the answering service to call in emergencies. Alternatively, the answering service may have a direct connection to the doctor's office, picking up calls after a certain number of rings day or night or during specific hours.

Although most answering services provide satisfactory, sometimes even outstanding, service, it is good practice to check up on the service every so often by calling it during its coverage hours. This quality check ensures that the service meets office standards and expectations.

Tips for the Office

Routing Calls Through an Automated Menu

An automated menu system answers calls for you and separates requests into categories so that you can deal with them efficiently. You may already be familiar with automated menus, which are widely used by many large businesses. Someone who calls an automated system hears a recorded message identifying the business. The message gives the caller a list of options from which to choose to identify the purpose of the call. The caller selects an option by pressing the corresponding button on her push-button telephone. If she does not have a push-button telephone, her call is automatically routed so that she can talk to a person or leave a voice-mail message.

How does an automated menu system save time and effort in a medical office? You don't have to answer calls as they come in but can instead reserve a block of time in which to listen and respond to messages. This system allows you to complete other work without interruption.

To set up an automated system, you need to plan specific categories from which patients can choose. Categories may include (1) making and changing appointments, (2) asking billing questions, (3) asking medical questions of the doctors or nurses, (4) reporting patient emergencies, and (5) calls from another doctor's office.

When the caller presses the code for a patient emergency, the call rings in the office because it needs to be answered immediately. You or other staff members can respond to calls in the other categories in a timely fashion. Questions for doctors or nurses can be routed immediately to the appropriate voice mail, bypassing you and the office receptionist.

Automated menu systems can be set up by telephone vendors listed in the yellow pages. When choosing an automated telephone system, be careful that callers do not become lost in the process. It is a good idea to set up a system that allows callers to return easily to the main menu. Be sure to build in an option for rotary dial telephones as well. Following up on messages promptly will also help callers feel comfortable with your voice-mail system, so you should check for messages at least once every hour.

Some answering services specialize in medical practices. These medical specialty services will ask the medical practice to give specific directives for the triage of calls. Always ask any service for references before signing a contract for service.

Pagers (Beepers)

Physicians often need to be reached when they are out of the office, so many carry pagers. Pagers or beepers are small electronic devices that give a signal to indicate that someone is trying to reach the physician.

Technology of Paging. Each paging device is assigned a telephone number. When someone calls that number, the pager picks up the signal and beeps, buzzes, or vibrates to indicate that a call has been made. Most pagers have a window that displays the caller's telephone number so that the person who has been paged can return the call promptly. Certain models display a short message. Some pagers store telephone numbers so that the receiver can return several calls without having to write down the numbers.

Paging a Physician. Many telephone messages can wait until the physician returns to the office or calls in for messages. When a message needs to be delivered immediately, however, paging is an efficient response. The paging process is as simple as making a telephone call.

1. A list of pager numbers for each physician in the practice should be kept in a prominent place in the office, such as by the main switchboard. Make sure you know where these numbers are kept. Look up the telephone number for the pager of the physician you need to contact.
2. Dial the telephone number for the pager.
3. You will hear the telephone ringing and the call picked up. Listen for a high-pitched tone, which signals the connection between the telephone and the pager.
4. To operate most pagers, you need to dial the telephone number you wish the physician to call, followed by the pound sign (#), located below the number 9 on a push-button telephone. (Some pager services have an operator and work much like an answering service. Give the operator a message, and the operator will contact the physician.)
5. Listen for a beep or a series of beeps signaling that the page has been transmitted. Then hang up the phone. The physician will call the number at his earliest convenience.

Interactive Pagers (I-Pagers)

Interactive pagers (I-pagers) are designed for two-way communication. The individual carrying the pager is paged in much the same way as the traditional pager. The pager can be set on "Audio" or "Vibrate" to alert the carrier that a message is coming in. However, the interactive pager screen displays a printed message and allows the physician to respond by way of a mini keyboard.

The physician can respond to the printed page by typing a return message (done by typing with the thumbs). The physician can respond back in real time to the office. The office computer and the physician enter into a conversation much like e-mail or an Internet chat room. Many problems can be handled quickly and efficiently in this manner. Additionally, because the I-pager can function silently, the physician can communicate with her office while in a meeting without disturbing others.

Each interactive pager has its own wireless Internet address. The user types in the receiving party's e-mail address and creates a message on a monitor screen. The interactive pager will give the sender the status of his message by indicating on the screen when the message has been sent, received, or read.

I-pagers can communicate with other I-pagers as well. I-pagers also have broadcast capability, meaning the sender can send to more than one receiver at a time. For this reason, practices with multiple physicians may find them very helpful.

Interactive pagers can also send messages to traditional telephones. The message is typed into the pager, and the system "calls" the telephone number. When answered, an electronic-type voice reads the message to the individual who has answered.

Facsimile Machines

Critical documents, such as laboratory reports or patient records, often need to be sent immediately to locations outside the office. Documents can be sent by means of a facsimile machine, or fax machine. A fax machine scans each page, translates it into electronic impulses, and transmits those impulses over the telephone line. When they are received by another fax machine, they are converted into an exact copy of the original document.

A fax machine in a medical office should have its own telephone line. A separate line ensures that transmission of incoming and outgoing faxes will not be interrupted and that the machine will not tie up a needed telephone line when sending or receiving information.

Benefits of Faxing. A fax machine can send an exact copy of a document within minutes. The cost for sending a fax is the same as for making a telephone call to that location. For a short document, this is usually less expensive than an overnight mail service.

Many fax machines have a copier function and can be used as an extra copy machine. This function may only be useful, however, if the machine uses plain paper. The telephone for the fax may also be used as an extra extension for outgoing calls, if needed.

Thermal Paper Versus Plain Paper. Some fax machines print on rolls of specially treated paper called electrothermal, or thermal, paper, which reacts to heat and electricity. Thermal paper tends to fade over time, so documents received on this type of paper may need to be photocopied. Many new models of fax machines use plain paper instead of thermal paper, avoiding the need for making copies. Information is transferred to the plain paper by either a carbon ribbon or a laser beam.

Sending a Fax. Sending a fax is a simple process. One or more pages of a document can be sent at any given time.

1. Prepare a **cover sheet,** which provides information about the transmission. Cover sheets can vary in appearance but usually include the name, telephone number, and fax number of the sender and the receiver; the number of pages being transmitted; and the date. Often medical practices use preprinted cover sheets, with blanks that can be filled in for each transmission. All cover sheets must carry a statement of disclaimer to guard the privacy of the patient. A **disclaimer** is a statement of denial of legal liability. (A sample cover sheet is shown in Figure 5-2.) A disclaimer should be included on the cover sheet and may read something like the following: "This fax or e-mail contains confidential or proprietary information that may be legally privileged. It is intended only for the named recipient(s). If an addressing or transmission error has misdirected the fax or e-mail, please notify the author by replying to this message. If you are not the named recipient, you are not authorized to use, disclose, distribute, copy, print, or rely on this fax or e-mail and should immediately shred it or delete it from your computer system."

2. Place all pages face down in the fax machine's sending tray or area. Dial the telephone number of the receiving fax machine, using either the telephone attached to the fax machine or the numbers on the fax keyboard.

3. If you use the fax telephone, listen for a high-pitched tone. Then press the "Send" or "Start" button, and hang up the telephone. Your fax is now being sent.

4. If you use the fax keyboard, press the "Send" or "Start" button after dialing the telephone number. This button will start the call.

5. Watch for the fax machine to make a connection. Often a green light appears as the document feeds through the machine.

6. If the fax machine is not able to make a connection, as when the receiving fax line is busy, it may have a feature that automatically redials the number every few minutes for a specified number of attempts.

City Medical Associates

555 London Street Strathspey, PA 19919

Janet Michaels, MD   INTERNAL MEDICINE   Scott J. Michaels, MD

FACSIMILE COVER SHEET

Date: _____

To: _____   From: _____

Fax #: _____   Fax #: _____

# of pages (including this cover sheet): _____

Message: _____

_____

Figure 5-2. Every document that is sent by fax transmission should include a cover sheet, which provides details about the transmission. A disclaimer should be included on the cover sheet.

7. When a fax has been successfully sent, most fax machines print a confirmation message. When a fax has not been sent, the machine either prints an error message or indicates on the screen that the transmission was unsuccessful.

Receiving a Fax. Faxes can be received 24 hours a day if the fax machine is turned on and has an adequate supply of paper. If the fax machine is not already sending or receiving a fax, the fax telephone rings briefly, signaling the start of a transmission. The transmission begins shortly thereafter, with the machine printing out the document as it is sent. When completed, the machine usually prints a transmission report, with the number of pages, the date and time, and the originating fax number.

Typewriters

Typewriters can be used to create correspondence, interoffice documents, medical forms brought in by patients or sent from insurance companies, and patient bills. Typewritten documents are easier to read than handwritten ones and project a more businesslike appearance.

Models and Features. Although typewriter models differ in features, all use a standard keyboard. Placement of the keys is identical on each typewriter. The arrangement is not alphabetic. Rather, the most frequently used keys are near the middle, where your fingers can most easily reach them, and the least used keys are toward the outside.

A wide variety of typewriter models are available. Most offices use electric or electronic models. Although both are powered by electricity, they differ in their ability to perform certain functions. For example, electronic typewriters can store limited amounts of information for further use, but electric typewriters cannot. Both electric and electronic typewriters provide a wide selection of features, including, but not limited to, automatic carriage return, automatic centering, self-correction, and changeable typefaces or fonts.

Typewriters Versus Word Processors. Typewriters should not be confused with word processors, which perform a similar function but are more sophisticated. Word processors can store entire documents in memory, thereby allowing much greater flexibility in manipulating material than do typewriters. Word processors display documents on a screen or monitor, and these documents can be revised as often as needed before being printed out. Word processors are typically more expensive than typewriters, but they are less expensive than computers and make it easy to generate perfect documents.

Today many medical practices use computers with word processing software. (Chapter 6 discusses the use of computers in a medical office.)

Office Automation Equipment

Using automated equipment enables you to perform a task more easily and quickly than doing it manually. For example, adding numbers on a calculator is a much faster process than doing it on paper. Many of the administrative tasks in a medical practice can be accomplished with automated equipment, giving you more time to perform other procedures.

Photocopiers

A photocopier, also called a copier or copy machine, instantly reproduces office correspondence, forms, bills, patient records, and other documents. Before photocopiers were available, offices used carbon paper to reproduce documents as they were being typed. The number of copies that could be made was limited.

A photocopier takes a picture of the document it is to reproduce and prints it on plain paper using a heat process. Photocopiers use either liquid or dry toner, a form of ink. They can make an unlimited number of copies. Photocopiers do not require treated or otherwise special paper. Various kinds of paper can be used in the machine, including office stationery and colored paper. Many photocopiers accept different sizes of paper, from the standard 8½- by 11-inch paper to 8½- by 14-inch legal paper and even larger.

Photocopiers come in many models, from desktop machines for limited use to industrial models for continual heavy use. The machines vary in features and speed. All styles of machines are available through purchase or lease.

Special Features. Copiers offer a wide range of special features. They may collate (assemble sets of multiple pages in order) and staple pages, enlarge or reduce images, and produce double-sided copies (print on both sides of the page). Some can also adjust contrast and even track the cost of a job via a specific code input into the machine. Although the majority of photocopiers used in medical offices produce black-and-white copies, photocopiers are available that make color copies. Some copiers can make transparencies (text and images printed on clear acetate), which physicians often use for presentations.

One of the more useful features of photocopiers is the help function. Selecting this function displays directions in plain English that explain how to fix a paper jam or deal with other routine copier problems. Some copiers are even programmed to indicate that service is needed.

Making Copies. Although the procedure for making copies differs slightly from machine to machine, most machines can be operated by following these basic steps.

1. Make sure the machine is turned on and warmed up. It will display a signal when it is ready for copying.

2. Prepare your materials, removing paper clips, staples, and self-adhesive flags.

3. Place the document to be copied in the automatic feeder tray as directed, or upside down directly on the glass. The feeder tray can accommodate many pages; you may place only one page at a time on the glass. Automatic feeding is a faster process, and you should use it when you wish to collate or staple packets. Page-by-page copying is advantageous if you need to copy a single sheet or to enlarge or reduce the image. To use any special features, such as making double-sided copies or stapling the copies, you have to press a button on the machine.

4. Set the machine for the desired paper size.

5. Key in the number of copies you want to make, and press the "Start" button. The copies are made automatically.

6. If necessary, press the "Clear" or "Reset" button when your job is finished to prepare the machine for the next user.

7. If the copier becomes jammed, follow the directions on the machine to locate the problem (for example, there may be multiple pieces of paper stuck inside the printer), and dislodge the jammed paper. Most copy machines will show a diagram of the printer and the location of the problem.

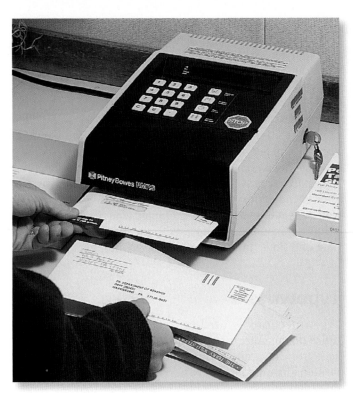

Figure 5-3. The postage meter is a convenient and cost-effective way to apply postage to office correspondence and packages.

Adding Machines and Calculators

For handling tasks such as patient billing, bank deposits, and payroll, medical practices depend on adding machines and calculators. The difference between the two types of machines is minimal. Adding machines typically plug into an outlet and produce a paper tape on which calculations are printed. Calculators are more often battery- or solar-powered, with memory to store figures. Calculators are portable and usually do not produce a paper tape.

Routine Calculations. Both adding machines and calculators are sufficient for routine office calculations. These machines perform basic arithmetic functions, such as addition, subtraction, multiplication, and division. Many of today's models perform such specialized functions as computing percentages and storing data. Some are even computerized.

Checking Your Work. It is easy to hit an incorrect key or to key in a number twice when using an adding machine or a calculator. Therefore, check all mathematical computations. An error on a bill causes problems for both the patient and the office.

If the machine produces a paper tape, check the numbers on the tape against the numbers you are adding. The paper tape is especially useful when adding a long series of numbers. Without a printed record, you must perform the same calculations again to make sure the total is correct.

Postage Meters

Every medical office uses the U.S. Postal Service. Patient bills, routine correspondence, purchase orders, and payments are just some of the items typically sent by mail. (See Chapter 7 for additional information on mailing correspondence.)

Although some medical offices use stamps, most use a postage meter. A postage meter is a machine that applies postage to an envelope or package, eliminating the need for postage stamps (Figure 5-3). There are often two parts to a postage meter: the meter, which belongs to the post office, and the mailing machine, which the practice can own. The meter actually applies the postage, and the mailing machine does the rest, such as sealing the envelope.

Benefits of Using a Postage Meter. There are several advantages to using a postage meter instead of purchasing stamps. It saves frequent trips to the post office. It also saves money for the office by providing the exact amount of postage needed for each item. When you have to use a combination of stamps, you may exceed the required postage. It is unlikely as well as impractical for a practice to keep every denomination of stamps on hand.

Some postage meters can imprint envelopes with the name of your medical practice or with a message at the same time postage is applied. The message appears immediately to the left of the postal mark, at the top of the envelope.

PROCEDURE 5.1

How to Use a Postage Meter

Objective: To correctly apply postage to an envelope or package for mailing, according to U.S. Postal Service guidelines

Materials: Postage meter, addressed envelope or package, postal scale

Method

1. For the postage meter to function, there must be money in your postal account. Contact the company that is managing your account or your local post office for more information.

2. Verify the day's date. U.S. Postal Service guidelines prohibit mailing envelopes and packages that are postmarked with an incorrect date. Check that the postage meter is plugged in and switched on before you proceed.

3. Locate the area where the meter registers the date. Many machines have a lid that can be flipped up, with rows of numbers underneath. Months are represented numerically, with 1 symbolizing January, 2 symbolizing February, and so on. Check that the date is correct. If it is not, change the numbers to the correct date.

4. Make sure that all materials have been included in the envelope or package. Weigh the envelope or package on a postal scale. Standard business envelopes weighing up to 1 oz require the minimum postage (the equivalent of one first-class stamp). Oversize envelopes and packages require additional postage. A postal scale will indicate the amount of postage required.

5. Key in the postage amount on the meter, and press the button that enters the amount. For amounts over $1, you may have to press a "$" button or the "Enter" button twice. This feature verifies large amounts, catching errors in case you mistakenly press too many keys.

6. Check that the amount you typed is the correct amount. Envelopes and packages with too little postage will be returned by the U.S. Postal Service. If you send an envelope or package with too much postage, your practice will not be reimbursed.

7. If you are applying postage to an envelope, hold it flat and right side up (so that you can read the address). Seal the envelope (unless the meter seals it for you). As you face the postage meter, locate the plate or area where the envelope can slide through. This feature is usually near the bottom of the meter. Place the envelope on the left side, and give it a gentle push toward the right. Some models hold the envelope in a stationary position. (If the meter seals the envelope for you, be sure to place it correctly to allow for sealing.) The meter will grab the envelope and pull it through quickly.

8. For packages, you need to create a postage label to affix to the package. Follow the same procedure for a label as for an envelope. Affix the postmarked label on the package in the upper right corner.

9. Check that the printed postmark has the correct date and amount and that it is legible.

Many types of postage meters are available, from basic models for a small office to advanced models for large businesses. The latest machines include automatic date setting, memory to program a large mailing, and display alerts for low postage or the need for ribbon replacement. Some models can apply postage to parcels without the use of labels or tape. Procedure 5-1 shows you how to use a postage meter.

Prepaying for Postage. To use a postage meter, you must prepay the postage. You can take your meter to the post office to add postage, or you can use a postage meter service. A service maintains the postal account for you. Although the money in each account is the property of the U.S. Postal Service, the provider manages the account and adds postage to the meter. Postage can also be added to the meter by telephone or by modem, with data sent directly to the meter over the telephone line. The process takes only a few minutes, and the call is often toll-free. Before postage can be added, however, money must be deposited into an account. Keeping the postage account current ensures that all mail is sent on a timely basis. This task may be one of your responsibilities.

On any meter, you can check the amount of postage used and the amount remaining with the touch of a button. On some models, the meter must have $10 or more for the machine to apply postage to an envelope or package.

Postage Scales

Besides the postage meter, you also need a scale. Postal scales are a good investment because they show both the weight and the amount of postage required. Some postage meters include an electronic scale. If you need a postal scale but one is not available, you can use any scale that weighs in ounces. You can then translate the weight into the correct postage by using a current postal rate chart, available from the U.S. Postal Service.

Posting Mail

Before you begin posting mail, make sure the envelope or package is complete, with all materials included. After applying the postage, place the postmarked envelope or package in the area of your office designated for mail pickup.

Dictation-Transcription Equipment

Physicians usually do not type their own correspondence, patient records, or other documents. Medical assistants, although not professional medical transcriptionists, may be asked to transcribe recorded words into written text. Using dictation-transcription equipment is the most efficient way to complete this task. *Dictation* is another word for speaking; *transcription* is another word for writing. Together they mean to transform spoken words into written form.

Medical assistants performing transcription often use a desktop dictation-transcription machine, a unit similar in size and appearance to a telephone. A smaller attachment

PROCEDURE 5.2

How to Use a Dictation-Transcription Machine

Objective: To correctly use a dictation-transcription machine to convert verbal communication into the written word

Materials: Dictation-transcription machine; audiocassette or magnetic tape or disk with the recorded dictation; typewriter, word processor, or computer; blank paper or stationery; medical dictionary; regular dictionary; pen; correction fluid or tape (for the typewriter)

Method

1. Insert the tape into the dictation-transcription machine (Figure 5-4). In front of you, next to the machine, will be a typewriter, word processor, or computer, on which you will type the information. Turn on the typewriter, word processor, or computer if it is not on already.

2. Place all materials, including a regular dictionary and a medical dictionary, within easy reach, and clear the area of items you will not use.

3. Choose the paper you will use, and insert it. Set the margins and line spacing. You can estimate the length of the document by using the scanning control.

4. Dictation-transcription machines use foot pedals to allow your fingers to remain on the keyboard. Press down the foot pedal to start and stop the dictation-transcription machine.

5. To rewind the tape, use the reverse foot pedal.

6. Pause the recording with the pause foot pedal, if your machine has one, or stop it with the stop/start pedal.

7. Adjust the speed and volume controls to help you work most efficiently.

8. Proofread the final document, and make any corrections directly on the document. Use correction fluid or correction tape as necessary. Make sure that the corrected document looks professional and businesslike. Retype it if necessary. Proofread the final copy once again. If possible, ask someone else to proofread it also.

9. Turn off all equipment that should not be left on.

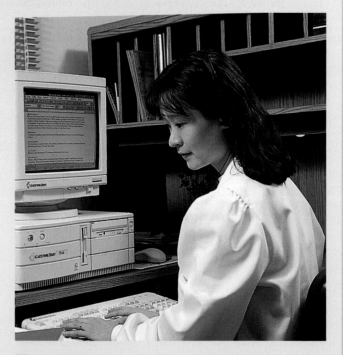

Figure 5-4. One of your responsibilities as a medical assistant may be to use dictation-transcription equipment.

resembles a handheld tape recorder. The machine includes special controls to record and play tapes.

Dictating and Transcribing.
Before a tape can be transcribed, it must be recorded. A doctor can take several steps during the recording process to make the job of transcribing the tape as easy as possible.

1. The doctor should indicate the date and the type of document being dictated and provide explicit instructions about the document. For example, the doctor should indicate that a particular document is a letter and that it is to be produced on office stationery and mailed to a patient.
2. The doctor should spell out all names and addresses as well as any unfamiliar terms.
3. Where possible, the doctor should dictate punctuation, by saying, for example, "comma" or "Begin new paragraph."
4. The doctor should speak clearly and slowly. The doctor should neither eat while dictating nor record in a noisy environment, such as the emergency room of a hospital, if at all possible.
5. By saving all dictation in the computer in an organized fashion, you can quickly cut and paste often-used phrases and addresses for fast and easy use again.

Procedure 5-2 shows you how to operate a dictation-transcription machine. Chapter 9 explains how to create accurate, complete transcriptions.

Special Controls.
Dictation-transcription machines often have special controls to streamline the transcription process. Volume and tone controls make dictation clearer, and speed controls separate words. Setting the speed to the rate at which you are comfortable typing also makes the transcription process more efficient. In addition, headphones allow you to concentrate on the recording, shutting out distracting office noise.

More specialized controls include scanning, which allows you to review a tape's contents quickly, and indicator strips, which mark important material. Some machines are also equipped with an automatic backspace control, which rewinds the tape slightly each time it is stopped, so that no words are missed. For the recording process, the machine may be equipped with an insert control, to allow someone to place additional dictation in the middle of existing dictation. The machine may also include a voice-activated sensor for hands-free recording. After a transcribed document has been approved, you may wish to use the machine's erase function to create a clean tape.

Check Writers

Medical practice personnel need to write checks to pay for equipment, supplies, and payroll. This common office procedure can be automated by using a check writer, which is a machine that imprints checks. The safety advantage of using such a machine is that the name of the payee (the person receiving the check) and the amount of the check, once imprinted, cannot be altered.

Producing a Check.
To produce a check using a check writer, you first put in a blank check or a sheet of blank checks. Then you key in the date, payee's name, and payment amount. The check writer imprints the check with this information and perforates it with the payee's name. The perforations are actual little holes in the paper, which prevent anyone from changing the name on the check. A doctor or another authorized person then signs the check. To complete the process, record the check in the office checkbook.

Voiding a Check.
If the information on an imprinted check is incorrect, it cannot be changed. Therefore, you must issue a new check and void the previous one. To void the check, write "VOID" in clear letters across it, or use a VOID stamp with red ink. Then file the check with the office bank records so that the practice's money manager is aware that it has been voided.

Paper Shredders

Paper shredders are usually associated with government offices but are also quite common in medical practices. A paper shredder, such as the one shown in Figure 5-5, is

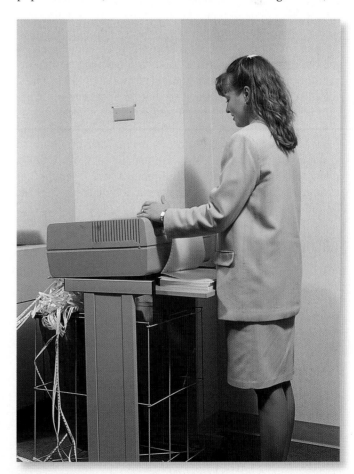

Figure 5-5. As a medical assistant, you may be asked to use a paper shredder to destroy confidential documents that are no longer needed by the practice.

often used when confidential documents, such as patient records, need to be destroyed. Paper shredders cut documents into tiny pieces to make them unreadable.

The most common type of shredder cuts paper into ribbonlike strips, which differ in width, depending on the model. Other shredders cut the paper in two directions, forming small pieces. Some paper shredders offer additional options, such as an electronic eye that automatically starts the machine when paper is inserted and stops when it is done. Other features available are paper jam detection, automatic reverse, and automatic shutdown when the machine gets too hot.

How to Shred Materials. A paper shredder is ready to use when it is turned on. To shred a document, insert it into the feed tray at the top of the shredder. The machine feeds the paper through hundreds of knifelike cutters, instantaneously shredding the paper. A basket attached beneath the shredder catches the bits of paper. Different models can accommodate different amounts of paper through the cutters. Shredder baskets must be emptied periodically to allow room for additional shredded paper. Some shredders signal when the basket is full. It is very important not to wear loose-fitting clothing while operating a shredder to avoid accident and personal injury.

When to Shred Materials. Medical practices often need to eliminate old patient records or other sensitive materials. These items cannot simply be thrown into the trash because of confidentiality problems. The shredder is an effective disposal solution. If records have incorrect information that has been corrected on subsequent documents, the old records are shredded so that the incorrect information is not mistakenly placed in the patient's folder.

A document that has been shredded cannot be put back together. Therefore, do not decide on your own to shred a document. The physician usually tells you when a document should be shredded. If you are not sure whether to shred a document, check with a senior staff member before beginning the process.

Microfilm and Microfiche Readers

If all information were stored on paper in file folders, medical offices would need additional rooms to hold it all. Therefore, some medical offices store information on microfilm or microfiche. **Microfilm** is a roll of film imprinted with information and stored on a reel. Film can also be stored in cartridges, to protect the film from being touched. **Microfiche** is film imprinted with information and stored in rectangular sheets.

Information stored on microfilm and microfiche is dramatically reduced in size. Because each roll or sheet can hold a large amount of material, less storage space is required than for comparable paper files. Because the information is so tiny, however, reading it requires special machines, such as those shown in Figures 5-6 and 5-7.

Even if your office does not store records on microfilm or microfiche, you may still need to have a reader because

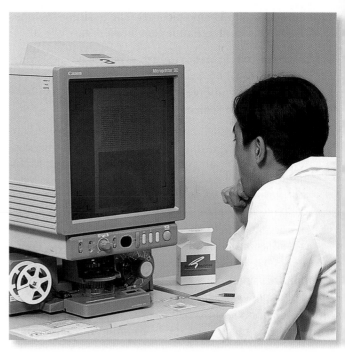

Figure 5-6. Storing information on microfilm helps reduce the amount of storage space needed by the practice.

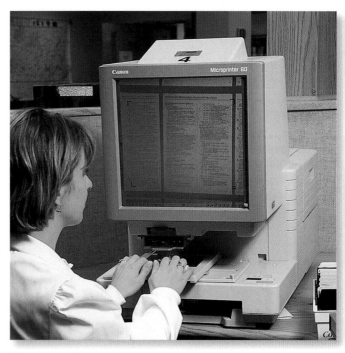

Figure 5-7. Special equipment must be used to read text that has been converted to microfiche.

back issues of medical journals and other publications are often available only in these formats.

Models and Features. Microfilm and microfiche machines come in many different sizes. Most medical offices use a desktop model to conserve space. The main difference between a desktop model and other models is size. The features and controls are similar.

Basic controls on microfilm and microfiche readers allow adjustment of the image—zooming into an area, focusing, and rotating it—and fast-forwarding to other parts of the film. Advanced controls include image editing, an odometer that measures the amount of film scanned, and search functions that can be connected to a computer to locate specific items.

Reading and Printing.   For ease of use, you should label and date each roll of microfilm or each microfiche sheet with the information it contains. Then you will be able to locate information easily when you need it.

Because the film is stored in different formats, microfilm and microfiche require different mechanisms to read them. For example, microfilm requires a roller attachment; microfiche requires a flat surface. Newer models can accommodate different formats with the use of detachable, interchangeable reading mechanisms.

Microfilm is inserted onto a rod and threaded onto the microfilm reader. Microfiche is placed directly on the glass tray of a microfiche reader. If you are unsure, check the directions in the manual for your reader.

The reading process is similar for all machines, with information displayed on a large screen. The screen displays only a small portion of the information stored on the film. You can fast-forward through the film to read additional information. Most machines allow you to print out the image on the screen.

Purchasing Decisions

As a medical assistant, you may be involved in making purchasing decisions for office equipment. For example, the physician or office manager may ask you to investigate whether the practice needs a certain piece of equipment, such as a new photocopier or microfiche reader. To make a sound decision about whether the office will benefit from such a purchase, you will need to conduct thorough research.

Evaluating Office Needs

The first step in the research process is to document the tasks that a piece of equipment can complete. In the case of a typewriter, for example, tasks include writing letters and bills, recording the staff's schedule, and preparing a fax cover sheet, as well as producing other office documents. To obtain a complete list of office needs, consult other staff members for their ideas.

If you are replacing an old piece of equipment, you will want to know what advantages the new piece of equipment offers over the current one. Next to each task on your list, indicate the benefits offered by the new product. For example, next to typing office correspondence, you might list several benefits of an electronic typewriter or a computer over a manual typewriter. Both the electronic typewriter and the computer are easy to use; they self-correct, making correction fluid or tape unnecessary; and they

store information, thus saving typing time. Some medical magazines, such as *Medical Economics* and *Professional Medical Assistant,* review medical office equipment periodically and are good resources to consult in making your purchasing decisions.

Contacting Suppliers.   Put together a list of the features you would like in your machine. Then contact suppliers who sell models that offer those features. You can call or e-mail the manufacturer directly to find out the name of a local vendor. Many manufacturers prepare brochures giving information about their products. If time allows, you can request that these be sent to you.

Go online and look in the yellow pages for office supply stores and other companies that sell office equipment. Obtain product and pricing information on each model. For certain equipment, such as photocopiers, a sales representative will come to your office to demonstrate and discuss the product.

Evaluating Warranty Options.   Most products come with a warranty. A **warranty** is a contract that guarantees free service and replacement of parts for a certain period, usually 1 year. Warranties are valid only for specified service and repairs. They usually do not cover accidents, vandalism, acts of God (such as damage caused by floods or earthquakes), or mistreatment of the machine. In most cases, warranty repairs must be made at an authorized service center.

If you want more coverage than the warranty allows, you can buy an extended warranty. Extended warranties increase the amount of time that equipment is covered. For expensive pieces of equipment or parts, the additional cost of an extended warranty may be justified.

After you purchase a product, you must fill out the warranty card and mail it to the manufacturer. File the receipt in a safe place in the office where it can easily be retrieved.

Preparing a Recommendation.   After you have obtained all the information, you are ready to evaluate it. To compare and contrast the different models, construct a chart. Place the product model names in columns across the top. Down the left side, list factors that will influence the purchase decision: cost, warranty options (including the length of the warranty and the price of an extended warranty), special features, and delivery time. Then fill in the information. This chart will provide an easy-to-use summary of your research.

Analyze the list, and choose the product you think will best meet the needs of the office. Then meet with the physician or office manager to discuss your recommendation.

Leasing Versus Buying Equipment

Once the product has been selected, there is one more decision to make: whether to lease or to buy the item. When buying a product, the purchaser becomes the owner of the product. Owners are free to do with the product anything they choose, which may include selling it to someone else.

Metropolitan Office Systems

Lease Agreement

Customer (Location)

Standard Education Corporation
Full Legal Name (Please Print)

119 Washington Blvd.
Address

Spokane,		*WA*	*98548*
City	County	State	Zip

Billing Contact

Dealer:

Customer (Billing address, if different)

Full Legal Name (Please Print)

Address

City	County	State	Zip

Phone

Quantity	Description: Make, Model, and Serial Number	Quantity	Description: Make, Model, and Serial Number
1	FT 6655 Copier AA3365430358		
1	Sorter A337502010902		
1	Document Feeder A338506		
1	RT 314 Large-capacity Tray		

Minimum Lease Term:	Payment Due:	Amount of Monthly Payment With Sales, Use, and Property Tax:	Advance Payment of _$965.56_ (Tax Included) by Check #_____	Documentation Fee
	__X__ Monthly ____ Quarterly ____ Annually ____ Other:		____ First Month's Rent __X__ First and Last ____ Security Deposit (Without Tax) ____ Other _____	
_60_ Months	$455.46	$482.78		$ _-0-_

Figure 5-8. Read lease agreements carefully.

For most large pieces of office equipment, such as photocopiers, there is also an option to **lease** the equipment. Leasing, or renting, usually involves an initial charge and a monthly fee. On average, the initial charge is equal to about two monthly payments.

Lease Agreement. A lease is for a specified time, after which time the equipment is returned to the seller (Figure 5-8). Some leases allow purchase of the equipment at the end of the rental period for an additional payment. The details of the purchase option are covered in the lease agreement.

Advantages of Leasing. When you lease a product, your office does not own it, but you have several advantages. Leasing allows purchasers to keep more of their money. The initial cost of obtaining the machine is a fraction of the full cost of purchasing it. Therefore, the remainder of the money can earn interest in the bank or be used for other expenses. Leasing is advantageous when you do not have enough money to buy the equipment but need the services it provides. In addition, leasing allows businesses to update equipment every few years at the end of each lease period. Updating may not be as affordable if you buy equipment. Often the company that leases the product is also responsible for servicing it. Finally, in most cases, businesses are able to take lease payments as a tax deduction each year.

Leasing is not the best solution for everyone. It is important to weigh the advantages of leasing against the advantages of buying equipment for your medical practice.

Negotiating. Whether you decide to lease or buy equipment, always ask whether the price is firm or if there is room for negotiation. Although most equipment prices are set, terms can sometimes be negotiated on more expensive pieces of equipment. Companies that lease office equipment are often flexible in determining the monthly payment. For example, many companies accept smaller payments to start out, with larger payments near the end, or vice versa.

Some suppliers will match their competitors' prices. Also, if you are purchasing several pieces of equipment at the same time, a supplier may be able to offer some savings on the total cost of the purchase or provide some service, such as delivery, free of charge.

Maintaining Office Equipment

Office equipment must be regularly maintained to provide high-quality service. Daily or weekly maintenance, such as cleaning the glass on the photocopier or replacing toner, can be performed by the office staff. However, more extensive maintenance should be done by the equipment supplier.

Equipment Manuals

The best source of information about maintaining a piece of equipment is the manual that comes with it. This booklet gives basic information about the equipment, including how to set it up, how it works, special features, and problems you may encounter. The information in an equipment manual is extremely valuable. If the manual is lost, call the manufacturer to obtain another one. Equipment manuals should be filed where they can be retrieved easily.

Maintenance and Service Contracts

Equipment suppliers provide standard maintenance contracts when office equipment is purchased. A **maintenance contract** specifies when the equipment will be cleaned, checked for worn parts, and repaired. A standard maintenance contract may include regular checkups as well as emergency repairs.

In addition, some suppliers offer a **service contract,** which covers services that are not included under the standard maintenance agreement. For example, a service contract may cover emergency repairs if they are not covered under standard maintenance. In some cases, service contracts are combined with maintenance contracts in one document.

It is important to keep track of all maintenance performed on your equipment. Many offices keep a maintenance log, where staff members record the date and purpose of each service call. This log is helpful in identifying whether equipment should be replaced because of its need for frequent servicing.

Troubleshooting

You can call a service supplier the minute a piece of equipment stops functioning properly, but you can also take steps to see whether you can determine and correct the problem yourself. This process is called **troubleshooting.** Resolving the problem can save you the cost of a service call that may not be covered by your standard agreement.

The first step in troubleshooting is to eliminate possible simple causes of a problem. For example, if the machine is powered by electricity, make sure that it is plugged into a functioning outlet and that it is turned on. Are all doors and other openings in their correct positions? Are all machine connections firmly in place?

If you cannot discover a simple cause for the problem, it is time to test the machine to determine what it is failing to do. In the case of a malfunctioning photocopier, for example, try making a copy, and note the response. Write down any error messages the machine provides.

Next, consult the equipment manual. Many manuals devote a section to troubleshooting. If you cannot find the solution after reading the manual, call the manufacturer or the place of purchase for additional assistance. Be prepared to explain the steps you have already taken toward resolving the problem.

Backup Systems

Occasionally, more than one piece of equipment can be affected by a problem. For example, if the electricity goes off, all electrical equipment will go out at once. To avoid losing important information and records, it is important to have backup systems in place.

Computers. Computers should be placed on a backup system. The company that services the computer system usually sets this up. Computer backup may occur either automatically off-site over the phone lines or on-site, which may require that a staff member manually plug in a backup tape every night before going home. Computer backup usually occurs at midnight, when the office is not using the system. Computer backup ensures that all information will be retrievable even if the computers suffer a catastrophic failure.

Telephones. The use of cell phones in addition to traditional phones offers a backup to communication in the event that phone service is interrupted. Cell phones are also helpful during emergency weather conditions.

Electricity. A backup generator may supply emergency power for lighting in key hallways and exam rooms. Interior rooms and halls can quickly become very dark and hazardous when the electricity is unexpectedly cut off.

Battery Power. Battery power backup is a key component of security and warning system backups. Audio warning signals sound when it is time to replace the batteries in smoke and security detectors. These systems should be checked every six months.

Fire Extinguishers. Fire extinguishers need to be serviced or replaced once a year to ensure maximum performance. The office may choose to contract with a local company to provide this annual maintenance evaluation.

Equipment Inventory

Each piece of equipment is an asset of a business. It is part of the business's net worth and should be listed on the medical practice's balance sheet. Therefore, taking inventory of office equipment provides relevant information for the practice's money manager. It may also indicate whether old machinery is due for replacement.

There is no set format for taking an office equipment inventory. Figure 5-9 shows one example. Many offices use a master inventory sheet to survey all equipment at a glance. The master sheet usually includes such general information as equipment names and the quantity of each type of equipment.

EQUIPMENT INVENTORY

ITEM	PURCHASE DATE	PURCHASE PRICE
1. TotalOffice oak desk	10/15/02	$295.00
2. TotalOffice rolling desk chair	10/15/02	$119.00
3. TotalOffice 4-drawer file cabinet	1/28/03	$150.00
4. TotalOffice 2-drawer file cabinet	1/28/03	$100.00
5. HYtech Pentium 100 computer	5/29/04	$1150.00
6. HYtech 14-inch monitor	5/29/04	$200.00

Figure 5-9. An equipment inventory sheet includes equipment names and the quantity of each type of equipment.

Many offices also keep more detailed information about each individual piece of equipment in files or on a single sheet of paper. Detailed information may include the following:

- Name of the equipment, including the brand name
- Brief description of the equipment
- Model number and registration number
- Date of purchase
- Place of purchase, including contact information
- Estimated life of the product
- Product warranty
- Maintenance and service contracts

All equipment inventories should be updated periodically.

Summary

In many ways, state-of-the-art office equipment is as important for a medical office as its medical equipment. Although every office does not have the same equipment, common machines include telephones, computers, pagers, fax machines, dictation-transcription equipment, photocopiers, adding machines and calculators, postage meters, check writers, paper shredders, and microfilm or microfiche readers.

As a medical assistant, you may be expected not only to operate this equipment but also to help make purchasing decisions by researching various options. This research includes obtaining information about product features, warranties, and maintenance. Yet another decision is whether to lease or buy the equipment.

Equipment is an asset for a medical office. The office staff needs to maintain a comprehensive inventory of the products leased and purchased. It is important to keep up to date with new technologies that will help the administrative office function smoothly and efficiently.

CASE STUDY QUESTIONS

Now that you have completed this chapter, review the case study at the beginning of the chapter and answer the following questions:

1. What factors might go into the choice of an answering machine over the use of an answering service?
2. What backups for system failure might be important for the equipment in a medical office?
3. How could a misdialed phone number on the fax machine impact the life of a patient?
4. Why is routine maintenance of all office equipment important?

Discussion Questions

1. Why is office equipment important to the medical office? Give at least three examples of pieces of typical office equipment, and describe their use in the medical office.
2. Compare and contrast the advantages and disadvantages of buying and leasing equipment.
3. What are some features of a standard product warranty?
4. Describe a scenario in which an interactive pager might be helpful in a medical office.

Critical Thinking Questions

1. Imagine that you are responsible for the maintenance of the office equipment in a busy medical practice. What weekly, monthly, and yearly checks might you perform? How would you document these checks?

2. You think that your office needs a new photocopier. Explain how you would justify this need to the office manager.
3. You have been asked to create a patient sign to hang on the wall over the courtesy phone. What will your sign say?
4. The fax machine in your office is malfunctioning. Explain the steps you might take to troubleshoot the problem.

Application Activities

1. Your office frequently uses temporary employees to help with copying. The office manager asks you to write directions for the use of the photocopier, to be posted near the machine. Using the computer, create a sign suitable for posting.
2. Your office is moving soon, and you have been asked to assist in the design of a new communication system for the practice. What features would you include in the new system?
3. You have been asked to design a cover sheet for the fax machine for your office. Using the computer, design a form with a disclaimer.
4. Go online and research three different types of photocopiers. Write a report describing each. Be sure to include the equipment name, manufacturer, warranty options, price, advantages to buying or leasing, features, and recommendations for use.

Using Computers in the Office

KEY TERMS

CD-ROM

central processing unit (CPU)

cursor

database

dot matrix printer

electronic mail

hard copy

hardware

icon

ink-jet printer

Internet

laser printer

modem

motherboard

multimedia

multitasking

network

random-access memory (RAM)

read-only memory (ROM)

scanner

screen saver

software

tower case

tutorial

AREAS OF COMPETENCE

2003 Role Delineation Study
GENERAL
Communication Skills
- Utilize electronic technology to receive, organize, prioritize, and transmit information

Operational Functions
- Apply computer techniques to support office operations

CHAPTER OUTLINE

- The Computer Revolution
- Types of Computers
- Components of the Computer
- Using Computer Software
- Selecting Computer Equipment
- Security in the Computerized Office
- Computer System Care and Maintenance
- Computers of the Future

OBJECTIVES

After completing Chapter 6, you will be able to:

6.1 List and describe common types of computers.

6.2 Identify computer hardware and software components and explain the functions of each.

6.3 Describe the types of computer software commonly used in the medical office.

6.4 Discuss how to select computer equipment for the medical office.

6.5 Explain the importance of security measures for computerized medical records.

6.6 Describe the basic care and maintenance of computer equipment.

6.7 Identify new advances in computer technology and explain their importance to the medical office.

Introduction

The practice of medicine today has grown to be increasingly complex:

- Never before has so much medical information been available for the physician.
- Never before has the practice of billing and collecting for medical services rendered and also the scheduling and coordinating of services among multiple providers been so complicated.

- Never before has a "super machine" been more needed to assist with all aspects of a busy practice. We live in the age of information. The need for a device to organize and correlate all this information has never been greater.

The computer has become an integral tool of the medical office. It is used to organize and categorize thousands of bits of information required to accurately record patient care, transmit information to others at distant points, and maintain an orderly record of all the activities of the business.

In this chapter you will learn about the many aspects of using a computer in a medical practice. Regardless of your past experience with computers, after you complete this chapter, you will have a growing awareness and respect for the marvelous technology it represents. You may even become enthusiastic about the possibilities of its many uses.

CASE STUDY

The big day has come at last! Today the new computer system will be installed. Everyone on staff will be involved in learning the new system and using it every day. For a while, everyone will be expected to learn the new system while continuing to maintain the old way of doing things. That will be no small effort for this busy medical office. Some of the office staff are nervous and edgy, while others are excited and looking forward to a new experience. Everyone agrees it is going to be a big change.

Chris is a medical assistant and is excited and eager to get started. She has been waiting for this day ever since she studied the use of computers in medical assisting school. She knows the next few weeks are going to be full of training and building data sets. She knows she is going to be an integral part of the creation of a new way of getting things done. Chris is excited.

Alicia, a medical assistant who works with Chris, thinks that life would be much easier if the administration had just chosen to leave things the way they were. Alicia is not alone in thinking that computers are just an unnecessary inconvenience. The truth is, Alicia is a little afraid that she will not be able to learn the new system. She has tried to ask questions and express her concerns about the new computer system. But each time she tried to talk to one of the computer specialists, she felt stupid and clumsy. They spoke in a language she didn't understand, and she was too intimidated to tell them she didn't understand what they were talking about. Alicia will go along with this new system just to keep her job. But she has decided that she is definitely not going to waste her time learning anything more than she absolutely has to.

As you read this chapter, consider the following questions:

1. Are you more like Chris or Alicia? What background do you bring to the study of computers that makes you feel the way you do?
2. Why is it important for an office to continue to use the manual system at the same time that it converts to a computerized system?
3. Who should be trained in the use of a new computer system in a medical practice? Why?
4. Which group do you think would be the most difficult to train in an average medical practice?
   a. Those who think like Chris?
   b. Those who think like Alicia?
   c. The physicians?

   What would be the best way to approach the group you just identified?

The Computer Revolution

Over the past decade computers have revolutionized the way we live and work. Computers make many tasks easier because they process information with great speed and accuracy. They are also capable of storing vast amounts of information in a small space.

In today's world computer skills are essential for most career choices, and medical assisting is no exception. Medical practices that have not yet made the switch to a computerized practice will most likely do so in the near future. As a medical assistant, you need to understand the fundamentals of computers and their uses. This knowledge will enable you to perform many office tasks with ease.

In addition, the more you know about computers, the more likely you will be able to solve or avoid computer problems.

A Brief History of the Computer

The computer is not new. The first known device used for basic arithmetic calculations was called an abacus and was in use 2000 years ago. In 1642, Blaise Pascal built the first digital calculating machine. The machine could add by adjusting a series of dials. Multiplication and addition became possible by machine in 1671. But there was no real commercial use of a mechanical device for maneuvering numbers or data until the 1850s and the availability of steam power to power great engineering feats. Between 1850 and 1900 there came a great need to produce a machine that could rapidly perform repetitive calculations.

In 1890 punch cards were used for the first time by the U.S. Census Bureau. A machine was built that could "read" information that had been punched into the cards, and the first modern computer was born. Because these calculations were being performed automatically, human error was eliminated from the process. Additionally, work could flow much faster and information could be stored on the cards. Now mathematical and numerical information was being maneuvered and stored.

The development of computers was enhanced by the advent of World War II and the development of vacuum tubes, which could be plugged together, and the program, which gave direction to the information and allowed it to flow. The first high-speed electronic digital computers were used in the late 1940s and early 1950s. Later improvements allowed instructions to be stored within libraries of memory for later use. The first generations of electronic computers were built in the late 1940s and were smaller in size than their predecessors. By today's standards, however, they were dinosaurs, averaging about the size of a grand piano.

The 1960s through the 1980s brought the space program and the microchip, which allowed for miniaturization of key components of the computer. Thousands of transmitters could be placed on a single chip, and multiple chips could be configured on a single circuit board. Today's technology, which allows the widespread computerization of information, would have been unimaginable just one generation ago. The computer on your desk today means the future has arrived!

Types of Computers

Four basic types of computers are used today: supercomputers, mainframe computers, minicomputers, and personal computers. Each type of computer is suitable for a certain type of work in a particular kind of workplace.

Supercomputers

Supercomputers are the biggest, fastest, and most complex computers in use today. They are primarily used in research in medicine and are considered to be the hope of the medicine of tomorrow. They are used for genetic coding and for DNA and cancer research.

Mainframe Computers

Often used by government facilities and large institutions, including universities and hospitals, mainframes can process and store huge quantities of information. Mainframe computers are used for large governmental service programs such as Medicare and Medicaid.

Minicomputers

Minicomputers are smaller than mainframes but larger than personal computers. Minicomputers have traditionally been used in network settings. A **network** is a system that links several computers together. In this environment a minicomputer typically functions as a server, which is a computer used as a centralized storage location for shared information. Today, however, personal computers are becoming as powerful as minicomputers and may eventually replace them.

Personal Computers

Also called microcomputers, personal computers can be found in homes, offices, and schools. They are ideal for these settings because they are small, self-contained units. Because users have different needs, personal computers are available in three different types: desktop, notebook, and palmtop.

Desktop. The most common type of personal computer, a desktop model fits easily on a desk or other flat surface. The system unit of many newer desktop models is housed in a **tower case,** which extends vertically instead of horizontally. A tower case—often placed on the floor next to the desk—allows more surface area at the workstation (see Figure 6-1). Both large and small medical offices commonly use desktop computers.

Notebook. A notebook computer (also called a laptop) is small—about the size of a thick magazine—and weighs only a few pounds. Notebooks operate either on battery power or on an AC adapter. As advances in technology make notebooks smaller, more powerful, and less expensive, they are expected to become more popular. Their portability makes them especially convenient for people who travel on business. Using notebook computers, physicians and other health-care professionals can communicate with the medical office computer from their homes or any other location.

Hardware

The computer's hardware serves four main functions: inputting data, processing data, storing data, and outputting data. Various hardware components are needed to perform each of these functions.

Input Devices. For a computer to handle information, such as patient records, the data must first be entered, or input. Several types of input devices may be used to enter data into the computer. Keyboards, pointing devices, modems, and scanners are input devices. After information is entered into the computer, it can be displayed on the monitor, processed, or stored.

Keyboard. The keyboard is the most common input device. The main part of a keyboard resembles a typewriter. Most keyboards have several additional keys, however. A typical keyboard contains the following:

- Standard typewriter keys to enter letters, numbers, symbols, and punctuation marks
- Separate numerical keypad for entering numbers faster and more easily
- Arrow keys to move the **cursor,** a blinking line or cube on the computer screen showing where the next character that is keyed will appear
- Function keys to perform such tasks as saving and printing files

When you use the keyboard, it is important to position your hands properly to avoid injury. The Diseases and Disorders section provides tips for preventing and coping with carpal tunnel syndrome, a condition resulting from repetitive motion.

Pointing Device. Many of today's sophisticated software programs need not only a keyboard but also a pointing device to enter information into the computer. When you move the pointing device, an arrow appears. You can point and click the arrow on various buttons that appear on the screen. The three types of pointing devices are the mouse, the trackball, and the touch pad.

1. A mouse, the most common pointing device, has two or three buttons on top and a rolling ball on the bottom. You move the mouse across a mouse pad until the arrow points at the desired button or object on the screen. Then, as shown in Figure 6-3, you push one of the buttons on the mouse to access a function, such as opening a file.
2. A trackball is similar to a mouse except that the rolling ball is on the top of the device instead of on the bottom. Rather than pushing a trackball across a pad, you roll the ball with your fingers while the trackball remains stationary.
3. A touch pad is the newest type of pointing device and is becoming popular, especially on notebook computers. It is a small, flat device that is highly sensitive to the touch. To move the arrow on the screen, you

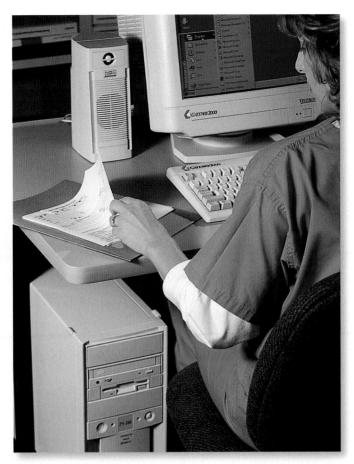

Figure 6-1. Offices can free up much-needed desktop space by using computers in tower cases, which can be kept on the floor.

Palmtop. As the name suggests, a palmtop computer is about the size of your palm and is extremely light. Because they are so small, palmtops generally cannot perform all the functions of desktop or even notebook computers. The keyboard of a palmtop does not contain all the extra function keys found on a standard keyboard, and the keys themselves are quite small. For these reasons, palmtops are usually not used for such tasks as word processing. They may, however, be useful for health-care professionals who need to enter patient data from locations outside the medical office.

Components of the Computer

Computer components are divided into hardware and software. **Hardware** comprises the physical components of a computer system, including the monitor, keyboard, and printer. **Software** is a set of instructions, or a program, that tells the computer what to do. Software includes both the operating system and applications that run on the operating system.

Carpal Tunnel Syndrome

As the number of computers used in the home and workplace has escalated in recent years, the number of cases of carpal tunnel syndrome has also risen dramatically. Carpal tunnel syndrome is a hand disorder that is often associated with computer use. The term for this condition comes from the name for a canal (the carpal tunnel) located in the wrist. Several tendons pass through this tunnel, allowing the hand to open and close.

Carpal tunnel syndrome results from repetitive motion, such as keyboarding, for hours at a time. This motion may cause swelling to develop around the tendons and carpal tunnel. The swelling compresses the nerve. The people most likely to develop carpal tunnel syndrome are workers whose jobs require them to perform repetitive hand and finger motions.

Symptoms

The symptoms associated with carpal tunnel syndrome include the following:

- Tingling or burning in the hands or fingers
- Weakness or numbness in the hands or fingers
- Hands that go to sleep frequently
- Difficulty opening or closing the hands
- Pain that stems from the wrist and travels up the arm

Tips for Prevention

If you use a keyboard for extended periods, you should practice proper techniques to prevent carpal tunnel syndrome.

- While seated, hold your arms relaxed at your sides, and check to make sure that your keyboard is positioned slightly higher than your elbows. As you input, keep your elbows at your sides, and relax your shoulders (see Figure 6-2).
- Use only your fingers to press keys, and do not use more pressure than necessary. Use a wrist rest, and keep your wrists relaxed and straight.

- When you need to strike difficult-to-reach keys, move your whole hand rather than stretching your fingers. When you need to press two keys at the same time, such as "Control" and "F1," use two hands.
- Try to break up long periods of keyboard work with other tasks that do not require computer use.

Tips for Relieving Symptoms

If you have symptoms of carpal tunnel syndrome, try these suggestions for relief.

- Elevate your arms
- Wear a splint on the hand and forearm
- Discuss your symptoms with a physician, who may prescribe medication

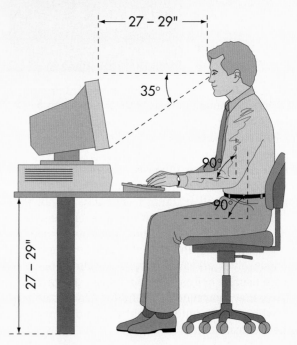

Figure 6-2. Maintaining proper posture and hand positions helps to avoid strain or injury of the back, eyes, neck, or wrist when keyboarding.

simply slide your finger across the touch pad. To click on an item, you push a button similar to that on a mouse or trackball, or you tap your finger on the touch pad.

Modem. This term **modem** is a shortened form of the words *modulator-demodulator.* A modem is used to transfer information from one computer to another over telephone lines. Because modems allow information to be transferred both to and from a computer, they are considered input/output devices. The speed at which a modem transfers data is called the baud rate. Although the current standard modem speed is 28,800 baud, modem speeds are continually being improved. Modems are essential for any medical office that needs to transfer files electronically, as when submitting insurance claim forms.

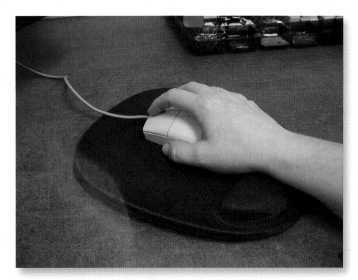

Figure 6-3. Using a mouse, you can point and click to access a variety of functions.

An advanced type of modem is a fax modem. This device allows the computer to send and receive files much as a fax machine does. A fax modem is not quite as versatile as a regular fax machine, however. The information being sent must first be input into the computer. You could not, for example, use a fax modem to send a patient record with handwritten notes on it.

Scanner. A **scanner** is a device used to input printed matter and convert it into a format that can be read by the computer. Scanners are useful in the medical office because patient reports from another doctor, a hospital, or another outside source can be easily entered into the computer. Scanners are also making it possible to move into a paperless medical system. Using a scanner is much faster than keyboarding, or inputting the information with a keyboard. Three types of scanners are available:

1. Handheld scanners are generally the least expensive but are more difficult to use and produce lower-quality results than the other two types.

2. A single-sheet scanner feeds one sheet of paper through at a time and looks similar to a single-sheet printer.

3. A flatbed scanner is the most expensive type of scanner but is the easiest to use and produces the highest-quality input. It works much like a small photocopier: the paper lies flat and still on a glass surface while the machine scans it.

Processing Devices. There are two major processing components inside the system unit, or computer cabinet. The **motherboard** is the main circuit board that controls the other components in the system. The **central processing unit (CPU),** or microprocessor, is the primary computer chip responsible for interpreting and executing programs.

How quickly the computer processes information depends on the type of microprocessor and its speed, which is measured in megahertz (MHz) or gigahertz (GHz). Most microprocessors are known by a number, such as 600 MHz or 3 GHz. A popular microprocessor is the Intel Pentium. Today's microprocessors are commonly measured in gigahertz. One gigahertz equals 1000 megahertz.

Storage Devices. One of the main tasks of a computer is to store information for later retrieval. The computer uses memory to store information either temporarily or permanently. Several types of drives are used for permanent information storage.

Memory. Computers use two types of memory to store data: **random-access memory (RAM)** and read-only memory (ROM). RAM is temporary, or programmable, memory. While you are working on a software program, the computer is accessing RAM. In general, the more RAM that is available, the faster the computer will perform. As software programs become more sophisticated, they require more RAM. Only a few years ago, 32 megabytes (MB) of RAM was the minimum amount needed to run most programs. (Megabytes are a measurement of memory space.) Today, however, many applications require much more RAM.

Read-only memory (ROM) is permanent memory. The computer can read it, but you cannot make changes to it. The purpose of ROM is to provide the basic operating instructions the computer needs to function.

Hard Disk Drive. The hard disk drive is where information is stored permanently for later retrieval. Software programs and important data are usually stored on the hard disk for quick and easy access. The amount of hard disk space needed to store software programs is increasing rapidly. The more software programs you want to store, the larger the hard disk you will need. Older computers have a 500- or 850-MB hard disk. Many newer computers have a hard disk capacity of 20 gigabytes (GB) to 250 gigabytes or more.

Diskette Drive. The diskette drive can read from and write to diskettes (also called disks). Flexible 5¼-inch disks, which were once commonly used, are now outdated. The standard diskette format in current use is 3½-inch disks, which are rigid. These disks are more compact and can store more information than the older, longer disks.

CD-ROM Drive. CD-ROMs look just like audio compact discs, but they contain software programs. The term **CD-ROM** stands for "compact disc—read-only memory." The main advantage of a CD-ROM over a diskette is its ability to store huge amounts of data.

CD-ROM drives have become standard equipment on most personal computers. Although many software packages are available on both CD-ROM and diskettes, some large programs are available only on CD-ROM. These programs include multimedia applications such as medical encyclopedias. **Multimedia** refers to software that uses more than one medium—such as graphics, sound, and text—to convey information.

Tape Drive. This storage device is used to back up (make a copy of) the files on the hard disk. The information is copied onto magnetic tapes that resemble audiotapes. If the hard drive malfunctions, you will have a copy of the information on these tapes. It is possible to back up the information onto diskettes. Most hard disks, however, contain so much information that a large number of diskettes would be required to back up all the data. With most tape drives, the entire contents of the hard disk can be stored on one or two tapes. Store these tapes at night in a fireproof container.

Output Devices. Output devices are used to display information after it has been processed. A monitor and a printer are two output devices needed in the medical office.

Monitor. A computer monitor looks like a television screen. It displays the information that is currently active, such as a word processing document, an Internet link, or e-mail. Monitors are available in color; all of the software programs that are used today, including multimedia applications, require a color monitor to run.

Color monitors vary in the number of colors they can display and in the resolution of the images. *Resolution* refers to the crispness of the images and is measured in dot pitch. The lower the dot pitch, the higher the resolution. For example, a monitor with a 0.26 dot pitch displays sharper images than a monitor with a 0.39 dot pitch. Using a high-resolution monitor can help you avoid eye strain.

Printer. A printer is required to produce a **hard copy,** which is a readable paper copy or printout of information (see Figure 6-4). You will need a printer to print out correspondence, patient reports, bills, insurance claims, and other documents. Printer resolution is noted in terms of dots per inch (dpi). The higher the dpi, the better the print quality. Printer output varies, depending on the type of printer and the model. The three most commonly used printers are dot matrix, ink-jet, and laser.

1. **Dot matrix printers** create characters by placing a series of tiny dots next to one another. The dot matrix printer is the only type that is an impact printer, which means that it makes an impression on the paper as it prints. Although it is the least expensive of the three types, the dot matrix printer is slower and noisier and produces a lower-quality output than the other types. Because it is an impact printer, however, it is the only type that is capable of producing multiple copies with carbon paper or other multicopy forms.

2. **Ink-jet printers** also form characters using a series of dots, but they are nonimpact printers in which the dots are created by tiny drops of ink. Many ink-jet printers are capable of printing in both black and color. Because of their high-quality output and affordable prices, ink-jet printers are popular for home and small-office use.

3. **Laser printers** are high-resolution printers that use a technology similar to that of photocopiers. Of the three printer types, laser printers are the fastest and produce the highest-quality output. Laser printers are more expensive than dot matrix or ink-jet printers. Prices have dropped significantly over the years, however, so laser printers may be affordable even for small medical offices.

Because each type of printer has advantages and disadvantages, some medical offices may purchase more than one type. For example, a medical office may have a dot matrix printer for creating internal memos and multipage insurance forms and a laser printer for creating documents whose quality resembles that of typeset documents.

A current trend in printers is the "all-in-one" model, which functions not only as an ink-jet printer but also as a fax machine, scanner, and photocopier. This type of machine may be convenient for a small medical office that requires each of these functions but does not have space for four separate devices. In addition, purchasing an all-in-one unit is usually more economical than purchasing the machines separately.

Software

Computer software is generally divided into two categories: operating system and application software. The operating system controls the computer's operation. Application software allows you to perform specific tasks, such as scheduling appointments.

Operating System. When you turn on a computer, the operating system starts working, providing instructions that the computer needs to function. Because most medical practices use IBM-compatible personal computers, the

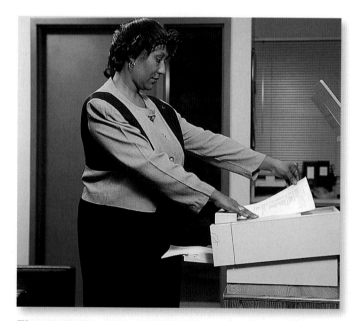

Figure 6-4. You may need to print out hard copies of documents to send to patients, vendors, insurance companies, or other doctors' offices.

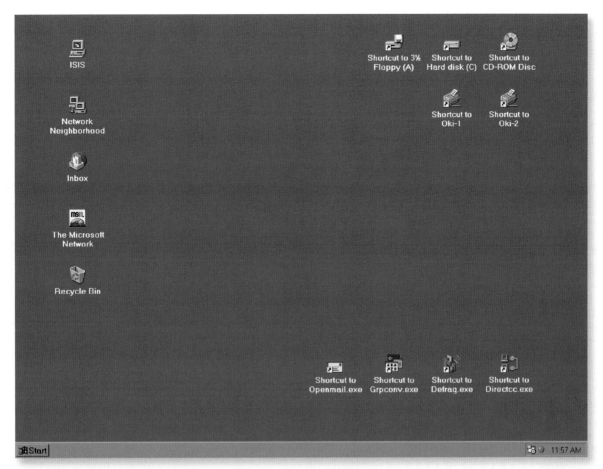

Figure 6-5. The Windows 2000 operating system employs a graphical user interface. Icons identify programs or other menu choices.

operating systems discussed here are DOS (disk operating system) and Microsoft Windows and Windows 2000. IBM-compatible computers are most suitable for businesses that use computers primarily to manipulate words. Apple computers are used by businesses, such as advertising agencies or design firms, that are extensively involved in graphics, visual images, or desktop publishing.

DOS. DOS is the original operating system created for IBM and IBM-compatible computers. It uses a command line interface—you must learn and use commands to perform certain tasks. For example, to copy a file from a hard drive to a diskette drive, you must type a command that instructs the computer to copy the file.

Windows. This operating system employs a graphical user interface (GUI) instead of a command line interface. With a GUI, menu choices are identified by **icons,** or graphic symbols. For example, the "Print" command is usually identified by a button with a tiny illustration of a printer on it. To print a document, you move the pointing device until the arrow is on the printer icon and then click the button.

An important advantage of the Windows operating system over DOS is that it is easier to learn because you do not have to remember commands. Another benefit of Windows is that it is a **multitasking** system—users can run two or more software programs simultaneously. You

could, for example, enter patient information into a **database,** a collection of records created and stored on the computer, while a word processing program is running in the background. DOS is not a multitasking system; you can run only one application at a time.

Windows 2000. This operating system, introduced in 2000, is similar to Windows but has many additional features (see Figure 6-5). In most businesses, Windows 2000 is quickly becoming the standard operating system for IBM and IBM-compatible computers. Most new computers are shipped with Windows 2000 preinstalled, and many software programs are being written to run exclusively under this operating system.

Applications. Most of the software sold in stores is application software. It is used for a specific purpose, or application. Word processing, database, and accounting software are just a few examples of the wide variety of applications available.

Using Computer Software

Computer software has been developed for nearly every office function imaginable. Using software, you can complete tasks with greater speed, accuracy, and ease than with a manual system. Learning how to use the software correctly, however, is the key to getting the most out of your computer system.

Word Processing

In the medical office, as in any office, word processing is a common computer application. It has replaced the typewriter for writing correspondence and reports, transcribing physicians' notes, and performing many other functions. Correcting errors is easy on a word processor, and you can save documents for later retrieval and modification. Procedure 6-1 shows you how to use a word processing program to create a form letter. A form letter can be merged with a patient mailing list to create letters that are personalized with patients' names.

Database Management

A database is a collection of records created and stored on a computer. In a medical office, databases are used to store patient records such as billing information, medical chart data, and insurance company facts. These records can be sorted and retrieved in many ways and for a variety of

purposes. You may be asked to find, add to, or modify information in a database. For example, you might use a database to determine all the patients covered by a particular insurance company.

Accounting and Billing

Accounting and billing software is extremely useful in an office environment. It enables you to perform many tasks, including keeping track of patients' accounts, creating billing statements, preparing financial reports, and maintaining tax records. (You will learn more about accounting and billing functions in Chapters 17 and 18.)

Appointment Scheduling

Instead of writing in an appointment book, you can use software to schedule appointments. Some scheduling packages allow you to enter patient preferences, such as day of the week and time, and then to list available appointments based on that information. If the office system is on a network, scheduling software is particularly valuable, because more than one user can access the appointment schedule at a time.

PROCEDURE 6.1

Creating a Form Letter

Objective: To use a word processing program to create a form letter

Materials: Computer equipped with a word processing program, printer, form letter to be input, 8½-by-11-inch paper.

Method

1. Turn on the computer. Select the word processing program.
2. Use the keyboard to begin entering text into a new document.
3. To edit text, press the arrow keys to move the cursor to the position at which you want to insert or delete characters, and enter the text. Use the "Insert" mode to add characters or the "Typeover" mode to type over and replace existing text.
4. To delete text, position the cursor to the left of the characters to be deleted and press the "Delete" key. Alternatively, place the cursor to the right of the characters to be deleted and press the "Backspace" key (the left-pointing

arrow usually found at the top right corner of the keyboard).

5. If you need to move an entire block of text, you must begin by highlighting it. In most Windows-based programs, you first click the mouse at the beginning of the text to be highlighted. Then you hold down the left mouse button, drag the mouse to the end of the block of text, and release your finger from the mouse. The text should now be highlighted. Choose the button or command for cutting text. Then move the cursor to the place where you want to insert the text, and select the button or command for retrieving or pasting text.
6. As you input the letter, it is important to save your work every 15 minutes or so. Some programs do this automatically. If yours does not, use the "Save" command or button to save the file. Be sure to save the file again when you have completed the letter.
7. Print the letter using the "Print" command or button.

Electronic Transactions

Using a computer equipped with a modem and communications software, you can perform several types of electronic transactions. This technology enables you to send and receive information instantaneously rather than waiting the days or weeks required for regular mail. Common electronic transactions include sending insurance claims and communicating with other computer users.

Sending Insurance Claims. Insurance claims can be submitted directly from the medical office to an insurance company. This procedure enables claims to be processed quickly and efficiently. (Processing insurance claims is discussed in Chapter 15.)

Communicating. The ability to communicate and share information with other computer users and systems is important in many medical offices. This communication may take place through electronic mail, online services, and the Internet. The Tips for the Office section gives ideas for saving time and money while you are online.

Electronic Mail. Commonly known as e-mail, **electronic mail** is a method of sending and receiving messages through a network. Through e-mail, you can communicate with computer users in your own office, across town, or on the other side of the world.

Online Services. These services, known as *servers*, provide a means for health-care professionals to communicate with one another. Most online services contain forums that

Tips for the Office

Saving Time and Money Online

If the medical office where you work is computerized, the system most likely has a modem for sending e-mail and transferring files electronically. The modem may also be used to access various online services and the Internet, a global network of computers. If this access is not currently available in the medical office, it probably will be in the near future. You may even be asked to help choose an online service or Internet provider for the office.

These services, known as *Internet Service Providers (ISPs)* allow access to a network of servers that provides a means for health-care professionals to communicate with one another. Unless the people using these services are careful, however, this access can be very costly. In general, the more time you spend online, the more expensive the service becomes. For this reason, knowing how to use these communications systems wisely is a valuable asset.

Choosing an Online Service

Compare several services for the following features:

- Free trial membership. Many services offer a free 1-month membership to try out the service. The trial periods enable office staff members to test several services to determine which one best suits their needs.
- Local access telephone number. Make sure the service provides an access number within the local dialing area of the office. If it does not, the office will be charged long-distance telephone rates each time someone goes online. These fees are separate from the online service's rates and can add up quickly.
- Volume discount plan. If the office will be using the online service often, find a provider that

offers a discount for frequent usage. Rather than charging a per-hour rate over the first 5 hours of use, for example, these services charge a flat rate for 20 or 30 hours of use per month. Some offer unlimited use for a flat rate.

- Extra fees. Although access to most of the information found in online services is included in the membership fee, some providers charge extra for premium or extended services. If you want to read or print out the full text of an article in a medical journal, for example, some providers charge an additional fee. Make sure you consider these extra fees when comparing costs of online services.
- Availability of health-care information. Some online services provide discussion groups (commonly known as chat rooms) and resources that would be useful to the medical office. Other services may not offer as much relevant information. By comparing several services, you can determine which service best meets the needs of the practice.

Sending and Receiving E-Mail

When using e-mail, follow these guidelines to manage your online time efficiently.

- Compose messages off-line. Most services allow you to write e-mail messages before you actually go online. When you have finished writing the message, you simply log onto the service and click a button to send the e-mail. This technique will save a great deal of online time, especially if you must frequently send lengthy messages.

continued ——→

offer information and discussion groups focusing on a wide range of medical topics. Health-care workers can learn about the latest medical research and technology or exchange ideas with others in their field. In addition, some online services provide access to medical databases such as MEDLINE, created by the National Library of Medicine. Users can search MEDLINE for records and abstracts from thousands of medical journals from around the world.

Internet. The **Internet** is a global network of computers. Through the Internet, you can communicate with millions of computer users around the world. In addition, many large medical facilities, universities, and other organizations—such as the National Institutes of Health and the Centers for Disease Control and Prevention—provide medical resources, databases, and other information on the Internet. Users can visit such Internet sites as the Virtual Hospital, sponsored by the University of Iowa, and the Cyberspace Hospital, sponsored by the National University of Singapore. At these sites you may find multimedia textbooks, presentations, and links to other related sites on the Internet. Table 6-1 describes these and other popular medical resources available on the Internet.

Research

The advent of CD-ROM technology has revolutionized the world of research. Not only can an immense amount of information be contained on one compact disc, but the CD-ROM usually provides additional information in the form of videos and sound (see Figure 6-6). A CD-ROM encyclopedia, for example, might also provide spoken pronunciations of medical terms. This type of software may help patients—especially children—understand the human body as well as various medical conditions.

Software Training

Software programs may seem quite complex. Most people need a period of training before they feel comfortable using the application. Several methods of training—some from outside sources and some provided by the software manufacturer—are available.

Classes. Many computer vendors offer training classes for the software packages they sell. In addition, community colleges and high schools sometimes offer adult education classes for a variety of applications, including word processing and communications. These classes may be at the beginner, intermediate, or advanced level.

Tutorials. Many software packages come with a **tutorial,** which is a small program designed to give users an overall picture of the product and its functions. The tutorial usually provides a step-by-step walk-through and exercises in which you can try out your newly acquired knowledge.

TABLE 6-1 Medical Resources on the Internet

Organization	Web Address	Description
American Medical Association	http://www.ama-assn.org	News announcements and press releases; articles from *JAMA* and other AMA journals; links to other medicine-related Internet sites
Cyberspace Hospital	http://ch.nus.sg	Various departments and services, organized like a real hospital; medical bulletins; capability for users to search for information on medical topics
HealthWeb	http://hsinfo.ghsl.nwu.edu/healthweb/index.html	Starting point for searching the Internet because it contains links to a wide variety of medical resources
National Institutes of Health	http://www.nih.gov	Medical news and current events; press releases; biomedical information about health issues; scientific resources; links to Internet sites of related government agencies
National Library of Medicine	http://www.nlm.nih.gov	Internet site for world's largest biomedical library; research and development activities; connections to online medical information services
New England Journal of Medicine	http://www.nejm.org	Articles and abstracts; archives of past issues
U.S. Department of Health and Human Services	http://www.os.dhhs.gov	Programs and activities of this agency; links to divisions of agency, including Centers for Disease Control and Prevention, Food and Drug Administration, and National Institutes of Health
Virtual Hospital	http://vh.radiology.uiowa.edu	Information on a variety of health issues, medical resources, tutorials, and multimedia textbooks

Documentation.   Nearly all software manufacturers provide some type of documentation with their programs. Documentation is usually in the form of written instruction manuals or online help that is accessed from within the program.

Manuals.   Some manuals provide detailed information on software operation and may include an index and sections on troubleshooting and commonly asked questions. Other manuals may simply give installation instructions and brief information on program basics. This type of manual may refer users to the software's online help.

On-Line Help.   In most software applications, users access the online help screen by clicking on a "Help" button or by pressing a certain function key, such as "F1." The online

help usually provides a "Contents" section (shown in Figure 6-7), in which you can browse for topics. An index, in which you can search for key words, is also provided.

Technical Support.   A software company's technical support service is designed to assist you with problems that go beyond the scope of the user's guide or manual. A call to technical support is important when you encounter a problem that cannot be solved by simple problem-solving techniques. By calling a toll-free number, you can access a knowledgeable team who will listen to the description of the problem and suggest solutions over the phone.

Before calling technical support:

- Check the system for errors to the best of your ability. Check your manual for answers. Ask your supervisor for assistance.

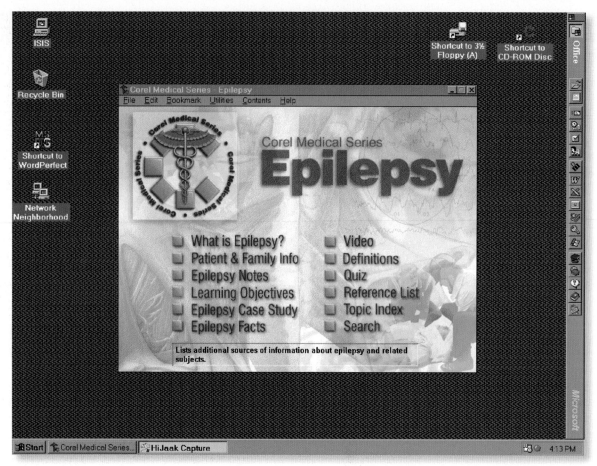

Figure 6-6. A CD-ROM provides features, such as video and sound, that are not possible in a standard printed book.

- Have the software registration number available.
- Be prepared to follow the instructions of the technical support personnel.
- Plan to call from a location that gives ready access to the computer with the problem.

Technical support is also helpful when you are upgrading software. Some software companies automatically notify their customers of available upgrades. The technical support service is always a good source of information regarding the latest products and their applications.

Selecting Computer Equipment

Perhaps you are working in a medical office that is not yet computerized. If the decision is made to convert to a computerized system, you may be asked to help select equipment. Even if your office already uses computers, the system will probably need to be upgraded at some point to provide more functions. In either situation, you may be asked for your input in selecting software, adding a network, or choosing a vendor.

The first step for helping in the selection process is to learn as much as you can about hardware and software. You can get information by taking an introductory computer class at an adult school or community college; by reading computer magazines or books; or by talking to friends, relatives, or coworkers who use computers.

Converting to a Computerized Office

When an office converts from a manual system to computers, staff members should determine how the new computer system will be used. The objective is to obtain a system that not only meets current office needs but that can also be expanded and upgraded to meet future needs. To get the longest use from a computer system, a good general guideline is to buy the most advanced system possible within the allowed budget.

Upgrading the Office System

Computer hardware is changing and improving at such a rapid pace that a new system seems to become outdated

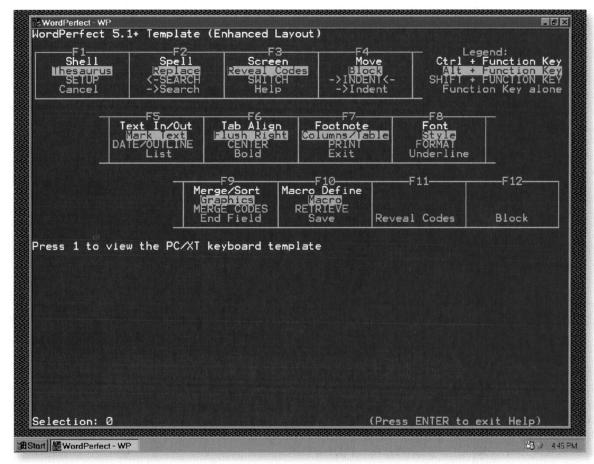

Figure 6-7. An online help system allows you to access helpful information when you are using a software program.

almost as soon as it is purchased. In addition, more-advanced software is introduced every day, and this software requires more-advanced hardware to run. Consequently, an office system purchased only a year or two ago may need to be upgraded. Sometimes an upgrade simply requires replacement or addition of certain components. For instance, a laser printer can take the place of a dot matrix printer, or a CD-ROM drive can be added. In other cases, such a solution is not possible or cost-effective, so an entirely new system must be purchased.

Selecting Software

After a decision is made regarding the type of software needed, such as an accounting program, a specific product must be chosen. To make an informed decision, you can read software reviews in computer magazines or trade publications. You might also check with other medical offices to get opinions on software packages. A crucial step in selecting software is to make sure the office computer system meets the minimum system requirements listed on the software box. For example, a medical encyclopedia may require a 486 SX processor, Windows 98, 16 MB of RAM, 30 MB of available hard disk space, and a CD-ROM drive.

Adding a Network

There are several advantages to adding a network to the computer system in a medical office. A computer network enables users to share software programs and files and allows more than one person to work on the same patient's information at one time. While you are working on a patient's insurance claim, for example, another assistant might be inputting billing information. Some medical offices are virtually paperless. They use a highly sophisticated network with a notebook or desktop computer in every examination room (Figure 6-8). Doctors input information into patients' computerized charts. If a doctor is in her office and a patient is waiting, a staff member at the front desk sends an e-mail message to the doctor's desktop computer, and a beep sounds as an alert. Networks also allow large medical facilities to communicate with employees via e-mail. For instance, an internal memo about changes in office policies may be sent by e-mail to all employees.

Choosing a Vendor

When purchasing computer equipment, you should look for a reputable vendor who not only offers a reasonable price but also provides training, service, and technical

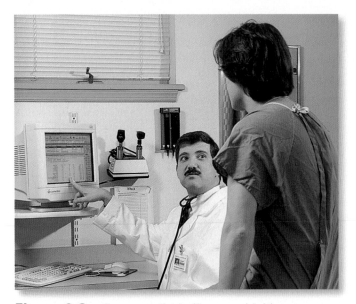

Figure 6-8. Some medical offices use highly sophisticated computer networks.

support. A first step might be to check with personnel in other medical offices that use a computer system. Find out which dealer they use and if they are satisfied with the system, salespeople, and support. You can also ask dealers for names of references—medical offices that have purchased systems from them. It is a good idea to get cost estimates from at least three vendors, and it is preferable to buy all hardware components from the same vendor.

Security in the Computerized Office

Although security measures are important in any office, they are especially important in a computerized medical office. Great care must be taken to safeguard confidential files, make backup copies on a regular basis, and prevent system contamination.

Safeguarding Confidential Files

Much of the information collected in a medical office is confidential. Just as with paper records, confidential information stored on the computer should be accessible only to authorized personnel. Two common ways to provide security in a computerized office are to employ passwords and to install an activity-monitoring system.

Passwords. In many hospitals and physicians' offices, each employee who is allowed access to computerized patient files is given a password. The employee must enter the password into the computer when using the files. Access codes or passwords only allow the user into approved areas according to the individual's job description. If you are given a password, do not divulge it to anyone else

unless your office manager asks you to do so. If an employee leaves or is fired, that person's password should be immediately erased from the system.

Activity-Monitoring Systems. In conjunction with passwords, some health-care facilities use a computer system that monitors user activity. Whenever someone accesses computer records, the system automatically keeps track of the user's name and the files that have been viewed or modified. In this way, problems or security breaches can be traced back to specific employees.

Making and Storing Backup Files

For securing important computer files, it is essential to routinely make diskette or tape backups of them (see Figure 6-9). How often backups are made varies among medical offices; your supervisor will tell you the policy for your office. Just as important as making the backups is storing them properly. Backup files should not be stored near the original files. Ideally, they should be kept outside the medical office—perhaps at the physician's home—so that they will be secure in case of fire, burglary, or other catastrophe at the office.

Preventing System Contamination

Another important security issue in the computerized medical office is computer viruses. Computer viruses are

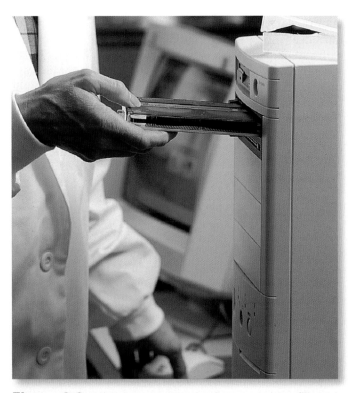

Figure 6-9. It is important to back up computer files and store them properly.

programs written specifically to contaminate the hard disk by damaging or destroying data.

One way that viruses can be passed from computer to computer is through shared diskettes that have been infected. Another way is through infected files retrieved from online services, the Internet, and electronic bulletin boards. Several software programs are available to detect and correct computer viruses. Most are fairly inexpensive but provide an invaluable service.

Computer System Care and Maintenance

Like a car, a computer needs routine care and maintenance to stay in sound condition. The computer user's manual outlines the steps required. Also, a good general rule is not to eat or drink near the computer. Crumbs and spilled liquids can damage the system components and storage devices.

System Unit

The system unit should be placed in a well-ventilated location, with nothing blocking the fan in the back of the cabinet. To keep the system's delicate circuitry from being damaged by an electrical power surge, you should use a power strip with a surge protector. You plug the computer into the power strip, and then plug the power strip into the electrical outlet.

Monitor

The computer monitor needs to be protected from screen burn-in, which may happen if the same image stays on the computer screen for an extended time. To prevent burn-in, you can use a **screen saver,** which automatically changes the monitor display at short intervals or constantly shows moving images. All Windows operating systems come equipped with screen savers. A wide variety of screen savers are also available as separate software packages.

To protect their screens, many newer monitors "power down" after a certain period of inactivity. If no one uses the computer for 30 minutes, for example, the monitor screen goes blank. To resume using the computer after the screen saver has been activated or the monitor has powered down, you simply touch any key or move the mouse.

Printer

Maintenance of a printer generally consists of replacing the ribbon, ink cartridge, or toner cartridge. You can tell when the ribbon or cartridge needs to be changed because the ink on your printouts becomes very light.

Replacement is usually a simple process, described in the printer manual.

Information Storage Devices

Diskettes, CD-ROMs, and magnetic tapes are highly sensitive devices. Even a small scratch may cause permanent damage or make it impossible to retrieve data. To avoid problems, handle and store disks and tapes properly.

Diskettes. Diskettes should be kept away from magnetic fields, such as a paper clip holder that has a magnet in it. They should also be kept out of direct sunlight and away from extreme temperatures. Although 3½-inch disks are sturdy they should be handled with care. They should be labeled appropriately and stored in a durable storage case.

CD-ROMs. Figure 6-10 shows the proper way to handle a CD-ROM. When you pick it up, touch only the edges or the edge and the hole in the center. CD-ROMs should be stored in the clear plastic case in which they are packaged, sometimes called a jewel case. If a CD-ROM becomes dusty or smudged with fingerprints, you can clean it by rubbing it gently with a soft cloth. Always rub from the center to the outside. *Never* rub in a circular motion.

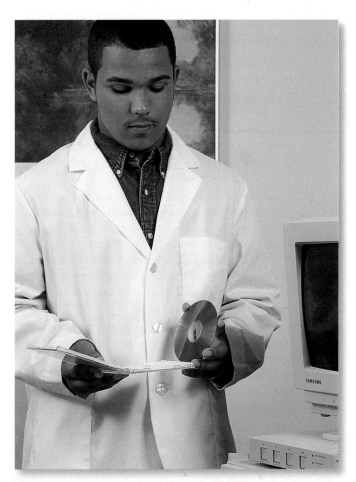

Figure 6-10. When handling a CD-ROM, be careful not to touch the flat surface of the disc.

Dental Office Administrator

To gain medical assistant credentials, you must fulfill the requirements of either the American Association of Medical Assistants (for a Certified Medical Assistant) or the American Medical Technologists (for a Registered Medical Assistant). After obtaining your medical assistant certification or registration, you may wish to acquire additional skills in specialty areas through course work or on-the-job training. Although this course work or training may not lead to an additional certification or degree, it will enable you to expand your role in the medical office and advance your career as the demand for skilled health professionals increases.

Skills and Duties

A dental office administrator carries out clerical and administrative duties for a dentist or a dental group. His duties may vary with the size of the practice. In a large practice he may oversee the clerical staff. In a small practice he may have more varied tasks, including staffing the reception desk, maintaining records, and performing other support services.

The duties of a dental office administrator mostly fall into the following six categories:

1. Communication. In many offices, this task is the administrator's main responsibility. He answers the telephones and manages the correspondence for the practice, which may include billing.
2. Reception. The office administrator greets and welcomes patients. He must have a knowledge of dental terminology in order to assist patients with dental paperwork.
3. Scheduling. The dental office administrator coordinates patient appointments and may schedule referrals with other specialists, such as orthodontists. He may also maintain the schedules of the dental hygienists and other office staff. Sometimes the administrator is responsible for calling patients to confirm appointments ahead of time.
4. Records and filing. The administrator may manage the patient records and other files. He attaches dental x-rays to the appropriate records and maintains up-to-date insurance information to ensure accurate billing.
5. Support duties. The dental office administrator has a range of other duties that vary from practice to practice. Typically, he is responsible for managing office supplies. He often needs to type or take shorthand. He also uses computer and word processing skills. Specialized skills, such as bookkeeping, may also be helpful.

6. Supervision. In a large dental practice, the administrator trains and oversees clerical staff and secretaries.

Workplace Settings

Dental office administrators may work in a private practice, a group practice, or a dental clinic.

Education

Dental office administrators often learn the dental and medical terminology they need on the job. They may acquire secretarial training by taking courses, either in a business/vocational school or in a junior or community college. A high school diploma is usually required. Further education may be necessary in a practice where the administrator must supervise other staff members.

Where to Go for More Information

American Academy of Dental Practice
  Administrators
1063 Whippoorwill Lane
Palatine, IL 60067
(312) 934-4404

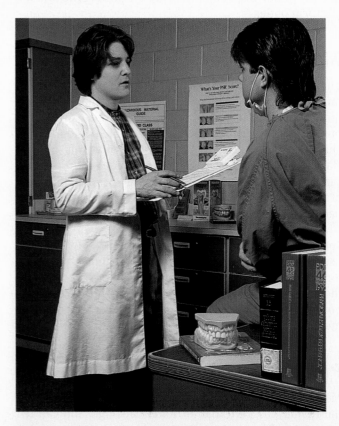

Communication is the dental office administrator's most important task.

Magnetic Tapes. These tapes should be treated much as you would treat audiotapes. They should be stored in a relatively cool, dry place, away from magnetic fields.

Computers of the Future

Computers are evolving at such a rapid pace that it is virtually impossible to predict the changes that will take place even in the next few years. Some important new technologies, however, have already been introduced in the medical office and will be improved in the near future. Telemedicine, CD-R technology, and speech recognition technology are only three examples of new computer technologies. Undoubtedly, more will be explored and developed every year.

Telemedicine

Telemedicine refers to the use of telecommunications to transmit video images of patient information. These images are already used to provide medical support to physicians caring for patients in rural areas. Some experts feel that telemedicine has great potential and that advancements in computer technology will make telemedicine more popular in the future.

CD-R Technology

While CD-ROMs can only be *read* by the computer, CD-R (compact disc–recordable) media can be read *and* written to. CD-R technology allows you to use compact discs like diskettes—to store data and information. Recordable CDs, however, can store much more information than diskettes can. Although CD-R technology is currently available, it is not yet widely used because it is still fairly expensive.

Speech Recognition Technology

This technology enables the computer to comprehend and interpret spoken words. The user simply speaks into a microphone instead of inputting information with a keyboard or a scanner. Because every human voice is different, however, and the English language is vast and complex, this technology is difficult to perfect. As speech recognition technology becomes more advanced, more accurate, and less expensive, it will most likely gain widespread acceptance. It has a great deal of potential, including the ability to virtually eliminate the need for medical assistants to transcribe physicians' notes.

Summary

Most medical offices have already converted from a paper-based system of record keeping to a computer-based one. You should familiarize yourself with the types of computers available and the hardware and software components that make up a computer system. A variety of software programs are used in the medical office, including word processing, database management, accounting and billing, appointment scheduling, and electronic transactions, such as submitting insurance claims. Other computer technology you need to know about includes modems, scanners, and CD-ROM software.

Whether you are converting to a computerized office or simply upgrading an existing system, learn the guidelines for selecting computer hardware and software. In a computerized office it is also important to know how to secure computerized files and to care for and maintain computer equipment.

REVIEW

CHAPTER 6

CASE STUDY *QUESTIONS*

Now that you have completed this chapter, review the case study at the beginning of the chapter and answer the following questions:

1. Are you more like Chris or Alicia? What background do you bring to the study of computers that makes you feel the way you do?
2. Why is it important for an office to continue to use the manual system at the same time that it converts to a computerized system?
3. Who should be trained in the use of a new computer system in a medical practice? Why?
4. Which group do you think would be the most difficult to train in an average medical practice?

   a. Those who think like Chris?
   b. Those who think like Alicia?
   c. The physicians?

   What would be the best way to approach the group you just identified?

Discussion Questions

1. Compare and contrast the three kinds of printers. What are the advantages of each?
2. What do you think is in the future in the development of computers? Describe your vision of the typical medical office and its use of computers 25 years from now.
3. A new computer system has just been installed at your office. How would you encourage and assist a fellow employee in learning the new system?

Critical Thinking Questions

1. A technical problem is detected on the computer at your desk. What would you do? Explain in detail.
2. A fellow employee asks to use your password to the computer because she has forgotten hers. How do you respond and why?
3. Summarize the proper care and maintenance of computer diskettes and CDs. How does proper care reduce problems?

Application Activities

1. Go online and research the purchase of a new software package for a medical encyclopedia. Which would you recommend for purchase by your office and why?
2. Look through computer magazines or trade journals for descriptions or reviews of the latest software upgrades for your computer system. Describe what new benefits the upgrades offer and how each feature would benefit a medical practice.
3. Research one of the technological advances mentioned in this chapter—telemedicine, CD-R technology, or speech recognition technology—to learn more about it. Find out how the technology benefits the medical office. Write and present a full report on your topic.

CHAPTER 7

Managing Correspondence and Mail

AREAS OF COMPETENCE

2003 Role Delineation Study

ADMINISTRATIVE

Administrative Procedures

- Perform basic administrative medical assisting functions

GENERAL

Communication Skills

- Recognize and respond effectively to verbal, nonverbal, and written communications
- Utilize electronic technology to receive, organize, prioritize, and transmit information

KEY TERMS

- annotate
- clarity
- concise
- courtesy title
- dateline
- editing
- enclosure
- full-block letter style
- identification line
- key
- letterhead
- modified-block letter style
- proofreading
- salutation
- simplified letter style
- template

CHAPTER OUTLINE

- Correspondence and Professionalism
- Choosing Correspondence Supplies
- Written Correspondence
- Effective Writing
- Editing and Proofreading
- Preparing Outgoing Mail
- Mailing Equipment and Supplies
- U.S. Postal Service Delivery
- Other Delivery Services
- Processing Incoming Mail

OBJECTIVES

After completing Chapter 7, you will be able to:

7.1 List the supplies necessary for creating and mailing professional-looking correspondence.

7.2 Identify the types of correspondence used in medical office communications.

7.3 Describe the parts of a letter and the different letter and punctuation styles.

7.4 Compose a business letter.

7.5 Explain the tasks involved in editing and proofreading.

7.6 Describe the process of handling incoming and outgoing mail.

7.7 Compare and contrast the services provided by the U.S. Postal Service and other delivery services.

Introduction

Communication skills are important in every profession. Written materials are tangible demonstrations of an office staff's ability to communicate and conduct business.

Others often evaluate the entire medical practice by the work of one employee. When a letter, form, or document is carelessly prepared and sent into the community, the physician may be judged as "careless." However, when a letter or general business correspondence is constructed in a neat, concise, and well-organized fashion, the physician is often judged to be organized and competent. The skill demonstrated in the creation of a simple business letter reflects on the medical skills of the physician and the practice. Professional image is conveyed in written correspondence.

Because written documents also serve as legal records, all documents must be prepared with great care and attention to detail. The administrative role of the medical assistant includes the creation of documents that are consistently accurate and clear.

In this chapter you will learn how to write effectively. You will develop skills in composing a business letter. You will learn different styles and formats of writing and will learn how to professionally manage all forms of correspondence commonly used in an ambulatory care setting.

CASE STUDY

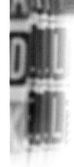

Paula and Tom are medical assistants whose duties include making sure the daily correspondence is created and on the physician's desk before they go home at the end of the day. Today, they are working together to complete these tasks.

Paula will key into the computer letters of referral to other physicians. She is using a template saved within the computer to easily and quickly turn out many different letters. She is simply keying in different fields of information with the specifics for each patient referral. She then prints out a draft copy for proofreading and review by the physician or office manager. Once reviewed, corrected, and approved, she will print out the final letters onto the more expensive letterhead of the office. She will also copy the address from the letters and complete a mailing envelope for each letter.

Tom is assisting as he takes each completed letter and attaches all materials noted as enclosures to each letter. He then folds each letter and its enclosures carefully and inserts them into the properly addressed envelope. Next, he determines the weight of each envelope and the best choice for mailing it. He sorts the mailing into separate piles for different mail handling. The routine mailing is run through the stamp machine. The appropriate forms for the specialty mailing are created and attached. Tom makes sure copies of all mailings are carefully placed in the patient's chart. Both Paula and Tom know the importance of careful and accurate handling of all patient correspondence.

As you read this chapter, consider the following questions:

1. Why is it important to accurately and carefully prepare correspondence for an ambulatory setting? What could the poor management of documents and correspondence mean to a medical practice?
2. What are the differences between the language used in an informal or casual letter and that used in a formal or professional business letter?
3. What are some appropriate shortcuts that can assist in the daily management of correspondence and mailing?
4. What are some factors to consider in choosing the best mode of delivery for letters and parcels?

Correspondence and Professionalism

As in any business, correspondence from health-care professionals to patients and colleagues must be handled carefully, with appropriate attention to content and presentation. By learning how to create, send, and receive correspondence and other types of mail, you can ensure positive, effective communication between your office and others. Well-written, neatly prepared correspondence is one of the most important means of communicating a professional image for the medical office (Figure 7-1).

Choosing Correspondence Supplies

The first step in preparing professional-looking correspondence is choosing the right supplies. Many offices already have most of these supplies on hand. However, you may

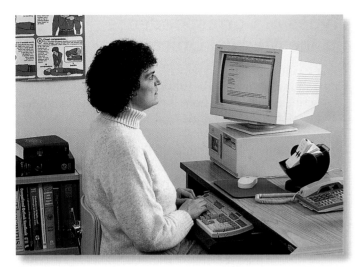

Figure 7-1. The correspondence that goes out of and comes into a medical office is vital to a well-run practice.

be responsible for choosing and ordering such supplies. You may need to make decisions about letterhead paper, envelopes, labels, invoices, and statements.

Letterhead Paper

Letterhead refers to formal business stationery on which the doctor's (or office's) name and address are printed at the top. In most cases, the office phone number is listed, along with the names of all the associates in the practice. Letterhead is used for correspondence with patients, colleagues, and vendors.

The fiber content of paper is the amount of wood pulp in the paper. Letterhead paper can be cotton fiber bond (sometimes called rag bond) or sulfite bond. Cotton fiber bond contains cotton pulp along with chemically treated wood pulp. It is usually more expensive than other types of paper. Cotton bond contains a watermark, which is an impression or pattern that can be seen when the paper is held up to the light. A watermark indicates that the paper is of high quality. The most popular cotton bond used for letterhead is 25% cotton because it is economical, but all higher grades can be used.

Sulfite bond is made from chemically treated wood pulp. It is smoother than cotton bond and less expensive. Sulfite bond comes in five grades, numbered one through five. Grade one is a cost-effective bond for letterhead. This grade of sulfite bond also has a watermark. You often cannot tell the difference between this grade of sulfite bond and cotton bond.

The finish of a paper refers to the paper's look and feel. Papers with a smooth finish are the most popular type for letterheads. They are less expensive and work well with most printers. Another type of finish used in high-quality letterhead is linen laid. This type has a rougher feel because it is embossed with a design, much like linen fabric.

Envelopes

Envelopes are used for correspondence, invoices, and statements. Typically, business letterhead, matching envelopes, and sometimes invoice and statement letterhead are printed together.

Familiarize yourself with the several types of envelopes used in the medical office.

- The most common envelope size used for correspondence is the No. 10 envelope (also called business size). It measures 4⅛ by 9½ inches.
- Envelopes used for invoices and statements can range from No. 6 (3⅝ by 6½ inches) to No. 10. These envelopes commonly have a transparent window that allows the address on the invoice or statement to show through, saving time and reducing the potential for errors involved in retyping the address.
- Smaller payment-return envelopes—preaddressed to the doctor's office—are often included along with a bill, for the patient's convenience.
- Tan kraft envelopes, also called clasp envelopes, are available in many sizes and are used to send large or bulky documents.
- Padded envelopes are used to send documents or materials, such as slides, that may be damaged in the normal course of mail handling.
- The stock and quality of the envelope should always match the stationery. An office typically has two grades of envelopes with a return address. One is a less expensive stock and quality of paper with a block format return address printed in black. The second is a more expensive stock and quality of paper with a block format return address printed in black or a dark color.

Labels

Address labels, printed from a computerized mailing list, can greatly speed the process of addressing envelopes for bulk mailings. For example, you may have to send a notice of a change in office hours or a quarterly office newsletter to a large number of patients in a practice.

You may choose to set up a system for frequently used labels. Many practices write referrals and other business letters to the same addresses again and again. For fast and easy access, it is helpful to print out labels a full page at a time of the same address. Pages of labels can then be stored in alphabetized folders near the transcription desk.

Invoices and Statements

There are several different types of invoices and statements in use today. They include:

- Preprinted invoices (used to send an original bill)
- Preprinted statements (used to send a reminder when an account is 30 or more days past due)

- Computer-generated invoices and statements
- Superbills (discussed in Chapter 17)
- Data mailers

Written Correspondence

A letter is a form of communication—much like holding a conversation in person. The recipient will form an impression of the physician or the office based on the letter. Therefore, letters must be clear and well written and must politely convey the appropriate information.

Commonly used paragraphs and even entire letter formats, or **templates,** are used repeatedly in some practices. It is handy to save these bodies of text in the computer for quick and easy repeated access. With very few keystrokes, the material can be selected and displayed quickly. Then minor changes specific to the letter or document can be added.

It is also helpful to use the cut, paste, and copy features in word processing software to quickly piece together a correspondence that uses sentences or paragraphs from other documents. Large and small bodies of text can easily be moved from document to document, saving time for the medical assistant.

Types of Correspondence in the Medical Office

As a medical assistant, you will be responsible for preparing routine letters at the physician's request. You may transcribe some letters from the physician's dictation and compose others from notes.

The purpose of most letters is to explain, clarify, or give instructions or other information. Correspondence includes letters of referral; letters about scheduling, canceling, or rescheduling appointments; patient reports for insurance companies; instructions for examinations or laboratory tests; answers to insurance or billing questions; and cover letters or form letters to order supplies, equipment, or magazine subscriptions.

Parts of a Business Letter

Figure 7-2 illustrates the parts of a typical business letter. Details about format may vary from office to office.

Dateline. The **dateline** consists of the month, day, and year. It should begin about three lines below the preprinted letterhead text on approximately line 15. The month should

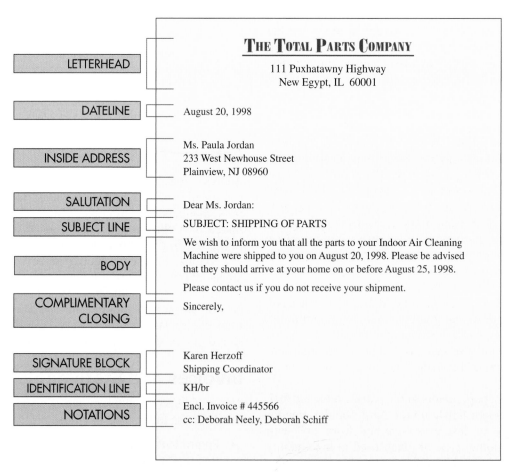

Figure 7-2. Knowing the parts of a typical business letter enables medical assistants to create written communications that reflect well on the office.

always be spelled out, and there should be a comma after the day.

Inside Address. The inside address contains all the necessary information for correct delivery of the letter. In general, you should:

- **Key,** or type, the inside address on the left margin. It should be two, three, or four lines in length.
- Include a **courtesy title** (Dr., Mr., Mrs., and so on) and the intended receiver's full name. Note: If Dr. is used, it is not followed by MD after the name. For example, either of these forms is acceptable: Dr. John Smith; John Smith, MD. This form is not acceptable: Dr. John Smith, MD.
- Include the intended receiver's title on the same line with the name, separated by a comma, or on the line below it.
- Include the company name, if applicable.
- Use numerals for the street address, except the single numbers one through nine, which should be spelled out—for example, Two Markham Place.
- Spell out numerical names of streets if they are numbers less than ten.
- Spell out the words *Street, Drive,* and so on.
- Include the full city name; do not abbreviate.
- Use the two-letter state abbreviation recommended by the U.S. Postal Service (USPS) (Table 7-1).

TABLE 7-1	USPS State Abbreviations		
State	**Abbreviation**	**State**	**Abbreviation**
Alabama	AL	Montana	MT
Alaska	AK	Nebraska	NE
Arizona	AZ	Nevada	NV
Arkansas	AR	New Hampshire	NH
California	CA	New Jersey	NJ
Colorado	CO	New Mexico	NM
Connecticut	CT	New York	NY
Delaware	DE	North Carolina	NC
District of Columbia	DC	North Dakota	ND
Florida	FL	Ohio	OH
Georgia	GA	Oklahoma	OK
Hawaii	HI	Oregon	OR
Idaho	ID	Pennsylvania	PA
Illinois	IL	Puerto Rico	PR
Indiana	IN	Rhode Island	RI
Iowa	IA	South Carolina	SC
Kansas	KS	South Dakota	SD
Kentucky	KY	Tennessee	TN
Louisiana	LA	Texas	TX
Maine	ME	Utah	UT
Maryland	MD	Vermont	VT
Massachusetts	MA	Virginia	VA
Michigan	MI	Washington	WA
Minnesota	MN	West Virginia	WV
Mississippi	MS	Wisconsin	WI
Missouri	MO	Wyoming	WY

- Leave one space between the state and the zip code; include the zip + 4 code, if known.

Attention Line.   An attention line is used when a letter is addressed to a company but sent to the attention of a particular individual. If you do not know the name of the individual, call the company directly to inquire the name of the appropriate contact person. A colon between the word *Attention* and the person's name is optional.

Salutation.   When addressing a person by name, use a **salutation,** a written greeting such as "Dear," followed by Mr., Mrs., or Ms., and the person's last name. The salutation should be keyed at the left margin on the second line below the inside address. A colon should follow. When you do not know the name, it is becoming common practice to use the business title or department in the salutation, as in "Dear Laboratory Director" or "Dear Claims Department." This also avoids confusion if you do not know the gender of a person with a name such as Pat or Chris.

Subject Line.   A subject line is sometimes used to bring the subject of the letter to the reader's attention. The subject line is not required. However, if it is used, it should be keyed on the second line below the salutation. The subject line may be flush with the left margin, indented five spaces, or centered to the page.

Body.   The body of the letter begins two lines below the salutation or subject line. The text is single-spaced with double-spacing between paragraphs.

   If the body contains a list, set the list apart from the rest of the text. Leave an extra line of space above and below the list. For each item in the list, indent five to ten spaces from each margin. Single-space within items, but leave an extra line between items. A bulleted list has a small, solid, round circle before each item.

Complimentary Closing.   The closing is placed two lines below the last line of the body. "Sincerely" is a common closing. "Very truly yours" and "Best regards" are also acceptable closings in business correspondence.

Signature Block.   The signature block contains the writer's name on the first line and the writer's business title on the second line. The block is aligned with the complimentary closing and typed four lines below it, to allow space for the signature.

Identification Line.   The letter writer's initials followed by a colon or slash and the typist's initials are sometimes included in the letter. These initials are called the **identification line.** This line is typed flush left, two lines below the signature block.

Notations.   Notations include information such as the number of **enclosures** that are included with the letter and the names of other people who will be receiving copies of the letter (sometimes referred to as cc's, or carbon copies).

If there are enclosures, a notation should appear flush left, one or two lines below the identification line (or one or two lines below the signature block, if no identification line is present). You may abbreviate the word *Enclosure* by typing "Enc," "Encl," or "Encs" (with or without punctuation, depending on the style of the letter you are writing). The copy notation, "cc," appears after the enclosure notation and includes one or more names or initials.

Punctuation Styles

Two different styles of punctuation are used in correspondence: open punctuation and mixed punctuation. A writer should use one punctuation style consistently throughout a letter.

Open Punctuation.   This style uses no punctuation after the following items when they appear in a letter:

- The word *Attention* in the attention line
- The salutation
- The complimentary closing
- The signature block
- The enclosure and copy notations

Mixed Punctuation.   This style includes the following punctuation marks used in specific instances:

- A colon after *Attention* in the attention line
- A colon after the salutation
- A comma after the complimentary closing
- A colon or period after the enclosure notation
- A colon after the copy notation

Letter Format

Follow these general formatting guidelines for all letters.

- With paper 8½ inches wide, it is common to use 1-inch margins on the left and right.
- Roughly center the letter on the page according to the length of the letter. (Most word processing programs can do this centering automatically.) For shorter letters, you can use wider margins and start the address farther down the page. For longer letters, use standard margins but start higher up on the page.
- Single-space the body of the letter. Double-space between paragraphs or parts of the letter.
- Use short sentences (no more than 20 words on average).
- Have at least two sentences in each paragraph.
- Divide long paragraphs—more than 10 lines of type—into shorter ones.

   For multipage letters, use letterhead for the first page and blank paper for the subsequent pages. (When you order letterhead, be sure to order blank paper of the same type as the letterhead for subsequent sheets.) Using a

1-inch margin at the top, include a heading with the addressee, date, and page number on all pages following the first one. Resume typing or printing the text about three lines below the heading.

Letter Styles

Different letter styles are used for different purposes. Your office is likely to have a preferred style in place. The four most common letter styles are full-block, modified-block, modified-block with indented paragraphs, and simplified.

Full-Block Style. The **full-block letter style,** also called block style, is typed with all lines flush left. Figure 7-3 shows an example of the block letter style. This style may include a subject line two lines below the salutation. Block-style letters are quick and easy to write because there are no indented paragraphs to slow the typist. Block style is one of the most common formats used in the medical office.

Modified-Block Style. The **modified-block letter style** is similar to full block but differs in that the dateline, complimentary closing, signature block, and notations are aligned and begin at the center of the page or slightly to the right. This type of letter has a traditional, balanced appearance.

Modified-Block Style With Indented Paragraphs. This style is identical to the modified-block style except that the paragraphs are indented.

Simplified Style. The **simplified letter style** is a modification of the full-block style and is the most modern letter style. Figure 7-4 shows an example of the simplified letter style. The salutation is omitted, eliminating the need for a courtesy title. A subject line in all-capital letters is placed between the address and the body of the letter. The subject line summarizes the main point of the letter, but does not actually use the word *subject*. All text is typed flush left. The complimentary closing is omitted, and the sender's name and title are typed in capital letters in a single line at the end of the letter. Note that this letter style always uses open punctuation, so it is both easy to read and quick to type. In most situations in a medical office, however, the simplified letter style may be too informal.

Effective Writing

To create effective, professional correspondence that reflects well on the practice, be sure that you use an appropriate style, clear and concise language, and the active voice. Following are some general tips to help you write effective letters.

- Before you write, know the type of person to whom you are writing. Is the letter to a physician, a patient, a vendor, or fellow staff members? Decide if the tone should be formal or more relaxed.

- Know the purpose of the letter before you begin, and make sure your letter accurately conveys that purpose.
- Be **concise.** Use short sentences. Be brief. Be specific. Do not use unnecessary words. Use the simplest way to say what you mean.
- Show **clarity** in your writing; state your message so that it can be understood easily.
- Use the active voice whenever possible. Voice shows whether the subject of a sentence is acting or is being acted upon. Here is an example of the active voice:

  "Dr. Huang is seeing 18 patients today."

  Here is an example of the same sentence, written in the passive voice:

  "Eighteen patients will be seen by Dr. Huang today."

  Note that the active voice is more direct and livelier to read.
- Use the passive voice, however, to soften the impact of negative news:

  "Your account will be turned over to a collection agency if we do not receive payment promptly."

  It would sound harsher to say:

  "We will turn over your account to a collection agency if we do not receive payment promptly."

- Always be polite and courteous.
- Always check spelling and the accuracy of dates and monetary figures.

Editing and Proofreading

Editing and proofreading take place after you create the first draft of a letter. Editing involves checking a document for factual accuracy, logical flow, conciseness, clarity, and tone. Proofreading involves checking a document for grammatical, spelling, and format errors. When possible, ask another person to proofread your work as well. *Never* skip over the very important steps of editing and proofreading!

Tools for Editing and Proofreading

Reference books can help you prepare letters that appear professional. Keep the following tools available.

Dictionary. An up-to-date dictionary gives you more than definitions of words. A dictionary tells you how to spell, divide, and pronounce a word and what part of speech it is, such as a noun or adjective.

Medical Dictionary. It is nearly impossible for even the most experienced health-care professional to be familiar with every medical term. A medical dictionary will serve as a handy reference for terms with which you are unfamiliar or about which you would like more information.

Becoming familiar with some of the prefixes and suffixes commonly used in medical terms can help you

ABC PUBLISHERS, INC.

July 10, 1998

Ms. Lara Erickson
2594 Hughes Boulevard
Hamilton City, NJ 08999

Dear Ms. Erickson:

SUBJECT: SHIPMENT DELAY

Thank you for contacting us regarding your order for *Smith and Doe's New Medical Dictionary*. Due to an unexpectedly heavy demand for the book, we are experiencing delays in processing and shipping orders.

We expect to ship your book in four weeks, around August 15. Because of this delay, we offer you the option of canceling your order with a full refund. If you would like to cancel at this point, please fill out and return the enclosed postcard. If we do not hear from you, your order will be shipped when ready.

We are sorry for any inconvenience this delay may cause you. Please be assured that ABC Publishers values its customers and always endeavors to fulfill orders in a timely fashion.

Sincerely yours,

Andrew Williams

Andrew Williams
Customer Service Manager

AW/cjc
Enclosure

117 New Avenue New York, NY 10000

Figure 7-3.   The full-block letter style is quicker and easier to type than other styles.

ABC PUBLISHERS, INC.

July 10, 1998

Ms. Lara Erickson
2594 Hughes Boulevard
Hamilton City, NJ 08999

SHIPMENT DELAY

Thank you for contacting us regarding your order for *Smith and Doe's New Medical Dictionary*. Due to an unexpectedly heavy demand for the book, we are experiencing delays in processing and shipping orders.

We expect to ship your book in four weeks, around August 15. Because of this delay, we offer you the option of canceling your order with a full refund. If you would like to cancel at this point, please fill out and return the enclosed postcard. If we do not hear from you, your order will be shipped when ready.

We are sorry for any inconvenience this delay may cause you. Please be assured that ABC Publishers values its customers and always endeavors to fulfill orders in a timely fashion.

Andrew Williams

ANDREW WILLIAMS, CUSTOMER SERVICE MANAGER

AW/cjc
Enclosure

117 New Avenue New York, NY 10000

Figure 7-4. The simplified letter style is considered by some executives to be the most readable style for correspondence.

understand the meanings of many words. Appendix B lists some common medical prefixes and suffixes.

Physicians' Desk Reference (PDR). The *PDR* may be thought of as a dictionary of medications. Published yearly, it provides up-to-date information on both prescription and nonprescription drugs. You can consult the *PDR* for the correct spelling of a particular drug or for other information about its usage, side effects, contraindications, and so on.

English Grammar and Usage Manuals. These manuals answer questions concerning grammar and word usage. They usually contain sections on punctuation, capitalization, and other details of written communication.

Word Processing Spelling Checkers. Most word processing programs used in medical offices have built-in spelling checkers. There are also programs designed specifically to check spelling in medical documents. These spelling checkers include most common medical terms that would not be found in a regular software program.

Spelling checkers pick up many spelling errors and often give you suggestions for correct spellings. If you indicate the choice you meant to input, the program automatically replaces the misspelled word. These programs may not detect all spelling errors, however. They should not be relied on as the only means of checking a document. For example, spelling checkers cannot tell you that you used the wrong word if you type the word *form* instead of *from,* because *form* is also a correctly spelled word.

You may be able to add words that are not currently recognized by the spelling checker in your computer. Use this feature to add medical terms. A word of caution is important here! Before you add the word to the computer's dictionary, be sure to look up the exact spelling in a medical dictionary. The computer will recognize only the spelling you add. If you place the *wrong* spelling in the computer, your spelling checker will not correct it.

When you type e-mails, take special care to use correct grammar and punctuation. Spelling checkers are available in most e-mail programs and should be used at the completion of the e-mail. The e-mail spelling checker does not automatically point out mistakes as you type.

Some software packages offer grammar-checking and style-checking features. These programs can identify certain problems, but the person using them still needs to know basic rules of grammar and style to correct errors.

Editing

The **editing** process ensures that a document is accurate, clear, and complete; free of grammatical errors; organized logically; and written in an appropriate style. It is a good idea to leave some time between the writing and editing stages so that you can look at the document in a fresh light. As you edit, you must examine language usage, content, and style.

Language Usage. Learn basic grammar rules. When in doubt, refer to a grammar handbook or reference manual. Make sure all sentences are complete. Ask yourself, Is this the best way to convey what I want to say? Do my word choices reflect the overall tone of the document? For example, in a business letter, you would avoid choosing phrases that are too colloquial or cute, such as "Thanks a million" or "Take it easy."

Content. A letter should contain all the necessary information the writer intends to convey. If you are editing someone else's letter and something appears to be missing, check with the writer. She may have omitted information by mistake.

The content of a letter should follow a logical thought pattern. Create a clean, concise letter by:

- Stating the purpose of the letter in the first sentence
- Discussing one topic at a time
- Changing paragraphs when you change topics
- Listing events in chronological order
- Sticking to the subject
- Selecting your words carefully
- Reading over what you have written before printing

Style. Use a writing style that is appropriate to the reader. A letter written to a patient is likely to require a different style than one written to a physician.

Proofreading

Proofreading means checking a document for errors. After you edit a document, put it aside for a short time before proofreading it. Ideally, have a coworker proofread your work. There are three types of errors that can occur when preparing a document: formatting, data, and mechanical.

Formatting Errors. These errors involve the positioning of the various parts of a letter. They may include errors in indenting, line length, or line spacing. To avoid these errors, take the following two steps:

1. Scan the letter to make sure that the indentions are consistent, that the spacing is correct, and that the text is centered from left to right and top to bottom.
2. Make sure you have followed the office style.

Data Errors. Data errors involve mistyping monetary figures, such as a balance on a patient statement. Verify the accuracy of all figures by checking them twice or by having one or two coworkers check them.

Mechanical Errors. Mechanical errors are errors in spelling, punctuation, spacing between words, and division of words. Mechanical errors also include reversing words or characters, typing them twice, or omitting them altogether. Here are some tips to help you avoid mechanical errors.

- Learn basic spelling, punctuation, and word division rules. When in doubt, be sure to check a manual on English usage. Table 7-2 presents some basic rules concerning the mechanics of writing. Figure 7-5 lists

Commonly Misspelled Medical Terms and Other Words

Medical Terms

abscess	dissect	leukocyte	prescription
aerobic	eosinophil	malaise	prophylaxis
anergic	epididymis	menstruation	prostate
anesthetic	epistaxis	metastasis	prosthesis
aneurysm	erythema	muscle	pruritus
anteflexion	eustachian	neuron	psoriasis
arrhythmia	fissure	nosocomial	psychiatrist
asepsis	flexure	occlusion	pyrexia
asthma	fomites	ophthalmology	respiration
auricle	glaucoma	oscilloscope	rheumatism
benign	glomerular	osseous	roentgenology
bilirubin	gonorrhea	palliative	scirrhous
bronchial	hemocytometer	parasite	serous
calcaneus	hemorrhage	parenteral	specimen
capillary	hemorrhoids	parietal	sphincter
cervical	homeostasis	paroxysm	sphygmomanometer
chancre	humerus	pericardium	squamous
choroid	ileum	perineum	staphylococcus
chromosome	ilium	peristalsis	surgeon
cirrhosis	infarction	peritoneum	vaccine
clavicle	inoculate	pharynx	vein
curettage	intussusception	pituitary	venous
cyanosis	ischemia	plantar	wheal
defibrillator	ischium	pleurisy	
desiccation	larynx	pneumonia	
diluent	leukemia	polyp	

Other Words

absence	assistance	controversy	eligible
accept	associate	corroborate	embarrass
accessible	auxiliary	counsel	emphasis
accommodate	balloon	courtesy	entrepreneur
accumulate	bankruptcy	defendant	envelope
achieve	believe	definite	environment
acquire	benefited	dependent	exceed
adequate	brochure	description	except
advantageous	bulletin	desirable	exercise
affect	business	development	exhibit
aggravate	category	dilemma	exhilaration
all right	changeable	disappear	existence
a lot	characteristic	disappoint	fantasy
already	cigarette	disapprove	fascinate
altogether	circumstance	disastrous	February
analysis	clientele	discreet	fluorescent
analyze	committee	discrete	forty
apparatus	comparative	discrimination	grammar
apparent	complement	dissatisfied	grievance
appearance	compliment	dissipate	guarantee
appropriate	concede	earnest	handkerchief
approximate	conscientious	ecstasy	height
argument	conscious	effect	humorous

(continued)

Figure 7-5. Familiarize yourself with these commonly misspelled words, and check their spelling carefully whenever you use them.

Other Words

hygiene	oscillate	privilege	stationery
incidentally	paid	procedure	stomach
indispensable	pamphlet	proceed	subpoena
inimitable	panicky	professor	succeed
insistent	paradigm	pronunciation	suddenness
irrelevant	parallel	psychiatry	supersede
irresistible	paralyze	psychology	surprise
irritable	pastime	pursue	tariff
its	persevere	questionnaire	technique
it's	persistent	rearrange	temperament
labeled	personal	recede	temperature
laboratory	personnel	receive	thorough
led	persuade	recommend	transferred
leisure	phenomenon	referral	truly
liable	plagiarism	relieve	tyrannize
liaison	pleasant	repetition	unnecessary
license	possession	rescind	until
liquefy	precede	résumé	vacillate
maintenance	precedent	rhythm	vacuum
maneuver	predictable	ridiculous	vegetable
miscellaneous	predominant	schedule	vicious
misspelled	prejudice	secretary	warrant
necessary	preparation	seize	Wednesday
noticeable	prerogative	separate	weird
occasion	prevalent	similar	
occurrence	principal	sizable	
offense	principle	stationary	

some of the most commonly misspelled medical terms and other words.

- Check carefully for transposed characters or words.
- Avoid dividing words at the end of a line. Most word processing programs automatically wrap words to the next line, so if you are writing on a computer, word division should not present a problem.

As you can see, creating a business letter involves many steps. Procedure 7-1 organizes these steps for you.

Preparing Outgoing Mail

After you have created, edited, and proofread a letter, you need to prepare it for mailing. This preparation includes having the letter signed, preparing the envelope, and folding and inserting the letter into the envelope. It will then be ready for postage to be calculated and affixed.

Signing Letters

After the letter is complete—it has been proofread and the envelope and enclosures have been prepared—it is ready for signing. Some doctors authorize other staff members to sign for them. If you have been authorized to sign letters, you should sign the doctor's name and place your initials after the doctor's signature.

If the doctor prefers to sign all letters, you should place the letter on the doctor's desk in a file folder marked "For Your Signature." If the letter is of an urgent nature, give it to the doctor as soon as possible. Otherwise, you can collect several letters in the folder and present the entire group for signing at one time. However, all prepared work should be given to the physician at the end of the day.

Preparing the Envelope

To ensure the quickest delivery of mail, the USPS has issued several guidelines for preparing envelopes. The USPS uses electronic optical character readers (OCRs) to help speed mail processing. OCRs read the last two lines of an address and sort the mail accordingly. To take advantage of this technology, envelopes must be no smaller than $3\frac{1}{2}$ by 5 inches and no larger than $6\frac{1}{8}$ by $11\frac{1}{2}$ inches. They must be addressed in a specific format that can be read by the OCR. Use USPS guidelines for addressing envelopes.

TABLE 7-2 Basic Rules of Writing

Word Division	Divide: • According to pronunciation • Compound words between the two words from which they derive • Hyphenated compound words at the hyphen • After a prefix • Before a suffix • Between two consonants that appear between vowels • Before *-ing* unless the last consonant is doubled; in that case, divide before the second consonant Do not divide: • Such suffixes as *-sion, -tial,* and *-gion* • A word so that only one letter is left on a line
Capitalization	Capitalize: • All proper names • All titles, positions, or indications of family relation when preceding a proper name or in place of a proper noun (not when used alone or with possessive pronouns or articles) • Days of the week, months, and holidays • Names of organizations and membership designations • Racial, religious, and political designations • Adjectives, nouns, and verbs that are derived from proper nouns (including currently copyrighted trade names) • Specific addresses and geographic locations • Sums of money written in legal or business documents • Titles, headings of books, magazines, and newspapers

Plurals	• Add *s* or *es* to most singular nouns (Plural forms of most medical terms do not follow this rule.)
	• With medical terms ending in *is,* drop the *is* and add *es:*
	    metastasis/metastases
	    epiphysis/epiphyses
	• With terms ending in *um,* drop the *um* and add *a:*
	    diverticulum/diverticula
	    atrium/atria
	• With terms ending in *us,* drop the *us* and add *i:*
	    calculus/calculi
	    bronchus/bronchi
	    (Two exceptions to this are virus/viruses and sinus/sinuses.)
	• With terms ending in *a,* keep the *a* and add *e:*
	    vertebra/vertebrae

Possessives	To show ownership or relation to another noun: • For singular nouns, add an apostrophe and an *s* • For plural nouns that do not end in an *s,* add an apostrophe and an *s* • For plural nouns that end in an *s,* just add an apostrophe
Numbers	Use numerals: • In general writing, when the number is 11 or greater • With abbreviations and symbols • When discussing laboratory results or statistics • When referring to specific sums of money • When using a series of numbers in a sentence Tips: • Use commas when numerals have more than three digits • Do not use commas when referring to account numbers, page numbers, or policy numbers • Use a hyphen with numerals to indicate a range

PROCEDURE 7.1

Creating a Letter

Objective: To follow standard procedure for constructing a business letter

Materials: Word processor or personal computer, letterhead paper, dictionaries or other sources

Method

1. Format the letter according to the office's standard procedure. Use the same punctuation style throughout.

2. Start the dateline three lines below the last line of the printed letterhead.

   (Note: Depending on the length of the letter, it is acceptable to start between two and six lines below the letterhead.)

3. Two lines below the dateline, type in any special mailing instructions (such as REGISTERED MAIL, CERTIFIED MAIL, and so on).

4. Three lines below any special instructions, begin the inside address.

   (Note: It is acceptable to start the inside address anywhere from 3 to 12 lines below the dateline, depending upon the length of the letter.)

   - Type the addressee's courtesy title (Mr., Mrs., Dr., and so on) and full name on the first line.
   - Type the addressee's business title on the second line.
   - Type the company name on the third line.
   - Type the street address on the fourth line, including the apartment or suite number.

   - Type the city, state, and zip code on the fifth line. Use the standard two-letter abbreviation for the state, followed by one space and the zip code.

5. Two lines below the inside address, type the salutation.

6. Two lines below the salutation, type the subject line, if applicable.

7. Two lines below the subject line, begin the body of the letter.
   - Single-space between lines.
   - Double-space between paragraphs.

8. Two lines below the body of the letter, type the complimentary closing.

9. Leave three blank lines (return four times), and begin the signature block. (Enough space must be left to allow for the signature.)
   - Type the sender's name on the first line.
   - Type the sender's title on the second line.

10. Two lines below the sender's title, type the identification line. Type the sender's initials in all capitals and your initials in lowercase letters, separating the two sets of initials with a colon or a slash.

11. One or two lines below the identification line, type the enclosure notation, if applicable.

12. Two lines below the enclosure notation, type the copy notation, if applicable.

13. Edit the letter.

14. Proofread the letter.

Address Placement. The address must be placed in a certain location on the envelope for reading by the OCR (Figure 7-6). The area the OCR can read has the following characteristics.

- It is bordered by a 1-inch margin on both the left and right sides of the envelope.
- It has a ⅝-inch margin on the bottom. The top of the city/state/zip code line (the last line in the address block) must be no higher than 2¼ inches from the bottom edge of the envelope.
- An area 4½ inches wide in the bottom right corner of the envelope should be left clear. The OCR reads the address and prints a bar code that corresponds to the zip code in this area.

Address Format. When you type an address, follow these format guidelines.

- Type or machine-print (for example, by computer) the address. (The OCR cannot read handwriting.) Avoid fancy script fonts.
- Use all-capital letters, and single-space the lines. Use only one or two spaces between numbers and words in the address.
- Use only USPS-approved abbreviations for location designations, as presented in Table 7-3.
- Put the addressee's name on the first line of the address block, the department (if any) on the second line, and the company name on the third line. If the letter is to go to someone's attention at a company, put

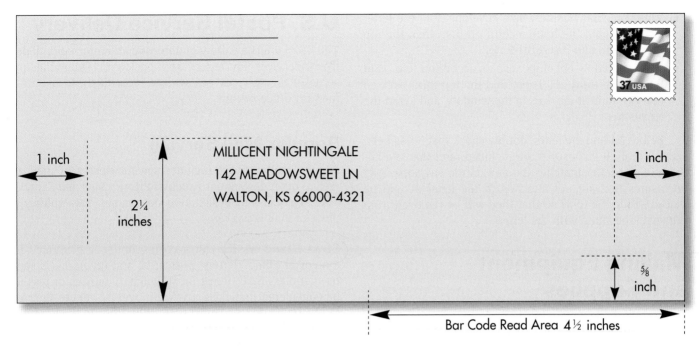

MILLICENT NIGHTINGALE
142 MEADOWSWEET LN
WALTON, KS 66000-4321

1 inch

1 inch

2¼ inches

⅝ inch

Bar Code Read Area 4½ inches

Figure 7-6. Following this format for typing an envelope ensures that it can be processed by USPS electronic equipment.

TABLE 7-3	USPS Abbreviations		
Word	**Abbreviation**	**Word**	**Abbreviation**
Avenue	AVE	Highway	HWY
Boulevard	BLVD	Junction	JCT
Center	CTR	Lane	LN
Circle	CIR	North	N
Corner	COR	Parkway	PKY
Court	CT	Place	PL
Drive	DR	Plaza	PLZ
East	E	South	S
Expressway	EXPY	West	W

the company name on the first line and "Attention: [Name]" on the second line.

- The line above the city, state, and zip code should contain the street address or post office box number. Include suite or apartment numbers on the same line as the street address.

- The last line of the address must include the city, state, and zip code. Use the zip + 4 code whenever possible.

- Include the hyphen in the zip + 4 code, for example, 08520-6142.

- Type any special notations (such as SPECIAL DELIVERY, CERTIFIED, or REGISTERED) two lines below the postage in all-capital letters. This information should appear outside the area the OCR can read.

- Type any handling instructions (such as PERSONAL or CONFIDENTIAL) three lines below the return address. This information should also be outside the area the OCR can read.

- Letters going to foreign countries should have the name of the country on the last line of the address block in all-capital letters.

Folding and Inserting Mail

Letters and invoices must be folded neatly before they are inserted into the envelopes. The proper way to fold a letter depends on the type of envelope into which the letter will fit.

- With a small envelope, fold the enclosure in half lengthwise, and insert it.

- With a regular business-size envelope, fold the letter in thirds. Fold the bottom third up first, then the top third down, and insert the letter.
- With a window envelope, use an accordion fold. Fold the bottom third up. Then, fold the top third back so that the address appears in the window, and insert the enclosure.

Before folding the letter, double-check that it has been signed, that all enclosures are included, and that the address on the letter matches the one on the envelope. Any enclosures that are not attached to the letter should be placed inside the folds so that they will be removed from the envelope along with the letter.

Mailing Equipment and Supplies

The proper equipment and supplies will help you handle the mail efficiently and cost-effectively. In addition to letterhead, blank stationery for multipage letters, and envelopes, you will need some standard supplies. The USPS provides forms, labels, and packaging for items that need special attention, such as airmail, Priority Mail, Express Mail, certified mail, or registered mail. Private delivery companies, such as United Parcel Service (UPS), also provide shipping supplies to their customers.

Airmail Supplies

In the past, any piece of mail that was transported by air was designated as airmail. Today nearly all first-class mail outside a local area is routinely sent by air. However, airmail services are still available for some packages and for most mail going to foreign countries.

If you are sending an item by airmail, attach special airmail stickers, available from the post office, on all sides. (The word *AIRMAIL* can also be neatly written on all sides.) Special airmail envelopes for letters can be purchased from the USPS.

Envelopes for Overnight Delivery Services

For correspondence or packages that must be delivered by the next day, a number of overnight delivery services are available through the USPS and private companies. Most companies require the use of their own envelopes and mailing materials. Make sure you keep adequate supplies on hand.

Postal Rates, Scales, and Meters

Postal rates and regulations change periodically, and every medical office should have a copy of the latest guidelines. These guidelines are available from the USPS. Postal scales and meters are described in Chapter 5.

U.S. Postal Service Delivery

The USPS offers a variety of domestic and international delivery services for letters and packages. Following are some of the services you will be most likely to use in a medical office setting.

Regular Mail Service

Regular mail delivery includes several classes of mail as well as other designations such as Priority Mail and Express Mail. The class or designation determines how quickly a piece of mail is delivered.

First-Class Mail. Most correspondence generated in a medical office—letters, postcards, and invoices—is sent by first-class mail. Items must weigh 11 ounces or less to be considered first-class. (An item over 11 ounces that requires quick delivery must be sent by Priority Mail, which is discussed later in the chapter.) The cost of mailing a first-class item is based on its weight. The standard rate is for items 1 ounce or less that are not larger than $6\frac{1}{8}$ inches high and $11\frac{1}{2}$ inches wide. Additional postage is required for items that are heavier or larger. Postage for postcards is less than the letter rate. First-class mail is forwarded at no additional cost.

Second-Class Mail. Second-class mail is not used by most medical offices. This class of mail is designed for the delivery of newspapers and periodicals only.

Third-Class Mail. Third-class mail is also known as bulk mail. It is not often used in medical offices. Bulk mail is used for the mailing of books, catalogs, and other printed material that weighs less than 16 ounces. This class of mailing is available only to authorized mailers.

Fourth-Class Mail. Fourth-class mail is also called parcel post. It is used for items that weigh at least 1 pound but not more than 70 pounds and that do not require speedy delivery. Rates are based on weight and distance. There is a special fourth-class rate for mailing books, manuscripts, and some types of medical information.

Priority Mail. Priority class is useful for heavier items that require quicker delivery than is available for fourth-class mail. Any first-class item that weighs between 11 ounces and 70 pounds requires Priority Mail service. Although the rate for Priority Mail varies with the weight of the item and the distance it must travel, the USPS offers a flat rate for all material that can fit into its special Priority Mail envelope. The USPS guarantees delivery of Priority Mail items in 2 to 3 days.

Express Mail. Express Mail is the quickest USPS service. Different types are available, including next-day and second-day delivery. Express Mail deliveries are made 365 days a year. Rates vary, depending on the weight and the specific service. A special flat-rate envelope is also available. Items sent by Express Mail are automatically insured against loss or damage. You can drop off packages at the post office or arrange for pickup service.

Special Postal Services

The USPS offers a variety of special mail delivery services in addition to the regular classes of mail. These services may require an additional fee above and beyond the cost of postage.

Special Delivery. Use special delivery if you want an item delivered as soon as it reaches the recipient's post office. Delivery of the item is typically made before the regularly scheduled mail delivery. Special delivery service is available within certain distance limits and during certain hours.

Certified Mail. Certified mail offers a guarantee that the item has been received. The item is marked as certified mail and requires the postal carrier to obtain a signature on delivery (Figure 7-7). The signature card is then returned to the sender. The card should be added to the patient's file. This documentation is evidence that the document was not only mailed but also received. The receiver's name is clearly printed along with the signature. The certified mail signature card becomes a legal document, which may be important in court.

Return Receipt Requested. You may request a return receipt to obtain proof that an item was delivered. The receipt indicates who received the item and when. You can obtain a return receipt for various types of mail.

Registered Mail. Use registered mail to send items that are valuable, irreplaceable, or otherwise important. Registered mail provides the sender with evidence of mailing and delivery. It also provides the security that an item is being tracked as it is transported through the postal system. Because of this tracking process, delivery may be slightly delayed.

To register a piece of mail, take it to the post office, and indicate the full value of the item. Both first-class mail and Priority Mail can be registered.

International Mail

The USPS offers both surface (via ship) and airmail service to most foreign countries. Information on rates and fees is available from the post office.

There are various types of international mail, which are similar to the domestic classes. The USPS also provides international Express Mail and Priority Mail services, along with special mail delivery services such as registered mail, certified mail, and special delivery.

Tracing Mail

If a piece of registered or certified mail does not reach its destination by the expected time, you can ask the post office to trace it (Figure 7-8). You will need to present your original receipt for the item.

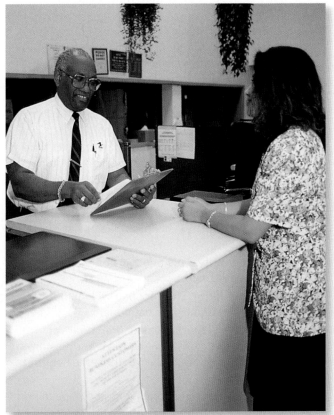

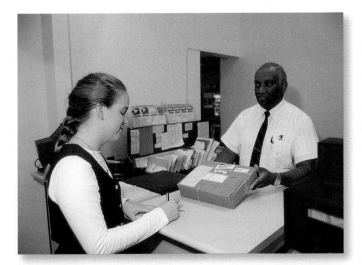

Figure 7-7. If no one is in the office when the mail is delivered, the medical assistant may need to go to the post office to sign for a certified letter or package.

Figure 7-8. Tracing an item is a service that post offices perform when important items are delayed or do not reach their destinations.

Other Delivery Services

In addition to the USPS, other companies provide mail and package delivery services. The costs and types of services vary.

United Parcel Service

United Parcel Service (UPS) delivers packages and provides overnight letter and express services. You can either drop off packages at a UPS location or have them picked up at your office. Fees vary with the services provided, such as ground or air. Packages are automatically insured against theft or damage.

Express Delivery Services

Companies such as Federal Express and Airborne Express provide several types of quick delivery services for letters

---

PROCEDURE 7.2

Sorting and Opening Mail

Objective: To follow a standard procedure for sorting, opening, and processing incoming office mail

Materials: Letter opener, date and time stamp (manual or automatic), stapler, paper clips, adhesive notes

Method

1. Check the address on each letter or package to be sure that it has been delivered to the correct location.

2. Sort the mail into piles according to priority and type of mail. Your system may include the following:
   - Top priority. This pile will contain any items that were sent by overnight mail delivery in addition to items sent by registered mail, certified mail, or special delivery. (Faxes and e-mail messages are also top priority.)
   - Second priority. This pile will include personal or confidential mail.
   - Third priority. This pile will contain all first-class mail, airmail, and Priority Mail items. These items should be divided into payments received, insurance forms, reports, and other correspondence.
   - Fourth priority. This pile will consist of packages.
   - Fifth priority. This pile will contain magazines and newspapers.
   - Sixth priority. This last pile will include advertisements and catalogs.

3. Set aside all letters labeled "Personal" or "Confidential." Unless you have permission to open these letters, only the addressee should open them.

4. Arrange all the envelopes with the flaps facing up and away from you.

5. Tap the lower edge of the envelope to shift the contents to the bottom. This step helps to prevent cutting any of the contents when you open the envelope.

6. Open all the envelopes. (It is more efficient to open all the envelopes first and then to remove the contents.)

7. Remove and unfold the contents, making sure that nothing remains in the envelope.

8. Review each document, and check the sender's name and address.
   - If the letter has no return address, save the envelope, or cut the address off the envelope, and tape it to the letter.
   - Check to see if the address matches the one on the envelope. If there is a difference, staple the envelope to the letter, and make a note to verify the correct address with the sender.

9. Compare the enclosure notation on the letter with the actual enclosures to make sure that all items are included. Make a note to contact the sender if anything is missing.

10. Clip together each letter and its enclosures.

11. Check the date of the letter. If there is a significant delay between the date of the letter and the postmark, keep the envelope. (It may be necessary to refer to the postmark in legal matters or cases of collection.)

12. If all contents appear to be in order, you can discard the envelope.

13. Review all bills and statements.
    - Make sure the amount enclosed is the same as the amount listed on the statement.
    - Make a note of any discrepancies.

14. Stamp each piece of correspondence with the date (and sometimes the time) to record its receipt. If possible, stamp each item in the same location—such as the upper right corner. (It may be necessary to refer to the date in legal matters or in cases of collection.)

How to Spot Urgent Incoming Mail

How can you tell if a piece of incoming mail is urgent? First-class mail marked "Urgent" tells you that it requires immediate attention. Here are some other signals to look for.

Overnight Mail

Any package that has been sent by an overnight carrier or by USPS Express Mail should be considered urgent and should be opened immediately.

Certified Mail

Certified mail requires your signature on delivery. The sender used certified mail to be sure that the item would be sent to the proper person.

Registered Mail

Items sent by registered mail typically are valuable, irreplaceable, or otherwise important. Registered mail provides the sender with evidence of mailing and delivery.

Special Delivery

An item sent by special delivery is likely to be delivered sometime before the normal mail delivery—possibly even on a Sunday or holiday. The sender requested special delivery to ensure that the item would be delivered promptly after it was received at the addressee's post office.

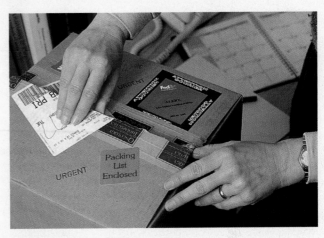

Figure 7-9. Urgent materials receive top priority upon arrival at an office.

and packages. Rates vary according to weight, time of delivery, and in some cases, whether you have the package picked up at your office or drop it off at one of the company's local branches.

Messengers or Couriers

When items must be delivered within the local area on the same day, local messenger services are an option. Many messenger companies are listed in the yellow pages of the telephone book.

Processing Incoming Mail

Mail is an important connection between the office and other professionals and patients. Often an office has an established procedure for handling the mail. It is best to set aside a specific time of the day to process all the incoming mail at once rather than trying to do a little bit at a time.

Although it sounds simple, processing mail involves more than merely opening envelopes. In general, it involves the following steps: sorting, opening, recording, annotating, and distributing.

Sorting and Opening

The first step in processing mail is to sort it. Mail is typically sorted according to its priority. Sort mail in an uncluttered area to avoid mixing it with other paperwork. Follow a regular sorting procedure each time so that you do not miss any steps. Procedure 7-2 outlines suggested steps for sorting and opening the mail. The Tips for the Office section discusses how to recognize urgent incoming mail.

Recording

It is a good idea to keep a log of each day's mail. This daily record lists the mail received and indicates follow-up correspondence and the date it is completed. This method helps in tracing items and keeping track of correspondence.

Annotating

Because you will be reading much of the incoming mail, you may also be encouraged to annotate it. To **annotate** means to underline or highlight key points of the letter or to write reminders, comments, or suggested actions in the margins or on self-adhesive notes. Annotating may involve

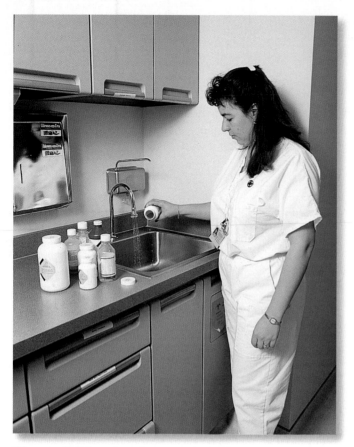

Figure 7-10. Certain nontoxic medical supplies must be carefully disposed of according to medical office policy.

pulling a patient's chart or any previous related correspondence from a file and attaching it to the letter.

Distributing

The next step is to sort letters into separate batches for distribution. These batches might include correspondence that requires the physician's attention, payments to be directed to the person in charge of billing, and correspondence that requires your attention. Each batch should be presented to the appropriate person in a file folder or arranged with the highest-priority items on top. You may be given specific instructions on how to distribute magazines, newspapers, and advertising circulars.

Handling Drug and Product Samples

Many physicians receive a number of drug and product samples in the mail. Handling procedures vary from office to office. Samples of nonprescription products, such as hand creams or cough drops, may be displayed in the patient treatment area for patients to take.

The physician may ask that you put samples of any new prescription drugs in the consultation room for him to evaluate. Store other drug samples in a locked cabinet reserved solely for such samples. Sort and label the samples by category, such as antibiotics, sedatives, painkillers, and so on. Never give samples to patients unless specified by the physician. If the physician directs you to give samples to a patient, make sure to write this information in the patient's chart and date the entry.

When a box of samples is half empty, it is common practice to destroy half of the remaining samples by pouring liquids down the drain and putting pills in a garbage disposal. Samples should not be put in the trash. (The remaining samples that have not been destroyed may be used at the physician's direction.) Once a month, any samples that are past their expiration date should be destroyed (Figure 7-10).

Summary

As a medical assistant, you are responsible for many of the tasks involved in writing correspondence and processing outgoing and incoming mail in the medical office. Proper and efficient management of correspondence and mail is essential to promoting a positive, professional office image.

Choosing the proper letterhead and envelopes helps to ensure professional-looking correspondence. Knowing the parts of a letter and the various letter styles and formats used in the business environment today helps you create effective correspondence. Knowing how to edit and proofread and how to use writing reference books helps ensure that your letters are understandable and well written.

Familiarity with the types of mail services available enables you to choose the proper services to meet the office's mailing needs. Following proper procedures and recommended USPS guidelines ensures that office mail will be received in the most timely manner.

Handling incoming mail is also an important responsibility. Following an established procedure allows you to process and route the mail efficiently.

CHAPTER 7

CASE STUDY *QUESTIONS*

Now that you have completed this chapter, review the case study at the beginning of the chapter and answer the following questions:

1. Why is it important to accurately and carefully prepare correspondence for an ambulatory setting? What could the poor management of documents and correspondence mean to a medical practice?
2. What are the differences between the language used in an informal or casual letter and that used in a formal or professional business letter?
3. What are some appropriate shortcuts that can assist in the daily management of correspondence and mailing?
4. What are some factors to consider in choosing the best mode of delivery for letters and parcels?

Discussion Questions

1. Why is it important to closely follow the basic rules of writing when creating a business letter?
2. Name and describe the five steps involved in processing incoming mail.
3. Explain the differences between certified mail, first-class mail, and registered mail.

Critical Thinking Questions

1. What is your weakest area in writing? How might you improve? Create and complete a project that helps you improve your weakest area.
2. The physician tells you to make sure that all patient letters that address withdrawing the services of the practice are "well documented." What does the physician mean? What would you do?
3. Imagine that your coworker is out sick. You must make sure all the work is handled. Which is more important—typing referral letters or sorting the mail? Why? How might you proceed if you are responsible for both but don't have the time to complete both?
4. Make flash cards from Table 7-1 and Table 7-3, and quiz one of your classmates. Which states or terms do you find difficult?

Application Activities

1. You are employed in Dr. Angelo Carillo's office. A young patient of yours, Rodney Sills, has broken his wrist, and Dr. Carillo says that Rodney will be unable to participate in gym class for 10 weeks. Create a letter notifying his gym instructor of the situation.
2. Prepare a No. 10 business envelope using the USPS guidelines for addressing envelopes. Include the following information.

Return address:
Dr. Angelo Carillo, 123 Winding Way, Suite 2, Rockland, NJ 09876

Mailing address:
ABC Insurance, 987 Hill Street, Marrakesh, CA 01234

Attention:
Susan Jones, Claims Department

Special Instructions:
Certified Mail

3. Using proper letter formatting technique and the basic rules of writing reviewed in this chapter, correct the following letter:

September 18th, 1997

Mountainside Hospital
Samuel Adams, Educational Coordinator
1 Mountainside Lane
San Francisco, California, 94112

Dear mr. Adams:
I am writing in response to your letter of the 10th. I am very interested in presenting a talk at your Health Fare in February. I am avialable to speak on either the 20th or the 21st.

If there is any flexibility in scheduling, I would prefer to present my talk in the afternoon. Also, please let me know how long I should prepare to speak. I am including a copy of an article I recently wrote on the same subject for the local paper.

I am looking forward to hearing from you.
Sincerly,
Enclosure
Dr. Angelo Carillo
AC/SCB

CHAPTER 8

Managing Office Supplies

KEY TERMS

disbursement
durable item
efficiency
expendable item
inventory
invoice
Material Safety Data
    Sheet (MSDS)
purchase order
purchasing group
reputable
requisition
unit price

AREAS OF COMPETENCE

2003 Role Delineation Study
GENERAL
Operational Functions
- Perform inventory of office supplies and equipment

CHAPTER OUTLINE

- Organizing Medical Office Supplies
- Taking Inventory of Medical Office Supplies
- Ordering Supplies

OBJECTIVES

After completing Chapter 8, you will be able to:

8.1 Give examples of vital, incidental, and periodic supplies used in a typical medical office.

8.2 Describe how to store administrative and clinical supplies.

8.3 Implement a system for tracking the inventory of supplies.

8.4 Schedule inventories and ordering times to maximize office efficiency.

8.5 Locate and evaluate supply sources.

8.6 Use strategies to obtain the best-quality supplies while controlling cost.

8.7 Follow procedures for ordering supplies.

8.8 Check a supply order and pay for the supplies.

Introduction

The purpose of a medical office or clinic is to deliver appropriate care to those in need. However, no medical office can function without adequate supplies. It is therefore essential that the medical assistant routinely evaluate and replenish the office's supplies before a shortage is noted.

In this chapter, you will focus on the importance of adequate administrative and clinical supplies in the daily operation of a typical medical practice. You learn to evaluate, replace, organize, and pay for expendable items used routinely in a practice.

The administration of the hospital where you are employed has made the decision to open a series of clinics across the city to provide ambulatory care to patients in their neighborhoods. As an experienced medical assistant, you have been asked to plan for the purchase of expendable items for stocking in the new clinics. What a task! How will you determine what items to provide for each clinic and the amount to order? Do you know where to go to get the best price for the best products? Who is the best vendor in each area? What about discounts for volume buying? Where do you start? You need a plan or a system to help organize your thoughts and then your actions.

As you read this chapter, consider the following questions:

1. What is an *expendable* item? What items would you list on the expendable administrative supply list? The clinical supply list? The general supply list?
2. What factors would you consider about each office as you determine the appropriate supplies?
3. How would you recommend that the supplies be stored with inventory management in mind?

Organizing Medical Office Supplies

Purchasing and maintaining administrative and medical supplies are essential skills that you will use in managing the office. You will be responsible for taking inventory of equipment and supplies, evaluating and recommending equipment and supplies, and negotiating prices with suppliers. When managing office supplies, your goal is to achieve **efficiency,** which is the ability to produce the desired result with the least effort, expense, and waste.

The word *supplies* refers to **expendable items,** or items that are used and then must be restocked, such as prescription pads (Figure 8-1). Ideally, office supplies are stored on labeled shelves. More **durable items,** or pieces of equipment that are used indefinitely—such as

telephones, computers, and examination tables—are not considered supplies. Also in the category of durable items is medical equipment, such as stethoscopes and reflex hammers. Ordering durable administrative items is discussed in Chapter 5.

Determining Responsibility for Organizing Supplies

It is recommended that the responsibility for organizing office supplies lie with at most one or two individuals. Often this responsibility is given to the medical assistant. In a small practice, one medical assistant may be able to handle this responsibility. A practice with several physicians may require two or three medical assistants to take care of supplies. When two medical assistants handle this responsibility, one is often assigned to handle administrative items and the other to handle clinical (medical) supplies. In a large practice, a third assistant might handle computer, copier, and fax supplies.

Categorizing Supplies

Most supplies in the medical office fall into two main categories: administrative and clinical. Examples of administrative supplies are those that keep the office running, such as stationery, insurance forms, pens, pencils, and clipboards. Clinical supplies are medically related and include alcohol swabs, tongue depressors, disposable tips for otoscopes, and disposable sheaths for thermometers.

There are also general supplies, which are used by both patients and staff. Examples of general supplies are paper towels, liquid hypoallergenic soap, and facial and toilet tissue.

The Supply List. You will need to determine what items in your office are used routinely and reordered

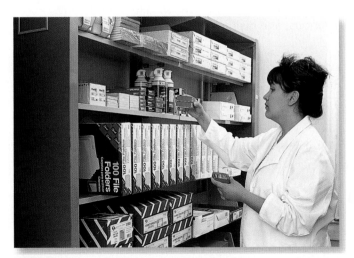

Figure 8-1. Making sure that supplies are in order is a continuous process that ensures an efficient, well-prepared office.

Typical Supplies in a Medical Office

Administrative Supplies

Appointment books, daybooks

Back-to-school/back-to-work slips

Clipboards

Computer supplies

Copy and facsimile (fax) machine paper

File folders, coding tabs

History and physical examination sheets/cards

Insurance forms: disability, HMO and other third party payers, life insurance examinations, Veterans Administration, workers' compensation

Insurance manuals

Local welfare department forms

Patient education materials

Pens, pencils, erasers

Rubber bands, paper clips

Social Security forms

Stamps

Stationery: appointment cards, bookkeeping supplies (ledgers, statements, billing forms), letterhead, second sheets, envelopes, business cards, prescription pads, notebooks, notepads, telephone memo pads

Clinical Supplies

Alcohol swabs

Applicators

Bandaging materials: adhesive tape, gauze pads, gauze sponges, elastic bandages, adhesive bandages, roller bandages (gauze and elastic)

Cloth or paper gowns

Cotton, cotton swabs

Culture tubes

50% dextrose solution

Disposable sheaths for thermometers

Disposable tips for otoscopes

Gloves: sterile, examination

Hemoccult test kits

Iodine or Betadine pads

Lancets

Lubricating jelly

Microscopic slides and fixative

Needles, syringes

Nitroglycerin tablets

Safety pins

Silver nitrate sticks

Suture removal kits

Sutures

Thermometer covers

Tongue depressors

Topical skin freeze

Urinalysis test sticks

Urine containers

Injectable medications: diazepam (Valium), diphenhydramine hydrochloride (Benadryl), epinephrine (Adrenalin), furosemide (Lasix), isoproterenol (Isuprel), lidocaine (Xylocaine: 1%, 2%, and plain), meperidine hydrochloride (Demerol), morphine, phenobarbital, sodium bicarbonate, sterile saline, sterile water

Other medicines, chemicals, solutions, ointments, lotions, and disinfectants, as needed

General Supplies

Liquid hypoallergenic soap

Paper cups

Paper towels

Tampons

Tissues: facial, toilet

Figure 8-2. Familiarize yourself with the typical supplies in a medical office.

systematically. Keep a list of these items, and update it as needed. This supply list is usually kept in the office procedures manual. Appropriate sections of the list may be posted on the cabinets where those items are stored.

To help keep track of supplies, categorize them according to the urgency of need. Although all supplies in your office are necessary, some supplies are more important than others. Figure 8-2 can help you determine vital, incidental, and periodic supplies for your office.

Vital Supplies. These items are absolutely necessary to ensure the smooth running of the practice. They include paper examination table covers and prescription pads. Without these items, the physician would be unable to work in a clean examination environment or to readily prescribe medication for patients during office visits. Another type of vital supply is an item that requires a special order, such as a printed form. Special orders take time to obtain, so they must be ordered well before supplies run low.

Incidental Supplies. These supplies are needed in the office but do not threaten the efficiency of the office if the supply runs low. Incidental supplies include staples and rubber bands, which can be purchased quickly and easily at a local stationery store.

Periodic Supplies. These supplies require ordering only occasionally. For example, you will order appointment books only once or twice a year, probably in small numbers. The urgency of ordering some periodic items can depend on the size of the office. A multiphysician office, for example, would require more appointment books than a single-physician office. Another example of a periodic item might be holiday cards to send to the physician's colleagues and patients.

Storing Office Supplies

Storing office supplies requires good organizational skills and attention to detail. Many people in an office use these supplies, so the items should be stored neatly and in an orderly way. In addition, it is important to store supplies safely to prevent loss or theft, damage, or deterioration.

Location. In a small medical office, supplies are generally kept near the areas of the office where they are used. Administrative supplies are usually stored behind or adjacent to the reception area, with clinical supplies stored near the examination rooms. If the practice has a laboratory, pertinent supplies are stored in or near the laboratory. Offices that have separate supply rooms offer more storage space.

Small medical offices may not have ample space for storage. It may be tempting to store boxes on the floor behind the air conditioning unit, stacked up close to the ceiling, or in potentially hazardous locations, such as near a source of heat. It is essential that supplies be stored according to the guidelines described by JCAHO (Joint Commission for Accreditation of Health Organizations).

Items may not be stored on the floor; instead, they must be raised off the floor, as on a crate or shelf, to avoid contamination by water. Items stored close to the ceiling are considered a fire hazard. JCAHO standards require that supplies stored on the top shelf of a closet or storage area be at least 18 inches below the ceiling.

Avoid storing any boxes or supplies near a water heater, air conditioning unit, heater, or stove. Many expendable items and their packaging are combustible and can quickly become a fire hazard. Air conditioning units may drip water on the floor. If boxes of expensive forms are stored nearby, they can quickly become ruined as water seeps unnoticed into the packaging.

Storage Cabinets. Each storage cabinet should be labeled with a list of its contents. Keep all stock of one item together. Store small items together according to type.

Finding supplies is easier if you keep small items at eye level. Put large, bulky goods, such as reams of stationery, on lower shelves. Label boxes and containers clearly so that all employees can readily find what they need and so that the inventory process is easier.

As you initially arrange items on storage shelves, label the shelves. Reserve enough space to completely stock each item. Do not put anything but the appropriate item in each designated space. This easy system allows for a quick review when you reorder supplies.

To reduce the risk of errors on reorders, keep each item's original label attached to it. Cover the label with clear tape, if necessary. If you must replace a worn label, do it immediately when needed, making sure the new label has the same detailed information as the old one. Bottles with pouring spouts should be labeled on the side opposite the spout to prevent the liquid from dripping onto the label. Use a laundry marking pen to label linens with the name of your office. Linen services usually premark linens with the name of the company or the practice.

Many items have a shelf life after which they are no longer usable. By not overordering and by rotating supplies—using older ones first—your office will be able to use items during their shelf life. This is true not only for perishable items such as medications, but also for linens and paper, which can deteriorate. Keep in mind when stocking medications or chemicals that a more recent shipment may have an earlier expiration date than a previous shipment. Always check expiration dates when storing supplies. Be careful to arrange them so that items with earlier expiration dates are in front of those with later dates.

Administrative Supplies. In addition to such expendable items as pens, pencils, and paper clips, paper products are important to a medical office. In general, paper products should be stored flat in their original boxes or wrappings to prevent pages from bending or curling. However, information booklets may be stored upright to save space. Envelopes and other paper goods with gummed surfaces must be kept dry to prevent them from sticking together.

Clinical Supplies. The rules of good housekeeping and asepsis apply to storage areas for clinical supplies. These areas must be kept clean and protected from damage and exposure to the elements.

All dressings and most bandaging materials must be kept sterile. For example, gauze that may be used to bandage an open wound must be sterile. Elastic rolled bandages, which do not touch open wounds, must be clean but not necessarily sterile.

Chemicals, drugs, and solutions should be kept in a cool, dark place because light causes some substances to deteriorate. Store all liquids in their original containers. Line cabinets with plastic-coated shelf paper, and wipe it frequently with a damp cloth.

Store poisons and narcotics separately from other products. Narcotics must be stored securely out of sight in a locked cabinet. Never store strong acids near alkaline solutions or flammable items near sources of heat. Solutions that will be stored for a considerable length of time should have a small amount of space at the top of the bottle to allow for heat expansion.

Some liquids should be stored in the refrigerator. Check each item for specific storage instructions. If storage space is limited, consider eliminating some items—especially bulky ones that are rarely used or items that patients can purchase at surgical supply stores.

Clinical refrigerators may be needed to store certain clinical supplies that require refrigeration. Never store food items and clinical items in the same refrigerator. A clinical refrigerator must be kept at a constant temperature to properly maintain the chemical integrity of lab supplies. Monitoring and recording the date and temperature of the clinical refrigerator should be completed once a week or per office protocol.

Taking Inventory of Medical Office Supplies

The list of supplies your office uses regularly and the quantities you have in storage constitute the office **inventory.** Keeping track of the office's inventory is a job that requires careful planning, attention to detail, and basic math skills. Accurate inventory activity ensures that the office never runs out of much-needed supplies.

Understanding Your Responsibilities

It is important to have an understanding with the doctor or doctors in the practice about the extent of your responsibilities for maintaining supplies. Some doctors are more involved with the details of running an office than others. Your responsibilities may grow as you become more experienced. The doctor, however, usually takes care of certain duties, such as meeting with drug company representatives or authorizing large purchases.

Generally you will be responsible for overseeing the flow of supplies bought and used, calculating the budget for supplies, selecting supplies and vendors, following correct purchasing and payment procedures, and storing the goods properly.

The Inventory Filing System. To oversee the flow of inventory efficiently, you will need a filing system (see Procedure 8-1). This system consists of several elements:

- The list of supplies (discussed earlier in the chapter)
- An itemized inventory
- An inventory card or record page for each item
- A list of the names and addresses of current vendors

- A file of current catalogs from vendors (including some vendors not currently used, for comparison shopping)
- A want list of brands or items that the office does not currently use but may want to try in the future
- Files for **invoices,** or bills from vendors, and completed order forms
- Reorder reminder cards to indicate when an in-stock item should be reordered
- Color-coded, removable self-adhesive flags to indicate "Need to Order" or "On Order"
- An inventory and ordering schedule
- Order forms for each vendor (may be multiple-copy forms, fax forms, electronic forms, or e-mail forms)

The Inventory Card or Record Page. The inventory card or record page for each item or category of items may be a 4-by-6-inch index card or a page in a loose-leaf binder (Figure 8-3). These separate cards or pages make it easy to group together the items that need to be ordered at any given time. Records kept on the card or page help you monitor how quickly items are used and how much should be ordered each time.

Some information may change. As you become more proficient at monitoring inventory or as the practice grows or diminishes in size, you may find that quantities, vendors, or reorder quantities need to be adjusted. With the help of the doctor, you will be able to determine the ideal quantity of each item to have on hand, depending on the size of the practice, the available storage space, and the ordering schedule.

It is important to check the storage areas regularly, preferably at specific times, and to count the items on hand. When the supply of an item begins to run low, you (or another staff member) should flag the inventory card or record page to indicate the need to reorder it at the next regular ordering time.

Color-coded, removable self-adhesive flags on the inventory card or record page are an efficient way to track inventory. A red flag, for example, might indicate that a supply needs to be ordered. A yellow flag might be substituted when the item has been ordered.

Reorder Reminder Cards. Reorder reminder cards (Figure 8-4) are usually brightly colored cards inserted directly into stock on the supply shelf to indicate when it is time to reorder an item. For example, if you have determined that four boxes of staples is a sufficient quantity to keep on hand and your office supply orders are filled in 2 business days, you might place the reorder reminder card between the third and fourth boxes of staples. The reorder quantity on the inventory card or record page for staples would indicate "four boxes."

The reorder reminder cards also remind other staff members to tell you when an item is in short supply. In some offices, the medical assistant labels the reminder card with the name and bar code number of the supply

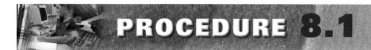

PROCEDURE 8.1

Step-by-Step Overview of Inventory Procedures

Objective: To set up an effective inventory program for a medical office

Materials: Pen, paper, file folders, vendor catalogs, index cards or loose-leaf binder and blank pages, reorder reminder cards, vendor order forms

Method

1. Define with your physician/employer the extent of your responsibility in managing supplies. Know whether the physician's approval or supervision is required for certain procedures, whether any systems have already been established, and if the physician has any preference for a particular vendor or trade-name item. If your medical practice is large, determine which medical assistant is responsible for each aspect of supply management.

2. Know what administrative and clinical supplies should be stocked in your office. Create a formal supply list of vital, incidental, and periodic items, and keep a copy in the office's procedures manual.

3. Start a file containing a list of current vendors with copies of their catalogs.

4. Create a want list of brands or products the office does not currently use but might like to try. Inform other staff members of the list so that they can make entries.

5. Make a file for supply invoices and completed order forms. (Keep these documents on file for at least 3 years.)

6. Devise an inventory system of index cards or loose-leaf pages for each item. List the following data for each item on its card:
   - Date and quantity of each order
   - Name and contact information for the vendor and sales representative
   - Date each shipment was received
   - Total cost and unit cost, or price per piece for the item
   - Payment method used
   - Results of periodic counts of the item
   - Quantity expected to cover the office for a given period of time
   - Reorder quantity (the quantity remaining on the shelf that indicates when reorder should be made)

7. Have a system for flagging items that need to be ordered and those that are already on order. For example, mark their cards or pages with a self-adhesive tab or note. Make or buy reorder reminder cards to put into the stock of each item at the reorder quantity level.

8. Establish with the physician a regular schedule for taking inventory. Every 1 to 2 weeks is usually sufficient. As a backup system for remembering to check stock and reorder, estimate the times for these activities. Mark them on your calendar, or create a tickler file on your computer.

9. Order at the same times each week or month, after inventory is taken. However, if there is an unexpected shortage of an item, and more than a week or so remains before the regular ordering time, place the order immediately.

10. Fill in the vendor's order form (or type a letter of request). Order by telephone, fax, or e-mail, if possible, to expedite the order. Be sure to follow procedures that have been approved by the physician or office manager. When placing an order, have all the necessary information at hand, including the correct name of the item and the order and account numbers. Record the order information in the inventory file for that item. Be sure to obtain from the vendor an estimated arrival time for the order, and mark that date and order number on your calendar.

11. When you receive the shipment, record the date and the amount received on the item's inventory card or record page. Check the shipment against the original order and the packing slip inside the package to ensure that the right items, sizes, styles, packaging, and amounts have arrived. If there is any error, immediately call the vendor, with the catalog page and the inventory card or record page at hand.

12. Check the invoice carefully against the original order and the packing slip, making sure that the bill has not already been paid. Sign or stamp the invoice to show that the order was received.

13. Write a check to the vendor to be signed by the physician. Be sure to show the physician the original order, packing slip, and invoice. Record the check number, date, and amount of payment on the invoice, and initial it or have the physician do so. Write the invoice number on the front of the check.

14. Mail the check and the vendor's copy of the invoice to the vendor within 30 days, and file the office copy of the invoice with the original order and packing slip.

(ITEM NAME)	Exam Table Paper 21"												

ORDER QUANTITY ___12___   **REORDER POINT** ___4___

ORDER	QTY	REC'D	UNIT COST	PRICE	PREPAID	ON ACCT.	ORDER	QTY	REC'D	UNIT COST	PRICE	PREPAID	ON ACCT.
1/4	12	1/8	$12.25	$147.00	Check 1214	X							
2/5	12	2/9	$12.25	$147.00	Check 2110	X							

INVENTORY COUNT

	JAN.	FEB.	MAR.	APR.	MAY	JUNE	JULY	AUG.	SEPT.	OCT.	NOV.	DEC.
DATE ___	7	10										
DATE ___												

ORDER SOURCE

Smith Physician's Supply Co.

493 Carlton Avenue

South Union, NJ 07422

908-899-6123   Contact: Martin Kohn

UNIT PRICE

12 – $147.00

36 – $441.00

Figure 8-3. The inventory card or record page is the primary inventory-tracking tool in managing medical office supplies.

item, such as "staples 002345." This method allows any staff member to pull the card when the last box of staples before the reminder card is taken from the supply shelf. The staff member can then place the card in a "To Be Ordered" envelope. Some offices can reorder simply by scanning the bar code. Staff members in some offices request supplies by writing them in an order book or on an order list.

Inventory Reminder Kits. Some mail-order supply vendors sell inventory kits, complete with cards and tabs or flags. Computerized inventory systems are also available. Shelves still need to be checked and counts logged on to the computer, however. Therefore, smaller offices generally do not benefit as much as larger ones from a computerized inventory system.

Scheduling Inventory and Ordering

Establish a regular schedule for counting the supplies in the office. Taking inventory every 1 or 2 weeks is usually sufficient. Estimating when you will probably need to reorder a particular item—and putting that date on your calendar or in your appointment book—is also helpful. You and the physician can determine how often storage areas should be checked.

Established Ordering Times. You should have established ordering times, such as the same day each week or month, after inventory is taken. For example, you might take inventory the first Tuesday of every month and order supplies the first Thursday of every month.

A regular schedule for taking inventory and ordering helps all staff members remember when they must give their requests to you. Although you may need to adjust the ordering time occasionally, try to adhere to the schedule to avoid the expense and inconvenience of rush orders.

When to Order Ahead of Schedule. When you take inventory, and the spare supply of an item has not reached but is close to the placement of the reorder reminder card, you must decide whether you should reorder then or wait until the next regular ordering time. You will probably find it is more efficient to go ahead and order rather than wait. Ordering early assures you that the supply will not be depleted before the next regular ordering time.

Ordering ahead of schedule can be especially important if there is a large demand for a particular product and manufacturers' production levels have not caught up with that demand. This situation can occur if there has been an outbreak of a particular flu or virus, or if the Food and Drug Administration has determined that a certain product is harmful, resulting in higher demand for an alternative product.

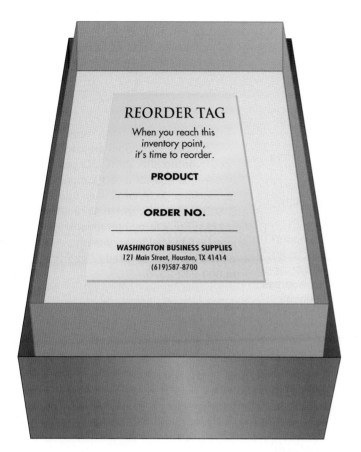

Figure 8-4. Reorder reminder cards are usually brightly colored cards inserted directly into the spare stock of an item on the supply shelf to indicate when it is time to reorder the item.

Unanticipated Shortage of a Supply Item. If the supply of an item reaches the reorder reminder card, and there is still a long time before the next regular ordering time, place the order immediately so that you do not risk running out of the item.

To help you oversee inventory effectively, finish one container before opening a new one. Keep all stock of the same item in one place. The need to count inventory of an item in more than one location or container increases the likelihood of errors. If an item is kept in more than one location, as in the case of multiple examination rooms, inventory is best maintained per room.

As a medical assistant, you want to be sure that there are always sufficient quantities of supplies to keep the office running efficiently. It is unwise to stock spare supplies in too great a quantity, however, because the administrative budget is not likely to support such expenditures. In addition, spare quantities of supplies can be a storage problem.

Ordering Supplies

Ordering supplies requires a procedure to deal with vendors and to order and check supplies. You can avoid common purchasing mistakes by understanding the most efficient way to order supplies for your office.

Locating and Evaluating Supply Vendors

A vendor will most likely already be in place when you join a practice. You should, however, be aware of competitors' prices, services, and other incentives intended to attract your office as a customer. Sometimes the incentives—such as bonus supplies with certain purchases—can represent sizable savings. Remember also that your time has a dollar value to the practice, and services that save you time are worth comparing when evaluating vendors.

Obtaining recommendations from other medical offices is a good way to locate office-supply dealers who sell items at reasonable prices and are also reputable. **Reputable** vendors fulfill orders accurately with quality items, deliver products in good condition, and charge fair prices. Keep in mind when evaluating vendors that the physician may have preferences for certain trade names or vendors.

Gathering Competitive Prices. The costs of maintaining a medical practice are continually rising. Saving money on supplies through careful purchasing strategies is one way to help your physician/employer reduce spending. The medical assistant is often largely responsible for comparison pricing, ordering, and establishing and maintaining relationships with vendors. Your awareness of the most up-to-date information about vendors and supplies is valuable to your physician/employer. Discuss prices with the physician, who in turn may want to discuss them with an accountant.

Setting Up a Supply Budget. The average medical practice spends 4% to 6% of its annual gross income on administrative, clinical, and general supplies. If an office is spending more than 6%, it may be time to reevaluate the office's spending practices. Remember, though, that any budget is only a guide. A budget is meant to serve your office, not the reverse. You and your physician/employer may need to adjust the supply budget based on prices and discounts available from vendors.

Comparing Vendors. To collect competitive data from vendors, contact them by telephone or in writing to request catalogs and other forms of product information. If you are not in charge of routing mail, make sure that supply-related mail, such as product catalogs and sale notices, is routed to you. Catalogs usually include basic information, such as the dealer's name, address, and telephone number, order numbers for items, and vendor policy (Figure 8-5). When investigating a vendor, obtain the following information:

- Prices—costs for supplies, delivery, and any other services; special discounts; minimum quantities applicable; bonus supplies with purchases

BY PHONE

Call our toll-free number:
(800) BIBBERO
(800-242-2376)
Monday thru Friday,
6:00 A.M. – 5:00 P.M. (PST)

BY MAIL

Complete order form and mail to:
Bibbero Systems, Inc.
1300 N. McDowell Blvd.
Petaluma, CA 94954-1180

BY FAX

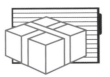

Complete order form and transmit via
FAX to : 800-242-9330
Our FAX line is open 24 hours daily.

Fill out the enclosed order form located in the center of this catalog, and return in the enclosed postage-paid envelope to:

Bibbero Systems, Inc.
1300 N. McDowell Blvd.
Petaluma, CA 94954-1180

If you are in a hurry, call us toll free at: 800-242-2376 or FAX us at 800-242-9330. Our Customer Service Department will be happy to assist you.

For items requiring custom imprinting, please enclose with your order the following information, either typed or printed: Name, Specialty, Address, City/State & Zip Code, Telephone Number and State License Number.

Send us your specifications for any type of special form - Patient Registration, History Forms, Dividers, Charts, etc. – and we will furnish quotes at no charge. We can print single page or multiple part forms.

Please Note: All custom printed orders are subject to an overrun or underrun variance of 10%.

TERMS

Full payment is due upon receipt of merchandise. Accounts are considered overdue after thirty (30) days and will be subject to a 1% monthly service charge. A service charge of $10.00 will be applied to all returned checks. For information regarding special financial arrangements, please contact our Credit Department at 800-242-2376.

GUARANTEE!

Your Satisfaction Guaranteed!

We guarantee our stock products. Return any of our stock products within 60 days of purchase for full credit, exchange or refund of your purchase price. After 60 days, your return will be subject to prior approval and a 15% restocking charge. All returns must have an authorization number. Call our Customer Service Department at 800-242-2376 for your authorization number and enclose it with your return. Opened and/or partially used packages cannot be returned. Personalized items, made to order, special orders and unlocked or opened software cannot be returned.

SHIPPING POLICY

Stock items are normally shipped the same day.

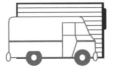

Stock orders received by 11:00 A.M. are normally shipped the same day. Out-of-stock items are automatically back ordered. Custom printed orders normally leave our plant within 10-15 working days after proof approval.

Combined stock and custom printed orders are shipped together, if requested. All orders are shipped via the best method available to your location. Common carriers are used for large volume orders. Overnight air and 2nd day delivery services are available on request.

FREE DELIVERY

Free delivery on pre-paid orders totaling $300.00 or more.

All orders prepaid by check, Visa, MasterCard or American Express totaling $300.00 or more will be shipped freight free within the continental U.S. This offer excludes furniture, cabinets, and special order items. We regret that the high cost of shipping outside the 48 contiguous states prohibits us from extending this service; we will use the most economical shipping method available to your location.

We accept Visa, MasterCard,
& American Express
for all your purchases.

BIBBᴱᴿᴼ **SYSTEMS, INC.**

Figure 8-5. Examine supply catalogs carefully to find out vendors' company policies.

- Quality—product descriptions, illustrations, trade names, recommendations for use, durability, guarantees
- Service—availability of products, delivery time and procedures, sales representative availability, damaged-goods policy
- Payment policies

Competitive Pricing and Quality

Part of your responsibility in managing office supplies is to stay informed about the pricing and quality of competitors to your vendors. Savings can add up quickly, and ongoing comparison pricing can save the practice hundreds of dollars a year.

Unit Pricing. Because many medical items come in a variety of package sizes, you need to be aware of how much the office is actually paying per item. To calculate an item's **unit price,** divide the total price of the package by the quantity, or number of items. For example, if a package of 12 pens costs $12, the unit price, or price per pen, is $1 ($12 divided by 12 pens). If another vendor provides the same type of pen in a package of 18 for $17.10, the unit price is 95 cents ($17.10 divided by 18 pens). The second set of pens is the better buy.

Unit prices are generally lower at larger quantities. Therefore, it makes sense to place one large order for a nonperishable item to cover the office until the next ordering time. Generally, however, you should not order more than a year's supply of any one item, particularly if the item is custom-printed. Addresses, insurance codes, or additions to medical staff can change. When placing quantity discount orders, always consider the following factors: whether the supply can be used within a reasonable time, the possibility of spoilage or deterioration, the amount of storage space in the office, and whether the doctor will continue to use the item. Avoid overspending by not ordering more of an item than is reasonable or necessary.

Rush Orders. Unexpected rush orders usually cost the office more money than regularly scheduled orders. (In some cases, a vendor may not charge extra to a steady customer, but these cases would be exceptions.) To avoid rush orders, be aware of approximately how long the vendor takes to deliver an order. You can obtain this information from the vendor policy and by keeping accurate records of your own experience with deliveries.

Mail-Order Companies. Using large, established mail-order companies often saves money for the medical office, but there may be less control over orders and a greater potential for hidden costs. The neighborhood pharmacy may also offer discounts, but ordering from wholesalers or directly from the manufacturer is usually more economical. The Tips for the Office section provides helpful information about cost-efficient ordering by telephone or fax or through an online service.

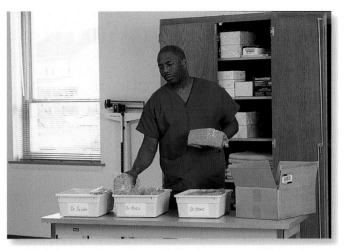

Figure 8-6. Ordering jointly with other offices can cut expenses for everyone.

Purchasing Groups. **Purchasing groups** are groups of physicians that order supplies together to obtain a quantity discount. For example, several medical offices associated with a nearby hospital may order through the hospital. In return for this convenience, the physicians pay dues and guarantee the vendors a certain amount of business. Some programs require members to spend a certain percentage of their supply budget through the group. Groups may also require that members not disclose the group's prices to other physicians. The larger medical practices that participate in these groups save an average of 20% on supplies. The savings are not usually significant for small offices.

Group Buying Pools. If a medical office wants to use local vendors instead of, or in addition to, a purchasing group or if it is too small to benefit from a purchasing group, it can still pool resources with other area offices to qualify for quantity discounts. Even if the offices are ordering different items, discounts are based on the total order, and savings can range from 10% to 20%. Under this arrangement the offices must usually take responsibility for distributing the items among themselves. A buying pool is convenient for medical practices that are in the same building or office complex (Figure 8-6).

Benefits of Using Local Vendors

There are many potential vendors, including local dealers, mail-order companies, and nearby pharmacies. Try to establish good credit and business relationships with reputable local vendors. These companies often charge a little more than mail-order companies. Still, spending most of the office's supply budget through one favored local dealer often results in discounts, special service in the event of an emergency, and information about upcoming sales and specials. Local dealers may also offer more personal assistance, perhaps even a salesperson's help with taking inventory, to compete with larger vendors whose business is

Tips for the Office

Ordering by Telephone or Fax or Online

You may occasionally purchase office supplies at a local retail outlet, but most often you will order them without leaving your office. Three common ways to do so are by telephone, by facsimile (or fax) machine, and through an online service. Here are tips to help make sure every order—no matter which option you choose—is successfully placed.

Ordering by Telephone

1. Clear communication is a must when ordering by telephone. Speak slowly, and enunciate your words carefully to make sure you are understood. It is also a good idea to spell each word of the practice's name and the address to ensure proper delivery. Use expressions like "S as in Sam, P as in people" to clarify your spelling.

2. Ask the representative taking your order to repeat the order. Check that every item is included with the appropriate price, quantity, style, and color.

3. Confirm the expected delivery date so that you will know if something is late. Also confirm how payment will be made, to prevent unexpected delays.

4. Record the name and telephone number of the person who takes the order in case there is a problem with the order. Get an order number (sometimes called a confirmation number) in case you have to call back with a question or a change in your order.

5. If possible, avoid placing telephone orders on Mondays and Fridays, when call volume is typically high.

Ordering by Fax

1. When ordering by fax, use the form provided by the vendor if one is available. This form uses the format to which the supply company is accustomed and will speed the processing of your order.

2. Type your order, or write it neatly and legibly, to prevent miscommunication. Fill out the form completely. Make sure you indicate quantities, descriptions, and prices (including shipping) for each item you order.

3. Proofread your order before you send it. Checking the accuracy of the order now will save time later.

4. Follow up by telephone to make sure your order was received and understood and to confirm the delivery date and payment requirements.

Ordering Online

1. Ordering online requires a computer and a modem connection to the Internet or to an online service. Before ordering online, make sure you are fully familiar with the equipment and the process, or have your supervisor or the supply company's sales representative oversee your initial orders.

2. Type your name and address accurately.

3. If pictures of supplies are not available online, consult the company's printed catalog or CD-ROM catalog. If you do not have access to a catalog, read the online text descriptions carefully, checking trade names and specifications, to select the appropriate merchandise. If you have questions, consult the supply company by telephone.

4. When you have completed the selections, the online service will display your order so that you can confirm it. Check that all the information is accurate, including your name, address, and telephone number.

5. If you have an account with the company, you may type in your account number to place the order. Otherwise, you may wish to arrange to make payment on delivery. If you prefer to pay by credit card, first make sure that the company is reputable and that it uses a security system that prevents your number from being read by anyone unauthorized to do so.

If, despite your best efforts, your order is processed incorrectly, take appropriate action immediately. Although ordering by telephone or fax or online is convenient, it still requires additional time to package items that must be returned.

By law, orders that you place must be fulfilled within a reasonable time. The Federal Trade Commission (FTC) monitors purchases by telephone, fax, and online services to protect consumers. The FTC requires supply companies to provide merchandise within 30 days or to give you the option of canceling the order and receiving a full refund.

based primarily on catalog sales. The extra service may be worth the higher cost.

Buying from local vendors can also provide a public relations benefit for physicians; it means keeping business in the community. However, specialty items may need to be ordered from other vendors. For example, letterhead should be ordered from a reliable printer, whether that printer is located in the community or out of state.

Payment Schedules

Another factor that affects the cost of supplies is the payment schedule. Many vendors do not charge for handling if an order is prepaid. Others offer a discount for enclosing a check with an order. Some delay billing for 30 to 90 days, allowing the physician to keep the money in the bank, collecting interest for a longer period.

The vendor's invoice usually describes payment terms. Two examples of payment terms are:

1. If the invoice says "Net 30," you have 30 days in which to pay the total amount.
2. "1% 10 Days Net 30" means that you will get a savings of 1% of the total price by paying within 10 days.

Copies of all bills and order forms for supplies should be kept on file for at least 7 years in case the practice is audited by the Internal Revenue Service (IRS).

Storage Space as a Cost Factor

When you plan purchases, you need to consider the available storage space. Ideally, there should be enough space in the office to allow occasional large purchases for quantity discounts. If there is not, a vendor might allow you to take partial shipments on a large order. The vendor might also allow you to pay for the partial shipments with partial payments, but you will probably have to request this plan.

Ordering Procedures

Ordering procedures for supplies vary from office to office but always involve these tasks: completing paperwork, checking orders received, correcting errors in shipments, and making payment.

Order Forms. Before ordering merchandise, you should inquire about a vendor's ordering options, discuss them with the physician, and determine which method is best for the office. Many vendors now accept telephone, fax, and e-mail as well as traditional written order forms. Many vendors will also send a sales representative to your office to help you decide which items to purchase and to show you how to complete an order form accurately. Sometimes the sales representative can give you better deals than those described in the catalog. Whatever form you use, be sure to keep a copy of each order you submit.

Before you place an order, gather all the necessary information, such as correct names of items, item numbers, and order and account numbers. This information helps ensure the accuracy of the order. Immediately after placing the order, note all order information on the inventory card or record page for that item.

Purchase Requisitions. You will need to follow any special ordering procedures established in your medical office. The specific procedures and the medical assistant's level of authority vary from one office to another. Sometimes placing an order requires a **requisition** (a formal request from a staff member or doctor), which is given to the medical assistant who does the actual ordering. The doctor's approval may be necessary for large purchases—for example, for orders that total more than $300. Recurring orders may not require the doctor's approval, but you may need to get approval before ordering a new brand or quantities of a particular item over a certain amount.

In a group practice where doctors order different items and several staffers are in charge of ordering, procedures for ordering can be complicated. One common way to simplify matters is to use **purchase orders,** forms that authorize a purchase for the practice. Figure 8-7 shows a sample purchase order. Purchase orders are usually preprinted with consecutive numbers. The medical assistant submits approved purchase orders to the vendor for fulfillment. This method is most often used for expensive items, such as office equipment, but some large practices also use purchase orders for supplies.

Checking Orders Received. When the shipment of supplies arrives, record on the inventory card or record page the date received as well as the quantity of each item. Check the shipment against the order form to make sure the correct items—in the correct sizes, styles, packaging, and quantity—have been delivered.

Then check the contents against the packing slip (a description of the package contents) enclosed in the package. This checking takes time, but catching even one error is worth the time taken. If several people on a staff have ordering responsibility, they can share the task.

Material Safety Data Sheets. Every chemical item ordered in a medical practice must have a **Material Safety Data Sheet (MSDS)** on file in the office. This sheet is provided by the manufacturer of the product and describes the chemical breakdown of the product as well as safety cautions and procedures to follow in using it. Items that require MSDS include, but are not limited to, all soaps, cleansers, waxes, reagents, clinical testing products, inks, toners, and any product that can be splashed or rubbed on the skin or eyes. JCAHO, OSHA (Occupational Safety Hazards Association), and other surveying organizations will require MSDS on all products used in the medical practice. The purpose of the sheet is to provide important

PURCHASE ORDER

Submitted by: _____
Order Number: _____
Date Ordered: _____
Date Required: _____

SHIP TO: Dr. Carlotta Montoni
201 Oak Walk, Suite 32
Gilead, PA 19034

PHONE: 215-610-4120

	ITEM	DESCRIPTION/MODEL	COLOR	SIZE	QUANTITY	PRICE EACH	TOTAL
1.							
2.							
3.							
4.							
5.							
6.							
7.							
8.							
						TOTAL	

Approved: _____   Date: _____

Figure 8-7. A purchase order, when approved by the physician or office manager, is an authorization from the practice for a purchase.

safety information about the item that may be critical in the event of unintended exposure or potentially dangerous reactions.

For fast and easy access, organize these sheets in a notebook in alphabetical order. As new items are ordered and delivered, add the MSDS into the master notebook. As a medical assistant, you must always check the MSDS notebook when stocking the supply shelves to ensure that all items stocked are included in the notebook. If MSDS information is not included with the item, either immediately request the information from the vendor or go online to print information directly from the product manufacturer.

Correcting Errors. All errors in a shipment should be reported immediately to the vendor so that the records can be corrected and missing supplies can be delivered. When you call to report errors, be sure you have all the paperwork in front of you. You will need the invoice number, order date, name of the person who placed the order, name of the person who took the order, and a list of questions or a description of the complaint. If a catalog was used in ordering, have it open to the appropriate page. Always record the name and title of the person you speak with when reporting the error.

Invoices. Typically the vendor sends an invoice to the medical office, either accompanying the merchandise or separately. This invoice also should be checked carefully against the original order and the packing slip. Be sure to check the arithmetic as well. Then sign or stamp the invoice to confirm that the order was received. If an item you order is temporarily out of stock, the vendor usually sends an invoice stamped "Back Ordered." Later, when the item is back in stock, the vendor will ship it to your office.

Make sure the invoice has not already been paid. It is a good habit to record the check number, date, and amount of payment on the invoice. You may initial it or have the doctor initial it.

Disbursements. An invoice is paid with a **disbursement** (payment of funds) to a vendor. Disbursements may be made in cash or by check or money order. Usually you will write a check to the vendor and have the physician sign it. Be sure to show the physician the original order, packing slip, and invoice. On the front of the check, record the invoice number. Finally, mail the check to the vendor with the vendor's copy of the invoice. File the office copy of the invoice, along with the original order and the packing slip, according to your inventory filing system (Figure 8-8).

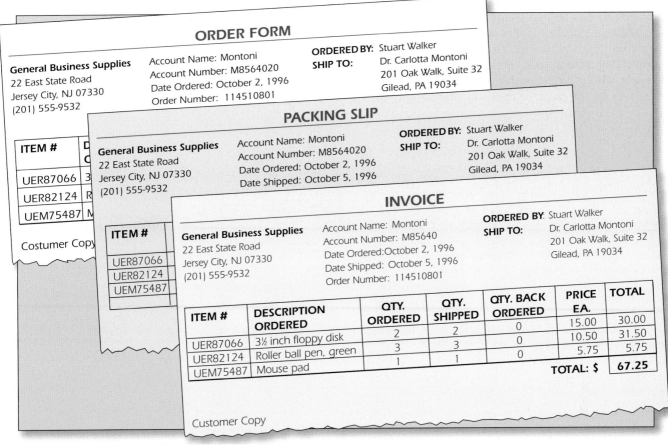

Figure 8-8. Check the information on the vendor invoice against the original order and the packing slip to make sure there are no errors.

If you make a cash disbursement, obtain a receipt to keep on file. If you are the one responsible for maintaining the practice's financial records and presenting them to the accountant, you may also be responsible for recording the payment information in the office's accounting books.

Avoiding Common Purchasing Mistakes

Even the most watchful professional can make purchasing mistakes. The best you can do is to educate yourself about common mistakes and try to avoid them. For example, be aware of the possibility of dishonest telephone solicitations. A caller may claim to be a sales representative for the manufacturer of the office photocopier, offering bargains on paper or toner. The caller may require advance payment to be sent to a post office box. The bargains may never arrive.

The best way to deal with these solicitations is to tell the caller that your office does not purchase supplies by telephone. If a telephone offer appears to be legitimate and to offer substantial savings, ask for the name and telephone number of the firm so that you can return the call at a more convenient time. Then you can verify the number with the telephone company and check the firm's name with the Better Business Bureau.

Another disreputable tactic some vendors use is bait and switch: the price of one item is lowered to attract the customer, but that item is always "sold out" and the customer is encouraged to buy a more expensive one. A vendor may also mislead you by raising the price of an item you have been ordering without informing you. Always confirm the current price, check invoices as they come in, and record everything in the item's file. Having your inventory card or record page open while ordering will prompt you to notice and question price changes. If there is an honest error, a reputable firm will readily and courteously correct it.

Problems can also be avoided by carefully supervising a new vendor's sales representative until a comfortable, professional rapport has been established. Discuss your inventory system with representatives, and ask them questions about their procedures.

Summary

A typical medical practice uses both administrative and clinical office supplies. Supplies can be categorized as vital, incidental, and periodic.

Keeping track of supplies involves creating supply lists and taking inventory. You must know the storage requirements for various kinds of supplies. An inventory filing system can help you organize office supply tasks. Maintaining adequate supplies and well-organized storage space contributes to the smooth running of the office.

You will also locate, evaluate, and establish and maintain working relationships with vendors. It is important to be adept at comparison pricing and to stay abreast of competitors' product quality, pricing policies, and services.

Just as cost-effectiveness is stressed in medical care, it is important to look for ways to control costs when ordering supplies. Checking orders carefully and avoiding dishonest telephone solicitations are two examples of ways to control costs.

CASE STUDY *QUESTIONS*

Now that you have completed this chapter, review the case study at the beginning of the chapter and answer the following questions:

1. What is an *expendable* item? What items would you list on the expendable administrative supply list? The clinical supply list? The general supply list?
2. What factors would you consider about each office as you determine the appropriate supplies?
3. How would you recommend that the supplies be stored with inventory management in mind?

Discussion Questions

1. As a new employee, what questions would you want to ask about the process of ordering supplies within the office?
2. What supplies do you think are the most important in a medical practice and why?

Critical Thinking Questions

1. During a routine inventory inspection, you notice that the supply of prescription pads is extremely low for typical office use. Could there be a problem within the office other than just the need to order more pads from the printer? What would you do?

2. You share the responsibility of ordering supplies with another medical assistant in the office. You are checking supplies and ordering regularly, but the other employee is allowing items to become completely depleted. What would you do?
3. The Sunday paper runs an ad indicating that a local supply vendor is going out of business soon. How do you shop for a new vendor? How could you make the most out of the closeout specials advertised?

Application Activities

1. Using vendor catalogs, make a list of ten typical office supply items for a medical practice. Create a fictional office supply list and ordering schedule (including quantities and prices) for the practice.
2. Select a supply company catalog, and become familiar with it. Imagine that you are a sales representative for that company, and make a presentation to your class as if it were a typical medical practice. Your goal is to have the medical office choose your company as its vendor. Be prepared to answer questions about how your company handles various customer concerns.
3. Make a diagram of an office supply cabinet, indicating how you would label and store items for maximum efficiency. Try to use several of the inventory elements discussed in the chapter.

CHAPTER 9

Maintaining Patient Records

KEY TERMS

documentation
informed consent form
noncompliant
objective
patient record/chart
POMR
sign
SOAP
subjective
symptom
transcription
transfer

AREAS OF COMPETENCE

2003 Role Delineation Study

ADMINISTRATIVE
Administrative Procedures
- Perform basic administrative medical assisting functions

CLINICAL
Patient Care
- Obtain patient history and vital signs
- Maintain medication and immunization records
- Coordinate patient care information with other health-care providers

GENERAL
Communication Skills
- Use medical terminology appropriately
- Utilize electronic technology to receive, organize, prioritize, and transmit information

Legal Concepts
- Prepare and maintain medical records
- Document accurately
- Implement and maintain federal and state health-care legislation and regulations

CHAPTER OUTLINE

- Importance of Patient Records
- Contents of Patient Charts
- Initiating and Maintaining Patient Records
- The Six Cs of Charting
- Types of Medical Records
- Appearance, Timeliness, and Accuracy of Records
- Medical Transcription
- Correcting and Updating Patient Records
- Release of Records

OBJECTIVES

After completing Chapter 9, you will be able to:

9.1 Explain the purpose of compiling patient medical records.
9.2 Describe the contents of patient record forms.
9.3 Describe how to create and maintain a patient record.
9.4 Identify and describe common approaches to documenting information in medical records.

9.5 Discuss the need for neatness, timeliness, accuracy, and professional tone in patient records.

9.6 Discuss tips for performing accurate transcription.

9.7 Explain how to correct a medical record.

9.8 Explain how to update a medical record.

9.9 Identify when and how a medical record may be released.

Introduction

The medical assistant plays a major role in writing and maintaining patient records. These records document the evaluation and treatment given to the patient. Patient records are critical to the care of the patient. Without accurate and complete patient records, medical care could easily be compromised.

Patient records have many parts or sections that describe these facets of every patient:

- Personal information or data
- Physical and mental condition
- Medical history
- Medical care
- Medical future if the patient is referred to other physicians

In this chapter you will learn how to carefully manage the records of the patient. You will understand that if the medical care is not documented, in a legal sense, the medical care did not occur at all.

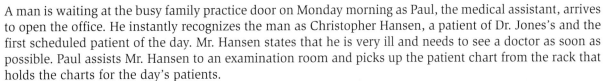

CASE STUDY

A man is waiting at the busy family practice door on Monday morning as Paul, the medical assistant, arrives to open the office. He instantly recognizes the man as Christopher Hansen, a patient of Dr. Jones's and the first scheduled patient of the day. Mr. Hansen states that he is very ill and needs to see a doctor as soon as possible. Paul assists Mr. Hansen to an examination room and picks up the patient chart from the rack that holds the charts for the day's patients.

As Paul begins to check the patient's vital signs, he asks Mr. Hansen what brings him to the doctor today. The patient grips his lower right side as he responds that his stomach hurts a lot. The patient also reports running a temperature between 100.5° and 101.3° for a full day and that he has not been able to eat in the last day because of his stomach pains. Paul knows that this information is important to chart in the permanent record as *subjective* information that has been stated by the patient.

Paul carefully writes down the vital signs for inclusion in the patient chart. He continues his evaluation with an abdominal exam to identify the exact area of tenderness. Paul knows that this information is important to chart in the permanent record as *objective* information that has been observed by the medical professional.

Paul is charting information in the patient record using the SOAP charting method:

- S for subjective
- O for objective
- A for assessment
- P for plan

Paul notifies the physician that the patient is ready for his exam. Dr. Jones completes the record after he evaluates the patient and makes entries to the chart for assessment and the plan for care. The medical record reflects the good clinical management that the patient receives.

As you read this chapter, consider the following questions:

1. Why is an accurate medical record important to the care of a patient?
2. Why is interviewing the patient important to the medical evaluation?
3. What are the six Cs of charting and what do they mean to you as a medical assistant?
4. What are the differences between the conventional and the POMR system of keeping charts?
5. What are some helpful tips you might use as you perform transcription?

Importance of Patient Records

One of your most important duties as a medical assistant will be filling out and maintaining accurate and thorough patient records. **Patient records,** also known as **charts,** contain important information about a patient's medical history and present condition. Patient records serve as communication tools as well as legal documents. They also play a role in patient and staff education and may be used for quality control and research.

These records provide physicians with all the important information, observations, and opinions that have been recorded about a patient. The health-care professional can read the complete patient medical history and information about treatment and outcomes. The information in the records can also be sent to other physicians or health-care specialists if the patient needs further treatment, changes physicians, or moves to a new location. Medical records include the following general information about the patient:

- Address and phone number
- Insurance coverage
- Name of the person responsible for payment
- Occupation
- Medical history
- Current complaint or condition
- Health-care needs
- Medical treatment plan or services received
- Radiology and laboratory reports (sometimes)
- Response to care

Legal Guidelines for Patient Records

Patient records are important for legal reasons. As a general rule, if information is not documented, no one can prove that an event or procedure took place. Medical records are used in lawsuits and malpractice cases to support a patient's claim of malpractice against a doctor and to support the doctor in defense against a claim.

All medical care, evaluation, and instruction given to the patient by the physician must be documented. Every chart entry must be clear, accurate, legible, dated, and per HIPAA guidelines, written in blue ink. The patient chart is a legal document. Always consider how the patient record would present if it was called into a court of law for review.

Additionally, it is very important to document when a patient is **noncompliant.** After a clear record has been made of the directions given to a patient for optimum health, it is essential to record the level of patient compliance. For example, after you have instructed a patient, you may write in her chart that "Patient stated she understood all direction. Written instruction given to patient." If it is determined that a patient did *not* follow the medical advice, it is then essential to chart this as well. The physician may wish to withdraw from the care of a patient because of the patient's noncompliance. Without a proper and accurate documentation of the patient's noncompliance, the physician may not be able to withdraw care without becoming legally liable.

Standards for Records

Records that are complete, accurate, and well documented can be convincing evidence that a doctor provided appropriate care. On the other hand, altered, incomplete, inaccurate, or illegible records may imply that a doctor's entire medical practice is below standard.

Additional Uses of Patient Records

Patient records serve as ongoing references about individual patients' medical care. They are also valuable for patient education, quality of treatment, and research.

Patient Education. Patient records can be used to educate patients about their own conditions and treatment plans. The physician can point out how test results have changed or how the patient's general health has improved or lessened. The physician can also emphasize the importance of following treatment instructions. The medical assistant in turn may use some of this information in educating the patient about his condition or its management. Records can also be used to educate the health-care staff about unusual medical conditions, patient progress, or results of treatment plans.

Quality of Treatment. Patient records may be used to evaluate the quality of treatment a facility or doctor's office provides. Auditing groups, such as peer review organizations or the Joint Commission on Accreditation of Healthcare Organizations (JCAHO), may review the charts to monitor whether the care provided and the fees charged meet accepted standards. Records also provide statistics for health-care analysis and future health-care plans and policy decisions.

Research. Patient records also play an important role in medical research. For example, a medical research team may be testing a new hypertension drug with volunteers who fit a certain medical category—perhaps men between the ages of 45 and 54 who have high blood pressure. Carefully kept records are valuable sources of data about patient responses, behavior, symptoms, side effects, and outcomes (see Figure 9-1).

Information in charts may spur researchers to begin a study. For example, the records may show that 80% of all patients taking a particular heart medication experience dizziness. Researchers can investigate why this reaction might be happening.

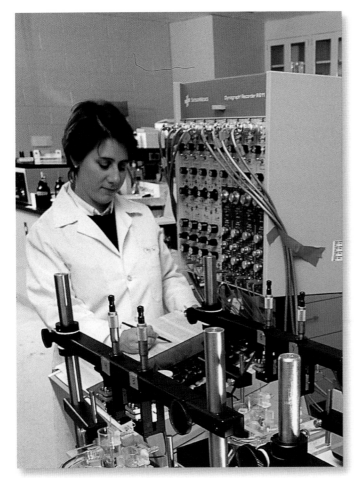

Figure 9-1. Medical researchers may rely on data gathered from patient records.

Contents of Patient Charts

You will fill out a record for each new patient who comes to the office. Although each physician's office has its own forms and medical charts, in general, all records must contain certain standard information.

Standard Chart Information

Standard chart information covers a spectrum of different, carefully detailed notes and facts about a patient, from his medical history to the doctor's diagnosis and comments on follow-up care. You must have an understanding of what each part means.

Patient Registration Form. The patient registration part of the record should list the date of the patient's current visit, the patient's age, address, Social Security number, DOB (date of birth), medical insurance, occupation, marital status, number of children, and the name of the person to contact in an emergency. Some patient registration forms include family medical history and a list of medical problems. This information is usually placed at the front or top half of the chart for easy reference. Figure 9-2 is an example of a patient registration form.

Patient Medical History. The medical history section includes the patient's past medical history (including illnesses, surgeries, known allergies, or current medications), family medical history, and social and occupational history (including diet, exercise, smoking, and use of alcohol or drugs). Usually, the history form ends with a section for the patient to describe the condition or complaint that is the reason for her visit. Medicare and managed care insurance now require that the patient's complaint be entered into the medical record. The complaint should be recorded in the patient's own words.

Physical Examination Results. Sometimes a form is used to record the results of a general physical examination. Figure 9-3 shows a combination medical history and physical examination form.

Results of Laboratory and Other Tests. Test results include findings from tests performed in the office and those received from other doctors, hospitals, or independent laboratories. Some offices use a laboratory summary sheet to help the doctor detect significant changes more easily.

Records From Other Physicians or Hospitals. Incoming records from other sources should be entered into the patient's chart. A copy of the patient's written request authorizing release of the records from the other sources should also be included.

Doctor's Diagnosis and Treatment Plan. The doctor's diagnosis must be recorded, along with the treatment plan, which may consist of treatment options, the final treatment list, instructions to the patient, and any medications prescribed. The doctor may also put specific comments or impressions on record.

Operative Reports, Follow-Up Visits, and Telephone Calls. Continuation of the record lasts as long as the patient is under the doctor's care. You should record and date all procedures, surgeries, follow-up care, and additional notes the doctor makes regarding the patient's case. You can use continuation forms to add more pages. In addition, you may keep a separate log of telephone calls to and from the patient.

Informed Consent Forms. **Informed consent forms,** such as the one shown in Figure 9-4, verify that a patient understands the treatment offered and the possible outcomes or side effects of the treatment. Consent forms may specify what the outcome might be if the patient receives no treatment. They may also describe alternative treatments and possible risks. The patient signs the consent form but may withdraw consent if she changes her mind.

Hospital Discharge Summary Forms. The discharge summary form generally includes information that summarizes the reason the patient entered the hospital; tests, procedures, or operations performed in the hospital;

Community Health Center • 6508 South Street • Kokomo, IN 46902
(317) 555-1234 • Fax: (317) 555-1245

Patient Registration
Patient Information

Name: _____ Today's Date: _____

Address: _____

City: _____ State: _____ Zip Code: _____

Telephone (Home): _____ (Work): _____ (Cell): _____

Birthdate: _____ Age: _____ Sex: M F No. of Children _____ Marital Status: M S W D

Social Security Number: _____ Employer: _____ Occupation: _____

Primary Physician: _____

Referred by: _____

Person to Contact in Emergency: _____

Emergency Telephone: _____

Special Needs: _____

Responsible Party

Party Responsible for Payment: Self   Spouse   Parent   Other

Name (If Other Than Self): _____

Address: _____

City: _____ State: _____ Zip Code: _____

Primary Insurance

Primary Medical Insurance: _____

Insured party: Self   Spouse   Parent   Other

ID#/Social Security No.: _____ Group/Plan No.: _____

Name (If Other Than Self): _____

Address: _____

City: _____ State: _____ Zip Code: _____

Secondary Insurance

Secondary Medical Insurance: _____

Insured party: Self   Spouse   Parent   Other

ID#/Social Security No.: _____ Group/Plan No.: _____

Name (If Other Than Self): _____

Address: _____

City: _____ State: _____ Zip Code: _____

Figure 9-2. The patient registration form is often the first document used in initiating a patient record.

The Medical Center at Springfield
Medical History

Name _____ Age _____ Sex _____ S M W D

Address _____ Phone _____ Date _____

Occupation _____ Ref. by _____

Chief Complaint _____

Present Illness _____

_____

_____

_____

_____

History —Military _____

    —Social _____

    —Family _____

    —Marital _____

    —Menstrual _____ Menarche _____ Para. _____ LMP _____

    —Illness   Measles   Pert.   Var.   Pneu.   Pleur.   Typh.   Mal.   Rh. Fev.   Sc. Fev.   Diphth.   Other

    —Surgery _____

    —Allergies _____

    —Current Medications _____

Physical Examination

Temp. _____ Pulse _____ Resp. _____ BP _____ Ht. _____ Wt. _____

General Appearance _____ Skin _____ Mucous Membrane _____

Eyes: _____ Vision _____ Pupil _____ Fundus _____

Ears: _____

Nose: _____

Throat: _____ Pharynx _____ Tonsils _____

Chest: _____ Breasts _____

Heart: _____

Lungs: _____

Abdomen: _____

Genitalia: _____

Rectum: _____

Pelvic: _____

Extremities: _____ Pulses: _____

Lymph Nodes: _____ Neck _____ Axilla _____ Inguinal _____ Abdominal _____

Neurological: _____

Diagnosis: _____

_____

Treatment: _____

_____

Laboratory Findings: _____

Date _____ Blood _____

_____

Date _____ Urine _____

_____

Figure 9-3. In some doctors' offices, the medical history form and the physical examination form are combined.

THE OAK HILLS MEDICAL CENTER
Oak Hills, MA

CONSENT TO OPERATION, ADMINISTRATION OF ANESTHETICS,
AND RENDERING OF OTHER MEDICAL SERVICE

Patient: _____ Age: _____

Date: _____ Time: _____

1. I AUTHORIZE AND DIRECT _____ , with the associates
    and assistants of his/her choice, to perform upon myself the following operation

    _____

    _____

    _____

    If any unforeseen conditions arise in the course of the operation or in the postoperative period, calling in their
    judgment for other operations or procedures, I further request and authorize them to do whatever is deemed
    advisable for my health and well-being.

2. The positive and negative aspects of autologous blood transfusions (receiving my own blood donated prior to
    surgery), designated blood transfusions (donated in advance by family/friends for my use), or homologous blood
    transfusions (from general donor population) have been explained to me. I understand autologous and designated
    transfusions can be accommodated only for nonemergency surgery.

6. I certify that I understand the above consent to operation and that the explanations referred to have been made.

    _____   _____
    Witness (of signature only)   Signature

Figure 9-4. Patients are asked to sign informed consent forms to confirm that they understand the treatment offered.

medications administered in the hospital; and the disposition, or outcome, of the case. Elements of the form may include the following:

- Date of admission
- Brief history
- Date of discharge
- Admitting diagnosis
- Operations and procedures or hospital course (course of action taken in the hospital)
- Complications
- Instructions to the patient for follow-up care after discharge from the hospital
- Physician's signature

Correspondence With or About the Patient.
All written correspondence from the patient or from other doctors, laboratories, or independent health-care agencies

should be kept in the patient's chart. Each piece of correspondence should be marked or stamped with the date the doctor's office received the document.

Information Received by Fax

Some information—such as laboratory results, physician comments, or correspondence—may be received by fax transmission. Always request that the original be mailed if possible. If the original is not available, make a photocopy of the fax. Fax copies made on thermal paper, as opposed to those made from a plain-paper fax, fade over time and may become unreadable.

Dating and Initialing

You must be careful not only to date everything you put into the patient chart but also to initial the entry. This system makes it easy to tell which items the assistant enters into the chart and which items others enter. In many practices the physician initials reports before they are filed to prove that he saw them.

Initiating and Maintaining Patient Records

Besides the receptionist, you will often be the first health-care professional that new patients talk with when they visit a doctor's office. During your first contact with a patient, you will initiate a patient record. Recording information in the medical record is called **documentation.** Complete, thorough documentation ensures that the doctor will have detailed notes about each contact with the patient and about the treatment plan, patient responses and progress, and treatment outcomes.

Initial Interview

You usually perform the following tasks on your own, depending on the doctor's practice and your experience and background. Familiarize yourself with each task.

Completing Medical History Forms. You will help new patients fill out medical history forms or questionnaires. You may retrieve current patients' records from the files to update them. Type the patient's name and other identifying information on the first page and on all subsequent pages of the form.

You may interview patients to fill in some of the remaining blanks about medical history. Some doctors prefer to ask patients questions themselves. Others believe that people sometimes talk more freely with an assistant than they do with the doctor.

Documenting Patient Statements. You will record any signs, symptoms, or other information the patient wishes to share. Document this information in the patient's words, not your interpretation of the words. Record these data in specific detail. For example, if the patient drinks alcohol, you should record the number of drinks per week, the type of liquor consumed, and whether the drinking has affected the patient's behavior and health.

Conduct the interview in a private room or in a semi-private office away from the reception area, as shown in Figure 9-5. Patients usually do not like to discuss their medical or personal problems in front of others. Your opinion of the patient, such as "the patient seems mentally unstable," is your own and should not be discussed or documented. The Tips for the Office section will help you take information from elderly patients.

Documenting Test Results. Put a copy in the chart of any test results, x-ray reports, or other diagnostic results that the patient has brought with him. You may also record this information on a separate test summary sheet in the chart.

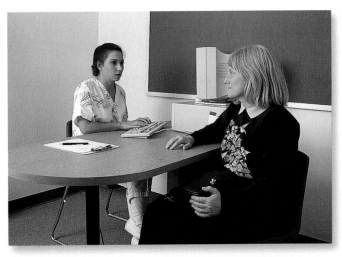

Figure 9-5. Conduct interviews with patients in a private or semiprivate room to make them feel more comfortable.

Examination Preparation and Vital Signs. In many instances, you will prepare patients for examination. You will record vital signs, medication the patient is currently taking, and any responses to treatment. Before you leave a patient, ask, "Is there anything else you would like the doctor to know?" The patient may be more comfortable sharing further information with you than with the doctor.

Follow-Up

After you record the initial interview and background information, the doctor decides what entries will be made regarding examinations, diagnosis, treatment options and plans, and comments or observations about each case. You then maintain the patient record by performing the following duties.

- Transcribe notes the doctor dictates about the patient's progress, follow-up visits, procedures, current status, and other necessary information.
- Post laboratory test results or results of examinations in the record or on the summary sheet.
- Record telephone calls from the patient and calls that the doctor or other office staff members make to the patient (Figure 9-6). Telephone calls can be an important part of good follow-up care. Calls must be dated, and the content of the conversations must be documented. You must initial the entry. Even if the doctor did not reach the patient, the call should be recorded and dated. State whether the doctor got an answer, left a message on an answering machine or with a person, and so on. Legally, if an item is not in the record, it did not happen.
- Record medical instructions or discharge instructions the doctor gives. At the doctor's request, you may counsel or educate the patient regarding treatment regimen or home-care procedures the patient must

Tips for the Office

Talking With the Older Patient

If you work in a practice that specializes in geriatrics or in any practice with older patients, certain communication skills will help you in your job. You may find yourself in various situations in which knowing how to talk with the older patient will be a necessary skill. Taking a medical history or helping a patient describe her symptoms are two such situations. The following tips will help you and the patient communicate with each other more effectively.

1. Make sure you select a private setting for the patient interview.

2. Many older patients are hard of hearing, but *not deaf.* Speak slightly more slowly than you normally would. Speak clearly and loudly (but do not shout—shouting will insult and anger an older patient who does hear well). Enunciate well, and use a lower tone of voice (elderly people lose the ability to hear high-frequency sounds first). If the patient asks you to repeat a question, rephrase it instead of repeating it verbatim.

3. Look at the patient directly so that she knows you care about what she has to say and so that you can make sure she understands what you tell or ask her.

4. You can show respect for the patient's age by addressing the patient with Mr., Mrs., Ms., or Miss, unless the patient asks to be called by his or her first name.

5. Be patient. Some older patients live alone or in relative isolation and may be out of practice with the two-way communication skills that make a conversation or interview go smoothly. The simple act of being interviewed, even for what may seem to you a straightforward medical history, may unsettle the older patient. For example, he may need to stop and think of a word here and there. Do not supply the word.

Wait and let the patient think of it on his own. Also, do not rush through your questions. Rushing will only make the patient feel anxious and incompetent if she feels she cannot keep up with you.

6. Practice active listening skills. Pay attention to the patient's verbal and nonverbal cues. Do not interrupt the patient. After the patient finishes giving each answer, repeat it, to give him a chance to correct you if you misheard or misunderstood.

7. If you are interviewing the patient to obtain a medical history, explain before you begin the type of questions you will ask and how the information will be used.

8. If you need to use medical terminology, try also to express the same information in lay terms. For example, you might ask, "Do you use a diuretic or pill to help you eliminate fluids?"

9. Be cheerful and friendly but not sugary-sweet. Do not talk down to older patients; they are not stupid.

10. Avoid sounding surprised or excited by any answer to a question or to any information the patient gives.

11. Under no circumstances use endearments such as dear, honey, or sweetie.

12. Look for ways to make a connection so that the patient feels relaxed and comfortable. In the course of taking a patient's history, you might find out that he enjoys swimming. Maybe you do, too—and you can describe a beautiful lake you once went swimming in.

13. Show an interest in the patient as a person. Ask about something she is interested in. For example, a patient might be wearing a piece of handmade jewelry. Ask where it came from. She might have a wonderful story to tell.

follow. This information must be entered into the record, dated, and initialed. Some offices make carbon copies or photocopies of patient instructions.

The Six Cs of Charting

To maintain accurate patient records, always keep these six Cs in mind when filling out and maintaining charts: Client's (patient's) words, Clarity, Completeness, Conciseness, Chronological order, and Confidentiality.

1. *Client's words.* Be careful to record the patient's exact words rather than your interpretation of them. For instance, if a client says, "My right knee feels like it's thick or full of fluid," write that down. Do not rephrase the sentence to say, "Client says he's got fluid on the knee." Often the patient's exact words, no matter how odd they may sound, provide important clues for the physician in making a diagnosis.

2. *Clarity.* Use precise descriptions and accepted medical terminology when describing a patient's condition.

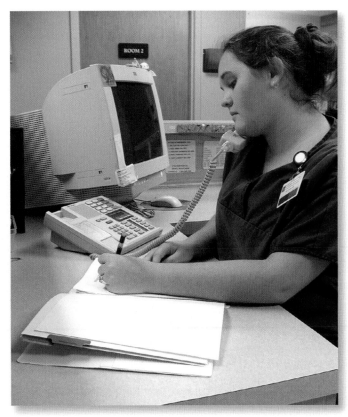

Figure 9-6. All telephone conversations to and from the patient must be logged in the patient record.

For instance, "Patient got out of bed and walked 20 feet without shortness of breath" is much clearer than "Patient got out of bed and felt fine."

3. *Completeness.* Fill out completely all the forms used in the patient record. Provide complete information that is readily understandable to others whenever you make any notation in the patient chart.

4. *Conciseness.* While striving for clarity, also be concise, or brief and to the point. Abbreviations and specific medical terminology can often save time and space when recording information. For instance, you can write "Patient got OOB and walked 20 ft w/o SOB." OOB and SOB are standard abbreviations for "out of bed" and "shortness of breath," respectively. Every member of the office staff should use the same abbreviations to avoid misunderstandings. Table 9-1 lists some common medical abbreviations.

5. *Chronological order.* All entries in patient records must be dated to show the order in which they are made. This factor is critical, not only for documenting patient care but also in case there is a legal question about the type and date of medical services.

6. *Confidentiality.* All the information in patient records and forms is confidential, to protect the patient's privacy. Only the patient, attending physicians, and the medical assistant (who needs the record to tend to the patient and/or to make entries into the record) are allowed to see the charts without the patient's written

consent. Never discuss a patient's records, forward them to another office, fax them, or show them to anyone but the physician unless you have the patient's written permission to do so.

Types of Medical Records

You should be familiar with the different approaches to documenting patient information. The most common methods are conventional/source-oriented and problem-oriented medical records.

Conventional, or Source-Oriented, Records

In the conventional, or source-oriented, approach, patient information is arranged according to who supplied the data—the patient, doctor, specialist, or someone else. The medical form may have a space for patient remarks, followed by a section for the doctor's comments.

These records describe all problems and treatments on the same form in simple chronological order. For example, a patient's broken wrist would be recorded on the same form as her stomach ulcer. Although easy to initiate and maintain, this system presents some difficulty in tracking the progress of a specific ailment, such as the patient's ulcer. The doctor has to search the entire record to find information on that one problem.

Problem-Oriented Medical Records

One way to overcome the disadvantages of the conventional approach is to use the problem-oriented medical record (POMR) system of keeping charts. This approach, developed by Lawrence L. Weed, MD, makes it easier for the physician to keep track of a patient's progress. The information in a POMR includes the database; problem list; educational, diagnostic, and treatment plan; and progress notes.

Database. The database includes a record of the patient's history; information from the initial interview with the patient (for example, "Patient unemployed—second time in past 12 months"); all findings and results from physical examinations (such as "Pulse 105 bpm, BP 210/80"), and any tests, x-rays, and other procedures.

Problem List. Each problem a patient has is listed separately, given its own number, and dated. You then identify a problem by its number throughout the record. You can also list work-related, social, or family problems that may be affecting the patient's health. For instance, the problem list for the example patient who is unemployed might include, "Severe stomach pain, worse at night and after eating."

You can alert the doctor to the fact that the patient has lost two jobs within 1 year. Such radical life changes can

TABLE 9-1　Common Medical Abbreviations

Abbreviation	Meaning	Abbreviation	Meaning
AIDS	acquired immunodeficiency syndrome	inj.	injection
a.m.a.	against medical advice	IV	intravenous
b.i.d./BID	twice a day	MI	myocardial infarction
BP	blood pressure	MM	mucous membrane
bpm	beats per minute	NPO	nothing by mouth
CBC	complete blood count	NYD	not yet diagnosed
C.C.	chief complaint	OOB	out of bed
CNS	central nervous system	OPD	outpatient department
CPE	complete physical examination	OR	operating room
CV	cardiovascular	PH	past history
D & C	dilation and curettage	PT	physical therapy
Dx	diagnosis	Pt	patient
ECG/EKG	electrocardiogram	q.i.d./QID	four times a day
ER	emergency room	ROS/SR	review of systems/systems review
FH	family history	s.c./subq.	subcutaneously
Fl/fl	fluid	SOB	shortness of breath
GBS	gallbladder series	S/R	suture removal
GI	gastrointestinal	stat	immediately
GU	genitourinary	t.i.d./TID	three times a day
GYN	gynecology	TPR	temperature, pulse, respirations
HEENT	head, ears, eyes, nose, throat	UCHD	usual childhood diseases
HIV	human immunodeficiency virus	VS	vital signs
I & D	incision and drainage	WNL	within normal limits
ICU	intensive care unit		

often provoke strong physical reactions. In this patient's case the elevated blood pressure may be related to the job losses, and stress may be causing the stomach pain.

When you document problems, be careful to distinguish between patient signs and symptoms. **Signs** are objective, or external, factors—such as blood pressure, rashes, or swelling—that can be seen or felt by the doctor or measured by an instrument. **Symptoms** are subjective, or internal, conditions felt by the patient, such as pain, headache, or nausea. Together, signs and symptoms help clarify a patient's problem.

Educational, Diagnostic, and Treatment Plan. Each problem should have a detailed educational, diagnostic, and treatment summary in the record. The summary

contains diagnostic workups, treatment plans, and instructions for the patient. Here is an example.

Problem 2, Stomach Pain, 2/2/XX [date]

- *Upper GI exam negative, CBC normal.*
- *Prescribed over-the-counter antacid, 2 tablets by mouth t.i.d. after each meal.*
- *Set up appointment for patient with Dr. R. Neil at stress-management clinic (Broughten Professional Center) for Monday, February 4, at 4:30 p.m.*
- *Patient's anxiety is high. Recheck in 1 week.*

Progress Notes. Progress notes are entered for each problem listed in the initial record. The documentation always includes—in chronological order—the patient's condition, complaints, problems, treatment, and responses to care. Here is an example.

> *Problem 2, Stomach Pain, 2/9/XX. Patient enrolled in stress-reduction class. Reports stomach pain has diminished—"I can eat without pain; only a little discomfort at night." Vital signs improved: pulse 85 bpm, BP 115/70, respiration 20. Reduced antacid to one tablet by mouth two times daily after meals. Anxiety much reduced. Recheck anxiety level in 2 weeks.*

SOAP Documentation

Many medical records, such as the POMR, emphasize the **SOAP** approach to documentation, which provides an orderly series of steps for dealing with any medical case. SOAP documentation lists the patient's symptoms, the diagnosis, and the suggested treatment. Information is documented in the record in the following order.

1. S: **Subjective** data come from the patient; they describe his or her signs and symptoms and supply any other opinions or comments.
2. O: **Objective** data come from the physician and from examinations and test results.
3. A: *Assessment* is the diagnosis or impression of a patient's problem.
4. P: *Plan* of action includes treatment options, chosen treatment, medications, tests, consultations, patient education, and follow-up.

Whether you keep conventional or POMR charts, you can include all these steps for each problem. Figure 9-7 shows an example of SOAP notes. If you abbreviate any term when entering data into the records, use only approved medical abbreviations. For example, use "5 g" instead of "5 grams." Several resources, including those published by JCAHO and the American Medical Association, list approved medical abbreviations for measurements, instructions for taking medication, and other topics. Keep these references readily available in the office.

Appearance, Timeliness, and Accuracy of Records

You must ensure that the medical records are complete. They must also be written neatly and legibly, contain up-to-date information, and present an accurate, professional record of a patient's case.

Neatness and Legibility

A medical record is useless if the doctor or others have difficulty reading it. You should make sure that every word and number in the record is clear and legible. Follow these tips to keep charts neat and easy to read.

- Use a good-quality pen that will not smudge or smear. Blue ink is required by HIPAA. Use highlighting pens to call attention to specific items such as allergies. Be aware, however, that unless the office has a color copier, most colored ink will photocopy black or gray. Highlighting-pen marks may not be visible on a photocopy.
- If you type notes, be sure the typewriter ribbon is dark enough to make clear letters, as shown in Figure 9-8.
- Make sure all handwriting is legible. Take time to write names, numbers, and abbreviations clearly.
- Never use correction fluid in medical records.

Timeliness

Medical records should be kept up to date and should be readily available when a doctor or another health-care professional needs to see them. Follow these guidelines to ensure that a doctor can find the most recent information on a patient when it is needed.

- Record all findings from examinations and tests as soon as they are available.
- If you forget to enter a finding into the record when it is received, record both the original date of receipt and the date the finding was entered into the record.
- To document telephone calls, record the date and time of the call, who initiated it, the information discussed, and any conclusions or results. You can either enter the telephone call directly into the record or make a note referring the doctor to a separate telephone log kept in the record.
- Establish a procedure for retrieving a file quickly in case of emergency. Should the patient be in a serious accident, for example, the emergency doctor will need the patient's medical history immediately.

Accuracy

The physician must be able to trust the accuracy of the information in the medical records. You must make it a priority always to check the accuracy of all data you will enter in a chart. To ensure accurate data, follow these guidelines.

- Never guess at or assume knowledge of names, procedures, medications, findings, or any other information about which there is some question. Always check all the information carefully. Make the extra effort to ask questions of the physician or senior staff member and to verify information.
- Double-check the accuracy of findings and instructions recorded in the chart. Have all numbers been copied accurately? Are instructions for taking medication clear and complete?
- Make sure the latest information has been entered into the chart so that the physician has an accurate picture of the patient's current condition.

OUTLINE FORMAT PROGRESS NOTES

Patient Name *Hansen* *Christopher* *M.* Date of Birth _3_ / _1_ / _65_ Chart # _H234_
         LAST   FIRST   MIDDLE

Prob. No. or Letter	DATE	S Subjective	O Objective	A Assess	P Plans	
						Page _1_
	6/16/04	*Patient complaining of pain in lower right quadrant. Has been running fever of between 100.5°F and 101.3°F since Sunday morning. Has queasy feeling in stomach and has been unable to eat since yesterday morning.*				
			BP 125/75. Temperature 101.2°F. Abdominal exam revealed rebound tenderness and distension in lower right quadrant.			
				Appendicitis		
					1. Admit to hospital	
					2. Surgically remove appendix.	
					Paul martin	

Start each Progress Note (Subjective, Objective, Assessment, and Plans) at the appropriate shaded column to create an outline form. Write through the intervening columns to the right margin of the page.

© 1976 BIBBERO SYSTEMS, INC., PETALUMA, CA

PROGRESS NOTES

TO REORDER CALL TOLL FREE: (800)BIBBERO (800 242-2376)
FORM # 26-7215-01

Figure 9-7. The SOAP approach to documentation is one way to organize information in a patient record.

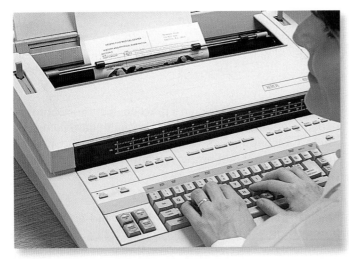

Figure 9-8. Typewritten notes and forms are clear and legible.

Procedure 9-1 explains how to correct a medical chart.

Professional Attitude and Tone

Part of creating timely, accurate records is maintaining a professional tone in your writing when recording information. Record information from the patient in his own words. Also record the doctor's observations and comments as well as any laboratory or test results. Do not record your personal, subjective comments, judgments, opinions, or speculations about a patient's words, problems, or test results. You may call attention to a particular problem or observation, for example, by attaching a note to the chart. Do not, however, make such comments part of the patient's record.

Computer Records

In some offices the computer is used for more than just storing financial, billing, and insurance information. Some hospitals, clinics, and even individual physicians use computer software to create and store patient records.

Advantages of Computerizing Records. In a setting in which several terminals in a network are connected to a main computer, computerizing medical records presents several advantages. A physician can call up the record on her own or another computer monitor whenever the record is needed, review or update the file, and save it to the central computer again (see Figure 9-9).

Computerized records can also be used in teleconferences, where people in different locations can look at the same record on their individual computer screens at the same time. Records can also be sent by modem to the physician's home computer so that the physician will have a patient's records on hand for calls after hours. Computer access to patient records is also helpful for health-care providers with satellite offices in different cities or different parts of a city.

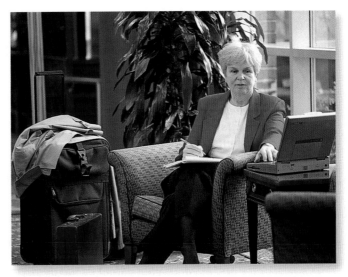

Figure 9-9. Computerized medical records, laptop computers, and the Internet provide physicians with easy access no matter where they are.

Computers are useful for tickler files (files that need periodic attention). For example, they can alert staff members about patients who are due for yearly checkups and patients who require follow-up care. Some hospitals have begun to use electronically scanned images of patients' thumbprints to keep track of records. This system saves time and helps maintain the security of patient records.

Security Concerns. Many health-care professionals have concerns about protecting the confidentiality of patient records in computer files. See Chapter 6 for more information on computer confidentiality.

Medical Transcription

Your knowledge of abbreviations, medical terminology, and medical coding will be invaluable when transcribing a doctor's notes or dictation (either recorded or direct). **Transcription** means transforming spoken notes into accurate written form. These written notes are then entered into the patient record. As is the case with information in medical charts, all dictated materials are confidential and should be regarded as potential legal documents. They are part of the patient's continuing case history. They often include findings, treatment stages, prognoses, and final outcomes. Always date and initial all transcription pages.

Strive to make transcribed material accurate and complete. Good grammar, spelling, and an accurate use of medical abbreviations and terminology are important in maintaining patient records. Use the medical dictionary and the medical computer spelling check to verify the spelling or meaning of words. Ask the physician only if you cannot find something in a reference source. Above-average typing or word processing accuracy and speed are also important.

Medical Transcriptionist

To gain medical assistant credentials, you must fulfill the requirements of either the American Association of Medical Assistants (for a Certified Medical Assistant) or the American Medical Technologists (for a Registered Medical Assistant). After obtaining your medical assistant certification or registration, you may wish to acquire additional skills in specialty areas through course work or on-the-job training. Although this course work or training may not lead to an additional certification or degree, it will enable you to expand your role in the medical office and advance your career as the demand for skilled health professionals increases.

Skills and Duties

A medical transcriptionist creates written health records for patients based on the physician's dictation or notes. The records may be typewritten or input on a computer. Some transcriptionists work for a single physician; others work for a small or large group.

To create a patient record, the transcriptionist listens to an audiocassette containing information dictated by the physician. Typical information on the tape includes the physician's diagnosis and treatment of the patient. Using dictation equipment, the transcriptionist can slow down or stop and start the cassette tape as she types.

The medical transcriptionist must have excellent typing skills and a good command of medical terminology to make sure that medical terms are used accurately and spelled correctly. She will often need to edit the physician's notes to make sure that the language follows Standard English grammar and usage. Sometimes she must also reorganize the physician's comments to create an understandable and easy-to-follow medical record. After she finishes transcribing the record, the medical transcriptionist checks it for correct spelling and punctuation. This last step is called proofreading.

Workplace Settings

Medical transcriptionists may work in the medical records department of a hospital or in a nursing home, clinic, laboratory, physician's practice, insurance company, or emergency or immediate health-care center. Some transcriptionists work for medical transcribing firms; others are self-employed and work out of their homes.

Education

Medical transcriptionists usually complete a training program at a 4-year college or university, junior or community college, vocational institute, or adult education center. They receive instruction in medical terminology, physiology, pharmaceuticals, laboratory procedures, and medical treatments. Some transcriptionists concentrate on a particular specialty area, such as pathology, and acquire specialized training in that area. Medical transcriptionists can become certified if they meet the qualifying standards of the American Association for Medical Transcription.

Where to Go for More Information

American Association for Medical Transcription
P.O. Box 576187
Modesto, CA 95355

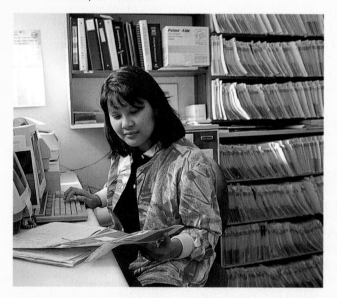

Transcribing Recorded Dictation

Often the doctor or another health-care provider dictates into a recording device or voice-mail dictation center. (This equipment is described in Chapter 5.) The following tips can help ensure fast, accurate transcription.

- Make sure that your workstation is free from clutter and that your desk and chair are at comfortable heights for proper support of your back, arms, and legs. Keep at hand all materials you may need for the transcription process—patient records, correspondence, and references for abbreviations and terminology.

- Adjust the transcribing equipment's speed, tone, and volume to obtain the best-quality sound at a rate of speed that matches your abilities.

- Listen once all the way through the dictation tape, noting instructions, corrections, or special cues. This step helps you plan how to put the material in the correct order. It also ensures accuracy.
- Write down the exact elapsed time on the transcribing equipment's digital counter where difficult phrases, garbled statements, or other problems occur on the tape. Then you can quickly find the problems again and seek the correct information from the doctor.
- While transcribing, listen carefully to the rise and fall of the doctor's voice, which can provide clues about where to place punctuation and where to end sentences.
- If a statement is particularly long or highly technical, simply transcribe it word for word. It may make sense in written form. Never try to guess at the meaning of a word or phrase.
- Finally, reread the finished transcription to make sure that all punctuation, capitalization, spelling of names and terms, and paragraph indentions have been done correctly. You should be able to arrange ideas in their logical order and ensure proper sentence structure. Note any items that are still unclear, and ask the doctor to check them as soon as possible. Never enter questionable material into patient records. Any incorrectly transcribed information can become a legal liability for the doctor should the records be used in a lawsuit.
- All transcribed doctor's notes for the patient's chart should be initialed by the doctor.

Transcribing Direct Dictation

At times the physician may wish to dictate material directly to you. He may want to get observations, comments, or treatment options into the record immediately rather than waiting until a more convenient time to dictate the material into a recorder. Follow these guidelines.

- Use a writing pad with a stiff backing or place the pad on a clipboard to make it easier to write quickly. Use a good ballpoint pen that will not smear or drag on the paper.
- Use incomplete sentences and phrases to keep up with the physician's pace. For example, say "Patient home Friday, recheck 2 wks" instead of "The patient is going home on Friday. We should see him again in 2 weeks."
- Use abbreviations for common phrases (*w/o* for "without," *s/b* for "should be," and so on); for medical terms (*q.d.* for "every day," *mg* for "milligrams," and so on); and for medications or chemicals.
- If a term, phrase, prescription, or name is unclear, ask for clarification right away (say "Excuse me, could you repeat that phrase, please?").
- If the physician speaks with a pronounced accent, ask her to speak more slowly than normal.

- Read the dictation back to the physician to verify all terms, names, figures, and other information for accuracy.
- Enter the notes into the patient record, and date and initial the notes.

Transcription Aids

Keep a library of medical, secretarial, and transcription reference books and medical terminology texts near the transcription workstation. Abbreviations can save time, but you should use only those that are accepted as standard. Reference books will help you find the correct word quickly and easily and help you apply proper grammar, style, and usage to the copy.

Correcting and Updating Patient Records

In legal terms, medical records are regarded as having been created in "due course." All information in the record should be entered at the time of a patient's visit and not days, weeks, or months later. Information corrected or added some time after a patient's visit can be regarded as "convenient" and may damage a doctor's position in a lawsuit.

Using Care With Corrections

If changes to the medical record are not done correctly, the record can become a legal problem for the physician. A physician may be able to more easily explain poor or incomplete documentation than to explain a chart that appears to have been altered after something was originally documented. You must be extremely careful to follow the appropriate procedures for correcting patient records.

Mistakes in medical records are not uncommon. The best defense is to correct the mistake immediately or as soon as possible after the original entry was made. Procedure 9-1 shows you how to correct the patient record.

Updating Patient Records

All additions to a patient's record—test results, observations, diagnoses, procedures—should be done in a way that no one could interpret as deception on the physician's part. In a note accompanying the material, the physician should explain why the information is being added to the record. In some cases the material may simply be a physician's recollections or observations on a patient visit that occurred in the past. Each item added to a record must be dated and initialed. Sometimes a third party may be asked to witness the addition.

Most hospitals and clinics have detailed guidelines for late entries to a patient's chart. You must follow these guidelines carefully to avoid potential legal problems (see Procedure 9-2).

PROCEDURE 9.1

Correcting Medical Records

Objective: To follow standard procedures for correcting a medical record

Materials: Patient file, other pertinent documents that contain the information to be used in making corrections (for example, transcribed notes, telephone notes, physician's comments, correspondence), good ballpoint pen

Method

1. Always make the correction in a way that does not suggest any intention to deceive, cover up, alter, or add information to conceal a lack of proper medical care.

2. When deleting information, never black it out, never use correction fluid to cover it up, and never in any other way erase or obliterate the original wording. Draw a line through the original information so that it is still legible.

3. Write or type in the correct information above or below the original line or in the margin. The location on the chart for the new information should be clear. You may need to attach another sheet of paper or another document with the correction on it. Note in the record "See attached document A" or similar wording to indicate where the corrected information can be found.

4. Place a note near the correction stating why it was made (for example, "error, wrong date; error, interrupted by phone call.") This indication can be a brief note in the margin or an attachment to the record. As a general rule of thumb, do not make any changes without noting the reason for them.

5. Enter the date and time, and initial the correction.

6. If possible, have another staff member or the physician witness and initial the correction to the record when you make it.

PROCEDURE 9.2

Updating Medical Records

Objective: To document continuity of care by creating a complete, accurate, timely record of the medical care provided at your facility

Materials: Patient file, other pertinent documents (test results, x-rays, telephone notes, correspondence), good ballpoint pen, notebook, typewriter/transcribing equipment

Method

1. Verify that you have the right records for the right patient. You do not want to record information on the wrong patient chart.

2. Transcribe dictated doctor's notes as soon as possible, and enter them into the patient record. Delays increase the chance of making errors in transcribing and recording the information. Also, for legal reasons, medical information should be entered into the record in a timely fashion.

3. Spell out the names of disorders, diseases, medications, and other terms the first time you enter them into the patient record, followed by the appropriate abbreviation (for example: "congestive heart failure [CHF]"). Thereafter, you may use the abbreviations. Using only abbreviations could cause confusion.

4. Enter only what the doctor has dictated. Do *not* add your own comments, observations, or evaluations. Use self-adhesive flags or other means to call the doctor's attention to something you have noticed that may be helpful to the patient's case. Date and initial each entry. Should the file be examined later in a legal proceeding, your notes and comments will be taken as part of the official record.

5. Ask the doctor where in the file to record routine or special laboratory test results. He may ask you to post them in a particular section of the

continued ⟶

Updating Medical Records (continued)

file or on a separate test summary form. If you use the summary form, make a note in the file that the results were received, and place the laboratory report in the patient's file with the record. Date and initial each entry. Whether or not test result printouts are posted in the record, always note in the chart the date of the test and the results.

6. Make a note in the record of all telephone calls to and from the patient. Date and initial the entries. These entries may also include the doctor's comments, observations, changes in the patient's medication, new instructions to the patient, and so on. If calls are recorded in a separate telephone log, you should note in the patient's record the time and date of the call and refer to the log.

It is particularly important to record such calls when the patient is resisting treatment or has not made follow-up appointments. These entries can demonstrate that a doctor made every effort to provide quality care and to advise the patient of the risks of not following the treatment plan or not scheduling follow-up appointments.

7. Read over the entries for omissions or mistakes. Ask the doctor to answer any questions you have.
8. Make sure that you have dated and initialed each entry.
9. Be sure that all documents are included in the file.
10. Replace the patient's file in the filing system as soon as possible.

Release of Records

All medical records, including x-rays and other test results, are created by the doctor and are considered the property of that doctor. The records and all they contain, however, are regarded as confidential. Even though the doctor owns the records, no one can see them without the patient's written consent. However, the law may require the doctor to release them, as in the case of a patient with a contagious disease or when the records are subpoenaed by a court.

Procedures for Releasing Records

Physicians often receive requests from lawyers, other physicians, insurance companies, government agencies, and the patient himself for copies of a patient's records. Follow these steps for releasing medical information.

1. Obtain a signed and newly dated release from the patient authorizing the **transfer** of information—that is, giving information to another party outside the physician's office. *Verbal consent in person or over the telephone is not considered a valid release.* The release form should be filed in the patient's record.
2. Make photocopies of the original material. Copy and send only those portions of the record covered by the release and only records originating from your facility (not records received from other sources). Do not send original documents. (If a record will be used in a court case, however, you must submit the original unless the judge specifies that a photocopy is acceptable.) If you cannot make copies, as in the case of x-rays, send the originals, and tell the recipient that they must be returned (see Figure 9-10). Follow up with the recipient until the originals have been returned and are placed in the patient's files.
3. Call the recipient to confirm that all materials were received. Avoid faxing confidential records. There is no way to tell who will see documents sent by fax.

Special Cases

It may not always be immediately clear who has the right to sign a release-of-records form. When a couple divorces, for example, both parents are still considered legal guardians of their children, and either one can sign a release form authorizing transfer of medical records. If a patient dies, the patient's next of kin or legally authorized representative, such as the executor of the estate, may see the records or authorize their release to a third party. When you are in doubt regarding who is authorized to sign, *always* ask your supervisor before releasing confidential medical records.

Confidentiality

When children reach age 18, most states consider them adults with the right to privacy. No one, not even their parents, may see their medical records without the children's written consent. Some states extend this right to privacy to emancipated minors who are under the age of 18 and living on their own or are married, a parent, or in the armed services.

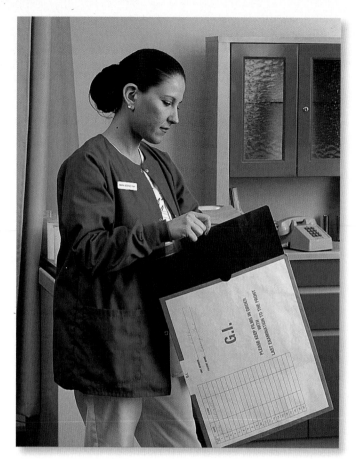

Figure 9-10. When you are preparing a patient record to be transferred, never send original material. One exception to this rule is x-rays, which should be sent with a request that the recipient return them as soon as possible.

The main legal and ethical principle to keep in mind is that you must protect each patient's right to privacy at all times.

Summary

The medical assistant must properly prepare and maintain patient records. Patient records, also known as charts, contain important information about a patient's medical history and present condition. Patient records serve as communication tools as well as legal documents. They also play a role in patient and staff education and may be used for quality control and research. The six Cs of charting are the client's words, clarity, completeness, conciseness, chronological order, and confidentiality.

You should be familiar with the most common methods for documenting patient information, which include the conventional, or source-oriented, and problem-oriented medical records approaches. You must ensure not only that the medical records are complete but also that they are neat and written legibly, contain up-to-date information, and present an accurate, professional record of a patient's case.

Part of maintaining patient records includes transcribing physician's notes—that is, transforming spoken notes into accurate written form. In addition, you must know the guidelines for how to correct and update a patient record and how to release it to a third party.

CASE STUDY QUESTIONS

Now that you have completed this chapter, review the case study at the beginning of the chapter and answer the following questions:

1. Why is an accurate medical record important to the care of a patient?
2. Why is interviewing the patient important to the medical evaluation?
3. What are the six Cs of charting and what do they mean to you as a medical assistant?
4. What are the differences between the conventional and the POMR system of keeping charts?
5. What are some helpful tips you might use as you perform transcription?

Discussion Questions

1. Who benefits from accurate medical charting? The patient? The doctor? The court? Divide into three teams and debate the issue.
2. Why is confidentiality regarding medical charting so difficult to maintain? Name three areas of concern in daily chart management that could lead to a loss of confidentiality, and discuss.
3. Medical transcription and medical charting are integral parts of daily medical records management. Which is more important? Why?

Critical Thinking Questions

1. A patient wants to take his medical records and x-rays to another physician's office. He insists that the records belong to him. How would you handle this situation?
2. Describe how a well-trained medical assistant could enhance the efficiency of a medical office's system of creating and maintaining patient records.

Application Activities

1. After reading the following description of a patient's condition, list the patient's signs and symptoms.

   A 72-year-old man with no history of gastrointestinal problems was complaining of fatigue, back pain, appetite loss, and nausea. The patient had a hemoglobin of about 7g, indicating marked anemia. His blood pressure was low (95/70), his heartbeat erratic—from 55 to 85 bpm—and his white blood cell count elevated.

   While in the office he experienced a headache and ringing in his right ear. A CT scan taken the next day revealed an abdominal aortic aneurysm containing a large clot. The scan also revealed a small lesion in the lining of the stomach.

2. Photocopy the blank patient registration form shown in Figure 9-2. With a partner, take each other's medical history and make appropriate notes on the form.

3. Photocopy the blank combination medical history and physical examination form shown in Figure 9-3. Fill out the form by using the following patient information.

   For medical history section: Date: 2/14/96; the patient is Heather R. MacEntee, age 35, living at 344 Westwind Lane, Apartment 28, Round Tree, IL 60012; telephone (708) 333-5555. She is a real estate broker, married, with a 6-year-old child. Her father died at age 55; her mother is 62 and has congestive heart disease. She has no siblings. The family has a history of heart disease and diabetes. The patient had chickenpox and mumps at age 7 and surgery for an ovarian cyst at 22. She has an allergy to ragweed but is not taking any medications at present.

   For physical examination section: Ms. MacEntee weighs 142 lb, is 5 ft 10 in tall, and her temperature and respiration are normal. Her pulse is 74, her blood pressure is 110/75, and her chest sounds are normal. Her chief complaint is discomfort in the area of the gallbladder. She has intense pain after eating. Blood tests are normal. The doctor's initial impression is suspected gallstones, and an ultrasound scan of the gallbladder is ordered. Treatment plan depends on the scan results.

4. Role-play with other students in your class, and compare the differences in charting methods.

   - Student 1 will play the role of the patient who is complaining of headaches.
   - Student 2 will chart using conventional charting methods.
   - Student 3 will chart the same information using the POMR method.

5. Go on the Internet and look up the *Medical Transcriptionists Bill of Rights* for discussion in your class.

Managing the Office Medical Records

KEY TERMS

- active file
- alphabetic filing system
- closed file
- compactible file
- cross-referenced
- file guide
- inactive file
- lateral file
- numeric filing system
- out guide
- records management system
- retention schedule
- sequential order
- tab
- tickler file
- vertical file

AREAS OF COMPETENCE

2003 Role Delineation Study

ADMINISTRATIVE

Administrative Procedures

- Perform basic administrative medical assisting functions

CHAPTER OUTLINE

- The Importance of Records Management
- Filing Equipment
- Filing Supplies
- Filing Systems
- The Filing Process
- File Storage

OBJECTIVES

After completing Chapter 10, you will be able to:

10.1 Describe the equipment and supplies needed for the filing of medical records.

10.2 List and describe the various types of filing systems.

10.3 Discuss the benefits of each type of system.

10.4 Discuss the advantages of color coding the files.

10.5 Explain how to set up and use a tickler file.

10.6 Describe each of the five steps in the filing process.

10.7 Explain the steps to take in trying to locate a misplaced file.

10.8 List and describe the basic file storage options and the advantages of each.

10.9 Identify criteria for determining whether files should be retained, stored, or discarded.

Introduction

The role of the medical assistant is both clerical and clinical in nature. The most important clerical function is the careful management of the patient chart, or record. The management of these individual files is vital to the care of each patient and to the smooth operation of the medical office.

In this chapter you will learn about various options for handling large volumes of patient records. As you work through this chapter, you will begin to have an appreciation for the very important task of chart management, and you will develop an organized approach to maintaining these critical documents. As you read, watch for helpful tips that teach you how to locate any patient chart quickly and efficiently.

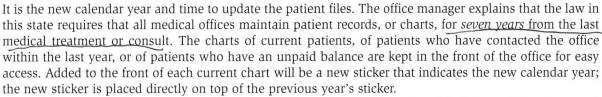

CASE STUDY

It is the new calendar year and time to update the patient files. The office manager explains that the law in this state requires that all medical offices maintain patient records, or charts, for *seven years* from the last medical treatment or consult. The charts of current patients, of patients who have contacted the office within the last year, or of patients who have an unpaid balance are kept in the front of the office for easy access. Added to the front of each current chart will be a new sticker that indicates the new calendar year; the new sticker is placed directly on top of the previous year's sticker.

All other charts will be moved to a separate chart storage room, organized alphabetically, and grouped according to the last year in which there was contact with the patient. These older charts must remain readily available in case:

- The patient returns to the practice
- Records are subpoenaed by a court of law
- Records are requested for a medical history

The office manager reminds the staff that all original charts belong to the physician who owns the practice. Copies can be made *only* when the patient signs a release authorizing the distribution to another party. When copies are made, a notation must be added to the chart that copying occurred and the date. In this state, even with a subpoena, physicians must have patient permission to release records to the court. Originals are *never* taken out of the medical office.

At this same time, the staff will purge the chart room and shred the oldest charts. All charts that have had no activity in the last eight years will be either pulled apart and shredded in a shredding machine in the office or picked up by a local company that will shred the documents for the physician. It is essential, the office manager points out, that all documents be shredded, not just thrown away, in order to guard the confidential content of the documents.

As you read this chapter, consider the following questions:

1. What are advantages and disadvantages of different file systems?
2. What security measures might be used to protect patient files?
3. What is a tickler system and how is it set up?
4. Identify several storage options for closed charts. Which is the most secure? The easiest? The most cost-efficient?

The Importance of Records Management

The information contained in the patient medical records is the most valuable information in a medical office. For a practice to operate smoothly and efficiently, it is critical that these records be organized in a way that makes them easily retrievable. Maintaining a well-organized, easy-to-use records management system is essential to providing good patient care. The **records management system** refers to the way patient records are created, filed, and maintained. When such a system is not in place, valuable time is wasted searching for important information. In addition, vital medical data can be lost.

Filing Equipment

Filing equipment generally refers to the place where records, or files, are housed. Although there are various types of equipment, two of the most common options are shelves and cabinets. The choice of whether to use filing shelves or filing cabinets is often made according to space considerations and personal preference.

Filing Shelves

Files can be kept on shelves, which resemble traditional shelves, as shown in Figure 10-1. Files are stacked upright on the shelves in filing containers such as boxes or large

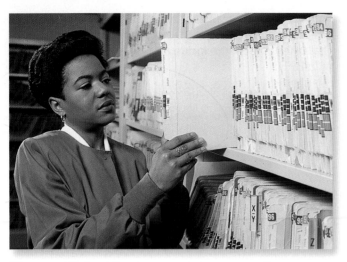

Figure 10-1. Files kept on shelves are easily accessible.

heavy-duty envelopes. Some shelf systems have doors that slide from side to side or above or below the files. These doors can be locked for security. Other shelf systems have no front covers. Filing shelves are often long, sometimes extending the full length and height of an office wall or room. An advantage of keeping files on shelves is that it allows several people to retrieve and return files at one time.

Filing Cabinets

Filing cabinets are sturdy pieces of office furniture, usually made of metal or wood. They contain a series of pullout drawers in which files are hung. Filing cabinets, unlike shelves, are best used by one person at a time because the drawer setup provides limited maneuvering room. In addition, cabinets require more floor space than filing shelves. About twice the depth of the file drawer is needed to allow it to fully open.

Although shelves are horizontal by design, filing cabinets can stand vertically or horizontally. You are probably familiar with the more traditional filing cabinet, the vertical file. A **vertical file** features pullout drawers that usually contain a metal frame or bar equipped to handle letter- or legal-size documents. Hanging file folders are hung on this frame, with identifying names facing out. Vertical files usually have two, four, or six drawers.

Horizontal filing cabinets, called **lateral files,** often feature doors that flip up and pullout drawers. Files are arranged with sides facing out. Lateral files require more wall space but do not extend as far into the room as vertical file drawers.

Compactible Files

Some offices have limited space in which to house filing cabinets or shelves. These offices use a variation of shelf filing, called compactible files. **Compactible files** are kept on rolling shelves that slide along permanent tracks in the floor.

When not in use, these files can be stored close together—even one on top of another—to conserve space. When needed, they are rolled out into an open area so that the staff can easily use them. Compactible files can be moved manually or automatically with the touch of a button.

Rotary Circular Files

Rotary circular files are another option to consider when space is limited. These files are stored in a circular fashion, similar to a revolving door, and are accessed by rotating the files. They also can be operated either manually or electronically.

Plastic or Cardboard Tubs or Boxes

Files may be suspended in hanging files in plastic or cardboard file boxes. While this system may be adequate for a small number of files, the system is less efficient for larger numbers of files because it would require numerous boxes.

Tubs or boxes resemble open drawers. They may have a lid or be open. When not in use, all tubs or boxes must be locked in a secure storage area to protect patient confidentiality. Additionally, open tubs or boxes collect dust and are inappropriate for storage in a dirty warehouse storage area. All tubs or boxes must be stored off the floor, either on shelves or on platforms, to avoid water damage. This is a JCAHO requirement and is routinely checked during a survey.

Tubs or boxes are often stacked to save space, which can make it very difficult to locate files. JCAHO also requires that nothing be stacked within 18 inches of the ceiling. Tubs and boxes appear portable, but are usually very heavy once filled. Care should be taken to avoid injury when moving these files.

Labeling Filing Equipment

Regardless of which type of filing equipment your office uses, files should be clearly labeled on the outside of the drawer so that you do not have to open doors or drawers to know the contents. Labeling allows you to go directly to the appropriate place when retrieving a file. The label lists the range of files the drawer or shelf contains. For example, if the drawer includes all the files of patients whose last names begin with the letters A, B, C, and D, the drawer should be labeled "A–D."

Security Measures

All filing equipment must be secure, to protect the confidentiality of medical records. *Never* place patient records in an unsecured filing system.

Most filing cabinets come with a lock and key. To protect filing shelves in a separate room, you can lock the file room. Security of the keys to that room then becomes an important issue. The number of staff members who have keys to that room should be limited—perhaps just the head doctor and the office manager. Every staff member does not need a key to the filing equipment. When the office manager comes into the office each morning, she can unlock the files. Because the files remain open during the day, it is important to make sure they are not placed in areas where unauthorized people can obtain access to them. Posting a sign on the file room door stating "Authorized Personnel Only" helps ensure that files remain secure. To ensure office security after hours, some practices install alarm systems.

Keep in mind that keys and locks bring a measure of security only when they are *used.* Many office staffs become lazy and routinely overlook locking file rooms and cabinets. Security survey teams will always ask to see the keys to any locked door or cabinet and ask the staff to demonstrate that they work. Within a medical office, conducting regular security drills at the same time that fire drills are held will aid staff in staying sharp and aware of security risks.

Equipment Safety

Safety is an important consideration for filing systems. For example, opening more than one drawer in a vertical file cabinet at the same time may cause it to fall forward. If the bottom drawer in a vertical file is left open, someone can easily trip over it. Shelves can be dangerous if staff members need to climb a ladder to retrieve files from the highest level.

Safety guidelines for each piece of equipment should be posted prominently in the office. Make sure that every staff member knows where the rules are posted. Then, make sure that everyone follows the rules to prevent possible injury.

Purchasing Filing Equipment

You may never have to buy filing equipment, because most medical offices already have filing systems in place. Occasionally, however, you may be responsible for setting up an office's filing system—for example, if your practice opens a new office. You may also need to buy equipment as the number of patients in the practice grows.

In either case you will need to determine where to position the files. When purchasing filing cabinets or shelves, you need to determine how much office space is available for files. This information, along with the number of file folders to be included, will help you figure out how many cabinets or shelves to purchase. An office-supply store or office-supply catalog can provide you with a list of available products.

Filing Supplies

Once you have chosen your filing equipment, you must select filing supplies. Figure 10-2 features an assortment of filing supplies commonly used by medical practices.

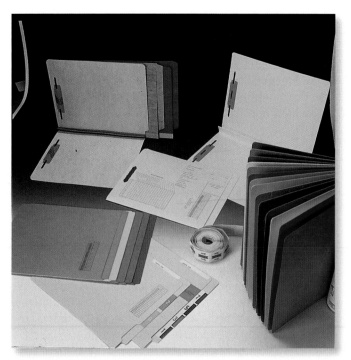

Figure 10-2. Medical offices use a wide variety of filing supplies.

File Folders

The most basic filing supply is the file folder, often referred to as a manila folder. This folder is made of heavy paper folded in half to form a pocket that can hold papers. File folders come in two sizes: letter size, which is 8½ by 11 inches, and legal size, which is 8½ by 14 inches.

Tabs. An important feature of file folders is the **tab,** the tapered rectangular or rounded extension at the top of the folder. Tabs may extend the full length of the folder, as with straight-cut folders, but they are usually cut to extend partway across a folder.

Using folders with a variety of tab cuts makes it easier to read the names on the tabs. One common type of folder is the third-cut folder. Tabs are one-third the width of the folder and appear at the left, center, or right side. Fourth-cut tabs are smaller. Tabs extend one-fourth the width of the folder and occupy one of four positions—left, left-center, right-center, or right.

Labels. The tabs on file folders are used to identify the contents of the individual folder. You can write directly on the tab area in pen or pencil, or you can type a label and affix it to the tab area for a more professional appearance. Tabs can be covered with transparent tape to prevent smudging.

No matter what filing system your office uses, it is important to be consistent in preparing file labels. If all the files are labeled with the patient's last name, followed by the patient's first name and middle initial (for example, Brown, Emma L.), you should not prepare a label for a new folder giving the patient's name in a different order (for example, James P. Regan). Each member of a family should have a separate file.

File Jackets

By themselves, file folders cannot be suspended inside filing cabinet drawers. They must be placed inside file jackets, or hanging file folders. These jackets resemble file folders but feature metal or plastic hooks on both sides at the top, which hook onto the metal bars inside the drawers. Like file folders, jackets come in letter and legal size.

Plastic tabs, either colored or clear, and blank inserts are supplied to identify the contents of hanging file folders. The information is typed on the insert and placed in the plastic tab, which is inserted into the hanging file folder. Again, all inserts should be prepared in a consistent style.

File Guides

To identify a group of file folders in a file drawer, you may use **file guides,** which are heavy cardboard or plastic inserts. For example, if a drawer contains the files for patients whose last names begin with the letters A through C, the guides might separate A from B and B from C.

Out Guides

Another filing supply is an **out guide,** which is a marker made of stiff material and used as a placeholder when someone takes a file out of the filing system. Some out guides include pockets that can hold the name of the file that belongs in that place or the name of the individual who took the file and its due date for return. On another type of out guide, you write the information on the out guide and cross it out when the file is returned. Out guides can be used for both shelf and cabinet filing.

Although out guides are not essential, they are extremely helpful in ensuring that files are returned to their proper places. Out guides also save the time and effort necessary to go through files to determine where a particular file belongs. Out guides work well when the entire staff, including the physicians, makes a dedicated effort to use the system.

File Sorters

File sorters are large envelope-style folders with tabs in which files can be stored temporarily. File sorters are used to hold patient records that will be returned to the files during the day or at the end of the day. The sorters help keep files in order and prevent them from being lost.

Binders

Some offices keep patient records in three-ring binders rather than in file folders. The binders are labeled on the outside spine. Documents are three-hole-punched and then placed inside the binder. Tab sheets are used to separate individual records. A binder can conveniently hold many records.

Purchasing Filing Supplies

Although you may never have to buy filing equipment, buying filing supplies may be one of your regular responsibilities as a medical assistant. (See Chapter 8 for a discussion of how to manage office supplies.)

Filing Systems

A filing system is a method by which files are organized. Any of a variety of filing systems may be used, but every system places patient records in some sort of **sequential order**—one after another in a pattern, or sequence, that can be predicted. It is important to find out which filing system your office is using and to follow it exactly. Any deviation can result in lost or misplaced records.

By far the most common filing system for maintaining patient files in sequential order is the alphabetic system. You would not, however, make any changes in your system without first consulting the doctors and other staff members in the practice.

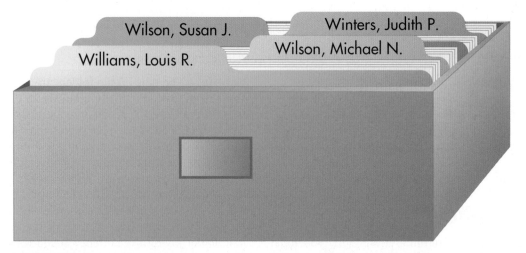

Figure 10-3. Most medical practices file patient records according to the alphabetic filing system.

Alphabetic

In the **alphabetic filing system,** files are arranged in alphabetic order, as shown in Figure 10-3. Files are labeled with the patient's last name first, followed by the first, or given, name and the middle initial.

There are specific rules to follow when filing personal names alphabetically (Table 10-1). If you have questions, consult a secretarial handbook or style manual. Although the alphabetic system is simple, you must know the exact spelling of a patient's name to retrieve a file.

Numeric

A **numeric filing system** organizes files by numbers instead of by names. In this system each patient name is assigned a number. New patients are assigned the next unused number in sequence. Then, instead of being filed by

TABLE 10-1	Rules for Alphabetic Filing of Personal Names			

In alphabetizing, treat each part of a patient's name as a separate unit, and look at the units in this order: last name, first name, middle initial, and any subsequent names or initials. Disregard punctuation.

Name	Unit 1	Unit 2	Unit 3	Unit 4
Stephen Jacobson	JACOBSON	STEPHEN		
Stephen Brent Jacobson	JACOBSON	STEPHEN	BRENT	
B. T. Jacoby	JACOBY	B	T	
C. Bruce Hay Jacoby	JACOBY	C	BRUCE	HAY
Kwong Kow Ng	NG	KWONG	KOW	
Philip K. Ng	NG	PHILIP	K	

Treat a prefix, such as the O' in O'Hara, as part of the name, not as a separate unit. Ignore variations in spacing, punctuation, and capitalization. Treat prefixes—such as De La, Mac, Saint, and St.—exactly as they are spelled.

Name	Unit 1	Unit 2	Unit 3	Unit 4
A. Serafino Delacruz	DELACRUZ	A	SERAFINO	
Victor P. De La Cruz	DELACRUZ	VICTOR	P	
Irene J. MacKay	MACKAY	IRENE	J	
Walter G. Mac Kay	MACKAY	WALTER	G	
Kyle N. Saint Clair	SAINTCLAIR	KYLE	N	
Peter St. Clair	STCLAIR	PETER		

Treat hyphenated names as a single unit. Disregard the hyphen.

Name	Unit 1	Unit 2	Unit 3	Unit 4
Victor Puentes-Ruiz	PUENTESRUIZ	VICTOR		
Jean-Marie Vigneau	VIGNEAU	JEANMARIE		

A title, such as Dr. or Major, or a seniority term, such as Jr. or 3d, should be treated as the last filing unit, to distinguish names that are otherwise identical.

Name	Unit 1	Unit 2	Unit 3	Unit 4
Dr. George B. Diaz	DIAZ	GEORGE	B	DR
Major George B. Diaz	DIAZ	GEORGE	B	MAJOR
James R. Foster, Jr.	FOSTER	JAMES	R	JR
James R. Foster, Sr.	FOSTER	JAMES	R	SR

Adapted from William A. Sabin, *The Gregg Reference Manual,* 8th ed. (Columbus, OH: Glencoe/McGraw-Hill, 1996), 288–295.

name, the files are arranged in numeric order—1, 2, 3, 4, and so on. The resulting files are sequential by the order in which patients have come to the practice.

Only the numbers are indicated on the files. Patient names are recorded elsewhere. Such a system is often used when patient information is highly confidential—as in the case of HIV-positive patients—and patients' identities need to be protected.

The numeric system can be expanded to indicate the location of files. For example, if the last three numbers represent the patient's number, the number 113306 may represent the file of the 306th patient, which can be found in the eleventh filing cabinet in the third drawer.

A numeric system must include a master list of patients' names and corresponding numbers. To ensure confidentiality, the office manager should keep the list in a secure place. The physician should hold a duplicate copy, which must also be kept under lock and key. Since folders are filed in numeric order, it should not be necessary for other staff members to have this list.

To find a patient's file number using a computer system, a staff member might input a password or access code, then type in the first three letters of the patient's last name. If the patient's last name were Mulligan, for example, the staff member would type in Mul. The computer would then show all patients whose last names begin with Mul. The staff member would scroll the names, find the patient, highlight the patient name, and hit the "Enter" key. The computer would then give the number of the patient's chart.

Color Coding

Color coding is used when there is a need to distinguish files within a filing system. For example, you may wish to find at a glance all the office's new patients, all patients on Medicare, or all patients whose last names begin with the letters WI. Coding by color can help you do so quickly and easily.

Patient records can be color-coded in a variety of ways. File folders are available in a range of colors, as are filing labels, plastic tabs, and stickers.

Using Classifications. To make the best use of color, you must first identify the classifications that are important to your office. For example, is it important to be able to identify all new patients easily? (A new patient is a patient who has never been seen in the practice or has not been seen at the practice in 3 years.) Once you select the classifications, choose a different color for each one.

Then file the information by color, within the filing system. For example, all new patients may be kept in red folders, or you can attach a red sticker or red filing label to the folders.

Some practices use the following color-coding system. Records of patients under the age of 18 are color-coded blue. Records of patients over the age of 65 are color-coded red. Records of patients who are insulin-dependent are color-coded green. Records of patients who are hemophiliacs are coded with a half-red/half-white sticker. In an emergency situation, as when a patient with diabetes passes out while in the office, the color coding gives staff members vital information at a glance.

After a color-coding system is finalized, the codes should be prominently posted on a chart in the file room so that all staff members are aware of them. This chart will help to ensure that records are filed correctly. Remember to update color-coded files consistently, coding new ones and revising older ones as a patient's status changes.

Using Color in an Alphabetic Filing System. One way to use color-coded filing is in conjunction with an alphabetic filing system. After files are organized alphabetically, each letter of the alphabet is assigned a color. Then the first two letters of each patient's last name are color-coded, usually with colored tabs.

The colored tabs are attached to the top of straight-edged or tabbed file folders. For example, if the letter S is coded as light blue and the letter M is coded as light green, all names starting with SM—like Smith—would have light-blue and light-green colored tabs at the top of the folders. The name Snyder would be filed under a different color combination, such as light blue (for S) and peach (for N). Because the colors will be the same in each segment of the file drawer, a color-coded system makes it easy to tell whether files are in their proper spots.

Using Color in a Numeric Filing System. Color can be used in a similar way with numeric systems. The numerals 1 to 9 may each be assigned a distinct color, as shown in Figure 10-4. Then, numerals 1, 21, 31, 41, and 51, for example, would share the same color in the ones place of their numeric designation.

As with the alphabetic system, color coding helps identify numeric files that are out of place. There are exceptions, however. For example, if a numeric system uses white stickers for the numeral 2 and red stickers for the numeral 3, the number 134 filed in place of 124 would be spotted immediately as a red sticker in a row of white, but

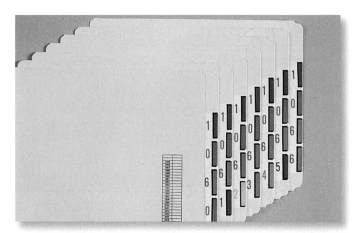

Figure 10-4. Color coding can make it easy to find a misfiled record.

PROCEDURE 10.1

Creating a Filing System for Patient Records

Objective: To create a filing system that keeps related materials together in a logical order and enables office staff to store and retrieve files efficiently

Materials: Vertical or horizontal filing cabinets with locks, file jackets, tabbed file folders, labels, file guides, out guides, filing sorters

Method

1. Evaluate which filing system is best for your office—alphabetic or numeric. Make sure the doctor approves the system you choose.

2. Establish a style for labeling files, and make sure that all file labels are prepared in this manner. Place records for different family members in separate files.

3. Avoid writing labels by hand. Use a typewriter or a label maker.

4. Set up a color-coding system to distinguish the files (for example, use blue for the letters A–C, red for D–F, and so on).

5. Use file guides to divide files into sections.

6. Use out guides as placeholders to indicate which files have been taken out of the system. Include a charge-out form to be signed and dated by the person who is taking the file.

7. To keep files in order and to prevent them from being misplaced, use a file sorter to hold those patient records that will be returned to the files during the day or at the end of the day.

8. Develop a manual explaining the filing system to new staff members. Include guidelines on how to keep the system in good order.

---

the number 128 misfiled in the same spot could go unnoticed. Procedure 10-1 explains how to use your knowledge of alphabetic and numeric filing and color coding to set up a patient records system.

Tickler Files

To avoid losing track of important dates, many medical practices use tickler files. A **tickler file** is a reminder file. Any activity that needs to be scheduled ahead of time can be noted and a reminder placed in the file. For example, reminders to order supplies or send patient checkup cards can be entered. When the task has been completed, the note can be crossed off the list or removed from the file and thrown away. In some offices these notes are dated and placed in a separate "Completed" file for future reference.

Tickler files should be located by themselves in a prominent place in the office, such as in a plastic box mounted on the wall near the receptionist's desk. Someone in the office should be assigned the responsibility of regularly checking the tickler files. Tickler files can be checked daily or, at a minimum, once a week. It is important to check tickler files frequently because they work only if they are used regularly.

You can organize tickler files in a variety of ways. The most common method, discussed in Procedure 10-2, is to allot one file folder to each month of the year. Tickler files can also be organized by day of the week or week of the month. This method is most useful if there are responsibilities that occur regularly on a certain day of the week or in a certain week within the month. If there are so many

notes in a monthly folder that it becomes cumbersome to deal with, it may be best to organize weekly files.

Tickler files are usually organized in file folders, but they can be set up in other ways. One way is to make notes on an office calendar or wall chart. Anyone walking by will be able to read the notes, however, and the number of activities you can include is limited by the space available.

Some offices keep their tickler files in three-ring binders, with tabs separating the months. Notes can be written on three-hole-punched sheets of paper, with pages added as needed. Binders offer essentially un-limited space.

Computers now offer tickler files. When the computer is turned on, it lists, for example, "Things to Do Today" with the tickler information posted for that date.

Supplemental Files

Occasionally you may need to set up additional files to supplement the medical records filing system. For example, you may wish to keep some information separate from the primary file, such as older patient records or insurance information. You may also be asked to create temporary files, such as copies of patient records in the primary files. In these cases you set up supplemental files. Supplemental files allow you to keep this additional information about each patient without cluttering up the primary filing cabinets and without making it difficult to find information.

Supplemental files are usually created using the same system as the primary files, but they are kept in a different location. Depending on frequency of use, they may be stored in a less accessible but equally secure area of the office.

PROCEDURE 10.2

Setting Up an Office Tickler File

Objective: To create a comprehensive office tickler file designed for year-round use

Materials: 12 manila file folders, 12 file labels, pen or typewriter, paper

Method

1. Write or type 12 file labels, 1 for each month of the year. Abbreviations are acceptable. Do *not* include the current calendar year, just the month.
2. Affix one label to the tab of each file folder.
3. Arrange the folders so that the current month is on the top of the pile. Months should follow in chronological order.
4. Write or type a list of upcoming responsibilities and activities. Indicate on the note the date by which the activity should be completed. Use a separate sheet of paper for each month.
5. File the notes by month in the appropriate folders.
6. Place the folders, with the current month on top, in a prominent place in the office, such as in a plastic box mounted on the wall near the receptionist's desk.
7. Check the tickler file at least once a week on a specific day, such as every Monday. Assign a backup person to check it in case you happen to be out of the office.
8. Complete the tickler activities on the designated days, if possible. Keep notes concerning activities in progress. Discard notes about completed activities.
9. At the end of the month, place that month's file folder at the bottom of the tickler file. If there are notes remaining in that month's folder, move them to the new month's folder.
10. Continue to add new notes to the appropriate tickler files.

If you are keeping supplemental files, it is important to distinguish their content from that of the primary files. For example, you may decide that all information pertaining to certain subjects—such as patient diagnosis and treatment—will be kept in the primary files and that all other information—such as insurance company payments for each patient—will be kept in the supplemental files. This designation will help you and other office staff members know exactly where to go to retrieve specific information.

The Filing Process

Pulling and filing patient records and filing individual documents may be among your responsibilities as a medical assistant. Some practices require that records be returned to the files as soon as they are no longer needed. In other practices the timing is up to you. Still other offices schedule a specific time at the end of each day to file the current day's records and pull those for the next day.

Records waiting to be filed should be placed temporarily in a file return area, as shown in Figure 10-5. To protect patient privacy, this place should be in a secure area of the office. Clear rules should designate who may handle these files and in what situations.

How to File

Essentially, you will be filing three types of items: new patient record folders, individual documents that belong in existing patient record folders, and patient record folders that have previously been filed. There are five steps involved in filing: inspecting, indexing, coding, sorting, and storing.

Inspecting. The first step in the filing process is to make sure the item is ready to be filed. Inspect the document or patient record folder for a mark, notation, or stamp indicating that it is ready to be filed. For example, it may be initialed by the physician or stamped with the word *File* on a self-adhesive flag attached to the upper right corner. Some offices have staff members simply place folders ready for filing in a specially designated box or bin.

At this point, remove paper clips, rubber bands, and any extraneous material that does not need to be filed. Staple papers to keep them together. Documents are less bulky when stapled than when held together by clips or rubber bands.

If the document to be filed is much smaller than standard size, it may become lost in the file or even fall out. You may want to use tape or rubber cement to attach it to a standard-size piece of paper before filing it within the folder. When small documents have wording on both sides of the paper, they can be placed in standard-size clear plastic envelopes and then filed.

Indexing. *Indexing* is another term for naming a file. Names should be chosen carefully because that is how the file will be known, retrieved, and replaced. Patient names are traditionally used as the file names for patient records.

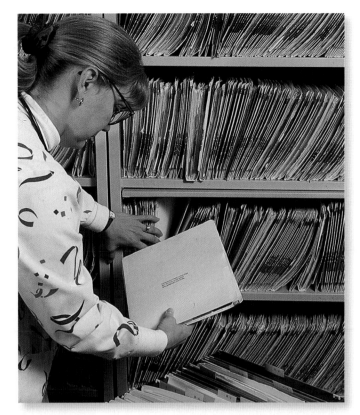

Figure 10-5. In some practices, patient records are filed once at the end of the day. Throughout the day, records are placed in a file sorter in a secure area of the office.

If you are using a numeric system, you can assign a number instead of a name. Most offices that use a numeric system use computer software to create new patient charts and assign numbers. As part of the indexing process, color-code the file (if you use color coding in your system).

Note that some files can logically be placed in more than one location. Such files should be **cross-referenced,** or filed in two or more places, with each place noted in each file. When cross-referencing a file, you may duplicate the exact contents of the file and place each file under a different heading, or you may create a cross-reference form that lists all the places to find the file. You would then place the form under any heading where it is appropriate to look for that file. You may wish to attach it to a blank file, cutting the file folder in half so that no other documents are mistakenly filed in it.

When filing folders that have previously been indexed, use this step as a way to check the indexing process. For example, take the opportunity to decide whether the name and color of the file folder are accurate or should be changed in any way.

Coding. This step can be skipped when filing patient record folders that have previously been filed. Coding means to put an identifying mark or phrase on a document to ensure that it is placed in the correct file. To code a record, simply mark the patient's name, the number, or the subject title of the file folder. If appropriate, you can underline or highlight key words on the document itself.

It is important to use a phrase or identifying code that anyone who will review the file can easily understand. Avoid medical jargon whenever possible because some terms may not be familiar to everybody. If you are unsure whether a code will be understood, attach a brief explanation to the front of the file folder for reference.

Sorting. If you have more than one folder to be filed, you must sort the files that have accumulated. Sort them in the order in which they are kept—such as alphabetically or numerically. Sorting saves you time later when you return the files to their proper places. If you will not be filing the folders immediately, store them in a temporary location, such as a file sorter.

Storing. The final step in the filing process is to store the files in the appropriate filing equipment. Documents should be stored neatly within their file folders in the proper sequence.

Careful attention to file storage will make your job easier in the long run. Make sure the folders are in good condition. Change them whenever they appear damaged or torn to prevent file contents from spilling out during the retrieval and filing process. If the file contains too many documents, divide it into two or more folders, and label each one (for example, Glass, Ann M.—Folder 1 of 2; Glass, Ann M.—Folder 2 of 2). Make sure to replace labels that are no longer legible.

Limiting Access to Files

Some offices restrict the number of people who can retrieve and return files. To obtain a file, staff members must fill out a requisition slip with their name and the name of the patient, as shown in Figure 10-6.

Springfield Medical Associates

Patient File Requisition Slip

Patient: _____

File Given to: _____

Date: _____

Time: _____

Due Back: _____

Figure 10-6. Some offices limit the personnel who have access to the file room. Staff members must fill out a requisition slip with their name and the name of the patient to obtain a patient record.

A record of who has the file is kept either in a notebook or on index cards in special boxes. The record includes the name of the file, the name of the borrower, the date the file was borrowed, and the date it is due back.

Under *no* circumstances should original patient medical records ever leave the practice. Photocopies can be made, if necessary. (Chapter 9 provides specific guidelines on releasing medical records to individuals and organizations outside your medical office.)

Filing Guidelines

There are specific rules for each filing system as well as general guidelines, or helpful hints, applicable to any system. Following these guidelines will help you file more efficiently.

- Each time you pull or file a patient record, glance at its contents. You should be familiar with the typical contents and the order of a patient record folder to help avoid filing errors.
- Keep files neat. Make sure that documents fit into the file folders and do not stick out or obscure file labels.
- Do not overstuff file folders. Folders should be able to stay closed when laid on a flat surface.
- When inserting documents into folders already in place in the drawer, lift the folders up and out of the drawer. Attempting to force documents into a folder inside the drawer can damage the documents or leave them sticking out of the folder.
- Do not crowd the file drawer. Leave extra space to allow for leafing through the files and for retrieving and replacing files easily.
- Where possible, use a combination of uppercase and lowercase letters to label folders. This format is easier to read than labels written completely in capital letters.
- Choose file guides with a different tab position than your folders to help them stand out. Do not place guides so close together that they hide one another. A good rule of thumb is to position guides at least 5 inches apart.
- If you are unsure whether to cross-reference a file, do it. It is better to err on the side of providing too many cross-references than too few.
- File regularly so that you are not overwhelmed with too many folders to file.
- Store only files in filing cabinets or on filing shelves. Do not store office equipment or supplies where files belong.
- Train all staff members who will retrieve and replace files to make sure they have a thorough understanding of the system. Update them on any changes.
- Periodically evaluate your office's filing system. The Tips for the Office section helps you with this task.

Locating Misplaced Files

Even in the best filing systems, there is a chance of temporarily misplacing or even losing patient medical records. No matter how good a system is, the people who do the filing are only human. If a file is misplaced, here are steps you can take to try to locate it.

1. Determine the last time you knew the file's location.
2. Go to that location, and retrace your steps. Look for the file along the way.
3. Look in the filing cabinet where the file belongs. Check neighboring files. Possibly the file was simply put in the wrong place.
4. Check underneath the files in the drawer or shelf to see if the file slipped out.
5. Check the pile of items to be filed or the file sorter envelope.
6. Consider possible cross-references or similar indexes (for example, similar patient names) for the file. Check those headings to see if the file was accidentally placed there.
7. Check with other staff members to determine if they have seen the file.
8. Check to make sure the missing file was not filed under the patient's *first* name instead of the last.
9. Stand back from the file cabinet and view the *top* of the folders looking at only the first three letters of the last names. A misfiled file will stand out.
10. If using a color-coded system, look for the color of the misfiled chart.
11. Even though files should always be kept in a secure area, occasionally individuals who are not part of the office staff, such as visiting physicians, may be in the area and may inadvertently pick up a file with their own materials. If you think someone could have taken the file, call the person immediately.
12. Ask another staff person to complete steps 1 through 7 to double-check your search.
13. Straighten the office, taking care to check through all piles of information where a file could be lodged.

If the misplaced file is not found within a reasonable time—24 to 48 hours—it may be considered lost. Losing a file has potentially devastating consequences. It may not be possible to duplicate the information within the file, but you can try to re-create it in a new file.

To do so, meet with the physician and office staff members to review the information needed. Record their recollections of information in the file. Note on the file document that it is a recollection and that the information is not official.

Then consult other office records that may include information related to the file. Contact insurance companies, laboratories, and other information providers for copies of original documents previously included in the lost file.

Evaluating Your Office Filing System

In a typical medical office, you retrieve and file documents daily using a filing system that may have been set up when the practice first opened. Now it is time to take a critical look at that system and determine how well it meets your needs.

The filing system you have probably does an adequate or better-than-average job of fulfilling the needs of the practice. Otherwise, retrieving and filing patient records would have become annoyingly inefficient. It is always beneficial to see where improvements can be made, however. Even a good filing system can be enhanced to increase office efficiency and save staff members valuable time.

Here are some simple guidelines for evaluating your filing system.

1. How well do you think your filing system meets your needs? Rate it on a scale of 1 to 10, with 10 representing the best. Survey staff members to determine their ratings, and calculate a composite number. *Based on this feedback, does your filing system seem to do a poor, adequate, or exceptional job?*

2. Note the type of system you use—for example, alphabetic or numeric. Then list the various reasons why files are retrieved from the system. *Would another system, a combination of systems (such as alphanumeric), or the addition* of color coding save time or offer other benefits?

3. Survey the office staff to determine whether there have been difficulties in retrieving or filing or problems with lost or misplaced files. Solicit suggestions for improvement. *If there have been problems, what steps can you take to avoid future difficulties?* (You might even ask your local office-supply representative for ideas.)

4. Consult personnel at other, similar medical practices to determine which filing system works for them. Compare and contrast their systems with yours. *How would their systems work in your office?*

Before making any major changes to your filing system, evaluate each idea in terms of the time and effort it will require and the benefits it will deliver. For example, changing from an alphabetic to a numeric system may provide a relatively small benefit to your office but require a great deal of time to prepare new files and re-file current documents. In that case implementing a numeric system is probably not worthwhile.

If you do make changes to your system, make sure that all staff members are retrained on how to file documents. It is well worth the extra time required at the start to prevent having to locate misplaced files in the future.

Place copies of those records in the new file, or excerpt information. If the physician considers it appropriate, tell the patient whose file has been misplaced about its status and the steps you have taken to re-create it.

Active Versus Inactive Files

At any given time, there are files that you use frequently and files that you use infrequently or not at all. Files that you use frequently are called **active files.** Files that you use infrequently are called **inactive files.** What constitutes an active, as opposed to an inactive, file? It depends on your individual practice. In a heart specialist's office, a patient who has not been seen for a year may be considered inactive, while in a dentist's office, a year may simply indicate one missed appointment.

There is a third category of files, called closed files. **Closed files** are files of patients who have died, have moved away, or for some other reason no longer consult the office. Although closed files could be moved immediately to storage, they are usually treated in the same manner as inactive files. That is, they are kept in the office for a certain length of time to make sure that there are no requests for the information in the file.

The physician must determine when a patient file is deemed inactive or closed. You and the physician can meet regularly, perhaps once a month or once a quarter, to review these files.

File Storage

No office has unlimited space. Therefore, you may regularly need to transfer inactive and closed files from the office's filing area to a storage area.

Basic Storage Options

Before you can transfer files, you need to determine how and where they will be stored. The design and layout of file storage should make even older stored files easily accessible so that they can be periodically evaluated for retention or elimination.

There are many ways to store inactive files. For example, they can be stored in their original paper state or transferred into another format, such as onto a computer disk or tape or into microfilm or microfiche. Files can even be electronically coded with bar codes for immediate retrieval with a computer system. Regardless of the medium chosen for storing and preserving documents, keeping related material together and retrieving it should be made as easy as possible. Inactive files also must be kept secure, just as active ones are.

Paper Storage. If you choose to store files in their original form, you will be storing them as paper files. Paper files are often stored in boxes labeled with their contents. Choose boxes that are uniform in size so that they will stack well. Lift-off lids enable easy access to the contents of the box.

Paper files are bulky to store. They require roughly the same amount of space as they occupied in the office's primary files. Paper files preserve the original documents, however, and these documents can be important when providing evidence of medical treatment in legal proceedings. If paper files start to become brittle, they should be transferred to another storage medium.

Computer Storage. If storage space is limited, there are a number of paperless options for storing files. One such option is storing files on computer tapes or floppy disks, as shown in Figure 10-7. To do so, the office needs a computer system that can transfer documents to tapes or disks, then read them when they are retrieved from storage.

The easiest way to transfer documents directly into the computer is to use a scanner. This device copies a document onto the computer's hard drive. This process saves countless hours of rekeying (reentering) documents into the computer. Many scanners also have the capability of copying graphics and handwritten notes.

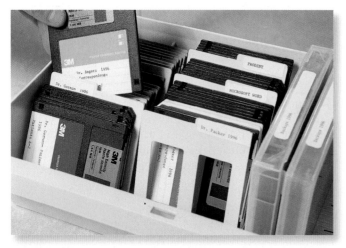

Figure 10-7. One paperless option for storing inactive files and closed files is on floppy disks.

The document is then saved on a disk or on computer tape. Disks or tapes are labeled with the range of contents they contain. If documents were originally created on the computer, they can be similarly transferred to disk or tape, then deleted from the hard drive. Disks and tapes are dated and stored in file boxes or other containers.

Documents can be stored on the hard drive of the computer. The information should also be stored on disks, however, as a backup in case the hard drive crashes and information is lost.

If documents are stored directly on the hard drive, a variety of computer software programs help in managing these records. This software checks files automatically using different criteria, such as the date the file was established or last updated. This software will help you make decisions about how long documents should be stored. When considering computer record management programs, look for user friendliness, speed and response time, and whether the features of the program meet your needs.

Microfilm, Microfiche, and Cartridges. Other paperless storage options include microfilm, microfiche, and film cartridges. (These storage options are discussed in Chapter 5.)

When considering transferring files to these formats, explore microfilm services, which index and transfer files for a fee. Using a service helps ensure that files are correctly indexed and thus easily found later on. Always have the microfilm service sign a confidentiality agreement.

Storage Facilities

Once you have determined the format for your stored files, you need to decide where to keep them. A number of options are available.

You may wish to store files in a remote area of your office building, such as an unused closet or office. Check to make sure that the area is secure, accessible, and safe for storing files (for example, do not store files where hazardous materials are stored). The practice may have to pay additional rent if the space is not within the confines of its office suite.

If there is no space in the building, consider a neighboring building, perhaps one in the same office complex. Many buildings rent space that can be used to store records. If you pursue this option, you will be responsible for managing the storage of records, including transporting them to the space, positioning them, and retrieving them as needed.

Certain storage facilities, called commercial records centers, will do some of the work for you (Figure 10-8). For a monthly fee, these centers typically house and manage stored documents. When evaluating commercial records centers, inquire about whether they will retrieve and/or deliver boxes or files and whether there is an on-site work area if someone needs to review the files at the storage location.

Beware of general storage facilities that are not specially equipped for document management. These facilities

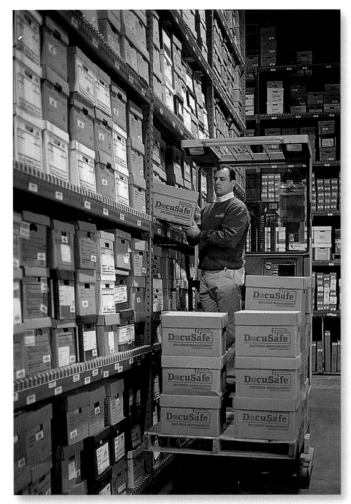

Figure 10-8. Commercial records centers manage stored documents for medical practices. Look for a center with personnel who retrieve and deliver boxes or files directly to your office.

may not address safety concerns by taking precautions for fire or floods, for example.

Maintain a separate list of files stored off-site. This list can save a wasted trip to the storage site if a needed file is not housed there. The list also provides a valuable record if files are damaged or destroyed. Remember to update the list as new files are moved into storage and old files are taken out of storage and destroyed.

Storage Safety

No matter where you store files, you must consider the issue of safety as well as security. Paper, computer, and film files are easily damaged and destroyed by fire, water, and extreme temperatures. Old, brittle paper files are particularly susceptible. Therefore, it is wise to evaluate the storage site and to take some basic precautions.

- Choose a site with moderate temperatures year-round and adequate ventilation.

- Select storage containers that can withstand intense heat and are waterproof. Look for metal or plastic boxes that are designated as fireproof and waterproof. Cardboard is not an option.
- Choose a site equipped with a smoke alarm, sprinkler system, and fire extinguishers.
- Select a site that is above ground and away from flood hazards. One way to find out if a site is susceptible to flooding is to inquire whether the facility has flood insurance, a requirement for sites at risk.
- Choose a site that is kept locked, is regularly patrolled, or has an alarm system, to prevent theft or vandalism.
- Remove old, brittle files as soon as possible, or transfer them into another format. They can then be placed in file storage again.
- Ask for references from people at other offices who have stored files at the site. Talk to these people about what they like and dislike about the storage facility and any problems they have had in storing or retrieving documents.
- If you are storing files in another form—on computer disk or microfiche—inquire about any special precautions the site owner takes to ensure safety.

Taking the time to thoroughly research storage options saves time and effort in the long run as you manage the stored files.

Retaining Files in the Office

Every office will develop a length of time appropriate for the long-term storage of files. Most practices develop a records retention program.

Typically the doctor decides—based on the potential need for the information—how long to keep inactive or closed patient files in the office before sending them to storage. Working with the doctor, you should prepare a retention schedule. A **retention schedule** specifies how long to keep different types of patient records in the office after files have become inactive or closed. The schedule also details when files should be moved to a storage area (if outside the office) and how long they should be kept in storage before being destroyed. The retention schedule should be posted in the file room to make certain that all staff members are aware of it.

Although the doctor decides how long to keep inactive or closed patient records in the office, there are legal requirements for retaining certain types of information, which determine how long these documents must be stored.

- According to the National Childhood Vaccine Injury Act of 1986, doctors must keep all immunization records on file in the office permanently. These records should not be put in storage.
- The Labor Standards Act states that doctors must keep employee health records for 3 years.
- The statute of limitations—the law stating the time period during which lawsuits may be filed—varies by

PROCEDURE 10.3

Developing a Records Retention Program

Objective: To establish a records retention program for patient medical records that meets office needs as well as legal and government guidelines

Materials: *Guide to Record Retention Requirements* (published annually by the federal government), names and telephone numbers of local medical associations and state offices (including the state insurance commissioner and the medical practice's attorney), file folders, index cards, index box, paper, pen or typewriter

Method

1. List the types of information contained in a typical patient medical record in your office. For example, a file for an adult patient may include the patient's case history, records of hospital stays, and insurance information.

2. Research the state and federal requirements for keeping documents. Consult the *Guide to Record Retention Requirements* for federal guidelines. Contact the appropriate state office (such as the office of the insurance commissioner) for specific state requirements, such as rules for keeping records of insurance payments and the statute of limitations for initiating lawsuits. If your office does business in more than one state, be sure to research all applicable regulations. Consult with the attorney who represents your practice.

3. Compile the results of your research in a chart. At the top of the chart, list the different kinds of information your office keeps in patient records. Down the left side of the chart, list the headings "Federal," "State," and "Other." Then, in each box, record the corresponding information.

4. Compare all the legal and government requirements. Indicate which one is for the longest period of time.

5. Meet with the doctor to review the information. Work together to prepare a retention schedule. Determine how long different types of patient records should be kept in the office after a patient leaves the practice and how long records should be kept in storage. Although retention periods can vary based on the type of information kept in a file, it is often easiest to choose a retention period that covers all records. For example, all records could be kept in the office for 1 year after a patient leaves the practice and then kept in storage for another 9 years, for a total of 10 years. Determine how files will be destroyed when they have exceeded the retention requirements. Usually, records are destroyed by paper shredding. Purchase the appropriate equipment, as necessary.

6. Put the retention schedule in writing, and post it prominently near the files. In addition, keep a copy of the schedule in a safe place in the office. Review it with the office staff.

7. Develop a system for identifying files easily under the retention system. For example, for each file deemed inactive or closed, prepare an index card or create a master list containing the following information:
   - Patient's name and Social Security number
   - Contents of the file
   - Date the file was deemed inactive and by whom
   - Date the file should be sent to storage (the actual date will be filled in later; if more than one storage location is used, indicate the exact location to which the file was sent)
   - Date the file should be destroyed (the actual date will be filled in later)

   Have the card signed by the doctor and by the person responsible for the files. Keep the card in an index box. This is your authorization to destroy the file at the appropriate time.

8. Use color coding to help identify inactive files. For example, all records that become inactive in 2002 could be placed in green file folders and moved to a supplemental file. Then, in January 2004 all the green files could be pulled and sent to storage.

9. One person should be responsible for checking the index cards once a month to determine which stored files should be destroyed. Before retrieving these files from storage, circulate a notice to the office staff stating which records will be destroyed. Indicate that the staff must let you know by a specific date if any of the files should be saved. You may want to keep a separate file with these notices.

10. After the deadline has passed, retrieve the files from storage. Review each file before it is

continued ⟶

Developing a Records Retention Program *(continued)*

destroyed. Make sure the staff members who will destroy the files are trained to use the equipment properly. Develop a sheet of instructions for destroying files. Post it prominently with the retention schedule, near the machinery used to destroy the files.

11. Update the index card, giving the date the file was destroyed and by whom.

12. Periodically review the retention schedule. Update it with the most current legal and governmental requirements. With the staff, evaluate whether the current schedule is meeting the needs of your office or whether files are being kept too long or destroyed prematurely. With the doctor's approval, change the schedule as necessary.

---

state for civil suits. The most common length of time is 2 years. If a case involves a child or someone mentally incompetent, the statute of limitations extends the deadline. Regardless of the statute of limitations, it is always advisable for doctors to seek legal advice before destroying any records.

- Many legal consultants advise that doctors maintain patient records for at least 7 years to protect themselves against malpractice suits.
- The Internal Revenue Service usually requires doctors to keep financial records for up to 10 years.
- Doctors are required to keep medical records of minors previously under their care for 2 to 7 years after the child reaches legal age, depending on the state. Some doctors keep these records indefinitely.
- The American Medical Association, the American Hospital Association, and other groups generally suggest that doctors keep patient records for up to 10 years after a patient's final visit or contact.

For a complete list of federal regulations, contact the U.S. Superintendent of Documents in Washington, D.C.,

and request a copy of the *Guide to Record Retention Requirements*. This guide is updated annually and can be purchased for a small fee.

State and local retention requirements can be obtained from offices with which you regularly conduct business, such as insurance companies, state and local agencies, and medical associations. If you do business in more than one state, follow the schedule that requires the longest retention time for materials.

When counting years in a retention schedule, remember not to count the year in which the document was produced but to begin counting with the following year. This way, documents produced near the end of a calendar year will be tracked more efficiently. Procedure 10-3 summarizes the steps for setting up a records retention program.

When records can finally be eliminated, they cannot simply be thrown away. Even old records hold confidential information about patients. Therefore, they must be completely destroyed by shredding. Be careful not to destroy records prematurely, because they often cannot be recreated. It is vital that you retain a list of documents that have been destroyed.

Career Opportunities

Medical Record Technologist

To gain medical assistant credentials, you must fulfill the requirements of either the American Association of Medical Assistants (for a Certified Medical Assistant) or the American Medical Technologists (for a Registered Medical Assistant). After obtaining your medical assistant certification or registration, you may wish to acquire additional skills in specialty areas through course work or on-the-job training. Although this course work or training may not lead to an additional

certification or degree, it will enable you to expand your role in the medical office and advance your career as the demand for skilled health professionals increases.

Skills and Duties

Also known as a medical record technician or a medical chart specialist, a medical record technologist (MRT) maintains patient records for a physician or group of

continued ⟶

Medical Record Technologist *(continued)*

physicians. The technician is responsible for ensuring that all medical information is accurate and complete. In a hospital, a medical record technologist deals strictly with health information and has no patient contact. In a small office, however, the technician may have additional clerical duties such as answering the telephone.

A patient's medical record includes a medical history and statement of symptoms as well as the re-sults of examinations, laboratory tests, and x-rays. The physician's diagnoses and treatment plans are also included. The information in the patient's record may be needed for insurance purposes or to aid in further diagnosis and treatment. In addition, it may be used for research purposes.

The medical record technologist checks all patient charts for completeness and accuracy. The MRT makes sure that all necessary forms related to the patient's care are included, properly filled out, and signed. The MRT checks to see that all reports and test results are attached to the chart. If necessary, the MRT speaks with the physician to clarify information about the patient's diagnosis or treatment.

The technologist must also code the medical record. The MRT assigns a code to each clinical procedure and diagnosis if this coding has not already been done by another member of the health-care team. In the hospital setting, the MRT assigns a diagnosis-related group (DRG) to the patient, using a special computer program. The DRG helps determine the reimbursement that the hospital will receive from Medicare or any other insurance provider that uses a DRG system. The medical record technologist may also use the coded records to set up a cross-reference index, a type of file that lists the same information under several different headings.

Some medical record technologists specialize in a particular area. Coding is one example. Another is registry, which involves keeping records of all occurrences of certain diseases like bone cancer. The information the registrar collects can be used by individual physicians or as part of a research study.

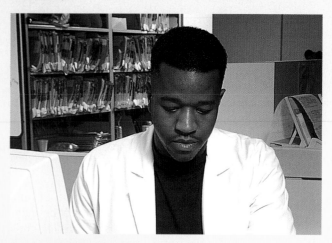

Workplace Settings

The majority of medical record technologists work in medical record departments of hospitals. Most of the rest work in nursing homes, group practices, and health maintenance organizations (HMOs). A few medical record technologists work in federal or state government offices, public health departments, health and property insurance companies, or accounting and law firms. Some record technologists are self-employed and work as consultants to nursing homes or physicians' offices.

Education

Most medical record technologists have completed a 2-year associate degree program at a junior or community college. Course work includes biology, anatomy and physiology, medical terminology, data processing, coding, and statistics. Record technologists can also be trained through the Independent Study Program in Medical Record Technology, a home-study program offered by the American Medical Record Association (AMRA).

To become certified as an Accredited Record Technician (ART), a technologist must take a written examination administered by the AMRA. In order to qualify for the examination, the technologist must be a graduate of a 2-year associate degree program accredited by the Commission on Accreditation of Allied Health Education Programs (CAAHEP), or must be a graduate of the Independent Study Program who has completed an additional 30 semester hours of academic credit.

Where to Go for More Information

American Health Information Management Association (formerly the American Medical Record Association)
919 North Michigan Avenue, Suite 1400
Chicago, IL 60611

Summary

The organization of a practice's filing system depends on how files need to be retrieved. Alphabetic systems are the most common. Numeric systems are sometimes used in practices with patients who require a high level of confidentiality, such as those who are HIV-positive.

Color coding may be used to further identify files. In addition, special types of files, such as tickler files or supplemental files, are sometimes used.

The five steps in the filing process are inspecting, indexing, coding, sorting, and storing. Failure to follow each of the steps in order can result in misplaced or lost files.

Typically, only active files are kept in the practice's main file area. When patient records are determined to be inactive or closed, they are transferred to storage—either elsewhere in the office or outside the practice in a special storage facility. Files may be stored in a variety of formats: paper, microfilm or microfiche, or on the computer. Wherever files are stored and in whatever format, they must be kept safe and secure.

The amount of time that stored files are retained depends on legal, state, and federal guidelines. Offices manage the storage and destruction of files by developing a records retention program. Because even old files contain confidential information, they must be destroyed in an approved manner, not simply thrown away.

REVIEW

CHAPTER 10

CASE STUDY QUESTIONS

Now that you have completed this chapter, review the case study at the beginning of the chapter and answer the following questions:

1. What are advantages and disadvantages of different file systems?
2. What security measures might be used to protect patient files?
3. What is a tickler system and how is it set up?
4. Identify several storage options for closed charts. Which is the most secure? The easiest? The most cost-efficient?

Discussion Questions

1. Why is it important to use a filing system to keep medical records? What could happen if a filing system is not instituted or not followed consistently in a medical practice?
2. Who is inconvenienced or even injured if a medical record is lost?
3. What important behaviors should an efficient medical record technologist demonstrate?
4. What skills are important for a staff member whose primary responsibility is to file medical records?

Critical Thinking Questions

1. You have been hired as part of a new staff in a start-up operation for a medical group that specializes in obstetrics/gynecology and fertility. What filing system will you implement and why?
2. What special concerns might arise when storing records on the computer rather than in traditional (hard copy) paper files? Why do you think major clinics such as the Mayo Clinic use a completely electronic or computerized file storage system?
3. What filing system would you choose for a series of numbered insurance claim forms for patients? Why?

Application Activities

1. Arrange these ten patient names in order as they would appear in an alphabetic filing system.
   Josephs, Leon S.
   Carl Jones
   Carly Jones
   Carl A. Jones
   Deirdre Anne Jones
   McCullough, Anthony L.
   E. Bruce Harrison
   Waters, Jamie H.
   Joan Carle
   James Waters
2. Using your class list, develop a numeric filing system and a master list that matches each number to a specific person. Then set up an alphabetic filing system based on students' last names. Discuss with your classmates which system is most useful in an educational setting and why.
3. Set up a personal tickler file for yourself, containing personal responsibilities—such as errands, appointments, and social engagements—for the coming week. Keep your notes in a file folder or on a calendar until all activities have been completed. At the end of the week, write a brief paragraph explaining whether you found the process helpful. Give several examples to support your answer.
4. Obtain an office-supply catalog that features filing supplies. Put together a product order to set up a patient records filing system for a midsized medical office serving approximately 100 patients. Assume that the practice has already purchased the appropriate equipment, such as filing cabinets or shelves.

SECTION 2

INTERACTING WITH PATIENTS

CHAPTER 11
Telephone Techniques

CHAPTER 12
Scheduling Appointments and Maintaining the Physician's Schedule

CHAPTER 13
Patient Reception Area

CHAPTER 14
Patient Education

Telephone Techniques

KEY TERMS

enunciation
etiquette
facsimile machine
pitch
pronunciation
telephone triage

AREAS OF COMPETENCE

2003 Role Delineation Study
GENERAL
Professionalism
- Prioritize and perform multiple tasks

Communication Skills
- Use professional telephone technique

CHAPTER OUTLINE

- Using the Telephone Effectively
- Communication Skills
- Managing Incoming Calls
- Types of Incoming Calls
- Using Proper Telephone Etiquette
- Taking Messages
- Telephone Answering Systems
- Placing Outgoing Calls
- Telephone Triage
- Telecommunications
- Facsimile (Fax) Machines

OBJECTIVES

After completing Chapter 11, you will be able to:

11.1 Explain how to manage incoming telephone calls.

11.2 Explain the importance of communication skills.

11.3 Compare the types of calls the medical assistant handles with those the physician or other staff members handle.

11.4 Describe how to handle various types of incoming calls from patients and from others.

11.5 Discuss the importance of proper telephone etiquette.

11.6 Describe the procedures for taking telephone messages.

11.7 Explain the basics of the Health Insurance Portability and Accountability Act (HIPAA).

11.8 Explain how to retrieve calls from an answering service.

11.9 Describe the procedures for placing outgoing calls.

11.10 Explain the function of telephone triage in the medical office.

11.11 Explain the uses of a facsimile machine in a medical office.

Introduction

In this chapter, you will learn key terms associated with telephone techniques. You will be able to utilize a telephone professionally and effectively while handing various types of calls that are either received or initiated by a medical office. These types of calls will vary and can include calls about patient illness and injury, prescription refills, or requests for test results; calls from other medical offices; or calls from sales representatives. After completing this chapter, you will understand which calls may be handled by the medical assistant and which require the physician's attention.

Most medical offices have policies and procedures on handling or routing incoming calls, especially emergency calls. This chapter helps you identify which calls are considered emergencies and how to properly route these calls.

In addition, after reading this chapter, you will be able to demonstrate proper telephone etiquette by using common courtesy, proper pronunciation, tone, and enunciation while speaking. You will learn how to effectively handle difficult telephone situations or complaints and how to properly document messages taken.

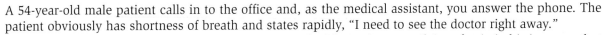

CASE STUDY

A 54-year-old male patient calls in to the office and, as the medical assistant, you answer the phone. The patient obviously has shortness of breath and states rapidly, "I need to see the doctor right away."

After you establish the patient's name, you learn that the patient complains of pain in his jaw area that lasts for about 5 minutes and then goes away. He also states that he was mowing the lawn when he started sweating heavily and having a little difficulty breathing. Once he was inside the house, he did have some nausea and vomited once.

As you read this chapter, consider the following questions:

1. What would your first response to the patient be?
2. Explain how you would handle this situation.
3. What type of incoming call was this?
4. What type of condition did this patient's symptoms indicate?
5. What are some other symptoms of this condition?

Using the Telephone Effectively

The telephone is an important tool for promoting the positive, professional image of a medical practice. When you answer the telephone, you may be the first contact a person has with the practice. The impression you leave can be either positive or negative. Your job is to ensure that it is positive.

Good telephone management leaves callers with a positive impression of you, the physician, and the practice. Poor telephone management can result in bad feelings, misunderstandings, and an unfavorable impression. The telephone image you present should convey the message that the staff is caring, attentive, and helpful. Showing concern for a patient's welfare is a quality that patients rate highly when evaluating health-care professionals. In addition, you must sound professional and knowledgeable when handling telephone calls. Learning and using proper telephone management skills will help keep patients informed and ensure their satisfaction with the medical practice.

Communication Skills

The telephone is a communication and public relations tool that is essential to the operation of the medical office. Good communication skills are important in telephone management—they help to project a positive image and to satisfy the needs and expectations of the patient. Individuals who engage in good and effective communication employ the following communications skills:

- Using tact and sensitivity
- Showing empathy
- Giving respect
- Being genuine
- Displaying openness and friendliness
- Refraining from passing judgment or stereotyping others
- Being supportive
- Asking for clarification and feedback
- Paraphrasing to ensure an understanding of what others are saying

- Being receptive to patients' needs
- Knowing when to speak and when to listen
- Exhibiting a willingness to consider other viewpoints and concerns

As a medical assistant, you can also apply the five Cs of communication to use the telephone effectively:

- Completeness—The message must contain all necessary information
- Clarity—The message must be legible and free from ambiguity
- Conciseness—The message must not include any unnecessary information
- Courtesy—The message must be respectful and considerate of others
- Cohesiveness—The message must be organized and logical

Managing Incoming Calls

Telephone calls must always be answered promptly. The procedures for answering calls may vary. Guidelines are usually presented in the office policy and procedures manual. In general, you should greet callers with your name and the office name. Some people may feel awkward using their own name when answering the telephone. Introducing yourself to callers, however, lets them know that they are speaking to a real person, not simply an anonymous voice.

No matter how hurried you are, you should be courteous, calm, and pleasant on the telephone, devoting your full attention to the caller. If the caller does not give a name, ask for it. Many calls result in pulling the patient's file, so it is important to obtain the correct name and date of birth of the patient.

Guidelines for Managing Incoming Calls

The following guidelines will help you manage incoming calls:

- Answer the telephone promptly by the second or third ring.
- Hold the mouthpiece about an inch away from your mouth and leave one hand free to write with.
- Greet the caller first with the name of the medical office and then with your name.
- Identify the caller. Demonstrate your willingness to assist the caller by asking, "How may I help you?"
- Be courteous, calm, and pleasant no matter how hurried you are.
- Identify the nature of the call and devote your full attention to the caller.

- At the end of the call, say goodbye and use the caller's name.

Following HIPAA Guidelines

As you learned in Chapter 3, the Health Insurance Portability and Accountability Act (HIPAA) was originally created in 1996 and has additions as recent as 2003. This act is concerned with the privacy and confidentiality of patient information, including information communicated via the telephone.

In compliance with HIPAA guidelines, all medical providers have standards or written policies that require the following to be in a secure area where no one can see or overhear:

- Medical records
- Clerical forms
- Financial forms and reports
- Computer monitors
- Conversations
- Verbal reports

All employees must comply with the guidelines to safeguard patient information, including when talking on the telephone with a patient.

Health-care providers are allowed to disclose patient information for the purpose of treatment, payment, and health-care operations. Any use of this information outside of these reasons would require a written authorization from the patient. Exceptions include emergency situations or information that is required by governmental agencies for compliance. Follow the medical provider's policy and procedures for disclosing patient information.

Screening Calls

Part of the responsibility of answering the telephone involves screening calls before you transfer them. Each office has its own policy about calls that should be put through right away, those that should be returned later, and those that should be handled by other staff members. The Tips for the Office section describes some guidelines for screening calls.

Routing Calls

In general, there are three types of incoming calls to a doctor's office: calls dealing mainly with administrative issues, emergency calls that require immediate action by the doctor, and calls relating to clinical issues that require the attention of the doctor, nurse, nurse practitioner, or physician assistant.

Calls Handled by the Medical Assistant. The most common calls to a medical office involve administrative and clinical issues. As a medical assistant, you will be

Tips for the Office

Screening Incoming Calls

Each medical office has its own policy about how to screen incoming calls before transferring them to the appropriate person. Calls come not only from patients but also from other physicians, hospital personnel, pharmacists, insurance company personnel, sales representatives, and family members and friends of patients. Here are some general tips for screening calls.

Find out who is calling. A polite way to do this is to say, "May I ask who is calling?" Another option is, "May I tell Dr. _____ who is calling?"

Ask what the call is in reference to. When a caller asks to speak with the physician, you should ask the purpose of the call. Depending on the answer, you may determine that you or someone else in the office can handle the situation without disturbing the physician. The response may be as simple as solving a billing problem or clarifying instructions. Remember, however, that emergency calls should be transferred to the physician right away.

Decide whether the call should be put through. Although most calls are routed to the appropriate person, any callers who refuse to identify themselves should not be put through. In such a case suggest that the caller write a letter to the physician and mark it "Personal."

Determine what to do if the matter is personal. The physician may ask you to take a message in these instances. Inform the caller that the physician will return the call as soon as possible.

---

able to handle most of these calls yourself. They will concern the following matters:

- Appointments (scheduling, rescheduling, canceling)
- Questions concerning office policies, fees, and hours
- Billing inquiries
- Insurance questions
- Other administrative questions
- X-ray and laboratory reports
- Reports from hospitals regarding a patient's progress
- Reports from patients concerning their progress
- Requests for referrals to other doctors
- Requests for prescription renewals, which must be approved by the doctor unless approval is indicated on the patient's chart
- Complaints from patients about administrative matters

Depending on the practice, the office manager or someone in the billing department may handle some administrative calls. The calls you handle may include scheduling appointments, receiving or requesting reports or information, insurance and billing questions, and general inquiries, such as those concerning office hours.

Calls Requiring the Doctor's Attention. Certain calls will require the doctor's personal attention. These include the following:

- Emergency calls
- Calls from other doctors
- Patient requests to discuss test results, particularly abnormal results

- Reports from patients concerning unsatisfactory progress
- Requests for prescription renewals (unless previously authorized on the patient's chart)
- Personal calls

Occasionally the patient may prefer to discuss symptoms only with the doctor. These requests should be honored. Depending on the doctor's preference and availability, you may call the doctor to the telephone to handle calls of this nature as they are received. Otherwise, the calls will be returned later that day when the doctor has time available. (Most doctors have a set time, such as a half hour in the late morning or at the end of the day, for returning nonemergency patient calls.)

In certain practices some of these calls may be handled by others on the staff, such as a nurse practitioner or physician assistant. For example, a nurse practitioner may be able to order a renewal of a regular prescription, provide advice for the care of a sprain, or answer well-baby questions or questions about the side effects of a drug.

The Routing List. Each medical office has a standard policy that documents how incoming telephone calls are to be routed and handled. A routing list, such as the one shown in Figure 11-1, specifies who is responsible for the various types of calls in the office and how the calls are to be handled. For example, the routing list indicates which calls should be put through to the doctor immediately and which ones can be returned later.

The routing procedure may simply identify the general title of the person responsible for handling a call. When more than one person in the office has the same

HANDLING INCOMING TELEPHONE CALLS

	Route to doctor immediately	Take message for doctor	Route to nurse or assistant
Emergencies: bleeding, drug/allergic reaction, difficulty breathing, injury, pain, poisoning, shock, unconsciousness, incoherence or hysteria	X		
Calls from other physicians	if possible		
Patient progress report		X	
Patient request for laboratory report		X (if abnormal)	Melissa (if normal)
Patient questions re medication		X	
Patient questions re billing or insurance			Jerry
Patient complaints			Melissa
Appointments			Melissa
Prescription renewals or refills		X	
Office business			Jerry
Personal business		X	
Salespeople			Jerry

Figure 11-1. A routing list identifies which office staff member is responsible for each type of incoming call.

title, however, the name of the individual who has that particular responsibility should be specified.

Types of Incoming Calls

In dealing with incoming telephone calls, you will encounter a variety of questions and requests from numerous people. Many incoming calls are from patients. You will also receive calls from other people, including attorneys, other physicians, pharmaceutical sales representatives, and other salespeople.

Calls From Patients

Patients call the medical office for a variety of reasons, including rescheduling appointments and requesting prescription renewals. If you will be discussing clinical matters over the telephone, it is a good idea to pull the patient's chart. The information in the chart may enable you to address any problems quickly. Having the chart handy also allows you to document the conversation immediately.

Always keep in mind that the physician is legally responsible for your actions, including relaying information to patients over the telephone. The office policy manual typically specifies what you may and may not discuss with patients. If you are uncertain about giving particular

information to a patient, it is best to have the physician return the patient's call.

Appointment Scheduling. Follow office procedures for making or changing appointment times over the telephone. (Scheduling appointments is discussed in Chapter 12.)

Billing Inquiries. If a patient calls about a billing problem, you will need to pull the patient's chart and billing information. With this information, you can compare the charges with the actual services performed.

If a patient claims to have been overcharged, check to see if the correct fee was charged. If you find that an error was made, apologize, and tell the patient the office will send a corrected statement. Ask the patient to wait for the new statement before sending payment. If in fact the proper fee was charged, it may be helpful to speak to the physician before responding to the patient. The physician may be able to tell you if there were special circumstances regarding the visit or charge in question. Allowing the patient to pay the bill in installments is usually an acceptable option.

If a patient is dissatisfied, document all comments, and relay the information to the physician. If a bill has not been paid, ask if there are special circumstances affecting the patient's ability to pay. Always give this information to the physician or office manager.

Requests for Laboratory or Radiology Reports.
If a patient calls the office requesting the results of tests, pull the patient's chart to see if the report has been received. If it has not, suggest that the patient call back in a day or two. Some offices will call the laboratory or radiology office for the results.

In some offices you may be authorized to give laboratory results by telephone if they are normal, or negative, so the patient does not have to wait for results to be mailed. Make a note on the patient's chart if you provide any information about test results. If a test result is abnormal, the physician will need to speak with the patient. In such a case tell the patient that the office has received the results and that the physician will call as soon as possible. Then place the patient's chart and the telephone message on the physician's desk.

Questions About Medications.
One of the most common types of calls from patients involves questions about medication. A patient may ask about using a current prescription or may want to renew an existing prescription.

Prescription Renewals.
Calls for prescription renewals occur frequently and may come from the patient's pharmacy or from the patient. A pharmacist usually calls to check before dispensing refills if more than a year has passed since the original prescription was written. If the physician has indicated on the patient's chart that renewals are approved, you may authorize the pharmacy to renew a prescription. In any other case, only the physician may authorize renewals. If the physician authorizes a renewal, you may be asked to telephone it in to the patient's pharmacy.

Old Prescriptions.
Patients may call to ask if they can use a medication that was prescribed for a previous condition. In these instances, recommend that the patient come in for an appointment. Explain why the medication should not be used: it may be old and no longer effective, the current problem may not be the same as the previous one, the medication may not be helpful, and using the medication may mask the current condition's symptoms and make a diagnosis difficult.

If the patient does not want to make an appointment, relay the information to the physician. The physician will probably want to speak with the patient.

Reports on Symptoms.
Sometimes patients call the office about symptoms they wish to discuss with the physician. Here are tips for handling such calls.

- Listen attentively to the patient.
- If the patient is in real distress, try to schedule an appointment that day or as soon as possible.
- Write down all the patient's symptoms completely, accurately, and immediately. In many instances the physician may be able to suggest simple emergency relief measures that you can relay to the patient. These measures may make the patient comfortable until the time of the appointment.

Progress Reports.
Physicians often ask patients to call the office to let them know how a prescribed treatment is working. In these instances route the call to the physician, and log the call in the patient's medical record immediately. You may also be responsible for making routine follow-up calls to patients to verify that they are following treatment instructions.

Requests for Advice.
Although a patient may ask you for your medical opinion, do not give medical advice of any kind. Explain that you are not trained to make a diagnosis or licensed to prescribe medication. Stress that the patient must see the physician. If the patient cannot come into the office, assure her that the physician will return the call or that you will call back after discussing the problem with the physician. Occasionally a patient wants to speak only with the physician, not other staff members. You must honor this request.

In some cases the physician may feel that a patient's symptoms warrant immediate attention and will insist on seeing the patient before prescribing any treatment. If the patient refuses to come to the office, note the reason on the chart, and suggest a visit to the emergency room or to a nearby physician. For legal reasons, it is important to document such conversations completely in the patient's chart, including the refusal of treatment.

Complaints.
Even when an office provides the highest-quality care, complaints still occur. When a patient calls with a complaint, such as a billing error, it is important to listen carefully, without interrupting. Take careful notes of all the details, and read them back to the caller to ensure that you have written them down correctly. Let the caller know the person to whose attention you will bring the complaint and, if possible, when to expect a response.

Always apologize to the caller for any inconvenience the problem may have caused, even if the problem occurred through no fault of the office. Make sure the proper person receives the information about the complaint.

Sometimes a patient who calls with a complaint is angry. Responding to this type of call can be difficult and uncomfortable. Your first priority is to stay calm and try to pacify the caller. Follow these guidelines when dealing with an angry caller.

- Listen carefully, and acknowledge the patient's anger. By understanding the problem, you will be better able to work toward a solution.
- Remain calm, and speak gently and kindly. Do not act superior or talk down to the patient. Do not interrupt the patient. Do not return the anger or blame.
- Let the patient know that you will do your best to correct the problem. This message will convey that you care.
- Take careful notes, and be sure to document the call.
- Do not become defensive.
- Never make promises you cannot keep.

- Follow up promptly on the problem.
- Inform the physician immediately if an angry patient threatens legal action against the office.

Emergencies. Emergency calls must be immediately routed to the physician. Emergency situations include serious or life-threatening medical conditions, such as severe bleeding, a reaction to a drug, injuries, poisoning, suicide attempts, loss of consciousness, or severe burns. Figure 11-2 lists symptoms and conditions that require immediate help.

Symptoms and Conditions That Require Immediate Medical Help

- Unconsciousness
- Lack of breathing or trouble breathing
- Severe bleeding
- Pressure or pain in the abdomen that will not go away
- Severe vomiting or bloody stools
- Poisoning
- Injuries to the head, neck, or back
- Choking
- Drowning
- Electrical shock
- Snakebites
- Vehicle collisions
- Allergic reactions to foods or insect stings
- Chemicals or foreign objects in the eye
- Fires, severe burns, or injuries from explosions
- Human bites or any deep animal bites
- Heart attack. Symptoms include chest pain or pressure; pain radiating from the chest to the arm, shoulder, neck, jaw, back, or stomach; nausea or vomiting; weakness; shortness of breath; pale or gray skin color.
- Stroke. Symptoms include seizures, severe headache, slurred speech.
- Broken bones. Symptoms include being unable to move or put weight on the injured body part. The injured part is very painful or looks misshapen.
- Shock. Symptoms include paleness; feeling faint and sweaty; weak, rapid pulse; cold, moist skin; confusion or drowsiness.
- Heatstroke (sunstroke). Symptoms include confusion or loss of consciousness; flushed skin that is hot and may be moist or dry; strong, rapid pulse.
- Hypothermia (a drop in body temperature during prolonged exposure to cold). Symptoms include becoming increasingly clumsy, unreasonable, irritable, confused, and sleepy; slurred speech; slipping into a coma with slow, weak breathing and heartbeat.

Figure 11-2. Emergency calls require swift but careful handling.

If someone calls the office on behalf of a patient who is experiencing any of these symptoms or conditions, you may instruct the caller to dial 911 to request an ambulance. Procedure 11-1 describes the steps for handling emergency calls. The physician should be called to the telephone immediately to offer assistance.

Other Calls

Besides calls from patients, a medical office receives many other types of calls. For example, family members and friends of patients may call the physician at the office. The physician will let you know how to handle these calls. Remember that a patient's information is confidential. HIPAA requires medical providers to obtain authorization from the patient before any information can be disclosed. This is usually in the form of a written authorization, signed by the patient, that indicates what type of information may be given out and to whom. The following are guidelines for managing calls from attorneys, other physicians, and salespeople.

Attorneys. Refer to the procedures listed in your practice's office policy manual regarding how to handle calls from attorneys. Follow the office guidelines closely, and ask the physician how to proceed if you receive a call that does not fall within the guidelines. Remember, never release any patient information to an outside caller unless the physician has asked you to do so.

Other Physicians. Patients at your practice may be referred to surgeons, specialists, and other physicians for consultations. Consequently, you may receive calls from those physicians' offices. Route those calls to the physician if the caller requests that you do so. Always remember to ask if the call is about a medical emergency. Also keep in mind that you may not give out any patient information—even to another physician—unless you have a written, signed release from the patient.

Salespeople. As a medical assistant, you will probably be the contact for salespeople, unless the office policy manual states that another staff member should handle this duty. On the telephone, ask the salesperson to send you information about any new products or equipment. Pharmaceutical sales representatives may want to meet with the physician. Forward such messages to the physician with a request to let you know when to schedule the appointment. Many physicians see pharmaceutical sales representatives on certain days at certain times. Sometimes they limit the number of representatives they will see in one day. Make sure you know your office policy.

Using Proper Telephone Etiquette

Handle all telephone calls politely and professionally. Use proper telephone **etiquette,** or good manners, so you feel confident in your role of providing quality care and

PROCEDURE 11.1

Handling Emergency Calls

Objective: To determine whether a telephone call involves a medical emergency and to learn the steps to take if it is an emergency call

Materials: Office guidelines for handling emergency calls; list of symptoms and conditions requiring immediate medical attention; telephone numbers of area emergency rooms, poison control centers, and ambulance transport services; telephone message forms or telephone message log

Method

1. When someone calls the office regarding a potential emergency, remain calm. This attitude will help calm the caller and enable you to gather necessary information in the most efficient manner.
2. Obtain the following information, taking accurate notes:
   a. The caller's name
   b. The caller's relation to the patient (if it is not the patient who is calling)
   c. The patient's name
   d. The patient's age
   e. A complete description of the patient's symptoms
   f. If the call is about an accident, a description of how the accident or injury occurred and any other pertinent information
   g. A description of how the patient is reacting to the situation
   h. Treatment that has been administered
   i. The caller's telephone number and the address from which the call is being made

It may be necessary for you to put the call on hold or to hang up so that you can call for medical assistance. Before you do so, however, be sure to read the information back to the caller to ensure that you have written it down correctly.

3. Read back the details of the medical problem to verify them.
4. If necessary, refer to the list of symptoms and conditions that require immediate medical attention to determine if the situation is indeed a medical emergency.

If the Situation Is a Medical Emergency

1. Put the call through to the doctor immediately, or handle the situation according to the established office procedures.
2. If the doctor is not in the office, follow established office procedures. They may involve one or more of the following:
   a. Transferring the call to the nurse practitioner or other medical personnel, as appropriate
   b. Instructing the caller to dial 911 to request an ambulance for the patient
   c. Instructing the patient to go to the nearest emergency room
   d. Instructing the caller to telephone the nearest poison control center for advice and supplying the caller with its telephone number
   e. Paging the doctor

If the Situation Is Not a Medical Emergency

1. Handle the call according to established office procedures.
2. If you are in doubt about whether the situation is a medical emergency, treat it like an emergency. It is better to be overly cautious than to let an emergency go untreated. The doctor should be the one to decide how to handle these situations. You must always alert the doctor immediately about an emergency call, even if the patient declines to speak with the doctor.

---

assistance. Adhering to the guidelines that follow will help ensure that your telephone conversations are pleasant and constructive.

Your Telephone Voice

When you speak on the telephone, your voice represents the medical office. It must effectively present your message. Because you cannot rely on body language or facial expressions to help you communicate over the telephone, it is important to make the most of your telephone voice. Use the following tips to make your voice pleasant and effective.

- Speak directly into the receiver. Otherwise, your voice will be difficult to understand.
- Smile. The smile in your voice will convey your friendliness and willingness to help.

- Visualize the caller, and speak directly to that person.
- Convey a friendly and respectful interest in the caller. You should sound helpful and alert.
- Use language that is nontechnical and easy to understand. Never use slang.
- Speak at a natural pace, not too quickly or too slowly.
- Use a normal conversational tone.
- Try to vary your pitch while you are talking. **Pitch** is the high or low level of your speech. Varying the pitch of your voice allows you to emphasize words and makes your voice more pleasant to listen to.
- Make the caller feel important.

Pronunciation. Proper **pronunciation** (saying words correctly) is one of the most important telephone skills. Sometimes last names are difficult to pronounce. Ask patients, "How do you pronounce your name?" to make them feel welcome and important. When clarifying the spelling of a word or name, it is common practice to state the letter and then a word that begins with the letter. Examples include D as in dog, V as in Victor, M as in Mary, N as in Nancy, and B as in balloon.

Enunciation. **Enunciation** (clear and distinct speaking) is the opposite of mumbling. Good enunciation helps the person you are speaking to understand you, which is especially important when you are trying to convey medical information.

Speaking clearly over the telephone is very important because the speaker cannot be seen. Correct interpretation of the message is determined by hearing the words precisely. Activities such as chewing gum, eating, or propping the phone between the ear and shoulder hinder proper enunciation.

Tone. Because you are not face-to-face with the caller, the most important measurements of good telephone communication are voice quality and tone. Always speak with a positive and respectful tone.

Making a Good Impression

In a sense your telephone duties include public relations skills. How you handle telephone calls will have an impact on the public image of the medical practice.

Exhibiting Courtesy. Using common courtesy is a characteristic of professional office personnel. Courtesy is expressed by projecting an attitude of helpfulness. Always use the person's name during the conversation, and apologize for any errors or delays. When ending the conversation, be sure to thank the caller before hanging up.

Giving Undivided Attention. Do not try to answer the telephone while continuing to carry out another task. This practice may lead to errors in message taking and may give the caller the impression that you are uncaring or uninterested. Give the caller the same undivided attention you would if the person were in the office. Listen carefully to get the correct information.

Putting a Call on Hold. Although you should try not to put a caller on hold, there will be times when it is unavoidable. You may receive a call on another line, or a situation in the office may prevent you from devoting your full attention to the caller. Sometimes you may have to check a file or ask someone else in the office a question on behalf of the caller. Before putting a call on hold, however, always let the caller state the reason for the call. This step is essential so that you do not inadvertently put an emergency call on hold.

The medical office may have a standard procedure for placing a call on hold. Typically you will ask the caller the purpose of the call, state why you need to place the call on hold, explain how long you expect the wait to be, and ask the caller if this wait is acceptable. If you think the wait will be long, offer to call back rather than asking the caller to hold. Being kept on hold too long or too often makes people think the staff is inattentive to their needs.

If you know you can return to the line shortly, you can put the caller on hold, then attend to the problem. If you need to answer a second call, get the second caller's name and telephone number, and put that call on hold until you have completed the first call. You can then return to the second call.

Handling Difficult Situations. At times it will be impossible to give your undivided attention to a caller because of a pressing issue or emergency in the office. If the call itself is not an emergency one, it is best to ask if you can call back. Explain that you are currently handling an urgent matter, and offer to return the call in a few minutes. Most people will appreciate your honesty. Return the call in a reasonable amount of time, and be sure to apologize for the inconvenience.

Remembering Patients' Names. When patients are recognized by name, they are more likely to have positive feelings about the practice. Using a caller's name during a conversation makes the caller feel important. If you do not recognize a patient's name, it is better to ask "Has it been some time since you've seen the doctor?" rather than to ask if the patient has been to the practice before.

Checking for Understanding. When communicating by telephone, you do not have visual signals to convey the caller's feelings and level of understanding of the information you are discussing. Consequently, you must ask certain questions in the right way. If a call is long or complicated, summarize what was said to be sure that both you and the caller understand the information. Ask if the caller has any questions about what you have discussed.

Communicating Feelings. Whenever information is conveyed over the telephone, feelings are also communicated. When dealing with a caller who is nervous, upset, or angry, try to show empathy (an understanding of the other person's feelings). Communicating with empathy helps the caller feel more positive about the conversation and the medical office.

Ending the Conversation. It is not useful to let a conversation run on if you can effectively complete the call sooner. Before hanging up, however, take a few seconds to complete the call so that the caller feels properly cared for and satisfied. You can complete the call by summarizing the important points of the conversation and thanking the caller. Then let the caller hang up first. When you put the receiver down, never slam it—even if the caller has already hung up. Remember that all your actions reflect the professional image of the medical practice. Patients in the waiting room may see you when you are talking on the telephone.

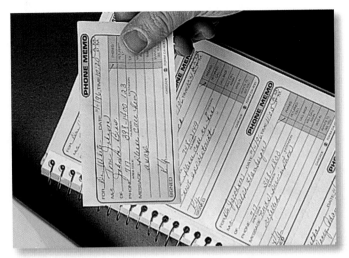

Figure 11-4. When using a telephone message pad or telephone log, be sure to fill out the form completely and accurately.

Taking Messages

Always have paper and a pen or pencil near the telephone so that you are prepared to write down messages (Figure 11-3). Proper documentation protects the physician if the caller takes legal action. A record of telephone calls should also be included in a patient's file as part of a complete medical history.

Documenting Calls

Documenting telephone calls is essential in a medical office. You can use telephone message pads or a telephone log book (Figure 11-4). Again, remember that many calls (for example, those concerning clinical problems or referrals)

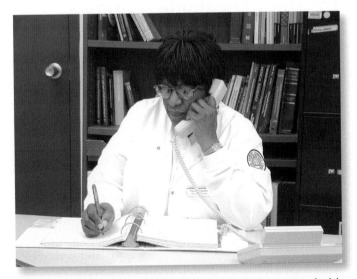

Figure 11-3. Use one hand or a telephone rest to hold the telephone so that the hand you write with is free to take messages.

and the actions or decisions they lead to need to be documented in patients' charts. Every entry into a patient's chart is considered a legal document; therefore the information must be accurate and legible. Accurate documentation helps guard against lawsuits.

Telephone Message Pads. You can use telephone message pads, which often come in brightly colored paper, to record the following information:

- Date and time of the call
- Name of the person for whom you took the message
- Caller's name
- Caller's telephone number (including area code and extension, if any)
- A description or an action to be taken, including comments such as "Urgent," "Please call back," "Wants to see you," "Will call back," or "Returned your call"
- The complete message, such as "Dr. Stephenson wants to reschedule the committee meeting."
- Name or initials of the person taking the call

The Telephone Log. Some medical offices use spiral-bound, perforated message books with carbonless forms to record messages. The top copy, or original, of each message is given to the appropriate person, and a copy is kept in the book for future reference.

Tips for Taking Messages. The following suggestions will help you provide accurate documentation for incoming messages:

- Always have a pen or pencil and paper on hand.
- Jot down notes as the information is given.
- Verify information, especially the spelling of patient or caller names and the correct spelling of medications.
- Verify the correct callback number.

PROCEDURE 11.2

Retrieving Messages From an Answering Service

Objective: To follow standard procedures for retrieving messages from an answering service

Materials: Telephone message pad or telephone log

Method

1. Set a regular schedule for calling the answering service to retrieve messages. Having a regular schedule ensures that you do not miss any messages.

2. Call at the regularly scheduled time(s) to see if there are any messages.

3. Identify yourself, and state that you are calling to obtain messages for the practice.

4. For each message, write down all pertinent information on the telephone message pad or telephone log. Be sure to include the patient's name and telephone number, time of call, message or description of the problem, and action taken, if any.

5. Repeat the information, confirming that you have the correct spelling of all names.

6. When you have retrieved all messages, route them according to the office policy.

- When taking a phone message for the physician, never make a commitment on behalf of the physician by saying, "I'll have the physician call you." An appropriate response would be, "I will give your message to the physician."

Ensuring Correct Information

When you are taking a message, be sure to get the proper spelling of the caller's name. Repeat the spelling to the caller to make sure it is correct. If it is necessary to pull the patient's chart, ask for the patient's date of birth, in case there are two patient's with the same name. When you have taken down all the necessary information, repeat the key points to the caller for verification.

Maintaining Patient Confidentiality

Do not repeat information over the telephone when the information is confidential. This point is especially important if patients or others in the office may overhear the conversation. You must also maintain patient confidentiality when handling written telephone messages. If a confidential message must be brought to the doctor's attention, do not leave it on the doctor's desk where it can be seen by someone else. Instead, put the message in a file folder marked "Confidential," and place the folder on the desk. Follow the same procedure when handling confidential faxes.

Telephone Answering Systems

An office telephone system can range from a single telephone line to a complex multiline system. Most medical offices use one or more of the following pieces of equipment

and services to provide efficient management of telephone calls: an automated voice mail system, an answering machine, and an answering service. These systems are described in Chapter 5. One of your telephone responsibilities may be to retrieve messages from the practice's answering service. Procedure 11-2 describes how to do so.

Placing Outgoing Calls

You will often be required to place outgoing calls on behalf of the medical office. You may need to return calls, obtain information, provide patient education, or arrange patient consultations with other physicians.

Locating Telephone Numbers

Before you can place an outgoing call, of course, you must have the correct telephone number. If you are calling a patient, the telephone number should be in the patient's chart. To find other telephone numbers, you may need to consult a telephone directory or call for directory assistance.

The medical office should have at least one telephone directory, or telephone book, for the local calling area and perhaps additional directories for surrounding areas. Use these books to locate telephone numbers for outside calls. The office may also have a card file with commonly used telephone numbers, as shown in Figure 11-5, or these numbers may be listed in the office policy manual.

If you need to find a long-distance telephone number, many offices use the directory assistance service. You can reach this service by dialing 1-[area code]-555-1212. Use directory assistance only when you have exhausted other options, however, because most long-distance carriers charge a fee each time you use the service.

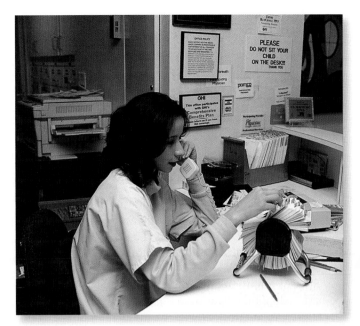

Figure 11-5. Keeping a card file on the desk allows you to easily find frequently used telephone numbers.

Applying Your Telephone Skills

You can apply the telephone skills you use for answering incoming calls when placing outgoing calls. Here are additional tips for handling outgoing calls.

- Plan before you call. Have all the information you need in front of you before you dial the telephone number. Plan what you will say, and decide what questions to ask so that you will not have to call back for additional information.
- Double-check the telephone number. Before placing a call, always confirm the number. If in doubt, look it up in the telephone directory. If you do dial a wrong number, be sure to apologize for the mistake.
- Allow enough time, at least a minute or about eight rings, for someone to answer the telephone. When calling patients who are elderly or physically disabled, allow additional time.
- Identify yourself. After reaching the person to whom you placed the call, give your name, and state that you are calling on behalf of the doctor.
- Ask if you have called at a convenient time and whether the person has time to talk with you. If it is not a good time, ask when you should call back.
- Be ready to speak as soon as the person you called answers the telephone. Do not waste the person's time while you collect your thoughts.
- If you are calling to give information, ask if the person has a pencil and piece of paper available. Do not begin with dates, times, or instructions until the person is ready to write down the information.

Arranging Conference Calls

It may be necessary for you to schedule conference calls with patients, hospitals, or other doctors to discuss tests or surgical results. When dealing with several people, suggest several time slots in case someone is not available at a particular time. Also keep in mind the various time zones in the country. Make sure that all the conference-call participants are given the proper time in their time zone to expect the call.

Telephone Triage

Some physicians delegate to other staff members some of the clinical decision making that is done over the telephone. In these instances, **telephone triage** is used as a process of deciding what necessary action to take. The word *triage* refers to the screening and sorting of emergency incidents. Performing triage correctly is an important skill. You should learn as much as possible about triage techniques.

Learning the Triage Process

Proper training of office staff is vital in providing safe, sound, and cost-effective medical care over the telephone. An increasing number of medical practices are preparing guidelines for the telephone staff to follow when patients call the office with specific medical problems or questions.

Guidelines are often written for common questions, such as how to deal with sniffles and fevers during cold and flu season or how to make a child with chickenpox more comfortable. Members of the telephone staff must realize, however, that their responsibility is to determine whether a caller needs additional medical care. They cannot diagnose or treat the patient's problem.

Office guidelines outline the specific information the telephone staff must obtain from the patient. In general, this information is the same type as that obtained during an office visit. It should include the patient's age, symptoms, when the problem began, and the patient's level of anxiety about the problem.

Categorizing Patient Problems and Providing Patient Education

After the patient information is obtained, the guidelines help the staff categorize the problem according to severity. The telephone staff then decides if the problem can be handled safely with advice over the telephone, whether the patient needs to come into the office, or whether the problem requires immediate attention at an emergency room.

If a problem is deemed appropriate for telephone management, the guidelines may include recommendations for nonprescription treatment that may relieve symptoms and anxiety. This information falls under the category of patient education. Advise the caller that recommendations are based on the symptoms and are not a diagnosis. Remember that only the doctor is authorized to make a diagnosis and prescribe medication. Ask the caller to repeat any instructions you give, and tell the patient to call back within a specified time if symptoms worsen. Be sure to document the conversation in the patient's chart.

Taking Action

Clinical triage involves determining the extent of medical emergencies and deciding on the appropriate action. If a caller is having chest pains, you would be performing a type of triage by instructing him to go to the emergency room as soon as possible. Telephone triage is also used in handling common minor medical problems and questions. Whatever the nature of the problem, the situation must be dealt with appropriately to protect the health and safety of the patient.

Telecommunications

An automated system is used in many hospitals and larger ambulatory care settings. When a call is answered, a recorded voice identifies departments or services the caller can reach by pressing a specified number on the telephone keypad. This telephone system and menu provides a convenient way for patients or callers to reach the direct service or department needed.

Facsimile (Fax) Machines

Facsimile machines, often referred to as fax machines, are commonly used in physicians' offices. A fax is sent over telephone lines from one fax modem to another. Fax machines may be used to send referrals, reports, insurance approvals, or medication refill approvals. Per HIPAA guidelines, a patient's confidentiality must be protected by placing the fax machine in a secure location that only authorized personnel can access. Federal and state laws also must be followed in maintaining or faxing medical records. The physician's office should develop guidelines to follow when faxing information about patients.

Summary

The telephone is an important communication tool in the medical office. Your telephone manner will reflect the professionalism of the office. Medical offices commonly receive several types of calls, and there are varying ways to handle these calls.

Special attention should be given to documenting incoming telephone calls and ensuring accuracy. HIPAA guidelines must be followed to maintain patient confidentiality. This applies to telephone conversations and computer monitors as well as medical records. Telephone etiquette involves practicing proper pronunciation and enunciation, using common courtesy and a respectful tone of voice, giving undivided attention to callers, and accommodating patients' requests and needs. Placing outgoing calls requires the same careful attention as taking incoming calls. Telephone triage is the art of determining the level of urgency of each call and how it should be handled or routed.

CASE STUDY *QUESTIONS*

Now that you have completed this chapter, review the case study at the beginning of the chapter and answer the following questions:

1. What would your first response to the patient be?
2. Explain how you would handle this situation.
3. What type of incoming call was this?
4. What type of condition did this patient's symptoms indicate?
5. What are some other symptoms of this condition?

Discussion Questions

1. What is the purpose of screening calls that come into the medical office?
2. Why is proper telephone etiquette so important in the medical office?
3. Name five of the most common types of calls received in the medical office that can be handled by the medical assistant. Name two that must be handled by the physician.
4. Describe what a routing list is and what it is used for.
5. Name five symptoms or conditions that require immediate medical help.
6. What is the best way to clarify the pronunciation or spelling of a patient's name?
7. What act does *HIPAA* stand for, and what is the purpose of the act?

Critical Thinking Questions

1. Outline the skills needed by a medical assistant who is responsible for answering incoming calls to a medical office.
2. Describe how you would handle a situation in which an angry patient calls to complain that he was overcharged for a recent office visit.

3. Imagine that you need to call a patient to tell her that she has to return to the office to have some blood redrawn because an insufficient amount of blood was drawn the first time. What would you say to the patient? What would you do if she refused to have the blood redrawn?
4. A 21-year-old female patient had lab tests performed. The patient's mother calls and requests to know her daughter's lab results. What should you do?
5. List the five Cs of communication and define what each means.

Application Activities

1. With a partner, role-play a scenario in which a patient calls the medical office to report symptoms. The patient then claims not to have time to come to the office for an appointment but instead asks for medical advice from the medical assistant. How should the medical assistant respond? When you have finished role-playing, discuss other ways the medical assistant could have dealt with the problem.
2. When speaking with patients on the telephone, how might you demonstrate the following qualities? Give several examples for each quality.
   a. concern
   b. attentiveness
   c. friendliness
   d. respect
   e. empathy
3. Create a one-page training sheet or chart for new personnel illustrating how to handle emergency calls coming into the medical office.
4. Define telephone triage. Give examples of three different patient calls and how you would triage each call.

CHAPTER 12

Scheduling Appointments and Maintaining the Physician's Schedule

KEY TERMS

advance scheduling
agenda
cluster scheduling
double-booking system
itinerary
locum tenens
matrix
minutes
modified-wave scheduling
no-show
open-hours scheduling
overbooking
time-specified scheduling
underbooking
walk-in
wave scheduling

AREAS OF COMPETENCE

2003 Role Delineation Study
ADMINISTRATIVE
Administrative Procedures
- Schedule, coordinate, and monitor appointments
- Schedule inpatient/outpatient admissions and procedures

GENERAL
Professionalism
- Prioritize and perform multiple tasks

CHAPTER OUTLINE

- The Appointment Book
- Appointment Scheduling Systems
- Arranging Appointments
- Special Scheduling Situations
- Scheduling Outside Appointments
- Maintaining the Physician's Schedule

OBJECTIVES

After completing Chapter 12, you will be able to:

12.1 Explain the importance of the appointment book in maintaining the schedule in the medical office.
12.2 Identify common scheduling abbreviations.
12.3 Identify and describe different types of appointment scheduling systems.
12.4 Discuss ways to arrange appointments for patients.
12.5 Explain how to handle special scheduling situations.
12.6 Explain how to properly document no-shows and late patients.
12.7 Describe how to schedule appointments that are outside the medical office.
12.8 Discuss ways to keep an accurate and efficient physician schedule.

Introduction

As a medical assistant, you need to know all aspects of how to create and utilize an appointment book. In this chapter you will learn to identify the different types of scheduling systems, how each is used, and which type of practice each system would work best in. You will also learn how to handle many types of scheduling situations within the office, including patient appointments, emergencies, pharmaceutical representatives, and the scheduling of outside appointments with other medical facilities. Legal aspects of the appointment book are discussed, and proper documentation is stressed. Additional topics include appointment cards, reminder mailings, reminder calls, and recall notices for patients.

CASE STUDY

A 71-year-old female patient has a routine follow-up appointment with the physician regarding her medications. Her appointment is at 9:00 A.M. and lasts about 15 minutes. As the patient is checking out at the reception desk, she trips and falls, hitting her head on the corner of the reception desk. There is a bleeding wound on her forehead, and she complains of a headache. The physician and another medical assistant obtain a stretcher and move the patient to an exam room to access her injuries. It is expected that this emergency will take at least 45 minutes to handle. You are managing the schedule for the day. The physician has a full schedule for this morning and has already worked in a couple of additional appointment times for patients who need to be seen this morning for acute problems.

The next scheduled appointment is for a 24-year-old male who needs an employment physical for a new job he is to start next week. He must have the physical performed prior to his first day. His appointment is scheduled for 9:15 A.M. and is expected to last 30 minutes. At 9:45 A.M., two patients are scheduled for the same 15-minute appointment. One has a sore throat, and the other is scheduled for a wound check. The afternoon schedule has two appointment openings: the first at 2:00 P.M., which is for 15 minutes, and the second at 4:15 P.M., also for 15 minutes.

As you read this chapter, consider the following questions:

1. How would you adjust the schedule to allow for the emergency without falling behind schedule?
2. If it is necessary to reschedule patients, who should be rescheduled and when?
3. Would you explain anything to the patients in the waiting room about the emergency? If so, what would you say?

The Appointment Book

Time is a treasured commodity for both patients and physicians. Scheduling appointments in an organized fashion shows respect for everyone's time and creates an efficient patient flow. A well-managed appointment book is the key to establishing this efficiency.

Although most patients understand that they will probably have to wait in the reception area before they are seen by the physician, few patients are willing to wait more than 20 minutes. Offices that routinely have long waiting times can end up with dissatisfied patients and other problems. Some patients, in an attempt to avoid a long wait, may deliberately arrive after their scheduled appointment times. Accommodating these latecomers can throw the office schedule off track. Other patients may become resentful and decide to seek medical care with a competing practice.

Even in a well-run office, however, unexpected events can disrupt the schedule. Some patients arrive early, some arrive late, and others do not arrive at all. Some appointments take longer than expected, for example, if the physician needs to spend extra time with a patient. In addition, emergency appointments sometimes need to be squeezed into the schedule. For these reasons, making an office schedule flow smoothly can be a challenge.

Preparing the Appointment Book

Before you can begin scheduling appointments, you need to prepare the appointment book. The first step is to establish the **matrix,** or basic format, of the appointment book. In order to create the matrix, you need to block off times on the schedule during which the doctor is not available to see patients. Time would be blocked off the schedule, for example, when the doctor was away for the following reasons.

- Hospital rounds
- Surgery
- Lunch

- Vacation days
- Holidays
- Scheduled meetings (for example, pharmaceutical, medical supply company, or in-service meetings)

The day's schedule is then built around this matrix. See Figure 12-1 for an example of a matrix.

Obtaining Patient Information

When the matrix has been established, you can begin scheduling appointments. You must obtain and enter certain patient information for each appointment. At some practices personnel enter the information into both traditional paper appointment books and computerized systems. Then, if the computer fails to work for some reason, the office has the book for reference. Some doctors who have been in practice for many years are used to the appointment book method and do not want to give it up for a computer system. Other offices are completely computerized. Using either the book or computer method, obtain the necessary patient information:

- Patient's full name. Obtain the correct spelling of the patient's name.
- Home and work telephone numbers. Repeat phone numbers to ensure accuracy.
- Purpose of the visit. Use a brief description and utilize approved abbreviations when possible. Do not create your own abbreviations.
- Estimated length of the visit.

Commonly Used Abbreviations

If you are the person who maintains the appointment book, you will find that certain procedures and conditions occur frequently. To save space and time when entering information, use these abbreviations:

BP	blood pressure check
can	cancellation
c/o	complains of
cons	consultation
CP	chest pain
CPE	complete physical examination
ECG	electrocardiogram
FU	follow-up appointment
GI	gastrointestinal
I & D	incision and drainage
inj	injection
lab	laboratory studies
N & V	nausea and vomiting
NP	new patient
NS	no-show patient
P & P	Pap smear (Papanicolaou smear) and pelvic examination
Pap	Pap smear
PMS	premenstrual syndrome
pt	patient
PT	physical therapy
re	recheck
ref	referral
RS	reschedule
Rx	prescription
sig	sigmoidoscopy
SOB	shortness of breath
S/R	suture removal
STD	sexually transmitted disease
surg	surgery
US	ultrasound

Determining Standard Procedure Times

If you are to schedule appointments efficiently, you must have an estimate of how long visits will take. Working with the physician or physicians in your practice, create a list of standard procedure times. Also indicate on the list how much time to allow for tests that are commonly performed in the practice. This list, kept beside the appointment book, helps you identify which openings are appropriate for the procedure or test involved. The lengths and types of tests and procedures will depend on the practice. Following are typical lengths of common procedures:

Complete physical examination	30–60 minutes
New patient visit	30 minutes or more
Follow-up office visit	5–10 minutes
Emergency office visit	15–20 minutes
Prenatal examination	15 minutes
Pap smear and pelvic examination	15–30 minutes
Minor in-office surgery, such as a mole removal	30 minutes
Suture removal	10–20 minutes

A Legal Record

The appointment book is considered a legal record. Some experts advise holding on to old appointment books for at least 3 years. Because the appointment book could be used as evidence in legal proceedings, entries must be clear and easy to read. Management consultants suggest that because the appointment book is a legal medical document, the schedule should be written in blue ink and never with a pencil. Never erase a name or use correction fluid to blot the name out. Instead, draw a single line through the name and beside it write "can" for canceled or "NS" for a no-show patient. Also write the date, time, and reason (if known) why the appointment was missed or canceled, then initial the entry. This information should also be documented in the patient's chart.

APPOINTMENT RECORD

	12 November Tuesday		DOCTOR	13 November Wednesday	
	Dr. Terrance	Dr. Hilbert		Dr. Terrance	Dr. Hilbert
			AM		
8	00 / 15 / 30 / 45				
9	00 / 15 / 30 / 45				
10	00 / 15 / 30 / 45				
11	00 / 15 / 30 / 45				
12	00 / 15 / 30 / 45				
			PM		
1	00 / 15 / 30 / 45				
2	00 / 15 / 30 / 45				
3	00 / 15 / 30 / 45				
4	00 / 15 / 30 / 45				
5	00 / 15 / 30 / 45				

REMARKS & NOTES _____

Figure 12-1. It is important to establish a matrix in the appointment book so that appointments are not scheduled for times when the doctor will be out of the office.

Some offices permit the use of pencil to allow for changes or corrections if necessary. If pencil is used, at the end of each day you or another designated staff member should write directly over the penciled entries in ink to create a permanent document.

Appointment Scheduling Systems

There are several possible appointment scheduling systems. The method chosen usually depends on the type of practice and the physician's preferences. No matter which method your office uses, it should be regularly reviewed to see whether it is meeting its goals: a smooth flow of patients and minimal waiting time.

Open-Hours Scheduling

In the **open-hours scheduling** system, patients arrive at their own convenience with the understanding that they will be seen on a first-come, first-served basis, unless there is an extreme emergency. Depending on how many other patients are ahead of them, they may have a considerable wait. The open-hours system eliminates the problems caused by broken appointments (because there are no appointments), but it increases the possibility of inefficient downtime for the doctor. In addition, with this system the medical assistant cannot pull patients' charts before they arrive.

Most private practices have replaced the open-hours system with scheduled appointments. Open-hours systems are sometimes still used by rural practices and by practices specializing in urgent care, such as emergency centers. An open-hours system still requires the use of an appointment book, to record patients as they come into the office. You must also still establish a matrix so that you will know when a doctor is out of the office.

Time-Specified Scheduling

Time-specified scheduling (also called stream scheduling) assumes a steady stream of patients all day long at regular, specified intervals. Most minor medical problems, such as sore throats, earaches, or blood pressure follow-ups, usually require only 10- to 15-minute appointment slots. More time may be required for appointments such as physical examinations, which usually require 60 minutes, or new patient visits, which usually require 30 minutes (Figure 12-2). When a visit requires more time, you simply assign the patient additional back-to-back slots.

Wave Scheduling

Wave scheduling works effectively in larger medical facilities that have enough departments and personnel to provide services to several patients at the same time. This method of scheduling is based on the reality that some patients will arrive late and that others will require more or less time than expected with the physician. Wave scheduling has the flexibility to allow for appointments that require more time than anticipated or for patients who miss appointments. The goal of wave scheduling is to begin and end each hour with the overall office schedule on track. You determine the number of patients to be seen each hour by dividing the hour by the length of the average visit. If the average is 15 minutes, for example, you schedule four patients for each hour. An example of wave scheduling would be:

10:00 A.M.	Patient A	555-5683	Sore throat
10:15 A.M.	Patient B	555-7322	Low back pain
10:30 A.M.	Patient C	555-4673	FU B/P
10:45 A.M.	Patient D	555-2854	B12 inj

You ask all four to arrive at the beginning of the hour and have the physician see them in the order of their actual arrival. The main problem with wave scheduling is that patients may realize they have appointments at the same time as other patients. The result may be confusion and possibly annoyance or anger.

Modified-Wave Scheduling

The wave system can be modified in several ways. With **modified-wave scheduling,** as shown in Figure 12-3, patients might be scheduled in 15-minute increments. Another option is to schedule four patients to arrive at planned intervals during the first half hour, leaving the second half hour unscheduled. Appointments that are anticipated to require more time should be scheduled at the beginning of the hour. Appointments that are expected to be less time-consuming should be scheduled in 10- to 20-minute time slots. This method allows time for catching up before the next hour begins.

Double Booking

With a **double-booking system,** two or more patients are scheduled for the same appointment slot. Unlike the wave or modified-wave system, however, the double-booking system assumes that both patients will actually be seen by the doctor within the scheduled period. If the types of visits are usually short (5 minutes, for example), it is reasonable to book two patients for one 15-minute opening. If both patients require the entire 15 minutes, however, the office falls behind schedule. Double-booking scheduling works most effectively in practices in which more than one patient can be attended to at a time.

Double booking can be helpful if a patient calls with a problem and needs to be seen that day but no appointments are available. You could double-book this patient with an already scheduled patient. In such cases you should explain that the caller might have to wait a bit before being seen by the doctor.

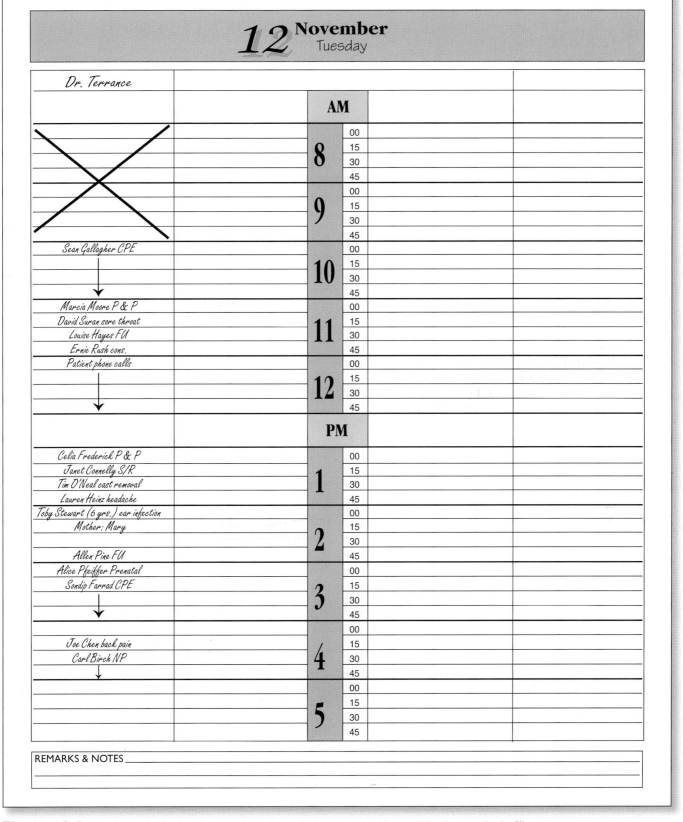

Figure 12-2. Time-specified appointment scheduling is commonly used in the medical office.

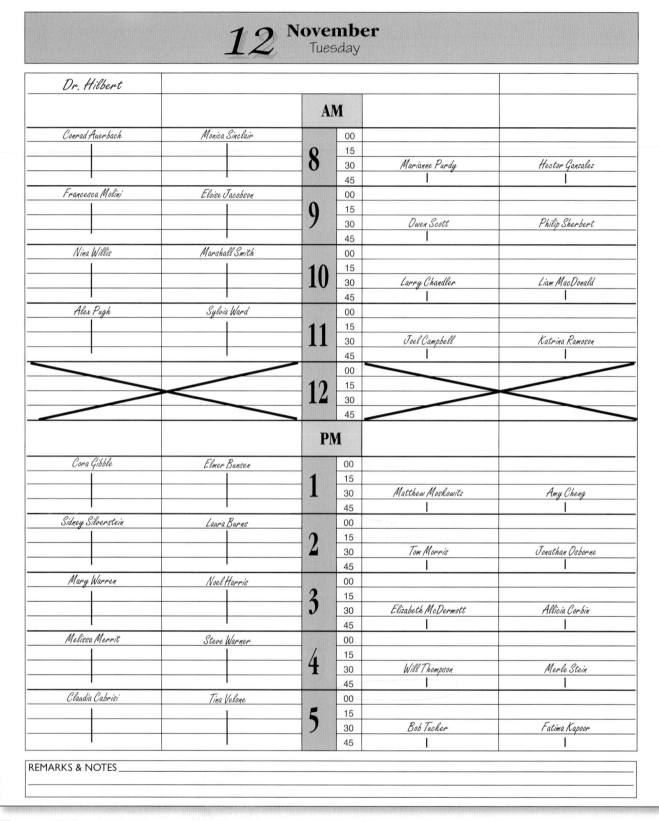

Figure 12-3. Modified-wave scheduling allows more flexibility than wave scheduling.

PROCEDURE 12.1

Creating a Cluster Schedule

Objective: To set up a cluster schedule

Materials: Calendar, tickler file, appointment book, colored pencils or markers (optional)

Method

1. Learn which categories of cases the physician would like to cluster and on what days and/or times of day.
2. Determine the length of the average visit in each category.
3. In the appointment book, cross out the hours in the week that the physician is typically not available (because of meetings, hospital rounds, lunch, teaching, days off, and so on).
4. Block out one period in midmorning and one in midafternoon for use as buffer, or reserve, times for unexpected needs.
5. Reserve additional slots for acutely ill patients. (The number of slots depends on the type of practice.)
6. Mark the appointment times for clustered procedures. If desired, color-code the blocks of time. For example, make immunization clusters pink, blood pressure checks green, and so forth.

Cluster Scheduling

As the name suggests, **cluster scheduling** groups similar appointments together during the day or week. (This system is also called categorization scheduling.) For example, you might cluster all physical examinations between 9:00 A.M. and 11:00 A.M. on Tuesdays and Thursdays. Cluster scheduling is also helpful in offices where specialized equipment or services (such as physical therapy or ultrasound) are available only at certain times. Procedure 12-1 explains how to create a cluster schedule.

Advance Scheduling

In some specialties patients might be booked weeks or months in advance, as for annual gynecologic examinations. In such practices **advance scheduling** is used. It is still advisable to leave a few slots open each day, however, for patients who call with unexpected or unusual problems.

Combination Scheduling

Some practices combine two or more scheduling methods. For example, they might use cluster scheduling for new patients and double booking for quick follow-ups.

Computerized Scheduling

Computerized scheduling systems are becoming more common in medical offices because they have several advantages over handwritten systems (Figure 12-4). For example, they can be programmed to "lock out" selected appointment slots so that those slots will always be available for emergencies. Another advantage of using a computerized system

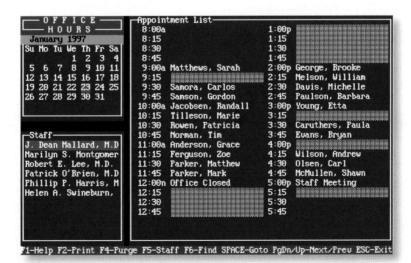

Figure 12-4. Many medical offices are now using computerized scheduling instead of or in addition to a traditional appointment book.

is that the scheduling information can be accessed from all terminals located within the practice. Computerized systems can also help staff members identify patients who often are late, forget their appointments altogether, or cancel. In addition, the computer can identify patients who may require additional time with the physician because of special needs.

Arranging Appointments

Whether you are arranging appointments in person or by telephone, be polite and courteous. In scheduling an appointment, try to offer the patient a choice between two different dates, with either a morning or afternoon time slot. Once the patient decides on the date and time, always confirm the appointment by repeating it to the person before printing it in the schedule. If you are scheduling the appointment in person, write the appointment date and time on an appointment card to give to the patient. Whenever possible, try to accommodate the patient's needs while still maintaining a smoothly flowing schedule.

New Patients

A patient who has not been established at a medical practice is considered a new patient. Appointments for new patients are most often arranged over the telephone. Be sure to obtain all the necessary information, including the correct spelling and pronunciation of the person's name, home address, daytime telephone number, and date of birth. When arranging the appointment, keep in mind that some physicians prefer to schedule new patients at certain times of the day, such as first thing in the morning. When scheduling an appointment for a new patient, make sure to allow enough time for filling out forms. Have the new patient arrive 15 to 30 minutes early to do this.

Return Appointments

It is always good practice to ask patients returning to the reception area if they need to schedule another appointment. Getting them to make the appointment then will save you from having to do so by telephone later on. When patients call to arrange appointments, use the telephone techniques outlined in Chapter 11.

Appointment Reminders

Some patients may have trouble remembering their next appointment, especially if they arrange it far in advance. To help patients keep track of their appointments, you can use several types of appointment reminders.

Appointment Cards. In many offices the medical assistant fills out and hands the patient an appointment reminder card, like the one shown in Figure 12-5. To reduce the chance of error, enter the appointment in the appointment book first, then fill out the card. Otherwise, when the

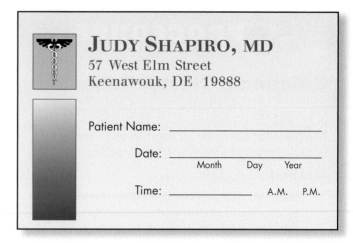

Figure 12-5. Before patients leave the office, be sure to give them an appointment card if they are scheduled to return to the office.

patient takes the appointment card, you have to rely on your memory when entering the appointment in the book.

Reminder Mailings. When making a follow-up appointment in person, you can ask the patient to address to himself a postcard on which you have written the next appointment's date and time. This postcard serves as a backup in case the patient loses the original appointment reminder card. Place the postcard in the tickler file under the day when it should be sent (usually a week before the appointment). Reminder mailings can also be sent to patients who make appointments over the telephone. In this case, of course, you must address the postcard for the tickler file yourself. Reminder mailings are useful when appointments are made many months in advance or are for geriatric patients.

Reminder Calls. Depending on office policy and available time, you might also call patients 1 or 2 days before their appointments to confirm the scheduled time. This technique can be especially helpful for patients with a history of late arrivals or for **no-shows** (patients who do not call to cancel and do not come to the appointment). Writing patients' phone numbers next to their names in the appointment book makes it convenient for you to make reminder appointment calls.

Recall Notices. Many offices book appointments no more than a few weeks in advance. If your office has such a policy, you need a way to make sure patients do not forget to call for appointments that are 6 months—or even a year—away from their last appointments.

Suppose, for example, that the physician tells a patient she should have an annual breast examination. How can you help her remember to call to schedule one at the appropriate time? One way is to use a system of recall notices. In a tickler file enter the patient's name under the month when she should call the office. When the time arrives, send a form letter reminding her that she will soon be due for a breast examination and asking her to call for an appointment.

Special Scheduling Situations

Although a great deal of scheduling is routine, creativity and flexibility are necessary for scheduling some special cases. These special situations often involve patients, but they may also involve physicians.

Patient Scheduling Situations

On some days all patients will keep their appointments and arrive on time. On many other days, however, patients may walk in without appointments, arrive late for scheduled appointments, or miss appointments entirely. Being prepared for these possibilities allows you to handle them better and to keep the office schedule running as smoothly as possible.

Emergencies. Your training as a medical assistant will help you recognize the signs of an emergency. In some instances you will refer the caller to the nearest hospital emergency room or instruct the caller to call Emergency Medical Services for an ambulance. In other instances you will ask the caller to come to the office right away. It is vital that doctors see emergency patients before patients who are already in the waiting area or on the schedule. It is best to explain to waiting patients that there has been an emergency (without giving details). This announcement helps them understand and accept the delay and also gives them an opportunity to reschedule their appointments. The Tips for the Office section provides guidelines for scheduling emergency appointments. Procedure 11-1 in Chapter 11 details how to handle emergency calls.

Referrals. Sometimes other doctors refer patients to the practice for second opinions or special consultations. Patients seeking second opinions before deciding on surgery should be fit into the schedule as soon as possible. Other referred patients should also be seen quickly, as a matter of professional courtesy to the referring doctor as well as good business practice.

If a physician in your office refers a patient to another doctor, your first step should be to check your office's policy and procedure manual. Many office manuals contain a

Tips for the Office

Scheduling Emergency Appointments

As a multiskilled medical assistant, you will be well prepared to tell the difference between acute conditions that are emergencies and those that are not. Guidelines on types of emergencies to be seen in the office and types to be referred elsewhere will vary. If you have any doubt, interrupt the physician to ask for instructions.

Even with buffer times built into the daily schedule, emergencies are still disruptive to most practices. Your ability to stay calm, respond quickly, and remain flexible will be of great comfort to the emergency patient and to others in the waiting area. Read the following story to see how an emergency situation can be handled skillfully.

The Situation

It is 4:15 P.M. in a busy family practice. The telephone rings. The caller is the father of a 10-year-old boy. Maria, the medical assistant, can hear the panic in his voice. His son Kyle has injured his knee while playing football with friends. Kyle cannot straighten the knee, and it is quite swollen.

Maria consults the physician, who suspects torn cartilage. The physician tells Maria to have the father wrap ice in a towel, apply it to Kyle's knee, and bring him in immediately. Maria relays this advice to the father and asks him how soon he can get to the office.

"It will take about 25 minutes," he replies.

The office schedule includes a buffer time opening at 4:30, but based on the father's estimate, Kyle cannot possibly arrive until 4:40. Maria notes that Mrs. Griffin, a good-natured retiree, is scheduled to come in for her weekly blood pressure check at 4:45 P.M. Hers is the last scheduled appointment of the day.

The Solution

Mrs. Griffin lives about 5 minutes from the office. Maria calls her home and explains that there has been an emergency. She offers Mrs. Griffin three choices: she can come in at 4:30 and be seen then; she can arrive at the usual time and expect to wait; or she can be rescheduled for tomorrow.

"No problem," Mrs. Griffin says cheerfully. "I'll come right over."

Mrs. Griffin arrives at 4:35. At 4:40, Kyle hobbles in, supported by his father. Maria greets them and offers Kyle a chair on which to prop his foot.

Mrs. Griffin's blood pressure check is complete at 4:45. Kyle waits only 5 minutes before he is seen.

Thanks to Maria's quick thinking, the office stays on schedule—essentially by switching one appointment for another.

listing of referral physicians and facilities, including the names of facilities or specialty physicians, their addresses, and their phone numbers. If possible, give the patient two referral names to choose from, along with the referral phone numbers and addresses. When choosing the referral names of either physicians or facilities, be sure that the facility accepts the patient's insurance.

Fasting Patients. Some procedures and tests require patients to fast (refrain from eating or drinking anything beginning the night before). Scheduling these patients as early in the day as possible shows consideration for their needs. When scheduling appointments that require the patient to fast, be sure to inform the patient of the need to fast and when fasting should start.

Patients With Diabetes. Like fasting patients, patients with diabetes can use extra consideration when you schedule their appointments. In general, patients who take insulin must eat meals and snacks at regular times. This routine keeps their blood sugar from dropping too low—a condition that can result in confused thinking or even loss of consciousness. Therefore, you might want to avoid scheduling patients with diabetes for slots in late morning, close to lunchtime. If the schedule is running late by the time these patients arrive, they will be waiting in your reception area at a time when they really need to eat.

If the physician sees several patients with diabetes, you might also ask him about keeping appropriate snacks on hand to offer these patients in emergencies. Most patients with diabetes, however, carry their own emergency snacks with them to treat low blood sugar.

Repeat Visits. Some patients need regular appointments, such as for prenatal checkups or physical therapy. If possible, schedule these appointments for the same day and time each week. Establishing a routine helps patients remember their appointments and simplifies the office schedule.

Late Arrivals. If the practice has patients who are routinely late and gentle reminders to be on time have not helped, you might try booking them toward the end of the day. Even if a patient arrives late for a late-afternoon appointment, the doctor has already seen most of the day's patients and the late patient will not disrupt the schedule. Document late arrivals or missed appointments in the patient's chart. With documentation, patients who are habitually late can be called to discuss the reasons for their lateness. The goal of the discussion should be to find a solution so that patients can make their appointments on time and the schedule will run smoothly.

Walk-Ins. From time to time, a patient (or a person who has not visited the practice before) may arrive without an appointment and still expect to see the doctor. These people are called **walk-ins.** Office policies on how to handle walk-ins vary. If the person is experiencing an emergency, handle the situation as you would handle any emergency. Otherwise, you might politely explain that the

doctor is fully booked for the day and offer to schedule an appointment in the usual manner. If, by chance, the doctor is available and willing to see the walk-in, you should still ask the person to call to schedule appointments in the future. If your physician's office has a policy of no walk-ins, post a sign in the lobby or waiting area stating that patients are seen by appointment only.

Cancellations. When patients call to cancel appointments, thank them for calling, and try to reschedule the appointment while they are on the telephone. If patients say they will call later to reschedule, note this information in the appointment book.

You should also write "canceled" in the appointment book and draw a single line through the patient's name. To avoid confusion, cancel the first appointment *before* entering the patient's rescheduled appointment. Remember that the appointment book is a legal record. If you forget to cross out the name at the time of the first appointment, it may later seem that the doctor saw the patient twice. It is also important to note the cancellation in the patient's medical record. This notation can protect the practice from possible legal action. For example, a patient whose incision became infected could not blame the doctor if the patient canceled an appointment for a dressing change.

You may be able to fill slots created by cancellations by calling patients who have appointments scheduled for later in the day or week. Some patients may be willing to come in earlier than planned. When you make appointments, you can ask patients if they would be interested in coming in earlier if openings occur. Placing the names of interested patients in a tickler file can save time later.

Missed Appointments. It is important for legal reasons to document a no-show in the appointment book and patient record. Always inform the physician of any missed appointments in case the patient's condition requires a follow-up. The physician may want you to call the patient with a polite reminder that the patient has missed an appointment and needs to reschedule. There may have been a misunderstanding about the time, or the patient may simply have forgotten the appointment. Some offices, especially ones that use computerized scheduling systems, send out form letters when patients miss appointments. If failure to keep the appointment could endanger the patient's health, mention this possibility to the patient, or ask the physician to tell the patient over the telephone.

Physician Scheduling Situations

Not all scheduling problems result from patients. Sometimes physicians disrupt the office schedule. They may be called away on an emergency, may be delayed at the hospital, or may simply arrive late. In any event, the appointment schedule may get off track.

Physicians are only human and may occasionally be late for appointments. Some physicians are frequently late, however, either when arriving in the morning or when returning from lunch or from regular meetings. If this situation occurs in your office, you might approach it in several ways.

At a staff meeting you could mention that the morning or afternoon schedule often seems to get off to a late start. Then you might ask if anyone has suggestions for improving this situation. The physician may recognize that she is the cause of the problem and decide to resolve it.

If the physician does not take responsibility for the problem, however, you may need to adjust the office schedule to handle the situation. Suppose, for example, that the first patient appointment slot is at 8:30 A.M., but the physician usually does not arrive until 8:35 A.M. You could simply avoid scheduling patients between 8:30 and 8:45 A.M. If a physician is often 15 minutes late returning from lunch or from meetings, you might leave open the first appointment slot after the normal arrival time. In effect, you build buffer time into the schedule.

Scheduling Outside Appointments

You may be responsible for arranging patient appointments outside the medical office. These appointments may include:

- Consultations with other physicians
- Laboratory work
- X-rays
- Other diagnostic tests
- Hospital stays
- Surgeries

Before scheduling these appointments, ask the doctor for an order that identifies the exact procedures to be performed and specifies when the results will be needed. Always verify the patient's type of insurance before choosing which facility or physician the referral will be sent to. Insurance companies that are HMOs (health maintenance organizations) often will arrange the referral themselves. The medical assistant or secretary sending the referral completes the necessary forms and faxes them to the insurance company. The insurance company will authorize the referral and notify the office when approved. Sometimes referrals, if not urgent, can take 30 days or longer to approve.

Once authorization has been obtained, then talk with the patient to find convenient appointment times. This habit is not only courteous but also gives patients a sense of control over situations they may find a bit frightening. Some doctors' offices may have you call the outside laboratory or hospital with all information concerning the patient and then give the patient the number to call to set up the appointment. This approach is often easier for patients. They then have the telephone number in case they need to reschedule.

If you are calling to make the appointment for the patient, tell the medical assistant, scheduling secretary, or admissions clerk what consultation, test, or procedure is required. Then find out what your office or the patient must do to prepare for the appointment. For example, the admitting doctor may need to complete a preadmission evaluation for a patient who is to be hospitalized.

When arrangements have been made, inform the patient, and note on the chart that you have done so. You may also provide the patient with a completed referral slip or, in the case of laboratory work, a laboratory request slip. Procedure 12-2 explains how to schedule and confirm

PROCEDURE 12.2

Scheduling and Confirming Surgery at a Hospital

Objective: To follow the proper procedure for scheduling and confirming surgery

Materials: Calendar, telephone, notepad, pen

Method

1. Elective surgery is usually performed on certain days when the doctor is scheduled to be in the operating room and a room and an anesthetist are available. The patient may be given only one or two choices of days and times. (For emergency surgery the first step is to reserve the operating room.)

2. Call the operating room secretary. Give the procedure required, the name of the surgeon, the time involved, and the preferred date and hour.

3. Provide the patient's name (including maiden name, if appropriate), address, telephone number, age, gender, Social Security number, and insurance information.

4. Call the admissions office. Arrange for the patient to be admitted on the day of surgery or the day before (depending on the surgery to be performed). Ask for a copy of the admissions form for the patient record.

5. Some hospitals want patients to complete preadmission forms. In such cases request a blank form for the patient.

6. Confirm the surgery and the patient's arrival time 1 business day before surgery.

appointments for surgery. (You will find additional information on preparing patients for surgery in Chapter 14.)

Maintaining the Physician's Schedule

The schedules of busy physicians are not limited to office visits with patients and hospital rounds. Physicians also need to attend professional meetings, travel to conferences, present speeches to colleagues, complete paperwork, and perform other duties. Your job is to help physicians make the most efficient use of their time.

One way is to avoid overbooking appointments with patients. **Overbooking** (scheduling more patients than can reasonably be seen in the time allowed) creates stress for the physician and eventually causes the office schedule to fall behind.

The opposite problem, **underbooking**—leaving large, unused gaps in the schedule—does not make the best use of the physician's time. Of course, you have no control over patients who cancel appointments. If you cannot reschedule another patient for the empty slot, the physician can use the time to catch up on telephone calls to patients or to attend to other matters.

At times you will have to cancel appointments because the physician has been delayed or called away by an emergency. Apologize to waiting patients on behalf of the physician, and offer them a choice. Explain that they can wait in the office (give an estimated waiting time), leave to run errands and return later, or reschedule their appointments for another day. Documentation should be noted in the patient's chart that because of an emergency in the office, the appointment had to be rescheduled. Be sure to write the date of the rescheduled appointment in the chart. Always make sure patients who need immediate attention are seen by another physician.

Reserving Operating Rooms

If the doctor in your office plans to perform surgery at a hospital, you will need to call the operating room secretary to reserve the facility. Give the preferred days and times, the type of surgery, and the length of time the doctor will need the operating room. After the day and time are set, provide the secretary with all relevant patient information. Relay any requests from the doctor, such as the blood type and units of blood that may be needed. It may also be your responsibility to make arrangements for surgical assistants, an anesthetist, and a hospital bed for the patient following surgery.

Stocking the Medical Bag

Some physicians see patients at skilled nursing facilities and elsewhere outside the office. You must enter these visits on the appointment schedule, taking into account

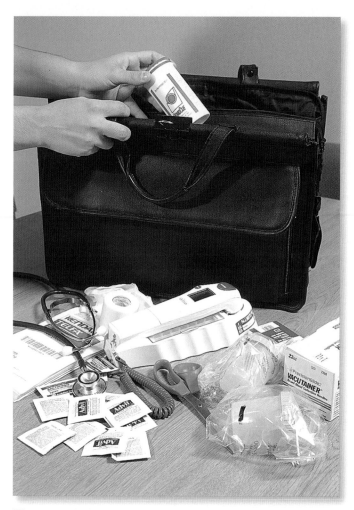

Figure 12-6. You may be responsible for keeping the physician's medical bag stocked with supplies.

the necessary travel time. For these visits, you may be responsible for stocking the physician's medical bag, as shown in Figure 12-6. The supplies vary depending on the practice, but the following items are commonly included:

- Adhesive tape, bandages, dressings
- Biohazard container
- Sphygmomanometer and blood pressure cuff
- Containers for specimens
- Medications—antibiotics, epinephrine, digitalis
- Microscope slides and fixative
- Ophthalmoscope
- Otoscope
- Penlight
- Personal protective equipment (for example, sterile latex gloves, protective face shield, and protective gown)
- Prescription pads and pens
- Scissors
- Sterile dressing forceps

- Sterile swabs
- Sterile syringes and needles
- Stethoscope
- Thermometers

Post a list of all the necessary items in the area where you check, clean, and restock the medical bag.

Scheduling Pharmaceutical Sales Representatives

Drug manufacturers often send pharmaceutical sales representatives into medical offices with printed information about new drugs as well as free samples that can be given to patients. These representatives are sometimes called detail persons. Some doctors do not want to meet with pharmaceutical representatives. Other doctors are willing to spend a few minutes if time permits and if the products are likely to be useful to the practice. Some doctors set aside a certain time 1 or 2 days a week to see detail persons. When a pharmaceutical representative who is unknown to you comes into the office, ask for a business card, and check with the doctor before scheduling an appointment (Figure 12-7). (Storing drug samples is discussed in Chapter 8.)

Making Travel Arrangements

You may be responsible for arranging transportation and lodging when physicians attend meetings, speaking engagements, and other events out of town. You may contact the airline, car rental agency, hotel, or other services yourself, or you may work through a travel agent. In either case request confirmation of travel and room reservations. You may also be responsible for picking up tickets or

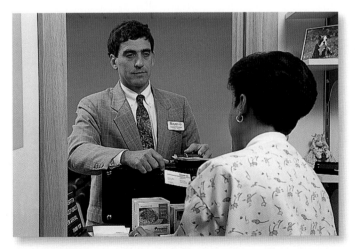

Figure 12-7. If pharmaceutical representatives come into the office without an appointment, you can ask them to leave a business card.

seeing that they are mailed to the office if time permits before the trip.

Before the day of departure, obtain an itinerary from the travel agent, or create one yourself. An **itinerary** is a detailed travel plan, listing dates and times of flights and events, locations of meetings and lodgings, and telephone numbers. Give several copies to the physician, and keep one for the office.

You must schedule and confirm professional coverage of the practice during the physician's absence. This coverage may be important for legal reasons. A **locum tenens,** or substitute physician, may be hired to see patients while the regular physician is away. (*Locum tenens* is Latin for "one occupying the place of another.") You may have more than one locum tenens on call, depending on the practice. In some areas special firms provide a locum tenens and other temporary medical and nursing help.

Planning Meetings

You may help the doctor set up meetings of professional societies or committees. To do so, you will need to know how many people are expected to attend, how long the meeting will last, and the purpose of the meeting. In addition, ask the doctor if a meal is to be served.

Some groups always meet at the same location. If there is no established meeting place, you must choose and reserve one. Select a location with an adequately sized meeting room, sufficient parking, and if needed, food services. Be sure also to arrange for necessary equipment, such as a microphone, podium, or overhead projector. Many conference centers and hotels have an on-site catering manager or conference manager to assist you with these arrangements. When the facility has been booked, mail a notice to all those expected to attend the meeting. On the notice provide the topic, names of the speakers, date, time, place, and admission costs or fees associated with attending.

With direction from the physician, you may also be responsible for creating the meeting's agenda. An **agenda** is a list of topics to be discussed or presented at a meeting in order of presentation. You may be asked to prepare the **minutes,** or the report of what was discussed and decided at the meeting.

Scheduling Time With the Physician

You and the physician should meet regularly to go through the tickler file and make sure necessary paperwork is prepared on time. Examples of recurring deadlines include those for state medical license renewal, Drug Enforcement Agency registrations, and documentation of the physician's continuing medical education (CME) requirements. Figure 12-8 lists items that are often part of a physician's schedule.

Common Items on a Physician's Schedule

Payments, Dues, and Fees
- Association dues
- Health insurance premium
- Payment for laundry service
- Liability insurance premium
- Life insurance premium
- Office rent
- Property insurance premium
- Paychecks for staff
- Payment for janitorial services
- Payment for leased equipment
- Taxes
  - *–Quarterly federal tax payments*
  - *–Quarterly state tax payments*
  - *–Annual federal and state tax filing deadline*

Time Commitments
- Committee meetings
- Conventions

Renewals and Accreditations
- Facility accreditation
  - *–State requirements*
  - *–Certificate of necessity*
  - *–Laboratory registration*
  - *–Federal requirements*
  - *–Ambulatory surgical centers*
  - *–Physician office laboratory*
- Medical license renewal
- Narcotics licenses renewal
- Drug Enforcement Agency registrations
- CME accreditations

Figure 12-8. Make time to meet with the physician regularly to review scheduling commitments.

Summary

Properly scheduling appointments in the medical office ensures a steady, efficient flow of patients. Setting up a matrix in the appointment book is the first step in scheduling appointments.

There are various appointment scheduling systems, including open-hours scheduling, wave scheduling, and cluster scheduling. Arranging appointments involves scheduling new and return patients and includes appointment reminder techniques. Special scheduling situations may occur, such as emergencies, referrals, and missed appointments. These situations may involve either patients or physicians. You may also be responsible for scheduling outside appointments for patients, as for testing or surgery.

Maintaining the physician's schedule includes such responsibilities as making travel arrangements and planning meetings. Meeting regularly with the physician helps ensure the smooth running of the office.

CASE STUDY QUESTIONS

Now that you have completed this chapter, review the case study at the beginning of the chapter and answer the following questions:

1. How would you adjust the schedule to allow for the emergency without falling behind schedule?
2. If it is necessary to reschedule patients, who should be rescheduled and when?
3. Would you explain anything to the patients in the waiting room about the emergency? If so, what would you say?

Discussion Questions

1. Describe situations that could cause the office to run behind schedule.
2. List the different types of appointment scheduling systems and briefly describe each.
3. Why is it important to note missed appointments and cancellations in the patient record and in the appointment book?
4. What is a matrix and why is it necessary?
5. List how long each of the following appointments should be scheduled for:
   a. earache
   b. CPE
   c. wound check
   d. Pap
   e. suture removal
   f. establish NP w/Rx prn
6. List the information that should be documented in the appointment book when scheduling.
7. Discuss how you would feel in a situation in which you had an extended wait in a physician's office. What could the medical assistant or office personnel do to ease your frustration?

Critical Thinking Questions

1. A patient has called to cancel her appointment for the third time. How should you handle this situation?
2. The physician is running about an hour and a half behind schedule and the schedule is completely filled. Describe how you would handle this problem.

3. Describe how you would handle a situation in which a patient calls for an appointment but is reluctant to disclose the purpose of the visit. What can you say to help the patient realize that it is advantageous to describe the nature of the visit?
4. Right after lunch, a patient walks into the office and requests to see the physician. The patient does not have an appointment and is complaining of pain in her stomach that will not go away. She has vomited a few times and looks very pale. How should you handle this situation?
5. Describe the best scheduling system for the following types of physician offices:
   a. A large practice with four physicians and with x-ray and lab facilities that are available anytime
   b. A small practice with two physicians and with lab facilities that are available only between 8:00 A.M. and 10:00 A.M.

Application Activities

1. A patient arrives at 10:00 A.M. for an appointment. When you check the schedule, the patient is not listed for an appointment for today. The patient produces an appointment card that clearly states that he has an appointment on this date at 10:00 A.M. You check tomorrow's schedule and realize that the patient is scheduled for the next day at 10:00 A.M. The medical office staff member who filled out the appointment card had made a mistake. The schedule for today is completely full and is already running behind. The patient is leaving the country for two months tomorrow morning and must see the physician today. What should you do?
2. A patient is a no-show for an appointment today. List where this should be documented. Discuss why it is important to document a no-show appointment.
3. Dr. Thompson, the only physician in your office, is out of town at a medical meeting. She is due back tomorrow morning. At 4:00 P.M., Dr. Thompson calls to say that a blizzard has closed the airport, and she will be forced to stay away for another day. You look at tomorrow's schedule. She has a full patient load. What should you do?

CHAPTER 13

Patient Reception Area

KEY TERMS

access

Americans With
    Disabilities Act

color family

contagious

differently abled

infectious waste

interim room

Older Americans Act of
    1965

teletype (TTY) device

AREAS OF COMPETENCE

2003 Role Delineation Study
GENERAL
Legal Concepts
- Implement and maintain federal and state health-care legislation and regulations
- Comply with established risk management and safety procedures

CHAPTER OUTLINE

- First Impressions
- The Importance of Cleanliness
- The Physical Components

- Keeping Patients Occupied and Informed
- Patients With Special Needs

OBJECTIVES

After completing Chapter 13, you will be able to:

13.1 Identify the elements that are important in a patient reception area.

13.2 Discuss ways to determine what furniture is necessary for a patient reception area and how it should be arranged.

13.3 List the housekeeping tasks and equipment needed for this area of the office.

13.4 Summarize the OSHA regulations that pertain to a patient reception area.

13.5 List the types of reading material appropriate to a patient reception area.

13.6 Describe how modifications to a reception area can accommodate patients with special needs.

13.7 Identify special situations that can affect the arrangement of a reception area.

Introduction

Going to the doctor's office can be an emotional and sometimes even a frightening event for many people. The office staff can do much to make the entry into the medical environment easier and less intimidating.

This chapter describes the patient reception area. As you look at the reception area and patient bathrooms through the eyes of patient needs, you begin to see ways to make the rooms both inviting and functional. Additionally, you will learn about the special needs of disabled patients. Well-planned and pleasant surroundings can do much to set the stage for a successful interaction between the patient and the doctor and other medical staff.

A 70-year-old patient has just arrived for his first appointment with his new primary care physician. He recently moved to Florida to be near his grown children, and today he meets his new doctor. He is apprehensive and concerned that he won't like this new doctor. He takes a deep breath and opens the door into the medical office reception room.

The first thing he notices is the cool air, which is in stark contrast to the hot humid air outside. As he enters the area, he sees a comfortable, spacious room decorated in soft color tones. The chairs and sofas are arranged in small conversational groupings. Neatly stacked on the tables is a colorful array of many different types of magazines. Playing softly in the corner of the room is a television tuned to a health channel. At the end of the room are a sliding glass window and a countertop with a sign-in clipboard. Crossing the room, he notices a family with small children playing with blocks in an adjoining room marked "Children's Reception Area." He sees a courtesy phone for patient use located in a nearby alcove. He adds his name to the list on the clipboard, noticing that all the patient names above his own have been blacked out. The glass window immediately opens and a neatly dressed medical assistant with a pleasant smile speaks to him, calling him by name. He is beginning to think this doctor might be all right after all.

As you read this chapter, consider the following questions:

1. What basic elements are *required* in every patient reception area? What other nonessential elements are nice to include as well?
2. Why is it important to think of the front patient area as the "patient reception area" and not the "waiting room"?
3. What special accommodations in the reception area are important to patients with disabilities?

First Impressions

The reception area plays a significant role in a patient's experience at the doctor's office. It is the first area patients see when entering the office. It is also a place where they have to spend time waiting for their appointments.

The appearance of the reception area creates an impression of the practice. Is the office bright and cheerful, cool and modern, or warm and cozy? The impression created by the reception area reflects on the quality of care patients can expect to receive. For example, old, tattered, or dirty furniture in the reception area will give patients the impression that the medical practice is unsuccessful and outdated. A carefully designed and well-maintained patient reception area, on the other hand, can attract and keep patients in the practice. It also ensures a pleasant and comfortable experience while they wait to receive medical care.

Reception Area

The reception area includes a reception window or desk, as shown in Figure 13-1, where patients check in for their appointments. It also includes chairs and couches for patients to sit on while waiting. Most patient reception areas are arranged using the same basic organizational concepts. The impressions they create can vary widely, however, depending on the elements chosen to enhance this part of the office.

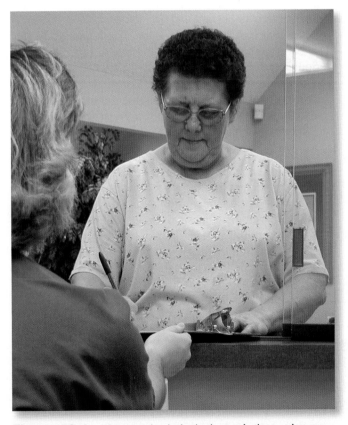

Figure 13-1. A receptionist's desk or window, where patients can check in, is part of every patient reception area.

Do not refer to the patient reception area as the "waiting room." The term has a negative connotation and implies that the patient and family members should expect a long wait. A more positive descriptive term to use is the "reception area."

Medical Office Contact Information.

As a convenience to patients, the business cards of all the physicians practicing at the location should be available. These cards are best placed at the reception window or desk, where patients can access them easily.

Lighting.

Most medical offices use fairly bright lighting in the reception area, allowing patients to see their surroundings easily. Subdued lighting, like that sometimes used in restaurants, could be hazardous because it could cause patients to trip over or bump into hard-to-see objects. In addition, bright lighting is essential for reading, which is a common activity in the patient reception area. Bright lighting also conveys an impression of cleanliness.

Lighting should not be so bright that it becomes bothersome, however. Extremely bright light can be harsh on the eyes and create an annoying glare. A specialist, such as an electrician or lighting showroom salesperson, can help determine the appropriate level of lighting for the patient reception area.

Room Temperature.

Patients will be uncomfortable if the reception area is too hot or too cold. In an uncomfortable setting, waiting time can seem much longer than it really is. Therefore, maintaining an average, comfortable temperature is important.

The thermostat should be kept at a temperature that feels comfortable to you and to the office staff. You might periodically survey patients to see if they are comfortable and adjust the setting accordingly. Many elderly people feel cold because of lowered metabolisms. You may want to increase the temperature setting for a geriatric practice or if the office sees a large number of elderly patients.

Music.

Many medical offices pipe music through speakers to the reception area as well as elsewhere in the office. The music provides a soothing background sound. Because the music is meant to calm patients, it should be chosen accordingly. Classical music, light jazz, and soft rock are appropriate choices, whereas heavy metal and rap music are not. Some offices use prepared tapes or compact discs. Others tune in to a local radio station.

The music should reflect the interests of the patients. If the office serves an older population, you might choose oldies or classical music. Try soft rock for an obstetrics/gynecology practice or children's folk music for a pediatric practice.

Decor

The patient reception area gets its distinctive look from the way it is decorated. With the appropriate elements, the decor can create whatever impression is desired—warm and friendly, modern and elegant, and so on. Some suggestions follow. It is wise to consult a professional decorator, if possible.

Colors and Fabrics.

Colors and fabrics are the primary elements that make up a room's decor. Colors can be used throughout the room—on walls, furniture, carpeting, and other items. Fabrics are used primarily on furniture and draperies.

When using several colors, it is important to decorate in color families to avoid a jarring, unprofessional look. A **color family** is a group of colors that work well together. Colors fall within two basic areas, cool and warm. Using all cool colors—like white, blue, and mauve—creates a more harmonious impression in the reception area than mixing cool colors with warm ones like red, orange, and hot pink. When choosing the color family, consider the mood you want to create. Bright colors produce a lively atmosphere, whereas softer, muted colors create a relaxing one.

Fabrics, too, add to the atmosphere in the room. Heavy fabrics like velvet or brocade are more formal, whereas lightweight or sheer fabrics create a soft, delicate appearance. Patterns on fabrics or wallpaper can immediately change the mood of the room. No matter what the design, fabrics should be easy to clean and maintain.

Many medical offices are carpeted, and carpets come in a variety of colors and patterns. Carpeting is attractive, and it helps reduce noise. Carpet also provides a comfortable cushion when people walk through the office.

Carpeting should be easy to clean and durable enough to handle a large volume of patient traffic. Wall-to-wall carpeting is preferable to scatter rugs, which can cause injuries if someone slips on or trips over them and falls.

Professional services can be contracted to deliver a clean, fresh entry carpet on a regular basis. These rubber-backed carpets lie directly on any floor surface and are commonly used at entranceways and hallways or areas of heavy traffic to catch soil from being "walked" into the rest of the office. Unlike scatter rugs, these heavyweight professional carpets lay flat and are not a hazard for tripping or falling. The service brings a fresh carpet and removes the soiled carpeting as scheduled.

Specialty Items.

Some offices include specialty items, or accessories, as part of the decor (Figure 13-2). Examples of such items include coatracks, aquariums, plants, paintings, sculptures, mobiles, and children's toys. Some items are meant to add a finishing touch, completing the desired atmosphere. Others may help to interest waiting patients by providing an activity, such as watching the fish in an aquarium.

Choosing Accessories. Although specialty items enhance the office decor, keep the number of accessories to a minimum. Too many pieces can give the room a cluttered look. Try to select specialty items that will be pleasing or helpful to patients. A clock is one example. Another useful item is a coatrack, which helps prevent clutter by providing a place for coats, umbrellas, and briefcases. Avoid accessories such as scented candles or potpourri that may be offensive to some people or cause allergic reactions.

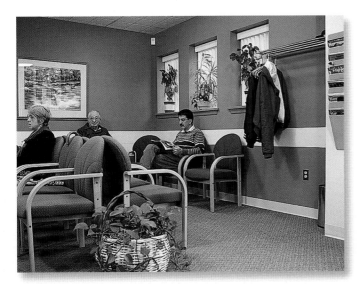

Figure 13-2. Specialty items—such as plants, paintings, and coatracks—enhance the patient reception area.

Keeping Safety in Mind. When selecting specialty items for the medical office, be sure to consider the issue of safety. Follow these guidelines to avoid potential hazards in the patient reception area.

- Do not include any item smaller than a golf ball. Small items present a choking hazard for young children.
- Avoid objects that can be easily pulled apart and then swallowed.
- Avoid easily breakable items, such as glass vases, that might cause cuts or other injuries to patients.
- Choose furniture with rounded, not sharp, corners. Coffee tables or other low tables with sharp corners can be a hazard especially to the elderly and to small children.
- Secure heavy wall hangings, shelves, and coatracks to the wall so that there is no risk of their falling.
- It is preferable to display artificial plants rather than living ones. Living plants may irritate patients who have allergies or present a poisoning hazard if parts of the plants are eaten by toddlers.
- If possible, build large, heavy items (such as fish tanks) into the wall to avoid climbing children and the danger of the items falling.
- Make sure all items in the reception area get a careful daily dusting before patients arrive. Artificial flowers and plants will need to be washed upside-down in soap and water occasionally to remove any potential allergens such as dust.

Furniture

Buying furniture for a patient reception room requires thoughtful planning. Although the office in which you work will no doubt be furnished already, it is a good idea to learn the steps and decisions involved in choosing furniture. You may be included in future purchasing decisions if the office expands or moves to a new location or if the doctor wants to redecorate.

Furniture styles vary to suit the office decor. Most important, seating furniture should be firm, comfortable, and easy to get in and out of. In addition, washable and fireproof fabric on the furniture minimizes care and maximizes safety.

The reception area should have enough furniture so that all patients and family members or friends who accompany them can sit, no matter how busy the office schedule. Forcing people to stand while they wait for an appointment makes the wait seem much longer. The American Medical Association (AMA) suggests that seating be sufficient to accommodate the number of patients, family members, and friends who may be in the office during a 2-hour time period. When calculating this number, be generous in allowing for family members. In some types of practices, such as pediatrics, all patients are accompanied by at least one parent or guardian and sometimes siblings as well.

Arranging Furniture. The furniture arrangement can make the office seem comfortable or uncomfortable. If furniture is too close together, patients do not have sufficient space to move around easily or to stretch their legs. They may feel cramped. To ensure that patients have adequate room, a good rule of thumb is to allow 12 square feet of space per person. By this measurement, a 120-square-foot room (10 feet by 12 feet) can accommodate ten people comfortably.

The furniture arrangement should allow maximum floor space. Patients should be able to stretch out their legs when seated and to walk around the waiting room if they wish (Figure 13-3). Placing chairs against the wall usually produces the greatest amount of floor area. Additional seating in the middle of the room can be placed back-to-back to conserve space. Seats should be grouped so that families or friends can sit together. Remember to reserve room for

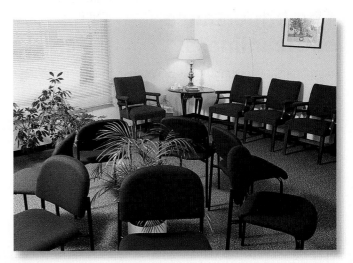

Figure 13-3. The furniture in a patient reception area can be arranged in a variety of ways.

patients in wheelchairs. This area should be carefully marked. Always allow enough space for wheelchairs with extended leg supports.

Ensuring Privacy. Some patients come to the office alone and value their privacy. Placing single chairs or small groups of chairs in corners of the room offers patients some measure of privacy.

Some medical offices offer more complete privacy in the form of an **interim room,** a room in which people can talk or meet without being seen or heard from the patient reception area. This interim room provides an ideal location for medical staff to confer privately with patients about appointments or bills. It also allows patients to make private telephone calls and allows people to feed or diaper babies in privacy. Not every office has the luxury of space for such a room, but it provides a valuable service to patients when it is possible.

Accommodating Children. A pediatric waiting room caters to a unique age group of patients. Reception areas for children usually have the same basic setup as those for adults, but special accommodations for children are also made.

In addition to regular chairs, for example, child-size chairs may be available. Some waiting rooms include playhouses or play furniture, such as small tables. The decor may also be made appealing to young children by the use of bright colors and storybook characters. It is important to make the setting feel familiar and comfortable. The reception desk may stock rolls of stickers or other inexpensive prizes to give to young patients after they have seen the doctor. Later in the chapter, you will learn how to set up a pediatric reception area.

Some pediatricians' offices have a well waiting room and a sick waiting room to separate children who are contagious from well children. **Contagious** means having a disease or condition that can easily be transmitted to others.

The Importance of Cleanliness

No matter how tastefully it is decorated, the reception area will be unappealing if it is not clean. Patients expect a physician's office to maintain a high standard of cleanliness. The perception is that a messy or dirty reception area or patient bathroom reflects a practice that does not meet minimum standards for cleanliness. A practice with a spotless, attractive reception area reassures patients that they have chosen a practice with high standards of cleanliness.

Housekeeping

Keeping the patient reception area clean usually falls within the duties of the medical assistant. In most cases you will be responsible for supervising the work of a professional cleaning service. In a small medical office you may be required to clean the area yourself.

Because professional services generally clean in the evening after business hours, you will probably not be present while the housekeeping staff is working. You may be asked to provide feedback to the cleaning company, however. It may also be your responsibility to outline the tasks you expect workers to complete, including any special requests.

One way of communicating with the cleaning staff is to create a Cleaning Communications Notebook. Arrange with the cleaning staff to leave the notebook open every evening in the same place. Date all entries. Write short, concise directions about any special requests for cleaning. Describe the nature of any stain so the service can best treat it. Sign each entry. Be sure to comment when something is done especially well. Like all of us, your cleaning staff likes to hear when they have done a particularly nice job!

Tasks. Although housekeeping tasks vary from office to office, basic routines are applicable to areas such as the patient reception room. The Caution: Handle With Care section gives more information about maintaining a clean reception area.

Whether or not the office employs a professional cleaning service, you or another staff member will need to check for cleanliness throughout the day. As patients spend time in the office, items may become dirty or be moved out of place. Taking time between patient appointments or at midday to spot-clean small areas that have become dirty and straighten items will help keep the patient reception area in good condition.

Equipment. If you, and not a professional service, are responsible for cleaning, the person in charge of the office budget will approve the purchase of cleaning equipment and supplies. Examples of cleaning equipment include handheld and upright vacuums, mops, and brooms. Supplies include trash bags, cleaning solutions, rags, and buckets. It is a good idea to have some basic cleaning materials on hand in case an emergency cleanup job is needed during office hours. Always wear gloves when doing cleaning of any kind.

Cleaning Stains

If furniture, carpet, or other items in the reception area become stained, it is important to remove the stains quickly. Follow these tips for stain removal.

- Try to remove the stain right away. The longer a stain remains, the more difficult it is to remove.
- Blot as much of the stain as possible before rubbing it with a cleaning solution.
- Take special precautions in handling stains involving blood, feces, and urine. Put on latex gloves before blotting or scraping up the stain.

CAUTION *Handle With Care*

Maintaining Cleanliness Standards in the Reception Area

Cleanliness is one of the hallmarks of a medical office. Not only is cleanliness required in the examination and testing rooms, it is also expected in the patient reception area. A messy patient reception area reflects poorly on the physician and on the practice. Maintaining standards of cleanliness helps ensure that the reception area is presentable at all times.

As a medical assistant, you may be involved—along with the physician, office manager, and other staff members—in setting cleanliness standards for the office. Standards are general guidelines. In addition to setting standards, you will need to specify the tasks required to meet each standard. A checklist of the tasks required to meet all standards is a helpful document to create as well.

The following list outlines standards you may want to consider. Specific housekeeping tasks for meeting those standards are included in parentheses.

1. Keep everything in its place. (Complete a daily visual check for items that are out of place. Return all magazines to racks. Push chairs back into place.)
2. Dispose of all trash. (Empty trash cans. Pick up trash on the floor or on furniture.)
3. Prevent dust and dirt from accumulating on surfaces. (Wipe or dust furniture, lamps, and artificial plants. Polish doorknobs. Clean mirrors, wall hangings, and pictures.)

4. Spot-clean areas that become dirty. (Remove scuff marks. Clean upholstery stains.)
5. Disinfect areas of the waiting room if they have been exposed to body fluids. (Immediately clean and disinfect all soiled areas.)
6. Handle items with care. (Take precautions when carrying potentially messy or breakable items. Do not carry too much at once.)

After the standards have been established, type and post them in a prominent place for the office staff to see. The checklist of cleaning activities may be posted, but the person responsible for cleaning the office should also keep a copy.

You should also produce a schedule of specific daily and weekly cleaning activities. Less frequent housekeeping duties, such as laundering drapes, shampooing the carpet, and cleaning windows and blinds, can be noted in a tickler file so that they will be performed on a regular basis.

It is always a good idea to have a second staff member responsible for periodically working with the medical assistant on housekeeping responsibilities. That person may also be responsible for handling cleaning duties when the medical assistant is away from the office.

- Wipe the area with a cleaning solution and water. Blood, urine, and feces may require special cleaners with an enzyme that breaks down organic waste.
- Use cold water instead of hot water because hot water often sets stains into the fabric.

Keep all cleaning materials within easy reach for quick action when a stain occurs.

Removing Odors

Odors are particularly offensive in a doctor's office because people expect a high level of cleanliness and cannot readily leave to escape the odor. Some odors that may occasionally be present in a medical practice include those of urine, feces, vomit, body odors, and laboratory chemicals. A good ventilating system with charcoal filters can help minimize odors. If the system has temporary high-speed

blowers, they can be activated as well. Disinfectant sprays and deodorant scents may also help.

One odor that can be prevented is smoke. Display "Thank You for Not Smoking" signs prominently in the patient reception area. Do not provide ashtrays, and ask smokers to leave the office if they insist on smoking. Not only does smoking produce an offensive odor, it also may affect the health of other patients in the waiting room. People who have asthma or other breathing disorders, or who are feeling unwell for any reason, are particularly sensitive to smoke and strong odors.

Infectious Waste

There may be times when you will need to clean up infectious waste. **Infectious waste** is waste that can be dangerous to those who handle it or to the environment. Infectious waste includes human waste, human tissue, and body fluids such as blood and urine. It also includes any potentially hazardous waste generated in the treatment of patients, such as needles, scalpels, cultures of human cells, and dressings.

Although infectious waste is not commonly generated in the patient reception area, it can be—as when a patient vomits or bleeds on the rug or on furniture. If that situation should occur, you must clean up the waste promptly.

Infectious waste must be handled in accordance with federal law. Your office may choose to purchase commercially prepared hazardous waste kits for use in cleaning up spills. After cleaning infectious waste from the patient reception area, deposit it in a biohazard container. Disinfect the site to eliminate possible contamination of other patients.

OSHA Regulations

Federal safety precautions for the workplace are mandated by the Occupational Safety and Health Administration (OSHA), a government agency. OSHA has developed general guidelines for most businesses as well as special rules for health-care practices. To determine whether the requirements are being met, OSHA periodically inspects medical offices. If the rules are not followed, medical offices may be required to pay penalties in addition to correcting the problem. All employees in a medical office must be thoroughly trained in following OSHA guidelines.

Among the OSHA requirements is regular cleaning of walls, floors, and other surfaces. OSHA requires the use of disinfectants to combat bacteria as part of a routine cleaning schedule. In addition, OSHA mandates that broken glass, which may be contaminated, be picked up using a dustpan and brush or tongs. It should not be picked up by hand, even if one wears gloves.

The Physical Components

No one arrangement of a reception area is necessarily better than another. As long as the arrangement provides clear pathways and comfortable places to sit, the reception area will be functional.

Office Access

The path patients must take to get from the parking area or street to the office and then back out again is called the office **access.** Some offices have easy access and some do not (Figure 13-4).

Parking Arrangements. Although some patients walk to the medical office or take public transportation, the majority of patients probably travel by car. Patients who drive to the office need a place to park.

The office can offer either on-street parking or a parking lot. On-street parking requires patients to fend for themselves. They may have to put money into parking meters, and parking spaces may be difficult to find. Both the money

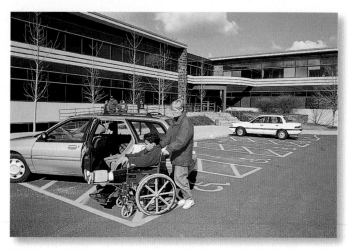

Figure 13-4. Patients should have easy, clear access from the parking lot to the medical office door.

required and the potential problems in finding parking spots limit the ease with which patients can gain access to the office.

A free parking lot improves office access. Parking lots should be well lit for safety. To determine the number of parking spaces the office needs, calculate the average length of time a patient spends in the office from arrival to departure and the number of appointments scheduled during that time period. Allow one parking spot per appointment if most patients drive to the office and fewer if many use public transportation. In your count be sure to include parking spaces for office staff. Periodically reevaluate the office's parking needs because they may change over time. All offices must also provide handicapped parking space for patients.

Entrances. The entrance to the office should be clearly marked so that patients can find the office easily. The name of the practice and of the doctor or doctors should be on the door or beside the door. Just outside the doorway should be a doormat to help control the amount of dirt tracked into the office. If the office door opens directly to the outside, people inside will feel a sudden change in temperature each time the door is opened in hot or cold weather. A foyer or double door arrangement helps minimize the effects of the weather and helps keep the office at a consistent, comfortable temperature.

Doorways must be wide enough to accommodate patients using wheelchairs and walkers. Hallways should be extra wide to allow patients in wheelchairs to turn around or to allow two wheelchairs to pass one another. The Americans With Disabilities Act, discussed later in this chapter, requires that doorways have a minimum width of 32 inches and that hallways have a minimum width of 5 feet. Well-lit hallways, without obstructions, are required.

Safety and Security

Safety and security are important concerns in any public building, and they are especially important in a doctor's office. To ensure safety of the patients and staff, such as protection from hazardous wiring or poorly lit hallways, there are guidelines for businesses, some of which pertain to the patient reception area. In addition, the medical office must be secure from burglary.

Building Exits. Make sure you and the office staff are familiar with all building exits. It may be necessary to leave the office quickly, as during a fire, flood, or other emergency. You and other staff members must be prepared to assist and direct patients toward the exits in such a situation.

Ideally, the office should have at least two doorways that lead directly to the outside or to a hallway that leads to stairs. This arrangement affords patients and staff members the speediest, most direct route outside in case of an emergency. All exits must be clearly labeled with illuminated red "Exit" signs. These signs normally have a backup power system, such as a battery, so that they will remain lit even during a power outage.

Having two or more exits also allows staff members to enter and leave the office during nonemergency situations without disrupting people in the patient reception area. Deliveries can be made at the second entrance, further minimizing interruptions.

Smoke Detectors. By law, a medical office is required to install smoke detectors that sound an alarm when triggered by heat or smoke. The office staff should be trained in the proper procedure if the smoke alarm sounds— including how to evacuate patients from the building efficiently. Smoke detectors must be checked regularly to ensure that they are operating properly.

Security Systems. No matter where the medical office is located, a security alarm system is a wise investment, even if the office building is patrolled by security personnel. A security alarm system offers valuable protection for the confidential patient information housed in a medical office. After the alarm system is installed, all office staff members should thoroughly familiarize themselves with it. They should be able to arm and disarm it easily and know what to do if it is accidentally activated. Each member of the staff should have her or his own individually assigned security access number. This number is required to authorize locking or unlocking the system. Like a credit card, bank, or other security PIN (personal identification number), it should never be shared.

Keeping Patients Occupied and Informed

Many patients who come into a medical office are ill, anxious, and concerned about their health. While they wait in the reception area, they need a way to stay occupied so that the time seems to pass quickly. In addition, patients may want to be informed about a particular medical condition or about general health issues. To meet these patient needs, most medical offices provide reading materials in the patient reception area. They may also offer television or educational videotapes.

Reading Materials

The most common activity in a patient reception area is probably reading. Although some patients bring their own books or magazines, most patients expect to find reading materials at the medical office (Figure 13-5). Magazines and books are probably the most popular types of reading materials, but a variety of others may also be available.

Magazines and Books. Choosing the right mix of reading material to interest all patients is a challenge. You may know doctors' offices that have a wonderful selection of magazines and books and others that have a poor selection. Your judgment of the selection, however, is based on how those publications match your interests. The Tips for the Office section gives guidelines on selecting magazines for the medical office. In addition to reading materials for adults, most offices also have children's books and magazines for younger patients and family members.

You or someone on the office staff should be sure to screen publications for medical content. You can then alert the doctors to articles that might stimulate patients' questions.

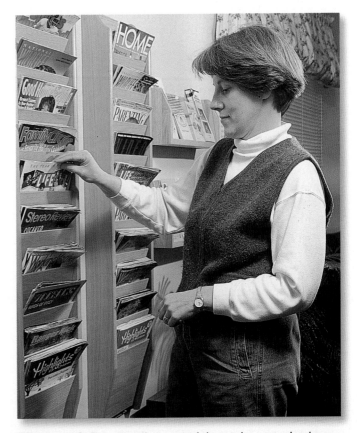

Figure 13-5. Reading materials can be organized on tables or in a wall rack.

Tips for the Office

Tailoring Office Magazines to Patient Interests

It is a common sight: patients waiting their turn for an appointment pick up one of the many magazines in the reception area. Sometimes it is hard to choose—because every magazine is interesting or because none of them are.

As a medical assistant, you may be responsible for selecting magazines for the office's reception area. The right selection can make the difference between a pleasant wait and a tedious one. Follow these guidelines to compile a suitable mix of magazines that will be of interest to a majority of patients.

1. Patients in some practices immediately share a common ground. They fall within the category of the practice's specialty—for example, geriatrics or pediatrics. Some magazines may be a natural fit for this category. A geriatric practice, for example, may provide publications geared toward senior citizens. A pediatric practice may offer parenting and children's magazines.

2. People waiting in a doctor's office usually have an interest in their health. Therefore, health magazines geared toward the general public are good choices. Of course, the reception area is not the place for the highly technical medical journals, with graphic pictures, that the doctor may receive.

3. Make sure the magazines cover a variety of interests. The more topics available, the greater the chance that someone will be interested in one of them. Instead of subscribing to several magazines on one topic, try to limit subscriptions to one magazine per topic, unless the topic is of special interest to most patients.

4. Choose magazines that cover topics in a general way—travel, news, sports, fashion, or entertainment. Delving into these areas too specifically—as in a tennis magazine rather than one on a variety of sports—may not interest many patients.

5. Remove torn or out-of-date magazines from the patient reception area. Replenish them with a fresh supply as soon as possible.

6. The best way to determine patients' interests is to ask for feedback. Develop a form on which patients can indicate their hobbies, interests, and favorite types of magazines. Periodically display the form in the reception area, and encourage patients to make suggestions.

Patient Information Packet. One type of reading material other than magazines is a patient information packet. This document is an easy way to inform patients about the practice. The packet can be designed in many ways, from a simple flyer to a formal folder with pockets to hold individual sheets of information. Topics covered in the packet can range from billing and insurance processing policies to biographical information on each physician in a group practice. Read Chapter 14 to learn more about how to develop the contents of a patient information packet.

Medical Information. Another type of reading material commonly found in reception areas is medical brochures. Patients may be interested in information that pertains to their general health or to a specific condition. Brochures on a variety of topics are available to medical offices either free of charge or for a nominal fee. These brochures are usually produced by nonprofit associations that specialize in a disease or condition, such as the American Cancer Society, and by pharmaceutical companies.

Before displaying pamphlets and brochures in the reception area, be sure to read them thoroughly. They should provide accurate information. The physician may also want to review them for medical accuracy.

Bulletin Board. Most patient reception areas feature a bulletin board. Bulletin boards often highlight area meetings, such as those of support groups, and offer other current information. To encourage patients to look at the bulletin board, change the format and content frequently. An interesting design with bright colors and bold headlines attracts readers. Depending on your time and inclination, you might change the bulletin board every week, month, or season.

Items on a reception area bulletin board should be tailored to patient interests. For example, an obstetrics/gynecology practice specializing in infertility might display recent birth announcements from its patients. The bulletin board might also feature support groups for parents trying to conceive, information on the latest medical studies of fertility drugs, and magazine clippings on parenting issues.

Other, more general items for display on any physician's bulletin board might include the following:

- Government reports on food and drugs
- Nutrition information

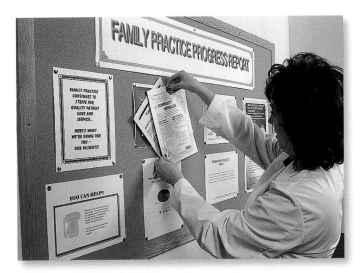

Figure 13-6. Check the office bulletin board frequently for outdated information.

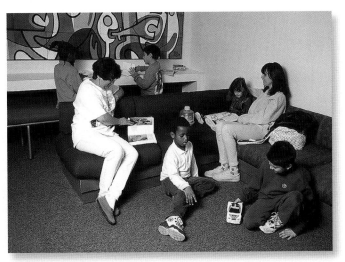

Figure 13-7. Toys and games that encourage quiet play are well suited to a reception area in a pediatric practice.

- Requests from the American Red Cross or the local blood bank for blood donors
- Pamphlets or flyers distributed by nonprofit health-care organizations, such as the American Heart Association
- Flyers on upcoming health fairs
- Blood pressure or other health screening notices
- Newspaper or magazine articles on interesting medical issues
- Community notices for food drives or similar charity events

The bulletin board might also feature information about staff members in the practice. Do not allow the bulletin board to become cluttered with advertising or business cards.

Finally, the bulletin board is an ideal place to display the office brochure. Put some extra copies of the brochure in an open envelope tacked to the bulletin board to encourage patients to take one home. To keep the bulletin board up to date, all time-sensitive materials, such as notices about a class or seminar, should be removed as soon as the date of the scheduled event has passed (Figure 13-6).

Television and Videotapes

Although reading remains the primary pastime in patient reception areas, watching television and videotapes is becoming a more common activity in physicians' offices across the country. Many patient reception areas now include a television, which can be tuned to regular stations or can play preselected videos. Physicians may provide informative health-care videos of general interest to their patients or videos that meet the more specific interests of the practice.

Items for Children

Many patient reception areas include items to occupy children while they wait. Because children—even sick ones—do not usually like to sit still for long periods, these items may include toys, games, videos, and books (Figure 13-7). If the pediatric reception area separates sick children from well children, the "well" side may include more active entertainment, such as an indoor slide or playhouse. The "sick" side may provide quieter games and activities, such as books and puzzles.

Choose toys carefully. You do not want children—even well ones—to be too active in the waiting room, because they might disrupt other patients and their families. Avoid balls, jump ropes, and other toys meant for outside use. Puzzles and blocks are good choices because they encourage quieter play. You might informally ask parents and children if they like the play items or if they would prefer other types of toys. Procedure 13-1 explains how to set up a pediatric playroom.

Patients With Special Needs

Some patients who come into the medical office will be disabled—that is, they were born with or have acquired a condition that limits or changes their abilities. A more positive way of referring to these patients is **differently abled.** For example, people who are paralyzed from the waist down are differently abled; so are people who are visually impaired. This does not mean that these people cannot perform the same tasks that other people can. They may simply need special accommodations to do so.

Americans With Disabilities Act

Differently abled individuals are often singled out for their differences and are sometimes discriminated against. For example, if a company building does not have access

PROCEDURE 13.1

Creating a Pediatric Playroom

Objective: To create a play environment for children in the patient reception area of a pediatric practice

Materials: Children's books and magazines, games, toys, nontoxic crayons and coloring books, television and videocassette recorder (VCR), children's videotapes, child- and adult-size chairs, child-size table, bookshelf, boxes or shelves, decorative wall hangings or educational posters (optional)

Method

1. Place all adult-size chairs against the wall. Position some of the child-size chairs along the wall with the adult chairs.

2. Place the remainder of the child-size chairs in small groupings throughout the room. In addition, put several chairs with the child-size table.

3. Put the books, magazines, crayons, and coloring books on the bookshelf in one corner of the room near a grouping of chairs.

4. Choose toys and games carefully. Avoid toys that encourage active play, such as balls, or toys that require a large area. Make sure that all toys meet safety guidelines. Watch for loose parts or parts that are smaller than a golf ball. Toys should also be easy to clean.

5. Place the activities for older children near one grouping of chairs and the games and toys for younger children near another grouping. Keep the toys and games in a toy box or on shelves designated for them. Consider labeling or color-coding boxes and shelves and the games and toys that belong there to encourage children to return the games and toys to the appropriate storage area.

6. Place the television and VCR on a high shelf, if possible, or attach it to the wall near the ceiling. Keep children's videos behind the reception desk, and periodically change the video in the VCR.

7. To make the room more cheerful, decorate it with wall hangings or posters.

---

ramps for wheelchairs, workers in wheelchairs cannot qualify for jobs there.

Preventing Discrimination. In 1990 a law was enacted to prevent certain types of discrimination. The **Americans With Disabilities Act** is a federal civil rights act forbidding discrimination on the basis of physical or mental handicap. This act maintains the rights of disabled people in many areas, including jobs, transportation, and access to public buildings. The act relates to medical practices (and reception areas) in that an office must be able to accommodate any patient who wants to see the physician.

Differently Abled Patients. Differently abled patients may have special needs. With some forethought and planning, the office can accommodate these needs. Ensuring wheelchair access through doors and hallways, as mentioned earlier, is just one way. Using ramps instead of steps, as shown in Figure 13-8, allows easier access not only for wheelchair users but also for others who have limited mobility. Allowing additional space in the waiting room for wheelchairs, walkers, crutches, and guide dogs accommodates several types of differently abled patients. Procedure 13-2 explains how to organize the patient reception area to meet the special needs of patients who are physically challenged.

Many offices do not make special accommodations for patients with vision or hearing impairments. Post prominent signs in the reception area with information that patients need to know. A staff member should offer to assist patients with hearing or vision impairments as needed from the reception area to the examination room when it is their turn to see the doctor.

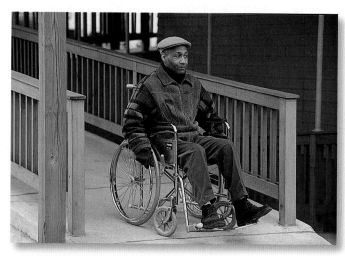

Figure 13-8. Ramps allow patients who use wheelchairs access to the medical office.

PROCEDURE 13.2

Creating a Reception Area Accessible to Differently Abled Patients

Objective: To arrange elements in the reception area to accommodate patients who are differently abled

Materials: Chairs, bars or rails, adjustable-height tables, doorway floor coverings, magazine rack, television/VCR, ramps (if needed), large-type and braille magazines

Method

1. Arrange chairs, leaving gaps so that substantial space is available for wheelchairs along walls and near other groups of chairs. Keep the arrangement flexible so that chairs can be removed to allow room for additional wheelchairs if needed.

2. Remove any obstacles that may interfere with the space needed for a wheelchair to swivel around completely. Also remove scatter rugs or any carpeting that is not attached to the floor. Such carpeting can cause patients to trip and create difficulties for wheelchair traffic.

3. Position coffee tables at a height that is accessible to people in wheelchairs.

4. Place office reading materials, such as magazines, at a height that is accessible to people in wheelchairs (for example, on tables or in racks attached midway up the wall).

5. Locate the television and VCR within full view of patients sitting on chairs and in wheelchairs so that they do not have to strain their necks to watch.

6. For patients who have a vision impairment, include reading materials with large type and in braille.

7. For patients who have difficulty walking, make sure bars or rails are attached securely to walls 34 to 38 inches above the floor, to accommodate requirements set forth in the Americans With Disabilities Act. Make sure the bars are sturdy enough to provide balance for patients who may need it. Bars are most important in entrances and hallways. Consider placing a bar near the receptionist's window for added support as patients check in.

8. Eliminate the sill of metal or wood along the floor in doorways. Otherwise, create a smoother travel surface for wheelchairs and pedestrians with a thin rubber covering to provide a graduated slope. Be sure that the covering is attached properly and meets safety standards.

9. Make sure the office has ramp access.

10. Solicit feedback from patients with physical disabilities about the accessibility of the patient reception area. Encourage ideas for improvements. Address any additional needs.

Patients who are hearing impaired may request that a certified sign language interpreter be present to assist in communicating with the medical staff. If requested, it is required by federal law that the physician provides and pays for this interpreter.

It is also helpful, but not required by law, to provide a **teletype (TTY) device** for hearing-impaired patients. This specially designed telephone looks very much like a laptop computer with a cradle for the receiver of a traditional telephone. The receiver is placed in the cradle, and the hearing-impaired patient can then type the communication on the keyboard. The message can be received by another TTY or relayed through a specialty relay service.

Some states offer a relay service for patients with hearing impairments or those with speech disabilities. When an individual accesses this service through the TTY, the service then places the call using voice. It is important to understand that a relay service could call a medical office to make an appointment for a patient. The medical assistant

needs to be careful to respond appropriately and not mistake the call as an unwanted marketing call.

Older Americans Act of 1965

A growing proportion of the American population is elderly. Like those who are disabled, many elderly people face discrimination. One reason for the discrimination may be that with age come medical conditions and disorders that create physical limitations.

The **Older Americans Act of 1965** was passed by Congress to eliminate discrimination against the elderly. Among other benefits, the act guarantees elderly citizens the best possible health care regardless of ability to pay, an adequate retirement income, and protection against abuse, neglect, and exploitation.

What does the Older Americans Act mean for the medical office reception area? If the practice serves elderly patients, the office staff must be sensitive to their special needs. The patient reception area should be as comfortable as possible for patients with arthritis, failing eyesight, and other common ailments of the elderly. Make sure there are a few straight-backed chairs, which are easier to get into and out of than soft sofas. Arms on chairs provide support when sitting and standing for patients who are unsteady. In addition, straight-backed chairs offer greater back support than low chairs or couches with sinking cushions. These chairs should be located near the front door and near the examination rooms.

Place reading materials within easy reach of the chairs so that elderly patients do not have to get up from their chairs for them. Have large-print books and magazines available, if possible, for patients with poor eyesight. You might also offer magnifying glasses for patients who like to use them. In addition, make sure that the print on all office signs is large and easy to read. The patient reception area and restrooms should be well lit to help everyone, including elderly patients, see more clearly.

Special Situations

Patients in a medical practice are usually a diverse group of people. Their interests, needs, and medical conditions can have an impact on the design of the reception area.

Patients From Diverse Cultural Backgrounds.
The United States has long been called a melting pot because of its mixture of people and cultures. Each culture lends its own special qualities, and together the cultures combine to create a unique blend of people called Americans.

You may work in a neighborhood that has a distinct culture or one in which many cultures are represented. To help patients feel comfortable, make the reception area reflect aspects of their cultural backgrounds whenever possible. This effort will help patients feel more welcome.

Suppose, for example, that the medical office where you work serves many Hispanic patients. Posting signs in Spanish and English acknowledges the fact that both languages are spoken in that neighborhood. Providing reading materials, such as newspapers and magazines, in a second language—for both adults and children—is another way to show respect and interest. Decorating the office for Spanish holidays in addition to American ones demonstrates that you care about what is important to patients. Displaying artwork created by local artists and artisans is another idea.

Patients Who Are Highly Contagious.
Patients may have to come into the physician's office when they are highly contagious. This fact is a concern for all patients, but it is especially critical for patients who are immunocompromised. Immunocompromised patients have an immune system—which protects against disease—that is not functioning at a normal level. Because these patients do not have the normal ability to fight off disease, they are at greater risk than the average person for becoming sick. Patients undergoing chemotherapy and patients with AIDS, for example, have compromised immune systems.

To protect patients who are immunocompromised, as well as other patients and staff members, you may need to separate a highly contagious patient from them. Instead of having contagious patients wait in the reception area, for example, you might bring them directly into an examination room to wait. By screening patients for highly contagious conditions and taking precautions, you can minimize the chances of exposing other people unnecessarily.

Summary

The patient reception area is where patients are received before they are seen by the physician. The area's appearance creates an immediate and lasting impression on patients. Patients may notice elements such as temperature, lighting, decor, and cleanliness, all of which influence their perception of the practice.

Offices with well-planned, pleasant reception areas provide a comfortable experience for waiting patients. Important elements include easy access from the outside, safety measures that meet federal requirements, and appropriate furnishings, reading material, and other entertainment to make the wait as enjoyable as possible. Special accommodations for patients who are young, elderly, differently abled, and from diverse cultural backgrounds help create a welcoming environment.

CASE STUDY QUESTIONS

Now that you have completed this chapter, review the case study at the beginning of the chapter and answer the following questions:

1. What basic elements are *required* in every patient reception area? What other nonessential elements are nice to include as well?
2. Why is it important to think of the front patient area as the "patient reception area" and not the "waiting room"?
3. What special accommodations in the reception area are important to patients with disabilities?

Discussion Questions

1. What is the Americans With Disabilities Act, and what impact does it have on the patient reception area and patient bathrooms?
2. What is the Older Americans Act, and what impact does it have on the patient reception area and patient bathrooms?
3. What psychological affect does a cheerful, inviting reception room have on the patient?

Critical Thinking Questions

1. What special difficulties might patients in wheelchairs have in a small, overcrowded reception area?
2. Who is responsible if a patient or family member or friend is hurt in the reception area or bathroom? What could be the possible consequences?
3. What would be the best design for a pediatric reception area and bathroom? Describe it.

Application Activities

1. Design a reception area bulletin board for a family practitioner's office. List at least six items to include, and draw a rough sketch for placing these items on a rectangular bulletin board.
2. Develop a daily checklist for closing down a patient reception area at the end of the day. Be sure to include any housekeeping chores.
3. Visit a patient reception area at a clinic or a doctor's or dentist's office. Notice the decor, furniture arrangement, specialty items, and reading materials. Note what you like and dislike about the area. Then write down suggestions for improvement. Compare your results with those of your classmates.

Patient Education

KEY TERMS

consumer education
dementia
modeling
philosophy
return demonstration
screening

AREAS OF COMPETENCE

2003 Role Delineation Study

GENERAL

Communication Skills

- Adapt communications to individual's ability to understand
- Use medical terminology appropriately

Instruction

- Instruct individuals according to their needs
- Explain office policies and procedures
- Teach methods of health promotion and disease prevention
- Locate community resources and disseminate information

CHAPTER OUTLINE

- The Educated Patient
- Types of Patient Education
- Promoting Good Health Through Education
- The Patient Information Packet
- Educating Patients With Special Needs
- Patient Education Prior to Surgery
- Additional Educational Resources

OBJECTIVES

After completing Chapter 14, you will be able to:

14.1 Identify the benefits of patient education.

14.2 Explain the role of the medical assistant in patient education.

14.3 Discuss factors that affect teaching and learning.

14.4 Describe patient education materials used in the medical office.

14.5 Explain how patient education can be used to promote good health habits.

14.6 Identify the types of information that should be included in the patient information packet.

14.7 Discuss techniques for educating patients with special needs.

14.8 Explain the benefits of patient education prior to surgery, and identify types of preoperative teaching.

14.9 List educational resources that are available outside the medical office.

Introduction

Health education should be a lifelong pursuit for all of us. The ultimate goal of all medical professionals is to encourage and teach healthy habits and behaviors to all patients. People first have to understand what is good for them, and then they have to make a decision to follow that advice. In patient education, the medical assistant both shares information and encourages patients to make good health decisions.

In this chapter you will learn about the medical assistant's role in patient education. You will sharpen your skills in recognizing and overcoming road blocks to education. You will become more comfortable with teaching and demonstrating procedures to others. Most importantly, you will begin to recognize the incredible responsibility of the medical assistant to correctly lead others to their highest level of health.

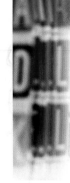

CASE STUDY

Laura is a 26-year-old pregnant patient with hypertension (high blood pressure). She is taking blood pressure medication, but her pressure is becoming increasing difficult to manage as she progresses with her pregnancy. The doctor has ordered a 24-hour urine collection test to help determine if Laura is in a dangerous state of preeclampsia. It is your task as medical assistant to explain to Laura the process of urine collection that she must follow. You know that she is not going to want to carry a large jug of urine to work with her and keep it on ice all day. You know that she is not likely to accurately follow the procedures of the test. But you also know it is imperative that the doctor accurately gather this test information for the health of this woman and the infant she carries.

After first reading the 24-hour urine collection procedure yourself and ensuring that you understand it thoroughly, you sit with Laura in a quiet place and explain the test and the need for accuracy. You then listen to her and evaluate her level of understanding. You listen for any cues she gives that indicate difficulties in completing the test as ordered. Thinking creatively, you suggest that Laura conduct the test on a Sunday when she can stay at home during the day and bring the specimen directly to the doctor's office early on Monday morning. You give her all the test lab items she will need, explaining each item. Additionally, you give her written instructions that she can take with her and a phone number to call with any questions she may have over the weekend. You encourage her as she leaves. By doing everything you can to ensure this patient's compliance, you contribute to the chances that both she and her baby will be strong and healthy throughout her pregnancy and delivery.

As you read this chapter, consider the following questions:

1. What might be important to consider when creating an educational plan for a patient? How might the plan vary according to the individual?
2. What factors could block effective patient education?
3. What specific behaviors do you associate with talking down to a patient?
4. Why are good listening skills an important part of teaching?

The Educated Patient

Patient education is an essential process in the medical office. It encourages patients to take an active role in their medical care. It results in better compliance with treatment programs. When patients are suffering from illness, disease, or injury, education can often help them regain their health and independence more quickly. Simply put, patient education helps patients stay healthy. Educated patients are more likely to comply with instructions if they understand the why behind the instructions. Also, educated patients are more likely to be satisfied clients of the practice.

Patients benefit from education, and the medical office benefits as well. Preoperative instruction of surgical patients, for example, lessens the chance that procedures will have to be rescheduled because surgical guidelines were not followed. Educated patients will also be less likely to call the office with questions. Thus, the office staff will have to spend less time on the telephone.

Patient education takes many forms and includes a variety of techniques. It can be as simple as answering a question that comes up during a routine visit. Patient education can involve printed materials. It can also be participatory, as with a demonstration of the procedure for changing a bandage or for giving oneself an insulin injection

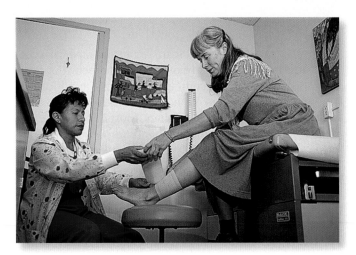

Figure 14-1. When helping patients learn through participation, you may demonstrate a technique, then ask the patient to demonstrate it for you.

(Figure 14-1). No matter what type of patient education is used, the goal is the same—to help patients help themselves attain better health. Procedure 14-1 will help you create a patient education plan.

As a medical assistant, you play a vital role in the process of patient education, primarily because of your constant interaction with patients in the office. Although the initial visit is a good time to assess the need for patient education, the educational process can and should be ongoing. Continue to assess patients' needs at every visit, and be aware of situations in which you can share meaningful and helpful information.

Types of Patient Education

Patient education can take many forms. Any instructions—verbal, written, or demonstrative—that you give to patients are a type of patient education. Most formal types of patient education involve some printed information. They may also include visual materials, such as videotapes. Patient educational materials inform patients and enable them to become involved in their own medical care.

Printed Materials

Printed educational materials come in a variety of formats. They can be as simple as a single sheet of paper, or they can be several sheets that are folded or stapled together to form a booklet.

Brochures, Booklets, and Fact Sheets. Many medical offices have materials available that explain procedures performed in the medical office or give information about specific diseases and medical conditions. For example, women who have had a cesarean section delivery may be given a fact sheet describing simple exercises

---

PROCEDURE 14.1

Developing a Patient Education Plan

Objective: To create and implement a patient teaching plan

Materials: Pen, paper, various educational aids

Method

1. Identify the patient's needs for education. Consider the following:
   a. The patient's current knowledge
   b. Any misconceptions the patient may have
   c. Any obstacles to learning (loss of hearing or vision, limitations of mobility, language barriers, and so on)
   d. The patient's willingness and readiness to learn (motivation)
   e. How the patient will use the information

2. Develop and outline a plan using the various educational aids available. Include the following areas in the outline:
   a. What you want to accomplish (your goal)
   b. How you plan to accomplish it

   c. How you will determine if the teaching was successful

3. Write the plan. Try to make the information interesting for the patient.

4. Before carrying out the plan, share it with the physician to get approval and suggestions for improvement.

5. Perform the instruction.

6. Document the teaching in the patient's chart.

7. Evaluate the effectiveness of your teaching session. Ask yourself:
   a. Did you cover all the topics in your plan?
   b. Was the information well received by the patient?
   c. Did the patient appear to learn?
   d. How would you rate your performance?

8. Revise your plan as necessary to make it even more effective.

they can do in bed to help regain strength in the abdominal muscles. Some printed materials provide information to help patients stay healthy, such as tips for eating low-fat foods. Many educational aids are prepared by pharmaceutical companies and are provided free of charge to medical offices. Others may be written by the physician or members of the office staff. You may be asked to help prepare some of these materials.

Educational Newsletters. A popular patient education tool is the medical office newsletter. Newsletters contain timely, practical health-care tips. Regular newsletters can also offer updates on office policies, information about new diagnostic tests or equipment, and news about the office staff. Newsletters are often written by the doctor or office staff. Some publishing companies and medical groups also offer newsletters that can be customized to a particular practice.

Community-Assistance Directory. Patients often require the assistance of health-related organizations within the community. For example, an elderly patient may need the services of a visiting nurse or a meals-on-wheels food program. Other patients may need the services of a day-care center, speech therapist, or weight clinic. A written community resource directory prepared by the office is a valuable aid for referring patients to appropriate agencies.

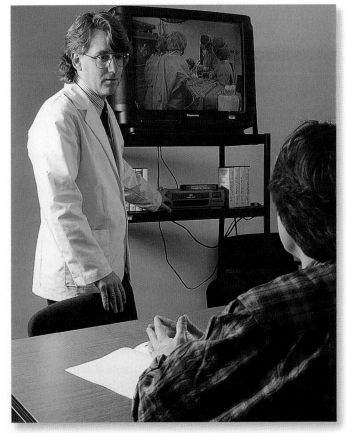

Figure 14-2. Videotapes are an excellent educational aid for the medical office because of their visual format.

Visual Materials

Many patients are better able to comprehend complicated medical information when it is presented in a visual format. When using visual educational materials, it is usually best to provide corresponding written materials that patients can keep for reference.

Videotapes. Videotapes are often used to educate patients about a variety of topics and to instruct them in self-care techniques (Figure 14-2). The use of videotapes is especially effective when teaching about complex subjects and procedures.

Seminars and Classes. Many physicians conduct or arrange educational seminars or classes for their patients. For example, an obstetrician might offer classes in childbirth preparation for patients and their partners.

Promoting Good Health Through Education

One of the most important goals of patient education is to promote good health. Health is not just the absence of illness. It is a complex concept that involves the body, mind, emotions, and environment. Health involves physical, mental, emotional, and social influences working together as a whole.

Maintaining or improving your health is the best way to protect yourself against disease and illness. **Consumer education**—education that is geared, both in content and language, toward the average person—has helped Americans become more aware of the importance of good health. As a result, many people are beginning to take greater responsibility for their own health and well-being.

There are many ways to achieve good health. You can develop healthful habits, take steps to protect yourself from injury, and take preventive measures to decrease the risk of disease or illness. Patient education in the medical office should help patients achieve these goals.

Healthful Habits

When educating patients about good health, you can recommend several specific guidelines. Encourage patients to incorporate the following healthful habits into their daily lives:

- Good nutrition, including limited fat intake and an adequate amount of fruits, vegetables, and fiber
- Regular exercise
- Adequate rest (7 to 8 hours of sleep a night)
- Not smoking and limiting alcohol consumption
- A balance of work and leisure activities (moderation)

Whenever possible, these guidelines should be recommended to patients of all ages. Good health should be a top priority in life. Although it is best to incorporate healthful behavior before illness develops, remind patients that it is never too late to work toward improving their health.

Protection From Injury

Many accidents happen because people fail to see potential risks and do not develop plans of action. Following safety measures at home, at work, at play, and while traveling can help prevent injury. A discussion of ways to avoid accidents and injury should be part of the educational process. Tips for preventing injury at home and at work are listed in Figure 14-3.

Facts from the latest National Safety Council data (2003) provide information on in-home deaths of people of all ages. These facts indicate that the home is not as safe as people think. According to this data, people are most likely to die in the home in the following ways:

- Falls (33%)
- Poisoning by solids (29%)
- Fires and burns (10%)
- Suffocation by ingestion (5%)
- Drowning (3%)
- Mechanical suffocation (2%)
- Poisoning by gases or vapors (1%)
- All other (15%)

Another essential aspect of educating patients about injury prevention is teaching them about the proper use of medications. A prescription includes specific instructions for taking the medication. Emphasize to the patient that these instructions must be followed exactly. In addition, the patient must not change the dosage or mix medications of any kind without first checking with the physician. Patients who do not adhere to these rules run the risk of potentially dangerous side effects. Tell patients to report to the physician any unusual reactions experienced when taking medications.

When providing a patient with a new prescription, always ask the patient if he has told the doctor about all the medications he is already taking, including herbs and over-the-counter (OTC) medications. If the patient tells you that he has not, immediately inform the physician before the

---

Tips for Preventing Injury

At Home

- Install smoke detectors, carbon monoxide detectors, and fire extinguishers.
- Keep all medicines, chemicals, and household cleaning solutions out of reach of children. Purchase products in childproof containers. Lock or attach childproof latches to all cabinets, medicine chests, and drawers that contain poisonous items.
- Keep chemicals in their original containers, and store them out of children's reach.
- Install adequate lighting in rooms and hallways. Install railings on stairs.
- Use nonskid backing on rugs to help prevent falls, or remove rugs altogether.
- In the bathroom use nonskid mats or strips that stick to the tub floor.
- Stay with young children when they are in the bathroom.
- Don't rely on bathseats or rings as a safety device for babies and children.
- Set the water temperature on the water heater at 120 degrees F.
- Practice good kitchen safety: Store knives and kitchen tools properly. Unplug small appliances when not in use. Wipe up spills immediately.
- Shorten long electrical cords and speaker wires, or secure them with electrical tape. Avoid plugging too many electrical appliances into the same outlet.
- Never use appliances in the bathtub or near a sink filled with water.
- Exercise caution when using electrical appliances. Use outlet covers when outlets are not in use.
- To reach high places, use proper equipment, such as stepladders, not chairs.
- Use child gates.

At Work

- Use appropriate safety equipment and protective gear, as required.
- Lift heavy objects properly: Bend at the knees, not at the waist. As you straighten your legs, bring the object close to your body quickly. That way, strong leg muscles do the lifting, not weaker back muscles. Never attempt to move furniture on your own. Request that a member of the office building maintenance staff be engaged to do so.
- Use surge protectors on computer equipment to prevent overloading outlets.
- Make sure hallways, entrance areas, work areas, offices, and parking lots are well lit.
- If your job involves desk work, practice proper posture when sitting. Do not sit for long periods of time. Get up and stretch, or walk down the hall and back.

Figure 14-3. You can help patients stay healthy by instructing them about ways to avoid injury.

patient leaves the office. Medications taken together can change the desired drug response. The physician needs to know about *all* drugs as well as herbal preparations and OTC medications that the patient is taking.

Preventive Measures

Preventive health care is an area in which patient education plays a vital role. Patients need to know that they can decrease their chances of getting certain illnesses and diseases by taking preventive measures and avoiding certain behaviors. Preventive techniques can be described on three levels: health-promoting behaviors, screening, and rehabilitation.

Health-Promoting Behaviors. The first level of disease and illness prevention involves adopting the health-promoting behaviors described in the section titled Healthful Habits. This primary level of prevention also includes educating patients about the symptoms and warning signs of disease. One example is informing patients about the warning signs of cancer. The first letters of these warning signs spell the word *caution*. They are as follows:

- **C**hange in bowel or bladder habits
- **A** sore that does not heal
- **U**nusual bleeding or discharge
- **T**hickening or lump in a breast or elsewhere
- **I**ndigestion or difficulty in swallowing
- **O**bvious change in a wart or mole
- **N**agging cough or hoarseness

Screening. The second level of disease prevention is screening. **Screening** involves the diagnostic testing of a patient who is typically free of symptoms. Screening allows early diagnosis and treatment of certain diseases. Examples of screening tests include mammography and Pap smears for women and prostate examinations for men.

Annual screening is important to health maintenance. Although the requirements may differ according to the age and condition of the patient, most annual screenings usually include:

- Routine blood work
- Urinalysis
- Chest x-ray
- EKG (electrocardiogram)
- Physical examination (PE)

Rehabilitation. The third level of disease prevention involves the rehabilitation and management of an existing illness. At this level the disease process remains stable, but the body will probably not heal any further. The objective is to maintain functionality and avoid further disability. Examples of this level of prevention include stroke rehabilitation programs, cardiac rehabilitation, and pain management for a condition such as arthritis.

The Patient Information Packet

When patients come to the medical practice, they need to learn not only about health and medical issues but also about the medical office itself. The patient information packet explains the medical practice and its policies. Unlike most other patient education materials, the patient information packet deals mainly with administrative matters rather than with medical issues.

The patient information packet may be as simple as a one-page brochure or pamphlet. It may be a multi-page brochure, however, or a folder with multiple-page inserts.

Benefits of the Information Packet

The patient information packet is a simple, effective, and inexpensive way to improve the relationship between the office and the patients. It provides important information about the practice and the office staff. This information helps patients feel more comfortable with the qualifications of the health-care professionals involved in their care. The packet may help clarify the roles that each office staff member has in patient care.

The information packet also informs patients of office policies and procedures. Patients will learn the doctor's office hours, how to schedule appointments, the office's payment policies, and other administrative details. This information helps limit misunderstandings about these procedures.

The patient information packet also benefits the office staff. It is both an excellent marketing tool and an aid to running the office more smoothly. Providing patients with a prepared information packet saves staff time by answering a number of potential patient inquiries. The information packet is also a good way to acquaint new office staff members with office policies.

Contents of the Information Packet

Regardless of what material the information packet contains, it must be written in clear language so that patients are able to read and understand it. All materials should be written at a sixth-grade level for reading ease of all patients. Information should not be presented in a technical medical style. Because you may be responsible for preparing portions of the policy packet, you should be familiar with the contents of a typical packet.

Introduction to the Office. A brief introduction serves to welcome the patient to the office. It may be helpful to summarize the office's philosophy of patient care. The office's **philosophy** means the system of values and principles the office has adopted in its everyday practices.

Physician's Qualifications. The packet commonly contains information about the physician's professional qualifications and training. It includes details about education, internship, and residency. It may list credentials such as board certification or board eligibility in a certain medical specialty. It may also list the physician's membership in professional societies. The information packet for a group practice may contain a paragraph or a page for each physician.

Description of the Practice. It is helpful to include a brief description of the practice, particularly if it is a specialty practice. Explaining the types of examinations or procedures that are commonly performed in the office may be useful. It may also be helpful to list any special services the office provides, such as physical examinations for employment, workers' compensation cases, or other occupational services. Be sure to make medical terms and specialties clear by avoiding the use of initials. Spell out everything the first time the reference is made and place the appropriate initials in parentheses.

Introduction to the Office Staff. Many patients are not familiar with the qualifications and duties of the various members of the office staff. It is a good idea, therefore, to identify the staff members according to their responsibilities and duties. Patients need to understand that some duties commonly thought to be a nurse's responsibilities may also be performed by a medical assistant. It may be helpful to include the professional credentials and licenses of key staff members.

Office Hours. This section should list the exact days and hours the office is open, including holidays. In addition, patients need to know what to do if an emergency occurs outside regular office hours. Tell the patient what number to call first (for example, the answering service, 911, or the hospital emergency room) and what to do next. Include the telephone number and address of the emergency room at the hospital with which the doctor is affiliated. Assure patients that the doctor can be reached at all times through the answering service. Some practices have multiple offices, and the physicians rotate from office to office on a regular schedule. List all office addresses and phone numbers along with directions to all office sites.

Appointment Scheduling. This section of the packet should explain the procedure for scheduling and canceling appointments. You might suggest that patients can benefit by scheduling routine checkups and visits as far in advance as possible. Also note if certain times of the day are reserved for sudden or unexpected office visits.

In this section encourage patients to be on time for appointments. Explain the problems that result from late or broken appointments. If the office charges a fee for breaking an appointment without advance notice, mention it here. Be careful to address these sensitive areas with a positive, nonthreatening tone. The office's written material should simply state the office policies and the problems that can result when functioning outside the policies.

Telephone Policy. Providing the office's telephone policies in the information packet can help reduce the number of unnecessary calls to the office and thus save time for the office staff. Explain which procedures can be handled over the telephone and which cannot. Explain procedures such as calling in for prescription renewals or laboratory test results. If the physician returns patients' calls at a certain time of day, mention that policy in this section. Some practices bill patients for telephone calls in which medical advice is given but not for follow-up calls. For example, if a parent of a child who was vomiting uncontrollably called the physician to get immediate medical advice, the call might be billed. If the physician called to inform a patient of test results, however, the call would not be billed.

Some offices (particularly pediatric offices) schedule a certain time of the day for patients (or parents and guardians) to call the physician for answers to their questions. This type of policy benefits both the office and the patients. The patients (or parents) have the assurance that they can speak with the physician about their concerns, and the office is spared interruptions during other times of the day.

Payment Policies. Inform patients of the office's policies regarding payment and billing. State whether payment is expected at the time of a visit or whether the patient can be billed. List accepted forms of payment (for example, cash, personal checks, and credit cards). It is not common practice to mention specific fees in an information packet.

Insurance Policies. Advise patients to bring proof of insurance coverage and the proper claim forms when they visit the office. State whether the office submits claim forms directly to the insurance company or whether the patient has this responsibility. Outline the practice's policy for handling Medicare coverage, including whether the office accepts patients who do not have supplemental insurance. Explain that the staff will help patients fill out insurance forms when necessary. Advise the patient of the office's policy for form completion. Include the amount of time that the patient should allow for completion and any fees that the office charges.

Patient Confidentiality Statement. The information packet must include a copy of the office privacy policy. Complete information regarding the privacy policy and HIPAA regulations can be found in Chapter 3 in the section titled HIPAA Privacy Rules. It is important to remember that the first step in informing patients of HIPAA compliance is the communication of patient rights. These rights are communicated through the Notice of Privacy Practices (NPP), which must adhere to the following specifications:

- Be written in plain, simple language.
- Include a header that reads "This notice describes how medical information about you may be used and disclosed and how you can get access to this information. Please review carefully."

- Describe the medical office's uses and disclosures of personal health information.
- Describe an individual's rights under the Privacy Rule.
- Describe the medical office's duties regarding patient privacy.
- Describe how patients can register complaints concerning suspected privacy violations.
- Specify a point of contract.
- Specify an effective date.
- State that the medical office reserves to right to change its privacy practices.

The information packet must also state that no information from patient files will be released without a signed authorization from the patient.

Other Information. The patient information packet may include the practice's policy on referrals. It may provide information about access to available community health resources or agencies. It may also include special instructions for common office procedures (for example, whether the patient needs to fast before a procedure or to avoid certain foods).

Distributing the Information Packet

For the information packet to be effective, you must make sure that new patients receive and read it. One way is to hand the packet to new patients at the time of their first office visit and briefly review the contents with them (Figure 14-4). Explain that they can find answers to many questions in the packet. Encourage patients to take the packet home, read the information, and keep it handy for future reference.

When new patients make an appointment, many offices send them a copy of the information packet if there is

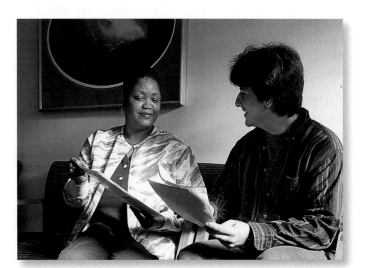

Figure 14-4. Give patients the patient information packet on their first visit to the office, or mail it prior to their first appointment.

enough time before the appointment to get it to them by regular mail. (It is a nice gesture to include a detailed map or written directions to the office for new patients who are not familiar with the area.) Patients can review the packet before coming to the office and can ask questions during the visit. Additional copies of the packet should be placed in an accessible area in the office so that patients can take them home.

Special Concerns

Some practices serve patients who cannot read well or who do not speak or understand English. It may be necessary to create a second information packet that is written in very simple terms and that presents information through pictures and charts. The information packet can also be translated into one or more languages.

It is important that patients understand the office's policies and procedures. Additional one-on-one explanations may be required. Patients should still receive the printed materials to take home, however. Family members or friends may be able to read the materials for them, reinforcing what they learned in the office.

Educating Patients With Special Needs

During your career as a medical assistant, you will probably encounter many patients with special needs. Each patient's individual circumstances will affect your approach to patient education. In all cases try to see situations from the point of view of the patient. In many instances you can enlist the support of family or friends to aid in the educational process.

Elderly Patients

You will probably be called on to provide care for more and more elderly patients as the number of older people continues to grow (Figure 14-5). Patient education for elderly patients is especially valuable because it can help them prevent or manage health problems and remain independent. You may need to educate some older people about the importance of taking measures to protect their health.

You may work with elderly patients who have hearing or vision problems or physical limitations that restrict their ability to perform certain tasks. Keep the following suggestions in mind when working with elderly patients.

- Treat each patient as an individual. This point is perhaps the most important to remember when dealing with elderly patients. Some older people have trouble understanding directions. Try to communicate with them at the highest level they can understand. Never talk down to patients.
- Put instructions in writing. Because some elderly patients have problems with memory, detailed written

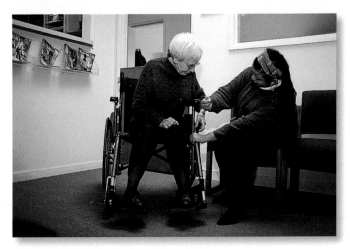

Figure 14-5. When instructing elderly patients, remember that each patient is an individual with unique needs.

instructions are an essential aspect of patient care. Patients can refer to the instructions as necessary or can ask a relative to do so.

- Adjust procedures as needed. When demonstrating a procedure to elderly patients, keep in mind any physical limitations they may have, and adjust the procedure accordingly. Make sure patients understand the instructions by asking them to perform the procedure for you.

Patients With Mental Impairments

Patients with impaired mental functions include those with **dementia,** Alzheimer's disease, mental retardation, drug addictions, and emotional problems. These patients can be challenging to deal with because communication may be difficult. Tact and empathy are important. A key to dealing with these patients is to speak at their level of understanding. Again, you must try to meet patients' needs without talking down to them.

Patients With Hearing Impairments

Patients with hearing impairments may have conditions ranging from mild impairment to total hearing loss. It is a common mistake to treat these patients as though they have mental impairments. Although you may have difficulty communicating with these patients, remember that their inability to hear has nothing to do with their level of intelligence. The Educating the Patient section provides techniques for educating patients who have hearing impairments.

Patients With Visual Impairments

As with hearing impairment, the level of visual impairment can vary significantly from patient to patient. Determining the severity of a patient's condition allows you to tailor your instruction to the patient's needs.

Educating the Patient

Instructing Patients With Hearing Impairments

Educating patients who have hearing impairments need not be difficult if you pay a little extra attention in the following areas.

- Try to eliminate all background noise. Talk in a quiet room, if possible.
- Make sure the room is well lit.
- Face the patient, and make sure the patient can see your mouth. Having the patient watch your mouth movements can help him understand what you are saying.
- Speak loudly and clearly, but do not shout.
- Use visual aids as necessary.
- Tell patients to let you know right away if they cannot hear you or do not catch something you have said. Even patients who do not have hearing impairments often appear to understand what a medical professional is saying rather than admit they are confused. It is a good idea to ask patients to repeat information to you to check their understanding. Also, periodically ask if they

would like you to go over any particular part of the explanation or instructions again.

An additional point to keep in mind when dealing with patients who have hearing impairments is that loss of hearing can cause them to withdraw and feel isolated. Being empathic and patient greatly enhances the educational process.

Elderly Patients With Hearing Loss

Most people experience a gradual loss of hearing as they get older. In addition to the preceding suggestions, try to talk in a lower pitch whenever possible. As people get older, they often have more trouble understanding higher tones.

Patients Who Wear Hearing Aids

When talking to a patient who wears a hearing aid, it is best to speak at a normal level. Many hearing aids make a normal voice louder but filter out loud noises. If you raise your voice, the hearing aid may filter it out. Consequently, the patient may hear only broken speech.

For those with mildly impaired vision, the approach may be as simple as providing instructional materials printed in large type. In addition, you can demonstrate procedures in a well-lit area and close to the patients. For more severe visual impairment, adjust the level of instruction appropriately. For example, to demonstrate how to use a particular knob on a wheelchair, you might actually place the patient's hand on the knob and discuss its function.

When speaking to someone who has a visual impairment, remember to use a normal tone of voice. A patient with a visual impairment does not necessarily also have a hearing impairment. Although you should never talk down to patients, you need to verify that they understand all verbal instructions. Have the patient repeat all instructions to you.

Giving procedural instructions may be a challenge, depending on the patient's ability to perform certain tasks. Suggest that patients ask a family member or friend to help them with procedures they have trouble doing on their own.

Multicultural Issues

Patients who come from diverse cultures often have different beliefs about the causes and treatment of illness. These differences may affect their treatment expectations and their willingness to follow instructions or agree to have certain procedures performed on them. There may also be communication problems if the patient does not understand English well. Communicating with patients in these situations is discussed in Chapter 4.

Patient Education Prior to Surgery

One instance in which patient education is vital to a successful outcome is the instruction given before a patient undergoes a surgical procedure. Although exact instructions vary according to the procedure, their purpose is to prepare the patient for the procedure and to aid the patient during the recovery period. Instructions may include verbal, written, and demonstrative techniques.

The Role of the Medical Assistant

Patients generally receive information about the need for surgery and its nature from the physician. Educating and preparing patients for surgery will probably be your responsibility, however. You may provide support and explanations to patients. You must verify that they understand any information they may have been given by other members of the health-care team. Preoperative instruction may include discussion of postoperative care issues, such as temporary dietary restrictions.

You may also be responsible for determining whether patients have all the information they need before surgery, from both an educational and a legal standpoint. All patients who are undergoing a surgical procedure must first sign an informed consent form. As stated in Chapter 9, this legal document provides specific information about the surgical procedure, including its purpose, the possible risks, and the expected outcome. The informed consent form, along with documentation of all preoperative instruction, must be put in the patient's chart.

Benefits of Preoperative Education

Preoperative education has many benefits. It increases patients' overall satisfaction with their care. It helps reduce patient anxiety and fear, use of pain medication, complications following surgery, and recovery time. Letting the patient know what to expect during the surgery and afterward allows the patient to participate in all aspects of the surgical procedure.

Types of Preoperative Teaching

Three types of teaching should occur during the preoperative period: factual, sensory, and participatory. The combination of these teaching methods gives the patient an overall understanding of the surgical procedure.

Factual. Factual teaching informs the patient of details about the procedure. You should tell the patient what will happen during the surgery, when it will happen, and why the procedure is necessary. Factual information also includes restrictions on diet or activity that may be necessary both before and after surgery. Procedure 14-2 describes how to inform patients of guidelines for surgery.

Sensory. Give patients a description of the physical sensations they may have during the procedure. All five senses may be involved: feeling, seeing, hearing, tasting, and smelling.

Participatory. Participatory teaching includes demonstrations of techniques that may be necessary or helpful during the postoperative period. Aspects of postoperative care include cleaning the wound, changing the dressing, and applying ice packs.

During this phase of teaching, you need to first describe the technique to the patient and then demonstrate it. The patient should repeat the demonstration for you. This practice is called **return demonstration**. If any aspects of the technique are unclear to the patient, you should demonstrate the technique again. The patient should be capable of performing the procedure properly. This process of teaching a new skill by having the patient observe and imitate is called **modeling.**

Using Anatomical Models

An anatomical model is a useful tool in preoperative education. As shown in Figure 14-6, looking at a lifelike model—and being able to see the actual body structures—helps patients better understand their condition. A model also allows patients to see how the surgical procedure will help correct their problem.

PROCEDURE 14.2

Informing the Patient of Guidelines for Surgery

Objective: To inform a preoperative patient of the necessary guidelines to follow prior to surgery

Materials: Patient chart, surgical guidelines

Method

1. Review the patient's chart to determine the type of surgery to be performed.
2. Tell the patient that you will be providing both verbal and written instructions that should be followed prior to surgery.
3. Inform the patient about policies regarding makeup, jewelry, contact lenses, wigs, dentures, and so on.
4. Tell the patient to leave money and valuables at home.
5. If applicable, suggest appropriate clothing for the patient to wear for postoperative ease and comfort.
6. Explain the need for someone to drive the patient home following an outpatient surgical procedure.
7. Tell the patient the correct time to arrive in the office or at the hospital for the procedure.

8. Inform the patient of dietary restrictions. Be sure to use specific, clear instructions about what may or may not be ingested and at what time the patient must abstain from eating or drinking. Also explain these points:
   a. The reasons for the dietary restrictions
   b. The possible consequences of not following the dietary restrictions
9. Ask patients who smoke to refrain from or reduce cigarette smoking during at least the 8 hours prior to the procedure. Explain to the patient that reducing smoking improves the level of oxygen in the blood during surgery.
10. Suggest that the patient shower or bathe the morning of the procedure or the evening before.
11. Instruct the patient about medications to take or avoid before surgery.
12. If necessary, clarify any information about which the patient is unclear.
13. Provide written surgical guidelines, and suggest that the patient call the office if additional questions arise.
14. Document the instruction in the patient's chart.

It may be difficult for a patient to visualize exactly what will take place in some surgical procedures. For example, think of arthroscopy of the knee. When told that the doctor will insert a viewing instrument into the knee, patients probably have no idea of the size of this scope. As a result, they may be particularly fearful of the procedure. Using a model to show exactly what will happen can ease patients' fears.

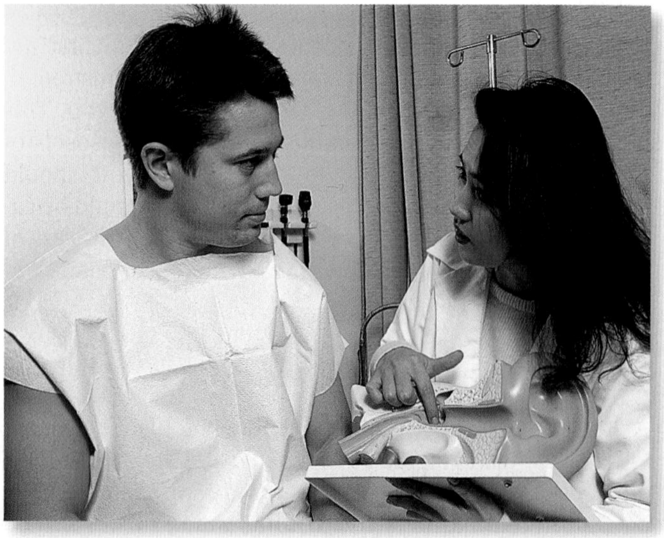

Helping Relieve Patient Anxiety

When you provide preoperative education, be aware that the fear and anxiety of patients who are about to undergo a surgical procedure can adversely affect the learning process. Consequently, allow extra time for repetition and reinforcement of material.

Always consider your choice of words carefully, stressing the positive rather than the negative whenever possible. Involving family members in the educational process is often beneficial, particularly if the patient is especially apprehensive about the surgery. Remember to present your instructions and explanations in straightforward language that they can understand. Family members can often help relieve the patient's anxiety.

Verifying Patient Understanding

The key to the success of any educational process is verifying that patients have actually understood the information. A good way to check for understanding is to have patients

Figure 14-6. An anatomical model can help patients visualize what will happen during surgery.

Alzheimer's Association
70 East Lake Street
Chicago, IL 60601-5997
(800) 621-0379
(800) 572-6037 (in Illinois)
(312) 335-8882 (hearing-impaired)

American Academy of Pediatrics
Publications Department
P.O. Box 927
Elk Grove, IL 60009-0927
(708) 228-5005

American Cancer Society
777 Third Avenue
New York, NY 10017
(212) 586-8700

American Diabetes Association
Two Park Avenue
New York, NY 10016
(800) ADA-DISC
(212) 683-7444

American Dietetic Association
216 West Jackson Boulevard, Suite 800
Chicago, IL 60606-6995
(800) 366-1655

American Heart Association
7272 Greenville Avenue
Dallas, TX 75231-4596
(800) 242-8721
(214) 750-5300

American Red Cross
17th and D Street, NW
Washington, DC 20006
(301) 737-8300

The Arthritis Foundation
1314 Spring Street, NW
Atlanta, GA 30309
(800) 283-7800
(404) 872-7100

Asthma and Allergy Foundation of America
1717 Massachusetts Avenue, Suite 305
Washington, DC 20036
(800) 7-ASTHMA
(202) 265-0265

National AIDS Hotline
215 Park Avenue South, Suite 714
New York, NY 10003
(800) 342-AIDS
(800) 344-SIDA (Spanish)
(800) AIDS-TTY (hearing-impaired)

National Cancer Institute
Cancer Information Clearinghouse
Office of Cancer Communications
Building 31, Room 10A18
9000 Rockville Pike
Bethesda, MD 20205
(800) 4-CANCER

National Clearinghouse for
Alcohol and Drug Information
P.O. Box 2345
Rockville, MD 20852
(301) 468-2600

National Health Information Center
P.O. Box 1133
Washington, DC 20013-1133
(800) 336-4797
(301) 565-4167 (in Maryland)
(The information specialists at this agency can provide
telephone numbers for associations that deal with
specific diseases or problems.)

National Kidney Foundation
30 East 33d Street
New York, NY 10016
(212) 889-2210

National Organization for Rare Disorders (NORD)
100 Route 37, P.O. Box 8923
New Fairfield, CT 06812
(800) 999-NORD

President's Council on Physical Fitness and Sports
Department of Health and Human Services
Washington, DC 20001
(202) 272-3421

Figure 14-7. The addresses and telephone numbers listed are for national headquarters. Check your telephone book for local listings.

explain in their own words what they have learned. In addition, have them engage in return demonstrations.

Additional Educational Resources

Besides the resources available in the medical office, a vast number of outside resources are available for patient education. You can use these resources to obtain information for your own use in patient education, or you can mention them to patients who are looking for additional information. Following are several sources of patient education materials:

- Libraries and patient resource rooms. Most public libraries have an assortment of books, magazines, and electronic databases pertaining to health and medical topics. Many hospitals provide patient resource rooms, which include a variety of educational materials—such as books, brochures, and videotapes—for public use.

- Computer resources. A great deal of up-to-date medical information can be accessed through online services and CD-ROMs. The Internet is another widely used source of medical information.

- Community resources. Many local social service agencies provide specialized health information related to such topics as nursing home care, visiting nurses' care, counseling, and rehabilitation. Most of these agencies are listed in the telephone book. Area hospitals, the library, and the local chamber of commerce are other good sources for these services.

- Associations. Thousands of health organizations and associations can be contacted for information about preventive health care and virtually every known disease or disorder. The names, addresses, and telephone numbers of these organizations are provided in several directories, which are available at most libraries. Figure 14-7 provides a sample list of patient resource organizations.

Career Opportunities

Occupational Therapy Assistant

To gain medical assistant credentials, you must fulfill the requirements of either the American Association of Medical Assistants (for a Certified Medical Assistant) or the American Medical Technologists (for a Registered Medical Assistant). After obtaining your medical assistant certification or registration, you may wish to acquire additional skills in specialty areas through course work or on-the-job training. Although this course work or training may not lead to an additional certification or degree, it will enable you to expand your role in the medical office and advance your career as the demand for skilled health professionals increases.

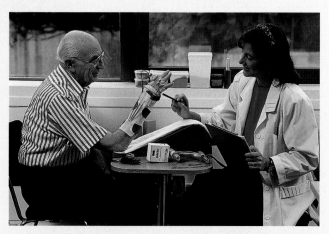

Skills and Duties

An occupational therapy assistant helps patients learn, or relearn, basic and special skills they need to function in their daily lives. Patient interaction is the focus of the occupational therapy assistant's job. An occupational therapy assistant works under the supervision of an occupational therapist.

Occupational therapists teach many different types of skills to many different types of patients. These skills include the following:

- Basic life skills, such as dressing and feeding oneself or moving about at home. For example,

patients with partial paralysis or nerve damage resulting from a stroke may need this type of help.

- Vocational skills, such as typing. These skills will help patients with disabilities get jobs to support themselves.

- Designing and supervising arts and crafts activities. These activities serve as recreation and help patients develop fine motor skills in a nonthreatening, pleasant atmosphere.

- Helping accident victims who have an injured limb or a prosthetic device learn new ways to

continued ⟶

Occupational Therapy Assistant *(continued)*

perform simple tasks. A patient with a prosthetic hand, for example, may need help learning to open jar lids.

- Working with patients who have behavioral or emotional disturbances. Occupational therapy may help these patients express their feelings in constructive ways, by building an interest in music, drama, or art.

The occupational therapy assistant also performs a number of clerical and administrative tasks. He checks inventories, orders supplies, and helps maintain the equipment in his workplace. He may also be responsible for paperwork, including writing reports on therapy sessions with patients.

Workplace Settings

Occupational therapy assistants often work in hospitals. They may also find work in clinics or long-term care facilities, such as retirement communities with assisted-care services, nursing homes, or rehabilitation centers. Some occupational therapists are employed in educational settings, including occupational workshops and schools for children with special needs.

Education

Community colleges and vocational schools offer 2-year programs for an associate degree in occupational therapy assisting. By completing a program approved by the American Occupational Therapy Association and passing a qualifying test, you can become a Certified Occupational Therapy Assistant (COTA).

Where to Go for More Information

The American Occupational Therapy Association
4720 Montgomery Lane
P.O. Box 31220
Bethesda, MD 20824-1220
(301) 948-9626

American Society of Hand Therapists
401 North Michigan Avenue
Chicago, IL 60611
(312) 321-6866

Summary

Patient education plays a key role in many aspects of patient care. Knowledgeable patients are able to take an active approach to their own medical care. They are also likely to be aware of the benefits of activities that promote and protect their health.

There are many reasons for patient education in the medical office. Patients need to understand their medical conditions and to be prepared for necessary procedures. Many opportunities exist to educate patients about the benefits of good health. In addition, patients need to be informed of the policies of the medical office.

Many educational resources are available to both medical assistants and patients. The key for medical assistants is to take advantage of all opportunities to educate patients and to match this teaching to the needs of individual patients.

REVIEW

CASE STUDY *QUESTIONS*

Now that you have completed this chapter, review the case study at the beginning of the chapter and answer the following questions:

1. What might be important to consider when creating an educational plan for a patient? How might the plan vary according to the individual?
2. What factors could block effective patient education?
3. What specific behaviors do you associate with talking down to a patient?
4. Why are good listening skills an important part of teaching?

Discussion Questions

1. Why is it important to educate patients about how to take care of themselves?
2. Patients spend less time in the hospital than ever before. How does this change the role of private medical offices and the role of medical assistants in those practices?
3. What are some good ways to get patients to read printed materials?

Critical Thinking Questions

1. A patient and her grown daughter meet with the physician in your medical office. She receives some bad news and is crying. The daughter is trying to comfort her. It is your job now to explain what will happen next in her care, including procedures and appointment schedules for some important tests in the hospital. How will you proceed?

2. You are measuring the vital signs of an overweight woman. She becomes visibly upset when you ask her to step on the scale. The office has many brochures with tips on promoting good health and exercise. How might you bring up the subject of proper diet and exercise?

Application Activities

1. Develop an educational plan for the overweight patient mentioned in the critical thinking questions. Have another student assume the role of the patient, and practice implementing your plan. Ask the other student to evaluate your teaching method.
2. Write the section of a patient information brochure that describes the general roles of the medical office staff. Exchange your writing sample with that of another student, and critique each other's work.
3. With a partner, role-play a medical assistant giving procedural instructions to a patient with a hearing impairment. Then switch roles, and offer suggestions for improving each other's teaching techniques.

SECTION 3

FINANCIAL RESPONSIBILITIES

CHAPTER 15
Processing Health-Care Claims

CHAPTER 16
Medical Coding

CHAPTER 17
Patient Billing and Collections

CHAPTER 18
Accounting for the Medical Office

CHAPTER 15

Processing Health-Care Claims

KEY TERMS

allowed charge
assignment of benefits
balance billing
benefits
birthday rule
capitation
Centers for Medicare and
    Medicaid Services
    (CMS)
CHAMPVA
clearinghouse
coinsurance
coordination of benefits
co-payment
deductible
disability insurance
electronic data
    interchange (EDI)
exclusion
fee-for-service
fee schedule
formulary
health maintenance
    organization (HMO)
liability insurance
lifetime maximum benefit
managed care
    organization (MCO)
Medicaid
Medicare
Medicare + Choice Plan
Medigap
Original Medicare Plan
participating physicians
preferred provider
    organization (PPO)
premium
referral
remittance advice (RA)
resource-based relative
    value scale (RBRVS)
third-party payer
TRICARE
X12 837 Health Care
    Claim

AREAS OF COMPETENCE

2003 Role Delineation Study

ADMINISTRATIVE

Administrative Procedures

- Understand and apply third-party guidelines
- Obtain reimbursement through accurate claims submissions
- Monitor third-party reimbursement
- Understand and adhere to managed care policies and procedures

CLINICAL

Patient Care

- Coordinate patient care information with other health-care providers

GENERAL

Communication Skills

- Utilize electronic technology to receive, organize, prioritize, and transmit information

Legal Concepts

- Follow employer's established policies dealing with the health-care contract
- Implement and maintain federal and state health-care legislation and regulations

CHAPTER OUTLINE

- Basic Insurance Terminology
- Types of Health Plans
- The Claims Process: An Overview
- Fee Schedules and Charges
- Preparing and Transmitting Health-Care Claims

OBJECTIVES

After completing Chapter 15, you will be able to:

15.1 List the basic steps of the health insurance claim process.
15.2 Describe your role in insurance claims processing.
15.3 Explain how payers set fees.
15.4 Define Medicare and Medicaid.
15.5 Discuss TRICARE and CHAMPVA health-care benefits programs.
15.6 Distinguish between HMOs and PPOs.

15.7 Explain how to manage a workers' compensation case.

15.8 Apply rules related to coordination of benefits.

15.9 Describe the health-care claim preparation process.

15.10 Complete a Centers for Medicare and Medicaid Service (CMS-1500) claim form.

15.11 Identify three ways to transmit electronic claims.

Introduction

Health-care claims are a critical part of the reimbursement process. Accurate claims sent to payers mean that physicians receive the maximum appropriate payment for the services they provide. Patients are also concerned with their health-care plans, asking "How much will my insurance pay?" "How much will I owe?" "Why are these doctor's fees different from my previous doctor's fees?"

You will handle questions such as these every day. Not only must you correctly prepare health-care claims, but you will also review patients' insurance coverage, explain the physician's fees, estimate what charges payers will cover, and prepare claims for patients. This chapter prepares you for these tasks by explaining the types of health-care insurance patients have, how payers set the charges they pay for providers' services, and how to transmit complete and accurate claims. This chapter also gives you the information you need about patients' financial responsibilities for services so that you can figure out how much patients should pay and how much will be billed to their health-care plans.

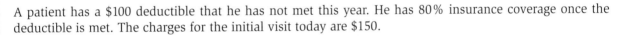

CASE STUDY

A patient has a $100 deductible that he has not met this year. He has 80% insurance coverage once the deductible is met. The charges for the initial visit today are $150.

As you read this chapter, consider the following questions:

1. How much should this patient pay?
2. How much will he owe for his next visit this year, which is expected to have a charge of $200?
3. Assuming that the patient in the case study has a managed care policy, what type of policy does he probably have?
4. What term would you use to describe the part of the payment that is based on 20% of the charges?
5. If you did not know whether the deductible had been met, what procedure would you follow?

Basic Insurance Terminology

The first step in understanding insurance is to learn some basic terminology. Medical insurance, which is also known as health insurance, is a written contract in the form of a policy between a policyholder and a health plan (insurance carrier). The policyholder may also be called the insured, the member, or the subscriber.

Under the insurance policy, the policyholder pays a **premium.** In exchange, the health plan provides **benefits**—payments for medical services—for a specified time period. The policy may cover dependents of the policyholder, such as a spouse or children. The contract may specify a **lifetime maximum benefit,** which is a total sum that the health plan will pay out over the patient's life.

There are actually three participants under insurance contracts. The patient (policyholder) is the *first party,* and the physician who provides medical services is the *second party.* A patient-physician contract is created when a physician agrees to treat a patient who seeks medical services. Through this unwritten contract, the patient is legally responsible for paying for services. The patient may have a policy with a health plan, the *third party,* which agrees to carry the risk of paying for those services and therefore is called a **third-party payer.**

Depending on the type of health plan, the policyholder may pay a **deductible**—a fixed dollar amount that must be paid or "met" once a year before the third-party payer begins to cover medical expenses. The patient may also have to pay **coinsurance,** a fixed percentage of coverage charges after the deductible is met. The coinsurance rate presents the health plan's percentage of the charge followed by the insured's percentage, such as 80-20. The patient often must pay a **co-payment,** a small fee that is collected at the time of the visit. The health plan then pays the covered amount of the charges.

Some expenses, such as routine eye examinations or dental care, may not be covered under the insured's contract. Uncovered expenses are **exclusions.** Many plans offer a prescription drug benefit. Such benefits usually require the use of drugs that are listed on the plan's **formulary,** a list of approved brands.

Two special types of insurance are liability insurance and disability insurance. **Liability insurance** covers injuries that are caused by the insured or that occurred on the insured's property. If an individual (or company) has home, business, automobile, or health liability insurance, the injured person can claim benefits under the insured's policy. To obtain details about coverage, contact the liability insurance company.

Disability insurance is a type of insurance that may be provided by an employer for its employees or purchased privately by self-employed individuals. Disability insurance is activated when the insured is injured or disabled. When the insured cannot work, the insurance company pays the insured a prearranged monthly amount that covers the insured's normal expenses. Generally, disability is far more expensive than life, home, or automobile insurance.

Types of Health Plans

All insurance companies have their own rules about benefits and procedures. Many companies also have their own manuals, printed or online, which you must keep handy in the office for reference. Representatives of the insurance companies are available to work with you, however, to answer questions and help ensure that claims are correctly filed. Their business depends on it. Never hesitate to contact an insurance company. Many have toll-free numbers and Web sites for just this purpose.

There are many sources of health plans in the United States. The majority of individuals with insurance are covered by group policies, usually through their employers. Some people have individual plans. Many are covered under a government plan. Still others—over 40 million Americans—have no health-care insurance.

Fee-for-Service and Managed Care Plans

There are two major types of health plans: fee-for-service plans and managed care plans. **Fee-for-service** plans, the oldest and most expensive type, repay policyholders for costs of health care due to illnesses and accidents. The policy lists the medical services that are covered. The amount charged for services is controlled by the physician who provides them. The benefit may be for all or part of the charges.

Managed care plans, in contrast, control both the financing and the delivery of health care to policyholders.

They enroll policyholders, and they also enroll physicians and other providers, controlling the delivery of health care. The **managed care organizations (MCOs)** that set up managed care health plans reach agreements with physicians and other health-care providers that control fees. Most people who are insured through their employers are covered by some form of a managed care plan.

Physicians who enroll in managed care plans are called **participating physicians.** They have contracts with the MCOs that stipulate their fees, the credentials they must have, and their responsibilities and that also explain the MCO's duties. For example, the MCO must usually publish the participating physicians' names in booklets and on a Web site so that policyholders can choose a provider from the list.

Managed care plans pay their participating physicians in one of two ways—either by contracted fees or a fixed prepayment called **capitation.** In a capitated managed care plan, providers are paid a fixed amount per month to provide necessary, contracted services to patients who are plan members. The rate the provider is paid is based on several factors, including the number of plan members in the insured pool and their ages. The capitated rate per enrollee is paid to the provider even if the provider does not provide any medical services to the patient during the time period covered by the payment. Similarly, the provider receives the same capitated rate if a patient is treated more than once during the time period. In other plans, negotiated per-service fees are paid. These fees are less than the regular rate for a service that the provider normally charges.

As shown in Figure 15-1, more than half of all health plans are **preferred provider organizations (PPOs).** A PPO is a managed care plan that establishes a network of providers to perform services for plan members. In exchange for the PPO sending them patients, the physicians agree to charge discounted fees. Plan members may usually choose to receive care from other doctors or providers outside the network, but they pay a higher charge for these visits.

Another common type of managed care system is a **health maintenance organization (HMO).** Physicians with HMO contracts are often paid a capitated rate, or they may be employees of the organization who are paid salaries. Patients who enroll in an HMO pay premiums and usually also pay a co-payment, oftentimes $10, at the time of the office visit. No other fees are required for any covered service that a member needs. In HMOs, patients must usually choose from a specific group of health-care providers for care. If they seek services from a provider who is not in the health plan, the HMO does not pay for the care. Patients also pay for excluded services.

Medicare

Several federal programs provide health care. The largest is **Medicare,** which provides health insurance for citizens aged 65 and older. Certain patients under the age of 65 may

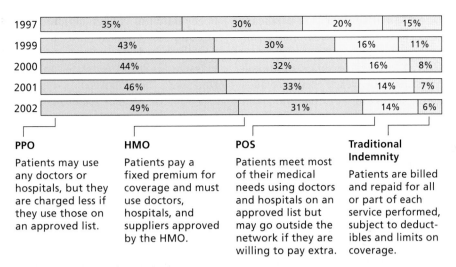

Figure 15-1. Types of health plans.

Source: Mercer's National Survey of Employer Sponsored Health Plans, 2003.
Copyright 2003, The Managed Care Information Center.

also be entitled to Medicare. Such patients include those who are blind or widowed or who have serious long-term disabilities, such as chronic joint pain or kidney failure. The Medicare program is managed by the **Centers for Medicare and Medicaid Services (CMS).**

Part A. Medicare has two parts. Part A is hospital insurance, which is billed by hospitals (or other health-care facilities). It pays most of the benefits for the following individuals:

- A patient who has been hospitalized (as an inpatient) up to 90 days for each benefit period. A benefit period begins the day a patient goes into the hospital and ends when that patient has not been hospitalized for 60 days.

- A patient who has been an inpatient in a skilled nursing facility (SNF) for no more than 100 days in each benefit period. A benefit period is usually 1 calendar year.

- A patient who is receiving medical care at home.

- A patient who has been diagnosed as terminally ill and needs hospice care. Medicare defines *terminally ill* as having a prognosis (prediction of the probable course of a disease in an individual and the chances of recovery) of 6 months or less to live. A hospice is a medical organization that provides pain relief to terminally ill patients and otherwise supports these patients and their families.

- A patient who requires psychiatric treatment. Currently Medicare covers only 190 days of psychiatric hospitalization in a patient's lifetime.

- A patient who requires respite care. Medicare provides for a respite, or short break, for the person who cares for a terminally ill patient at home. The terminally ill patient is moved to a care facility for the respite.

Anyone who receives Social Security benefits is automatically enrolled in Part A and does not have to pay a premium. Individuals aged 65 or older who are not eligible for Social Security benefits may enroll in Part A, but they must pay premiums for the coverage.

Part B. Part B helps pay for a wide range of procedures and supplies. For example, it covers physician services, outpatient hospital services, diagnostic tests, clinical laboratory services, and outpatient physical and speech therapy as long as these services are considered medically necessary. Individuals entitled to Part A benefits automatically qualify for Part B benefits. In addition, U.S. citizens and permanent residents over the age of 65 are also eligible. Part B is a voluntary program; eligible persons may or may not take part in it. However, those desiring Part B must enroll, because coverage is not automatic. Unlike Part A, Part B coverage is not premium-free. In 2003, Part B coverage cost $58.70 per month, and the premium usually increases annually.

Each Medicare enrollee receives a health insurance card. This card lists the beneficiary's name, sex, effective dates for Part A and Part B coverage, and Medicare number. The Medicare number is assigned by CMS and usually consists of the Social Security number followed by a numeric or alphanumeric suffix.

Types of Medicare Plans. Medicare beneficiaries can choose from among a number of insurance plans, including traditional fee-for-service and Medicare + Choice, which consists of a group of different plans.

Fee-for-Service: The Original Medicare Plan. The Medicare fee-for-service plan, referred to by Medicare as the **Original Medicare Plan,** allows the beneficiary to choose any licensed physician certified by Medicare. Each time the beneficiary receives services, a fee is billable. Part of this fee is generally paid by Medicare and part is due from the beneficiary. An annual deductible of $100 is the patient's responsibility. Medicare then pays 80% of approved charges and the patient is responsible for the remaining 20%.

To pay these bills, individuals enrolled in Medicare Part B Original Medicare Plan often buy additional insurance called a **Medigap** plan. These plans frequently reimburse the patient's Part B deductible and additional procedures that Medicare does not cover. If Medicare does not pay a claim, Medigap is not required to pay the claim either. Although private insurance carriers offer Medigap plans, coverage and standards are regulated by federal and state law. In exchange for Medigap coverage, the policyholder pays a monthly premium. A number of different options are available. These choices are labeled A through J. Monthly premiums vary widely across the different plan levels as well as within a single plan level, depending on the insurance company selected. While coverage varies from policy to policy, a set of core benefits is common to all Medigap plans, including the Part B coinsurance amount (usually 20% of approved charges) after the deductible ($100).

Medicare + Choice Plans.   Medicare also offers a group of plans called the **Medicare + Choice Plans.** Beneficiaries can choose to enroll in one of three major types of plans instead of the Original Medicare Plan:

1. Medicare Managed Care Plans
2. Medicare Preferred Provider Organization Plans (PPOs)
3. Medicare Private Fee-for-Service Plans

Medicare Managed Care Plans charge a monthly premium and a small co-payment for each office visit, but not a deductible. Like private payer managed care plans, Medicare managed care plans often require patients to use a specific network of physicians, hospitals, and facilities. Some plans offer the option of receiving services from providers outside the network for a higher fee. However, they offer coverage for services not reimbursed in the Original Medicare Plan, such as physical examinations and inoculations. Participants are generally required to select a primary care provider (PCP) from within the network. The PCP provides treatment and manages the patient's medical care through referrals.

In the *Medicare Preferred Provider Organization Plan (PPO)*, patients pay less to use doctors within a network, but they may choose to go outside the network for additional costs, such as a higher co-payment or higher coinsurance. Patients do not need a PCP, and referrals are not required.

Under a *Medicare Private Fee-for-Service Plan*, patients receive services from the provider they choose, as long as Medicare has approved the provider or facility. The plan is operated by a private insurance company that contracts with Medicare to provide services to beneficiaries. The plan sets its own rates for services, and physicians are allowed to bill patients the amount of the charge not covered by the plan. A co-payment may or may not be required.

Medicaid

Medicaid, also run by CMS, is a health-benefit program designed for low-income, blind, or disabled patients; needy families; foster children; and children born with birth defects. Medicaid is a health cost assistance program, not an insurance program. The federal government provides funds to all 50 states to administer Medicaid, and states add their own funds. Every state has a program to assist with medical expenses for citizens who meet its qualifications. Such programs may have different names and slightly different rules, but they provide basically the same assistance. This assistance includes:

- Physician services
- Emergency services
- Laboratory services and x-rays
- SNF care
- Early diagnostic screening and treatment for minors (those aged 21 and younger)
- Vaccines for children

Accepting Assignment.   A physician who agrees to treat Medicaid patients also agrees to accept the established Medicaid payment for covered services. This agreement is called accepting assignment. If the physician's fee is higher than the Medicaid payment, the patient cannot be billed for the difference. The physician can bill the patient for services that Medicaid does not cover, however.

Medi/Medi.   Older or disabled patients who have Medicare and who cannot pay the difference between the bill and the Medicare payment may qualify for Medicare and Medicaid. This type of coverage is known as Medi/Medi. In such cases, Medicare is the primary payer, and Medicaid is the secondary payer.

State Guidelines.   Medicaid benefits can vary greatly from state to state. It is important to understand the Medicaid guidelines in your state so that your office's Medicaid reimbursement is prompt and trouble-free. Here are some suggestions:

- Always ask for a Medicaid card from all patients who state that they are entitled to Medicaid. Do not submit a claim to Medicaid if the patient cannot prove Medicaid membership. Doing so may constitute fraud. You may contact Medicaid to verify eligibility.
- Check the patient's Medicaid card, which is issued monthly and shows the patient's eligibility for services or procedures (Figure 15-2). Eligibility is based on how much income the patient reported for the previous month.
- Ensure that the physician signs all claims. Then send them to the state's Medicaid-approved contractor (which pays on behalf of the state) or to the state department that administers Medicaid (for example, the state department of social services or public health). Check the regulations with the state Medicaid office if you are unsure where to send the claim.
- Unless the patient has a medical emergency, Medicaid often requires authorization before services are

INDIANA MEDICAID
AND OTHER MEDICAL ASSISTANCE PROGRAMS

100341842799   001

Danny L Owens
07/19/62

Figure 15-2. A Medicaid card gives the patient's name and identification (or Social Security) number.

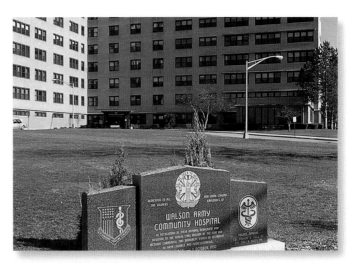

Figure 15-3. TRICARE covers health-care services for family members of military personnel and military retirees at facilities such as the military base hospital pictured here.

performed. Authorization must be obtained from the state Medicaid office in advance.

- Check the time limit on claim submissions. It can be as short as 2 months or as long as 1 year. Verify deadlines with your local Medicaid office.
- Meet the deadlines. If a Medicaid claim is submitted after the time limit, the claim may be rejected.
- Treat Medicaid patients with the same professionalism and courtesy that you extend to other patients. Simply because a patient qualifies for Medicaid assistance does not mean that the patient is in any way inferior to those with private insurance.

TRICARE and CHAMPVA

The U.S. government provides health-care benefits to families of current military personnel, retired military personnel, and veterans through the TRICARE and CHAMPVA programs. Unless you work in a military-related facility, you will probably see TRICARE and CHAMPVA patients only for emergency services or for nonemergency care that a military base cannot provide.

TRICARE. Run by the Defense Department, **TRICARE** is not a health insurance plan. Rather, it is a health-care benefit for families of uniformed personnel and retirees from the uniformed services, including the Army, Navy, Marines, Air Force, Coast Guard, Public Health Service, and National Oceanic and Atmospheric Administration (Figure 15-3). TRICARE offers families three choices of health-care benefits:

1. TRICARE Prime, a health maintenance organization
2. TRICARE Extra, a managed care network of health-care providers that families can use on a case-by-case basis without a required enrollment
3. TRICARE Standard, a fee-for-service plan

Another program, TRICARE for Life, is aimed at Medicare-eligible military retirees and Medicare-eligible family members. TRICARE for Life offers the opportunity to receive health care at a military treatment facility to individuals aged 65 and older who are eligible for both Medicare and TRICARE.

In the past, individuals became ineligible for TRICARE once they reached age 65, and they were required to enroll in Medicare to obtain any health-care coverage. Beneficiaries could still seek treatment at military treatment facilities, but only if space was available. Under TRICARE for Life, enrollees in TRICARE who are aged 65 and older can continue to obtain medical services at military hospitals and clinics as they did before they turned 65. TRICARE for Life acts as a secondary payer to Medicare; Medicare pays first, and the remaining out-of-pocket expenses are paid by TRICARE.

CHAMPVA. **CHAMPVA** (Civilian Health and Medical Program of the Veterans Administration) covers the expenses of the families (dependent spouses and children) of veterans with total, permanent, service-connected disabilities. It also covers surviving spouses and dependent children of veterans who died in the line of duty or as a result of service-connected disabilities.

TRICARE and CHAMPVA Eligibility. You must verify TRICARE eligibility. All TRICARE patients should have a valid identification card. To receive TRICARE benefits, eligible individuals must be enrolled in the Defense Enrollment Eligibility Reporting System (DEERS), a computer database.

Eligibility for CHAMPVA is determined by the nearest Veterans Affairs medical center. Contact this center if any questions arise. Patients can choose the doctor they wish after CHAMPVA eligibility is confirmed.

Under TRICARE and CHAMPVA, participating doctors have the option of deciding whether to accept patients on a case-by-case basis. Make sure you know the policy of the doctor or doctors in your office on this issue.

Blue Cross and Blue Shield

Many people think that Blue Cross and Blue Shield (BCBS) is one large corporation. Rather, it is a nationwide federation of nonprofit and for-profit service organizations that provide prepaid health-care services to BCBS subscribers. Each local organization operates under its own state laws, and specific plans for BCBS can vary greatly.

Workers' Compensation

Workers' compensation insurance covers accidents or diseases incurred in the workplace. Federal law requires employers to purchase and maintain a certain minimum amount of workers' compensation insurance for their employees. Workers' compensation laws vary from state to state. In most states, workers' compensation includes these benefits:

- Basic medical treatment.
- A weekly amount paid to the patient for a temporary disability. This amount compensates workers for loss of job income until they can return to work.
- A weekly or monthly sum paid to the patient for a permanent disability.
- Death benefits.
- Rehabilitation costs to restore an employee's ability to work again.

Not all medical practices accept workers' compensation cases. Make sure you know your office's policy. Records management of workers' compensation varies by state. Typically, you will be responsible for the following administrative tasks when a workers' compensation patient contacts the practice for the first time.

- Call the patient's employer and verify that the accident occurred on the employer's premises.
- Obtain the employer's approval to provide treatment.
- Ask the employer for the name of its workers' compensation insurance company. (Employers are required by law to carry such insurance. It is a good policy to notify your state labor department about any employer you encounter that does not have workers' compensation insurance, although you are not required to do so.) You may wish to remind the employer to report any workplace accidents or injuries that result in a workers' compensation claim to

the state labor department within 24 hours of the incident.
- Contact the insurance company and verify that the employer does indeed have a policy with the company and that the policy is in good standing.
- Obtain a claim number for the case from the insurance company. This claim number is used on all bills and paperwork.

At the time the patient starts treatment, create a patient record. If the patient is already one of the practice's regular patients, create a separate record for the workers' compensation case.

The Claims Process: An Overview

From the time the patient enters a doctor's office until the time the insurer pays the practice for that office visit and associated services, several steps are carried out. In brief, the doctor's office performs the following services:

- Obtains patient information
- Delivers services to the patient and determines the diagnosis and fee
- Records payment from the patient and prepares health-care claims
- Reviews the insurer's processing of the claim, remittance advice, and payment

Most medical assistants use a medical billing program to support administrative tasks such as:

- Gathering and recording patient information
- Verifying patients' insurance coverage
- Recording procedures and services performed
- Filing insurance claims and billing patients
- Reviewing and recording payments

Billing programs streamline the important process of creating and following up on health-care claims sent to payers and bills sent to patients. For example, a large medical practice with a group of providers and thousands of patients may receive a phone call from a patient who wants to know the amount owed on an account. With a billing program, the medical assistant can key the first few letters of the patient's last name and the patient's account data will appear on the screen. The outstanding balance can then be communicated to the patient.

Billing programs are also used to exchange health information about the practice's patients with health plans. Using electronic data interchange (EDI), similar to the technology behind ATMs, information is sent quickly and securely.

Abbreviations Related to Diagnosis

AHF	Acute heart failure
Ca	Cancer
CC	Chief complaint
CHF	Congestive heart failure
CO	Complains of
COPD	Chronic obstructive pulmonary disease
CVA	Cerebrovascular accident
DJD	Degenerative joint disease
DVT	Deep vein thrombosis
Dx	Diagnosis
ESRD	End-stage renal disease
ESRF	End-stage renal failure
FAS	Fetal alcohol syndrome
FBD	Fibrocystic breast disease
FM	Fibromyalgia
FUO	Fever of unknown origin
Fx	Fracture
GI	Gastrointestinal
HA	Headache
HPV	Human papillomavirus
Hx	History
JRA	Juvenile rheumatoid arthritis
RO	Rule out
SOM	Serous otitis media

Abbreviations Related to Procedures

AKA	Above-knee amputation
BKA	Below-knee amputation
Bx	Biopsy
CABG	Coronary artery bypass graft
CT	Computed tomography
CXR	Chest x-ray
D & C	Dilation and curettage
ERCP	Endoscopic retrograde cannulation of pancreatic (duct)
I & D	Incision and drainage
IF	Internal fixation
IVP	Intravenous pyelogram
MRI	Magnetic resonance imaging
PE	Physical examination
PET	Positron emission tomography
PFT	Pulmonary function test
PTCA	Percutaneous transluminal coronary angioplasty
T & A	Tonsilectomy and adenoidectomy
TKA	Total knee arthroplasty
Tx	Treatment

Figure 15-4. Common abbreviations used in claim forms processing.

Obtaining Patient Information

You will need certain information to be able to complete insurance claims for the patients of the medical practice where you work. This information is usually completed on a patient registration form, as shown in Chapter 9.

Basic Facts. When the patient first arrives, obtain or verify the following personal information:

- Name of patient
- Current home address
- Current home telephone number
- Date of birth (month, day, and the four digits of the year)
- Social Security number
- Next of kin or person to contact in case of an emergency

Obtain the following insurance information:

- Current employer (may be more than one)
- Employer address and telephone number
- Insurance carrier and effective date of coverage
- Insurance group plan number
- Insurance identification number (frequently the patient's Social Security number)
- Name of subscriber or insured

Depending on state law, obtain the following release signatures:

- Patient's signature on a form authorizing release of information to the insurance carrier
- Patient's signature on a form for assignment of benefits

Eligibility for Services. After you obtain personal and insurance information and release signatures from the patient, scan or copy the patient's insurance card, front and back, to include in the patient's record. Also verify the effective date of insurance coverage because services performed before this date may be excluded from claims. To reduce possible payment problems, remind the patient before a service is performed if it might not be covered.

Coordination of Benefits. **Coordination of benefits** clauses are legal clauses in insurance policies that prevent duplication of payment. These clauses restrict payment by insurance companies to no more than 100% of the cost of covered benefits. In many families, husband and wife are both wage earners. They and their children are frequently eligible for health insurance benefits through both employers' plans. In such cases the two insurance companies coordinate their payments to pay up to 100% of a procedure's cost. A payment of 100% includes the policyholder's deductible and co-payment. The *primary,* or main, plan is the policy that pays benefits first. Then the *secondary,* or supplemental, plan pays the deductible and co-payment. To determine which plan is the primary, the **birthday rule** is followed. It states that the insurance policy of the policyholder whose birthday comes first in the calendar year is the primary payer for all dependents.

For example, suppose a husband and wife are both employed and have work-sponsored insurance plans that cover their spouses and their three children. The husband's birthday is July 14 and the wife's birthday is June 11. Because of the birthday rule, the wife's insurance plan is the primary payer, and the husband's is the secondary payer. If a husband and wife were born on the same day, the policy that has been in effect the longest is the primary payer.

The birthday rule is applied in most states in which dependents are covered by two or more medical plans. Different states may have different rules, however. You should check with your state's insurance commission whenever you are in doubt. Table 15-1 describes widely used guidelines.

Delivering Services to the Patient

To ensure accuracy in claims processing, any services delivered to the patient in the office by the physician or other members of the health-care team must be entered into the patient record. **Referrals** to outside physicians or specialists must be entered into the record.

Physician's Services. The physician who examines the patient notes the patient's symptoms in the medical record. The physician also notes a diagnosis and treatment plan (including prescribed medications) and specifies if and when the patient should return for a follow-up visit.

TABLE 15-1 Determining Primary Coverage
• If the patient has only one policy, it is primary.
• If the patient has coverage under two plans, the plan that has been in effect for the patient for the longest period of time is primary. However, if an active employee has a plan with the present employer and is still covered by a former employer's plan as a retiree or a laid-off employee, the current employer's plan is primary.
• If the patient is also covered as a dependent under another insurance policy, the patient's plan is primary.
• If an employed patient has coverage under the employer's plan and additional coverage under a government-sponsored plan, the employer's plan is primary. An example of this is a patient enrolled in a PPO through employment who is also on Medicare.
• If a retired patient is covered by the plan of the spouse's employer and the spouse is still employed, the spouse's plan is primary, even if the retired person has Medicare.
• If the patient is a dependent child covered by both parents' plans and the parents are not separated or divorced (or have joint custody of the child), the primary plan is determined by which parent has the first birth date in the calendar year (the birthday rule).
• If two or more plans cover the dependent children of separated or divorced parents who do not have joint custody of their children, the children's primary plan is determined in this order: 1. The plan of the custodial parent   2. The plan of the spouse of the custodial parent (if the parent has remarried)   3. The plan of the parent without custody

Patient's Name	Insurance Company	Claim Filed		Payment Received		Difference (owed by patient)
		Date	Amount	Date	Amount	

Figure 15-5. After submitting a claim to an insurer, track each claim in an insurance claim register, such as the one pictured here.

After completing the visit with the patient, the physician writes the diagnosis, treatment, and sometimes the fee on a charge slip and instructs the patient to give you the charge slip before leaving.

Medical Coding. The next step is to translate the medical terminology on the charge slip into precise descriptions of medical services and procedural and diagnostic codes on the health-care claim. This step, which is critical to the provider and to reimbursement, is the topic of Chapter 16.

Referrals to Other Services. You may be asked to secure authorization from the insurance company for additional procedures. If so, contact the insurance company to explain the procedures and obtain approval and an authorization number. Enter this referral number in the billing program.

Frequently you will be asked to arrange an appointment for the referred services, particularly if the physician believes they are urgently needed. For example, a physician may send a patient for a specialist's evaluation or x-ray on the same day the patient visits your office.

Preparing the Health-Care Claim

Everyone who receives services from a doctor in the practice where you work is responsible for paying the practice for those services. When the patient brings you the charge slip from the doctor, you may perform one or more of the following procedures, depending on the policy of your practice:

- Prepare and transmit a health-care claim on behalf of the patient directly to the insurance company.
- Accept payment from the patient for the full amount. The patient will submit a claim to the insurance carrier for reimbursement.
- Accept an insurance co-payment.

Filing the Insurance Claim. If you are going to transmit the claim directly to the payer, you will prepare an insurance claim, usually electronically. After the physician reviews the claim, you will transmit the claim to the insurance carrier for payment. The billing program will create a log of transmitted claims, or a register such as the one shown in Figure 15-5 may be maintained.

Time Limits. Claims must be filed in a timely manner. Time limits for filing claims vary from company to company. For example, some insurers will not pay a claim unless it is filed within 6 months of the date of service. The limits for commercial payers such as Blue Cross and Blue Shield vary from state to state.

Medicare states that for services rendered from January 1 to September 30, claims must be filed by December 31 of the following year; for services rendered from October 1 through December 31, claims must be filed no later than December 31 of the second year following the service.

Medicaid states that claims must be filed no later than 1 year from the date of service. The time frame for refiling rejected claims varies by state. In Indiana, for example, if you filed a claim for a service performed on January 2, 2006, and the claim was rejected on May 31, 2006, you would have until May 31, 2007, to refile the claim.

Although Medicare and Medicaid allow quite a long time for claims to be filed, it is poor business practice to wait so long. In the typical medical practice, claims are transmitted within a few business days after the date of service. Many large practices file claims every day or twice a week.

Insurer's Processing and Payment

Your transmitted claim for payment will undergo a number of reviews by the insurer. Currently, much of the review process occurs electronically.

Review for Medical Necessity. The insurance carrier reviews each claim to determine whether the diagnosis and accompanying treatment are compatible and whether the treatment is medically necessary, as explained in Chapter 16.

Review for Allowable Benefits. The claims department also compares the fees the doctor charges with the benefits provided by the patient's health insurance policy. This review determines the amount of deductible or coinsurance the patient owes. This amount—that is, what the patient owes—is called subscriber liability.

Payment and Remittance Advice. After reviewing the claim, the insurer pays a benefit, either to the subscriber (patient) or to the practice, depending on what recipient the claim requested. With the payment, the insurer sends **remittance advice (RA),** also called an explanation of benefits. A patient who receives the payment gets the original RA, and the practice receives a copy (and vice versa). For each service submitted to an insurer, the RA form gives the following information:

- Name of the insured and identification number
- Name of the beneficiary
- Claim number
- Date, place, and type of service (coded)
- Amount billed by the practice
- Amount allowed (according to the subscriber's policy)
- Amount of subscriber liability (co-payment or deductible)
- Amount paid and included in the current payment
- A notation of any services not covered and an explanation of why they were not covered (for example, many insurance plans do not cover a woman's annual gynecologic examination and only a certain dollar amount of well-baby visits for infants)

Reviewing the Insurer's RA and Payment

Verify all information on the RA, line by line, using your records for each patient represented on the RA. In a large practice, you will frequently receive payment and an RA for several patients at one time. An example of a Medicare RA, which is called a Medicare Remittance Notice, is shown in Figure 15-6.

If all numbers on the RA agree with your records, you can make the appropriate entries in the insurance follow-up log for claims paid. In a small practice, the insurance follow-up log is used to track filed claims, using such information as patient name, date the claim was filed, services the claim reflects, notations about the results of the claim, and any balance due from the patient. Larger practices tend to track claims on computer in a file called, for example, "Unpaid Claims." If all the numbers do not agree, you will need to trace the claim with the insurance company.

When a claim is rejected, the RA states the reason. You will need to review the claim, examining all procedural and diagnosis codes for accuracy and comparing the claim with the patient's insurance information. You will probably need to contact the insurance company by telephone to resolve the claim problem.

Fee Schedules and Charges

Physicians establish a list of their usual fees for the procedures and services they frequently perform. The usual fees are those that they charge to most of their patients most of the time under typical conditions. These fees are listed on the office's **fee schedule.**

Medicare Payment System: RBRVS

Third-party payers also set the fees they are willing to pay providers, and often these fees are less than the physician's fee schedule. Most payers base their fees on the amounts that Medicare allows because the Medicare method of fee setting takes into account important factors other than only the usual fees.

The payment system used by Medicare is called the **resource-based relative value scale (RBRVS).** The RBRVS establishes the relative value units for services, replacing providers' consensus on fees (the "usual" or historical charges) with amounts based on resources (what each service really costs to provide).

There are three parts to an RBRVS fee:

1. The nationally uniform relative value. The relative value of a procedure is based on three cost elements: the physician's work, the practice cost (overhead), and the cost of malpractice insurance. For example, the relative value for a simple office visit, such as to administer a flu shot, is much lower than the relative value for a complicated encounter such as planning the treatment of uncontrolled diabetes in a patient.

2. A geographic adjustment factor. A geographic adjustment factor is used to adjust each relative value to reflect a geographical area's relative costs, such as office rents.

3. A nationally uniform conversion factor. A uniform conversion factor is a dollar amount used to multiply the relative values to produce a payment amount. It is used by Medicare to make adjustments according to changes in the cost-of-living index.

When RBRVS fees are used, providers receive considerably lower payments than when usual fees are used. Each part of the RBRVS—the relative values, the geographic adjustment, and the conversion factor—is updated each year by CMS. The year's Medicare fee schedule (MFS) is published by CMS in the *Federal Register.*

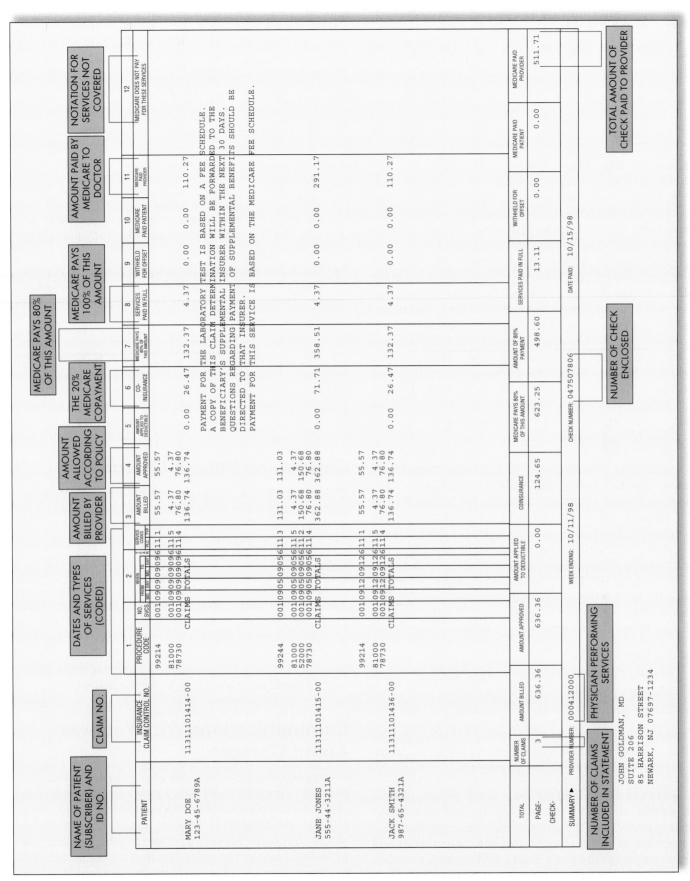

Figure 15-6. The insurer sends the remittance advice form to the medical practice.

Payment Methods

Most third-party payers use one of three methods for reimbursing physicians:

1. Allowed charges
2. Contracted fee schedule
3. Capitation

Allowed Charges. Many payers set an **allowed charge** for each procedure or service. This amount is the most the payer will pay any provider for that work. The term *allowed charge* has many equivalent terms, including *maximum allowable fee, maximum charge, allowed amount, allowed fee,* or *allowable charge.*

The physician's usual charge is often greater than a plan's allowed charge. If the physician participates in the plan, only the allowed charge can be billed to the payer. The plan's rules govern whether the provider is permitted to bill a patient for the part of a usual charge that the payer does not cover. Billing a patient for the difference between a higher usual fee and a lower allowed charge is called **balance billing.** Under most contracts, participating providers may not bill the patient for the difference. Instead, the provider must write off the difference, meaning that the amount of the difference is subtracted from the patient's bill and never collected.

For example, Medicare-participating providers may not receive an amount greater than the Medicare-allowed charge that is based on the Medicare fee schedule. The Original Medicare Plan is responsible for paying 80% of this allowed charge (after patients have met their annual deductible). Patients are responsible for the other 20%.

Here is an example of a Medicare billing. A Medicare-participating provider reports a usual charge of $200 for a service, and the Medicare-allowed charge is $84. The provider must write off the difference between the two charges. The patient is responsible for 20% of the allowed charge, not of the provider's usual charge:

Provider's usual fee:	$200.00
Medicare-allowed charge:	$84.00
Medicare pays 80%	$67.20
Patient pays 20%	$16.80

The total that the provider can collect is $84. The provider must write off the difference between the usual fee and the allowed charge, or $116.00 in this example.

Contracted Fee Schedule. Some payers, particularly PPOs, establish fixed fee schedules with their participating physicians. The terms of the plan determine what percentage of the charges, if any, the patient owes and what percentage the payer covers. Participating providers can typically bill patients their usual charges for procedures and services that are not covered by the plan.

Capitation. The fixed prepayment for each plan member in capitation contracts is determined by the managed care plan that initiates contracts with providers. The plan's contract with the provider lists the services and procedures that are covered by the cap rate. For example, a typical contract with a primary care provider might include the following services:

- Preventive care, including well-child care, adult physical exams, gynecological exams, eye exams, and hearing exams
- Counseling and telephone calls
- Office visits
- Medical care, including medical care services such as therapeutic injections and immunizations, allergy immunotherapy, electrocardiograms, and pulmonary function tests
- The local treatment of first-degree burns, the application of dressings, suture removal, the excision of small skin lesions, the removal of foreign bodies or cerumen from the external ear

These services are covered in the per-member charge for each plan member who selects the PCP. Noncovered services can be billed to patients using the physician's usual rate. Plans often require the provider to notify the patient in advance that a service is not covered and to state the fee for which the patient will be responsible.

Calculating Patient Charges

The patients of medical practices have a variety of health plans, so they have different financial responsibilities. In addition to premiums, patients may be obligated to pay deductibles, co-payments, coinsurance, excluded and over-limit services, and balance billing.

All payers require patients to pay for excluded (non-covered) services. Physicians generally can charge their usual fees for these services. Likewise, in managed care plans that set limits on the annual usage (or other period) of covered services, patients are responsible for usage beyond the allowed number. For example, if one preventive physical examination is permitted annually, additional preventive examinations are paid for by the patient.

Communications With Patients About Charges

When patients have office visits with a physician who participates in the plan under which they have coverage, such as a Medicare-participating (PAR) provider, they generally sign an **assignment of benefits** statement. When this occurs, the provider agrees to prepare health-care claims for patients, to receive payments directly from the payers, and to accept a payer's allowed charge. Patients are billed for charges that payers deny or do not pay. When patients have encounters with nonparticipating (nonPAR) providers, the procedure is usually different. To avoid the difficulty of collecting payments at a later date from a patient, practices may require that the patient either (1) assigns benefits or (2) pays in full at the time of services.

Many times patients want to know what their bills will be. For example, suppose a patient receives a bill for $100 from your practice. She calls to say that she has paid her deductible for the year, so her insurance company should have paid 80% of the bill. You call the patient's insurance company and learn that she still has to pay $100 to meet her deductible. If she pays the $100 bill in full, her deductible will then be met. You would have to explain these facts to the patient.

To estimate patients' bills, you should check with the payer to find out:

- The patient's deductible amount and whether it has been paid in full, the covered benefits, and coinsurance or other patient financial obligations
- The payer's allowed charges for the services that the provider anticipates providing

If the patient's request comes after the appointment, the encounter form can be used to tell the payer what procedures are going to be reported on the patient's claim to determine the likely payer reimbursement.

Patients should always be reminded of their financial obligations under their plans, including claim denials, according to practice procedures. The practice's financial policy regarding payment for services is usually either displayed on the wall of the reception area or included in a new patient information packet. The policy should explain what is required of the patient and when payment is due. For example, the policy may state the following:

- For unassigned claims: Payment for the physician's services is expected at the end of your appointment, unless you have made other arrangements with our practice manager.
- For assigned claims: After your insurance claim is processed by your insurance company, you will be billed for any amount you owe. You are responsible for any part of the charges that are denied or not paid by the carrier. All patient accounts are due within 30 days of the date of the invoice you receive.
- For managed care members: Co-payments must be paid before patients leave the office.

It is also a good practice to notify patients in advance of the probable cost of procedures that are not going to be covered by their plan. For example, many private plans as well as Medicare do not pay for most preventive services, such as annual physical examinations. Many patients, however, consider preventive services a good idea and are willing to pay for them. Patients should be asked to agree in writing to pay for any noncovered services. A letter of agreement should also specify why the service will not be covered and the cost of the procedure. In the case of Medicare, a form called the Advance Beneficiary Notice (Figure 15-7) is given to the patient to sign. It explains the charges that the patient is likely to have to pay.

Preparing and Transmitting Health-Care Claims

Health-care claims are a critical communication between medical offices and payers on behalf of patients. Processing claims is a major task in most offices, and the numbers can be huge. For example, a 40-physician group practice with 55,000 patients served annually typically processes 1000 claims daily!

HIPAA Claims and Paper Claims

Two types of claims are in use: (1) the predominant HIPAA electronic claim transaction and (2) the older CMS-1500 paper form. The electronic claim transaction is the HIPAA Health-Care Claim or Equivalent Encounter Information; it is commonly referred to as the "HIPAA claim." Its official name is **X12 837 Health Care Claim.** The paper format is the "universal claim" known as the CMS-1500 claim form (or the HCFA-1500).

As of October 2003, Medicare mandates the X12 837 transaction for all Medicare claims except those from very small practices. Third-party payers may continue to accept paper transactions. But practices that elect to use paper claims must have two versions of their medical billing software: one to capture the necessary data elements for HIPAA-compliant electronic Medicare claims and an older version to generate CMS-1500 claims. Also, under HIPAA regulations, only medical offices that do not handle any other HIPAA-related transactions can still use paper claims. It is anticipated that eventually, for cost reasons, all payers will require electronic submissions and add this provision to their contracts with providers.

Preparing HIPAA Claims. The information entered on claims is called data elements. Many elements, such as the patient's personal and insurance information, are entered in the billing program before patient's appointments, based on forms patients fill out and on communications with payers. After patients' office visits, their claims are completed when the medical assistant enters the billing transactions—the services, charges, and payments—as detailed on the superbill (encounter form). The medical assistant then instructs the software to prepare claims for editing and transmission.

Follow these tips when entering data in medical billing programs:

- Enter data in all capital letters
- Do not use prefixes for people's names, such as Mr., Ms., or Dr.
- Unless required by a particular insurance carrier, do not use special characters such as hyphens, commas, or apostrophes
- Use only valid data in all fields; avoid words such as "same"

Patient's Name: _____   Medicare # (HICN): _____

ADVANCE BENEFICIARY NOTICE (ABN)

NOTE: You need to make a choice about receiving these health care items or services.

We expect that Medicare will not pay for the item(s) or service(s) that are described below. Medicare does not pay for all of your health care costs. Medicare only pays for covered items and services when Medicare rules are met. The fact that Medicare may not pay for a particular item or service does not mean that you should not receive it. There may be a good reason your doctor recommended it. Right now, in your case, **Medicare probably will not pay for –**

Items or Services:
Because:

The purpose of this form is to help you make an informed choice about whether or not you want to receive these items or services, knowing that you might have to pay for them yourself. Before you make a decision about your options, you should **read this entire notice carefully**.

- Ask us to explain, if you don't understand why Medicare probably won't pay.
- Ask us how much these items or services will cost you (**Estimated Cost: $_____**), in case you have to pay for them yourself or through other insurance.

PLEASE CHOOSE **ONE** OPTION.   CHECK **ONE** BOX.   **SIGN & DATE** YOUR CHOICE.

☐ **Option 1. YES.   I want to receive these items or services.**
I understand that Medicare will not decide whether to pay unless I receive these items or services. Please submit my claim to Medicare. I understand that you may bill me for items or services and that I may have to pay the bill while Medicare is making its decision. If Medicare does pay, you will refund to me any payments I made to you that are due to me. If Medicare denies payment, I agree to be personally and fully responsible for payment. That is, I will pay personally, either out of pocket or through any other insurance that I have. I understand I can appeal Medicare's decision.

☐ **Option 2. NO.   I have decided not to receive these items or services.**
I will not receive these items or services. I understand that you will not be able to submit a claim to Medicare and that I will not be able to appeal your opinion that Medicare won't pay.

_____   _____
     Date   **Signature of patient or person acting on patient's behalf**

NOTE: Your health information will be kept confidential. Any information that we collect about you on this form will be kept confidential in our offices. If a claim is submitted to Medicare, your health information on this form may be shared with Medicare. Your health information which Medicare sees will be kept confidential by Medicare.

OMB Approval No. 0938-0566   Form No. CMS-R-131-G   (June 2002)

Figure 15-7. Advance Beneficiary Notice.
Source: Centers for Medicare and Medicaid Services.

The X12 837 transaction requires many data elements, and all must be correct. Most billing programs or claim transmission programs automatically reformat data such as dates into the correct formats. These data elements are reported in five major sections:

1. Provider
2. Subscriber (the insured or policyholder)
3. Patient (who may be the subscriber or another person) and payer
4. Claim details
5. Services

Not all data elements are required. Some are considered situational and are required only when a certain condition applies. When it does apply, then that data element also becomes required. For example, if a claim involves pregnancy, the date of the last menstrual period is required. If the claim does not involve pregnancy, that date should not be reported.

Before the HIPAA mandate for standard transactions, some payers required additional records, such as their own information sheet, when providers billed them. Some payers also used their own coding systems. The HIPAA Electronic Health Care Transactions and Code Sets (TCS) mandate means that health plans are required to accept the standard claim submitted electronically.

Other standard transactions also support the claim process, such as advising the office of claim status, payment, and other key information. These transactions standards apply to the treatment, payment, and operations information that is exchanged between medical offices and health plans. Each electronic transaction has both a title and a number. Each number begins with X12, which is the number of the EDI format, followed by a unique number that stands for the transaction. Here are some examples of titles and numbers that medical assistants may encounter while processing X12 837 health-care claims:

Number	Title
X12 276/277	Claim status inquiry and response
X12 270/271	Eligibility inquiry and response
X12 278	Referral authorization inquiry and response
X12 835	Payment and remittance advice
X12 820	Health plan premium payments
X12 834	Enrollment in and withdrawal from a health plan

Preparing Paper Claims. The process for preparing paper claims is similar to the X12 837 claim. Usually, the medical billing program is updated with information about the patient's office visit. Then the program is instructed to print the data on a CMS-1500 paper form, shown in Figure 15-8. This claim may be mailed or faxed to a third-party payer.

Because of the HIPAA mandate, the paper claim is not widely in use; however, the information it contains is essentially very similar to the X12 837. For this reason, you should study Procedure 15-1, Completing the CMS-1500 Claim Form. This exercise will give you a good understanding of the data elements needed on all claims.

The CMS-1500 contains 33 form locators, which are numbered items. Form locators 1–13 refer to the patient and the patient's insurance coverage. Form locators 14–33 contain information about the provider and the transaction information, including the patient's diagnoses, procedures, and charges.

Transmission of Electronic Claims

Practices handle the transmission of electronic claims—which may be called electronic media claims, or EMC—in a variety of ways. Some practices transmit claims themselves; others hire outside vendors to handle this task for them.

Claims are prepared for transmission after all required data elements have been posted to the medical billing software program. The data elements that are transmitted are not seen physically, as they would be on a paper form. Instead, these elements are in a computer file.

Three major methods are used to transmit claims electronically: direct transmission to the payer, clearinghouse use, and direct data entry.

Transmitting Claims Directly. In the direct transmission approach, medical offices and payers exchange transactions directly. To do this, providers and payers need the necessary information systems, including a translator and communications technology, to conduct **electronic data interchange** (EDI).

Using a Clearinghouse. Many offices whose medical billing software vendors do not have translation software must use a **clearinghouse** in order to send and receive data in the correct EDI format. Clearinghouses can take in nonstandard formats and translate them into the standard format. To ensure that the standard format is compliant, the clearinghouse must receive all the required data elements from the physician. Clearinghouses are prohibited from creating or modifying data content.

Medical offices may use a clearinghouse to transmit all their claims, or they may use a combination of direct transmission and a clearinghouse. For example, they may send claims directly to Medicare, Medicaid, and a few other major commercial payers, and use a clearinghouse to send claims to other payers.

Using Direct Data Entry. Online direct data entry (DDE) is offered by some payers. It uses an Internet-based service into which employees key the standard data elements. Although the data elements must meet the HIPAA standards requirements regarding content, they do not have to be formatted for EDI. Instead, they are loaded directly in the health plans' computer.

PLEASE
DO NOT
STAPLE
IN THIS
AREA

CARRIER →

[ ] PICA

HEALTH INSURANCE CLAIM FORM

PICA [ ]

1. MEDICARE [ ] (Medicare #) MEDICAID [ ] (Medicaid #) CHAMPUS [ ] (Sponsor's SSN) CHAMPVA [ ] (VA File #) GROUP HEALTH PLAN [ ] (SSN or ID) FECA BLK LUNG [ ] (SSN) OTHER [ ] (ID)

1a. INSURED'S I.D. NUMBER   (FOR PROGRAM IN ITEM 1)

2. PATIENT'S NAME (Last Name, First Name, Middle Initial)

3. PATIENT'S BIRTH DATE MM DD YY   SEX M [ ] F [ ]

4. INSURED'S NAME (Last Name, First Name, Middle Initial)

5. PATIENT'S ADDRESS (No., Street)

6. PATIENT RELATIONSHIP TO INSURED Self [ ] Spouse [ ] Child [ ] Other [ ]

7. INSURED'S ADDRESS (No., Street)

CITY   STATE

8. PATIENT STATUS Single [ ] Married [ ] Other [ ] Employed [ ] Full-Time Student [ ] Part-Time Student [ ]

CITY   STATE

ZIP CODE   TELEPHONE (Include Area Code) (   )

ZIP CODE   TELEPHONE (INCLUDE AREA CODE) (   )

9. OTHER INSURED'S NAME (Last Name, First Name, Middle Initial)

10. IS PATIENT'S CONDITION RELATED TO:

11. INSURED'S POLICY GROUP OR FECA NUMBER

a. OTHER INSURED'S POLICY OR GROUP NUMBER

a. EMPLOYMENT? (CURRENT OR PREVIOUS) YES [ ] NO [ ]

a. INSURED'S DATE OF BIRTH MM DD YY   SEX M [ ] F [ ]

b. OTHER INSURED'S DATE OF BIRTH MM DD YY   SEX M [ ] F [ ]

b. AUTO ACCIDENT?   PLACE (State) YES [ ] NO [ ]

b. EMPLOYER'S NAME OR SCHOOL NAME

c. EMPLOYER'S NAME OR SCHOOL NAME

c. OTHER ACCIDENT? YES [ ] NO [ ]

c. INSURANCE PLAN NAME OR PROGRAM NAME

d. INSURANCE PLAN NAME OR PROGRAM NAME

10d. RESERVED FOR LOCAL USE

d. IS THERE ANOTHER HEALTH BENEFIT PLAN? YES [ ] NO [ ] If yes, return to and complete item 9 a-d.

READ BACK OF FORM BEFORE COMPLETING & SIGNING THIS FORM.
12. PATIENT'S OR AUTHORIZED PERSON'S SIGNATURE I authorize the release of any medical or other information necessary to process this claim. I also request payment of government benefits either to myself or to the party who accepts assignment below.

SIGNED _____   DATE _____

13. INSURED'S OR AUTHORIZED PERSON'S SIGNATURE I authorize payment of medical benefits to the undersigned physician or supplier for services described below.

SIGNED _____

14. DATE OF CURRENT: MM DD YY ◄ ILLNESS (First symptom) OR INJURY (Accident) OR PREGNANCY(LMP)

15. IF PATIENT HAS HAD SAME OR SIMILAR ILLNESS. GIVE FIRST DATE MM DD YY

16. DATES PATIENT UNABLE TO WORK IN CURRENT OCCUPATION MM DD YY FROM   TO   MM DD YY

17. NAME OF REFERRING PHYSICIAN OR OTHER SOURCE

17a. I.D. NUMBER OF REFERRING PHYSICIAN

18. HOSPITALIZATION DATES RELATED TO CURRENT SERVICES MM DD YY FROM   TO   MM DD YY

19. RESERVED FOR LOCAL USE

20. OUTSIDE LAB? $ CHARGES YES [ ] NO [ ]

21. DIAGNOSIS OR NATURE OF ILLNESS OR INJURY. (RELATE ITEMS 1,2,3 OR 4 TO ITEM 24E BY LINE)

1. |___.__   3. |___.__

2. |___.__   4. |___.__

22. MEDICAID RESUBMISSION CODE   ORIGINAL REF. NO.

23. PRIOR AUTHORIZATION NUMBER

24. A DATE(S) OF SERVICE						B Place of Service	C Type of Service	D PROCEDURES, SERVICES, OR SUPPLIES (Explain Unusual Circumstances) CPT/HCPCS | MODIFIER	E DIAGNOSIS CODE	F $ CHARGES	G DAYS OR UNITS	H EPSDT Family Plan	I EMG	J COB	K RESERVED FOR LOCAL USE
From MM	DD	YY	To MM	DD	YY										
1															
2															
3															
4															
5															
6															

25. FEDERAL TAX I.D. NUMBER SSN [ ] EIN [ ]

26. PATIENT'S ACCOUNT NO.

27. ACCEPT ASSIGNMENT? (For govt. claims, see back) YES [ ] NO [ ]

28. TOTAL CHARGE $

29. AMOUNT PAID $

30. BALANCE DUE $

31. SIGNATURE OF PHYSICIAN OR SUPPLIER INCLUDING DEGREES OR CREDENTIALS (I certify that the statements on the reverse apply to this bill and are made a part thereof.)

SIGNED _____   DATE _____

32. NAME AND ADDRESS OF FACILITY WHERE SERVICES WERE RENDERED (If other than home or office)

33. PHYSICIAN'S, SUPPLIER'S BILLING NAME, ADDRESS, ZIP CODE & PHONE #

PIN#   GRP#

(APPROVED BY AMA COUNCIL ON MEDICAL SERVICE 8/88)

PLEASE PRINT OR TYPE

FORM HCFA-1500 (12-90)
FORM OWCP-1500   FORM RRB-1500

790-0115 (12/90) (OCR) 1 pt.

PATIENT AND INSURED INFORMATION

PHYSICIAN OR SUPPLIER INFORMATION

Figure 15-8. The CMS-1500 is a paper health insurance claim form.

PROCEDURE 15.1

Completing the CMS-1500 Claim Form

Objective: To complete the CMS-1500 claim form correctly

Materials: Patient record, CMS-1500 form, typewriter or computer, patient ledger card

Method

The numbers below correspond to the numbered fields on the CMS-1500.

Patient Information Section

1. Check the appropriate insurance box.
1a. Enter the insured's insurance identification number as it appears on the insurance card.
2. Enter the patient's name in this order: last name, first name, middle initial (if any).
3. Enter the patient's birth date using two digits each for the month and day. For example, for a patient born on February 9, 1954, enter 02-09-1954. Indicate the sex of the patient: male or female.
4. If the insured and the patient are the same person, enter SAME. If not, enter the policy-holder's name. For TRICARE claims, enter the sponsor's (service person's) full name.
5. Enter the patient's mailing address, city, state, and zip code.
6. Enter the patient's relationship to the insured. If they are the same, mark SELF. For TRICARE, enter the patient's relationship to the sponsor.
7. Enter the insured's mailing address, city, state, zip code, and telephone number. If this address is the same as the patient's, enter SAME.
8. Indicate the patient's marital, employment, and student status by checking boxes.
9. Enter the last name, first name, and middle initial of any other insured person whose policy might cover the patient. If the claim is for Medicare and the patient has a Medigap policy, enter SAME.
9a. Enter the policy or group number for the other insured person. If this is a Medigap policy, enter MEDIGAP before the policy number.
9b. Enter the date of birth and sex of the other insured person (field 9).
9c. Enter the other insured's employer or school name. (Note: If this is a Medicare claim, enter the claims-processing address for the Medigap insurer from field 9. If this is a Medicaid claim

and other insurance is available, note it in field 1a and in field 2, and enter the requested policy information.
9d. Enter the other insured's insurance plan or program name. If the plan is Medigap and CMS has assigned it a nine-digit number called PAYERID, enter that number here. On an attached sheet, give the complete mailing address for all other insurance information, and enter the word ATTACHMENT in 10d.
10. Check the appropriate YES or NO boxes in a, b, and c to indicate whether the patient's place of employment, an auto accident, or other type of accident precipitated the patient's condition. For PLACE, enter the two-letter state postal abbreviation.

    For Medicaid claims, enter MCD and the Medicaid number at line 10d. For all other claims, enter ATTACHMENT here if there is other insurance information. Be sure the full names and addresses of the other insurers appear on the attached sheet. Also, code the insurer as follows:

MSP	Medicare Secondary Payer
MG	Medigap
SP	Supplemental Employer
MCD	Medicaid

11. Enter the insured's policy or group number. For Medicare claims, fill out this section only if there is other insurance primary to Medicare; otherwise, enter NONE.
11a. Enter the insured's date of birth and sex as in field 3, if the insured is not the patient.
11b. Enter the employer's name or school name here. This information will determine if Medicare is the primary payer.
11c. Enter the insurance plan or program name.
11d. Check YES or NO to indicate if there is another health benefit plan. If YES, you must complete 9a through 9d. Failure to do so will cause the claim to be denied.
12. Have the patient or an authorized representative sign and date the form here. If a representative signs, have the representative indicate the relationship to the patient.
13. Have the insured (the patient or another individual) sign here.

continued ⟶

Completing the CMS-1500 Claim Form *(continued)*

Physician Information Section

14. Enter the date of the current illness, injury, or pregnancy, using eight digits.

15. *Do not complete this field.* Leave it blank for Medicare.

16. Enter the dates the patient is or was unable to work. This information could signal a workers' compensation claim.

17. Enter the name of the referring physician, clinical laboratory, or other referring source.

17a. Enter the referring physician's unique physician identifier number, or UPIN.

18. Enter the dates the patient was hospitalized, if at all, with the current condition.

19. Enter the date the patient was last seen by the referring physician or other medical professional.

20. Check YES if a laboratory test was performed outside the physician's office, and enter the test price. Ensure that field 32 carries the laboratory's exact name and address and the insurance carrier's nine-digit provider identification number (PIN). Check NO if the test was done in the office of the physician who is billing the insurance company.

21. Enter the multidigit *International Classification of Diseases, 9th edition, Clinical Modification* (ICD-9-CM) code number diagnosis or nature of injury (see Chapter 16). Enter up to four codes in order of importance.

22. Enter the Medicaid resubmission code and original reference number.

23. Enter the prior authorization number if required by the payer.

24A. Enter the date of each service, procedure, or supply provided. Add the number of days for each, and enter them, in chronological order, in field 24G.

24B. Enter the two-digit place-of-service code. For example, 11 is for office, 12 is for home, and 25 is for birthing center. Your office should have a list for reference.

24C. Leave this field blank.

24D. Enter the CPT/HCPCS codes with modifiers for the procedures, services, or supplies provided (see Chapter 16).

24E. Enter the diagnosis code that applies to that procedure, as listed in field 21.

24F. Enter the dollar amount of fee charged.

24G. Enter the days or units on which the service was performed, using three digits. If a service took 3 days, as listed in 24A, enter 030. Note that 1 unit or service would be 010, 5.5 services 055, and 10 services 100.

24H. This field is Medicaid-specific.

24I. If the service was performed in an emergency room, check this field.

24J. Some plans require a check mark here if the patient has coverage in addition to the primary plan.

24K. Enter the insurance-company-assigned nine-digit physician PIN. For TRICARE, enter the physician's state license number.

25. Enter the physician's or care provider's federal tax identification number or Social Security number.

26. Enter the patient's account number assigned by your office.

27. Check YES to indicate that the physician will accept Medicare or TRICARE assignment of benefits.

28. Enter the total charge for the service.

29. Enter the amount already paid by the patient or insurance company.

30. Enter the balance due your office (subtract field 29 from field 28 to obtain this figure).

31. Have the physician or service supplier sign and date the form here.

32. Enter the name and address of the organization or individual who performed the services. If performed in the patient's home or the physician's office, leave this field blank.

33. List the billing physician's or supplier's name, address, zip code, and phone number.

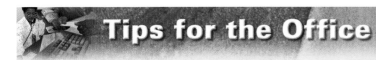

Data Elements for HIPAA Electronic Claims

The X12 837 health-care claim has many of the same data elements as are required to correctly complete a paper claim, but some elements require understanding new terms. Here are tips for locating these types of information.

Reporting Provider Information

The *billing provider* is the entity that is transmitting the claim to the payer. Medical offices often use a billing service or a clearinghouse to serve as the billing provider and transmit their claims. When this is done, the outside organization is the billing provider, and the practice is the *pay-to provider* that receives the payment from the insurance carrier. If an office sends claims directly to the payer, it is the billing provider and there is no additional pay-to provider to report.

Another term associated with claim preparation is *rendering provider*. It is common to have a billing provider (such as a clearinghouse), a pay-to provider (the office), and a rendering provider, the physician who, as a member of the practice, treats the patient.

Reporting Taxonomy Information

A *taxonomy code* is a 10-digit number that stands for a physician's medical specialty. Physicians select the taxonomy code that most closely matches their education, license, or certification. The code is reported on claims because payment for some services is impacted by the particular specialty of the doctor performing them and by payers' contracts. For example, nuclear medicine is usually a higher-paid specialty than internal medicine. An internist who also has a specialty in nuclear medicine would report the nuclear medicine taxonomy code when billing for that service and use the internal medicine taxonomy code when reporting internal medicine claims. Many medical billing programs store the necessary taxonomy codes. The user selects the correct specialty, and the code is correctly selected for reporting on the claim.

Reporting HIPAA National Identifiers

HIPAA *national identifiers* must be established for the following:

- Employers
- Health-care providers
- Health plans
- Patients

Identifiers are numbers of predetermined length and structure, such as a person's Social Security number. As the HIPAA rules establishing these identifiers are passed, the correct data elements must be reported on the claim. For example, the employer identifier has been adopted; it is the Employer Identification Number (EIN) issued by the Internal Revenue Service.

Until the identifiers for the three other entities are adopted, these rules are in effect:

- For health care providers, report the tax identification number or Social Security number
- For health plans, report the appropriate code; here are some common codes

Code	Definition
09	Self-pay
12	Preferred provider organization (PPO)
15	Indemnity insurance
BL	Blue Cross/Blue Shield
CH	TRICARE
CI	Commercial insurance company
HM	Health maintenance organization
MB	Medicare Part B
MC	Medicaid
WC	Worker's compensation health claim

- For patients, report the policyholder's health plan identification number

Generating Clean Claims

Although health-care claims require many data elements and are complex, often simple errors prevent you from generating "clean" claims—that is, those accepted for processing by the payer. Claims should be carefully checked before transmission or printing (Figure 15-9). Be alert for these common errors:

- Missing or incomplete service facility name, address, and identification for services rendered outside the

office or home. This includes invalid ZIP codes or state abbreviations.
- Missing Medicare assignment indicator or benefits assignment indicator.
- Missing part of the name or the identifier of the referring provider.
- Missing or invalid subscriber's birth date.
- Missing information about secondary insurance plans, such as a spouse's payer.

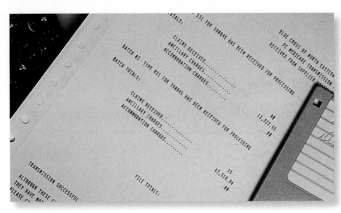

Figure 15-9. Print out the claims report to check for any errors that might make the payer reject a claim.

• Missing payer name and/or payer identifier, required for both primary and secondary payers.

Many offices use a specialized software program called a "claim scrubber" to check claims before they are released and to allow errors to be fixed. Clearinghouses also apply software checks to claims they receive and transmit back reports of errors or missing information to the sender.

Claims Security

Electronic data about patients are stored on a computer system. Most medical offices use computer networks in which personal computers are connected to a local area network (LAN), so users can exchange and share information and hardware. The LAN is linked to remote networks such as the Internet by a router that determines the best route for data to travel across the network. Packets of data traveling between the LAN and the Internet—such as electronic claims—must usually pass through a firewall, a security device that examines information (for example, e-mails) that enter and leave a network, determining whether to forward them to their destination.

The HIPAA rules set standards for protecting individually identifiable health information when it is maintained or transmitted electronically. Medical offices must protect the confidentiality, integrity, and availability of this information. A number of security measures are used:

• Access control, passwords, and log files to keep intruders out

• Backups (saved copies of files) to replace items after damage to the computer

• Security policies to handle violations that do occur

Medical assistants participate in the protection of patients' health information. One way is to select a good password for your computer. Here are tips:

• Always use a combination of letters and numbers that are not real words and also not an obvious number string such as 123456 or a birth date.

• Do not use a user ID (log-on or sign-on) as a password. Even if it has both numbers and letters, it is not secret.

• Select a mixture of both upper case and lower case letters if the system can distinguish between them, and if possible, include special characters such as @, $, or &.

• Use a minimum of six or seven alphanumeric characters. The optimal minimum number varies by system, but most security experts recommend a length of at least six or seven characters.

• Change passwords periodically, but not too often. Forcing frequent changes can actually make security worse because users are more likely to keep passwords written down.

Summary

Part of your responsibilities as a medical assistant will be to make sure that health-care claims are processed accurately. When accurate claims are sent to payers, physicians receive the maximum appropriate payment for the services they provide.

As a medical assistant, you will handle patients' questions about their health-care plans and claims. You will review patients' insurance coverage, explain the physician's fees, estimate what charges payers will cover, estimate how much patients should pay, and prepare complete and accurate health-care claims for patients.

CASE STUDY QUESTIONS

Now that you have completed this chapter, review the case study at the beginning of the chapter and answer the following questions:

1. How much should this patient pay?
2. How much will he owe for his next visit this year, which is expected to have a charge of $200?
3. Assuming that the patient in the case study has a managed care policy, what type of policy does he probably have?
4. What term would you use to describe the part of the payment that is based on 20% of the charges?
5. If you did not know whether the deductible had been met, what procedure would you follow?

Discussion Questions

1. How do HMOs and PPOs compare?
2. What are the differences between Medicare Part A and Part B?
3. Why do insurers coordinate benefits?
4. What is the difference between TRICARE and CHAMPVA?

Critical Thinking Questions

1. How is the increasing cost of medical procedures affecting the insurance industry?
2. How does managed care help control the cost of health insurance?
3. What are the advantages of electronic claims?

Application Activities

1. Apply the birthday rule in this situation:
   Both parents of the patient have health-care coverage through their employers. The father's birthday is October 6 and the mother's is November 23. Which plan is primary for the child?
2. A patient's insurance policy states:
   Annual deductible: $300
   Coinsurance: 70-30
   This year, the patient has made payments totaling $533 to all providers. Today, the patient has an office visit (fee: $80). The patient presents a credit card for payment of today's bill. What is the amount that the patient should pay?
3. A patient is a member of an HMO with a capitation plan and a $10 copay. The usual charges for the day's services would be $480. What does the patient pay?
4. A patient is a member of a PPO health plan that has a 20% discount from the provider and a 15% co-payment. If the day's usual charges are $210, what are the amounts that the plan and the patient each pay?

Internet Activities

1. Visit the BCBS Internet site. Use e-mail to post a question about insurance processing. Check back in a couple of days and report to the class.
2. Visit the CMS Web site and research the current plans available to Medicare beneficiaries.

Medical Coding

KEY TERMS

add-on code

Alphabetic Index

code linkage

compliance plan

conventions

cross-reference

Current Procedural Terminology (CPT)

diagnosis (Dx)

diagnosis code

E code

E/M code

established patient

global period

HCPCS Level II code

Health Care Common Procedure Coding System (HCPCS)

International Classification of Diseases, Ninth Revision, Clinical Modification (ICD-9)

modifier

new patient

panel

procedure code

Tabular List

V code

AREAS OF COMPETENCE

2003 Role Delineation Study

ADMINISTRATIVE

Administrative Procedures

- Understand and apply third-party guidelines
- Obtain reimbursement through accurate claims submission

Practice Finances

- Perform procedural and diagnostic coding

CHAPTER OUTLINE

- Diagnosis Codes: The ICD-9-CM
- Procedure Codes: The CPT
- HCPCS
- Avoiding Fraud: Coding Compliance

OBJECTIVES

After completing Chapter 16, you will be able to:

16.1 Explain the purpose and format of the ICD-9-CM volumes that are used by medical offices.

16.2 Describe how to analyze diagnoses and locate correct codes using the ICD-9-CM.

16.3 Identify the purpose and format of the CPT.

16.4 Name three key factors that determine the level of Evaluation and Management codes that are selected.

16.5 Identify the two types of codes in the Health Care Common Procedure Coding System (HCPCS).

16.6 Describe the process used to locate correct procedure codes using CPT.

16.7 Explain how medical coding affects the payment process.

16.8 Define fraud and provide examples of fraudulent billing and coding.

Introduction

In order to correctly report on health-care claims the conditions that patients have and the services they receive during office visits, medical assistants need to understand the basics of medical coding. Medical coding is the translation of medical terms for diagnoses and procedures into code numbers selected from standardized code sets. Codes on health-care claims explain to payers that the services patients received were medically necessary and complied with the payer's rules. Finding the correct codes can require detective work! The reward is accurate claims that bring the maximum appropriate reimbursement to the physicians in your medical office.

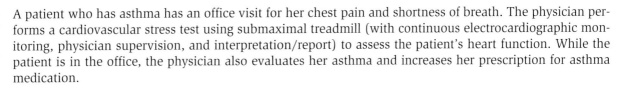

CASE STUDY

A patient who has asthma has an office visit for her chest pain and shortness of breath. The physician performs a cardiovascular stress test using submaximal treadmill (with continuous electrocardiographic monitoring, physician supervision, and interpretation/report) to assess the patient's heart function. While the patient is in the office, the physician also evaluates her asthma and increases her prescription for asthma medication.

As you read this chapter, consider the following questions:

1. How would you select the ICD-9 and CPT codes for a health-care claim for this visit?
2. What diagnosis and procedure codes will result in the correct payment for these services?
3. How should the claim show the medical necessity of the procedures?
4. Locate the ICD-9 code for the patient's asthma. How many digits are required? What code did you assign?
5. Locate the CPT code for the cardiovascular stress test. What information did you use to select it from the list of related codes?

Diagnosis Codes: The ICD-9-CM

Patients present to physicians with a description of their medical problems, called their chief complaints (CC) in the documentation of their visits. To diagnose a patient's condition, the physician follows a complex process of decision making based on the patient's statements, an examination, and the physician's evaluation of this information. The physician establishes a **diagnosis (Dx)** that describes the primary condition for which a patient is receiving care. Additional conditions or symptoms, called coexisting conditions, which are either treated or related to the patient's current illness, may also be noted in the chart.

The diagnosis is communicated to the third-party payer through a **diagnosis code** on the health care claim. The diagnosis codes used in the United States are found in the *International Classification of Diseases, Ninth Revision, Clinical Modification,* commonly referred to as the **ICD-9.** This code set is based on a system maintained by the World Health Organization of the United Nations.

The use of the ICD-9 codes in the health-care industry is mandated by HIPAA for reporting patients' diseases, their conditions, and their signs and symptoms. The codes are updated every year. Medical offices should have the current year's reference book and should update office forms that contain diagnosis codes.

Using the ICD-9

To find the correct diagnosis codes, you follow a five-step process, working with the diagnostic information and the ICD-9. Coding becomes easier with practice, but do not be tempted to take shortcuts. Every case is different, and additional terms or digits may be necessary to make a diagnosis code as specific as possible. If a step is skipped, important information may be missed. If more than one diagnosis is described in a patient's chart, work on only one diagnosis at a time to avoid coding errors.

The ICD-9-CM used in medical offices has two parts, the Tabular List and the Alphabetic Index.

Diseases and Injuries: Tabular List, Volume 1. The **Tabular List** has 17 chapters of disease descriptions and codes, with two additional types of codes and five appendixes.

Diseases and Injuries: Alphabetic Index, Volume 2. The **Alphabetic Index** provides the following:

- An index of the disease descriptions in the Tabular List
- An index in table format of drugs and chemicals that cause poisoning
- An index of external causes of injury, such as accidents

Diagnoses are listed two ways in the ICD-9, as illustrated in Figure 16-1. In the Alphabetic Index, diagnoses appear in alphabetic order with their corresponding diagnosis codes. In the Tabular List, the diagnosis codes are listed in numerical order with additional instructions. Both the Alphabetic Index and the Tabular List are used to find the right code. The Alphabetic Index is never used alone, because it does not contain all the necessary information. After you locate a code in the index, look it up in the Tabular List. Notes in this list may suggest or require the use of additional codes, or indicate that conditions should be coded differently because of exclusion from a category.

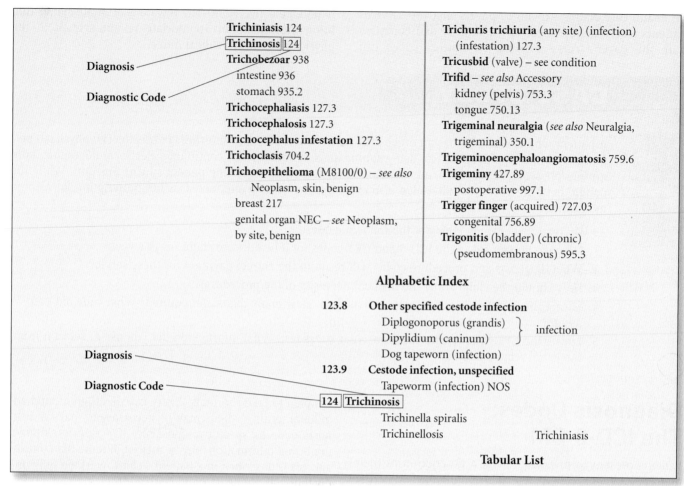

Figure 16-1. ICD alphabetic index and tabular list.

Source: International Classification of Diseases, Ninth Revision, Clinical Modification, 2004, Volumes 1 and 2.

Although the official order of the volumes puts the Tabular List before the Alphabetic Index, the correct use is to examine the Alphabetic Index when you are researching a term and then to verify your selection in the Tabular List. For this reason, commercial printers usually reverse the order, printing the Alphabetic Index at the front and the Tabular List behind it.

The Alphabetic Index

The Alphabetic Index contains all the medical terms in the Tabular List. For some conditions, it also has common terms that are not found in the Tabular List. The index is organized by the condition, not by the body part in which it occurs. For example, you would find the term *wrist fracture* by looking under *fracture* (the condition) and then, below it, *wrist* (the location), rather than by looking under *wrist* to find *fracture*.

The assignment of the correct code begins with looking up the medical term that describes the patient's condition in the Alphabetic Index. The following example illustrates the index's format. Each main term is printed in boldface type and is followed by its code number. For example, if the diagnostic statement is "the patient presents with blindness," the main term *blindness* is located in the Alphabetic Index.

Blindness (acquired) (congenital) (Both eyes) 369.00
 blast 921.3
  with nerve injury—see Injury, nerve, optic
 Brightis—see Uremia
 color (congenital) 368.59
  acquired 368.55
  blue 368.53
  green 368.52
  red 368.51
  total 368.54
 concussion 950.9
 cortical 377.75

Any other terms that are needed to select correct codes are printed after the main term. These terms may show the cause or source of the disease, or describe a particular type or body site for the main term. In this shortened example, the main term *blindness* is followed by five additional terms, each indicating a different type—such as color blindness—for this medical condition.

Other helpful terms may also be shown. In the example, any of the terms *acquired, congenital,* and *both eyes* may be in the diagnostic statement, such as "the patient presents with blindness acquired in childhood."

Some entries use **cross-references.** If the cross-reference *see* appears after a main term, you *must* look up the term that follows the word *see* in the index. The *see* reference means that the main term where you first looked is not correct; another category must be used. In the previous example, to code *Brightis,* the term *Uremia* must be located.

The Tabular List

The diseases and injuries in the Tabular List are organized into chapters according to the source or body system. There are also two kinds of supplementary codes. The organization of the Tabular List and the ranges of codes each chapter covers are shown in Table 16-1.

Code Structure.   ICD-9-CM diagnosis codes are made up of three, four, or five digits, and a description. The system uses three-digit categories for diseases, injuries, and symptoms. Many of these categories are divided into four-digit codes. Some codes are further subdivided into five-digit codes. For example:

415 Acute pulmonary heart disease *[three digits]*

  415.1 Pulmonary embolism and infarction *[four digits; more specific]*

    415.11 Iatrogenic pulmonary embolism and infarction *[five digits; most specific]*

When listed in the ICD-9, four- and five-digit diagnosis codes should be reported on claims because they represent the most specific diagnosis documented in the patient medical record. If available, the use of fourth and fifth digits is not optional; payers require them. For example, Centers for Medicare and Medicaid Services (CMS) rules state that a Medicare claim will be rejected when the most specific code available is not used.

TABLE 16-1   Tabular List Organization

Classification of Diseases and Injuries

Chapter	Categories
1 Infectious and Parasitic Diseases	001–139
2 Neoplasms	140–239
3 Endocrine, Nutritional, and Metabolic Diseases, and Immunity Disorders	240–279
4 Diseases of the Blood and Blood-Forming Organs	280–289
5 Mental Disorders	290–319
6 Diseases of the Central Nervous System and Sense Organs	320–389
7 Diseases of the Circulatory System	390–459
8 Diseases of the Respiratory System	460–519
9 Diseases of the Digestive System	520–579
10 Diseases of the Genitourinary System	580–629
11 Complications of Pregnancy, Childbirth, and the Puerperium	630–679
12 Diseases of the Skin and Subcutaneous Tissue	680–709
13 Diseases of the Musculoskeletal System and Connective Tissue	710–739
14 Congenital Anomalies	740–759
15 Certain Conditions Originating in the Perinatal Period	760–779
16 Symptoms, Signs, and Ill-Defined Conditions	780–799
17 Injury and Poisoning	800–999
Supplementary Classifications	
V Codes—Supplementary Classification of Factors Influencing Health Status and Contact with Health Services	V01–V83
E Codes—Supplementary Classification of External Causes of Injury and Poisoning	E800–E999

V Codes and E Codes. Two additional types of codes follow the chapters of the Tabular List:

1. **V codes** identify encounters for reasons other than illness or injury, such as annual checkups, immunizations, and normal childbirth. A V code can be used either as a primary code for an encounter or as an additional code.

2. **E codes** identify the external causes of injuries and poisoning. E (for external) codes are used for injuries resulting from various environmental events, such as transportation accidents, accidental poisoning by drugs or other substances, falls, and fires. An E code is never used alone as a diagnosis code. It always supplements a code that identifies the injury or condition itself. E codes are often used in collecting public health information.

Both V and E codes are alphanumeric; they contain letters followed by numbers. For example, the code for a complete physical examination of an adult is V70.0. The code for a fall from a ladder is E881.0.

ICD-9-CM Conventions

A list of abbreviations, punctuation, symbols, type faces, and instructional notes appears at the beginning of the ICD-9. These items, called **conventions,** provide guidelines for using the code set. Here are some important conventions:

NOS—This abbreviation means "not otherwise specified," or "unspecified." It is used when a condition cannot be described more specifically. In general, codes with *NOS* should be avoided. The physician

PROCEDURE 16.1

Locating an ICD-9-CM Code

Objective: To analyze diagnoses and locate the correct ICD code.

Materials: Patient record, ICD-9-CM

Method

1. Locate the statement of the diagnosis in the patient's medical record.
   First, find the diagnosis. This information may be located on the superbill (encounter form) or elsewhere in the patient's chart.

   Example: A patient's medical record reads:
   CC: Chest and epigastric pain; feels like a burning inside. Occasional reflux. Abdomen soft, flat without tenderness. No bowel masses or organomegaly.
   Dx: Peptic ulcer.

   The diagnosis is peptic ulcer.

   Then, if needed, decide which is the main term or condition of the diagnosis.

   Example: In the above diagnosis, the main term or condition is *ulcer.* The word *peptic* describes the type of ulcer.

2. Find the diagnosis in the ICD's Alphabetic Index. Look for the condition first. Then find descriptive words that make the condition more specific. Read all cross-references to check all the possibilities for a term and its synonyms.

   Example: The diagnosis is sebaceous cyst. Look under *cyst,* the condition, rather than *sebaceous,* the descriptive word. Many entries

   in the Alphabetic Index are cross-referenced. For example, *sebaceous* is followed by instructions in parentheses that say "(*see also* Cyst, sebaceous)." Observe all cross-reference instructions.

3. Locate the code from the Alphabetic Index in the ICD's Tabular List.
   Remember, the number to check is a code number, not a page number. The Tabular List gives codes in numerical order. Look for the number in bold-faced type.

4. Read all information to find the code that corresponds to the patient's specific disease or condition.
   Study the list of codes and descriptions. Be sure to pick the most specific code available. Check for the symbol that shows that a five-digit code is required.

5. Record the diagnosis code on the insurance claim and proofread the numbers.
   Enter the correct diagnosis code on the health-care claim, checking that

   • The numbers are entered correctly. If two numbers are transposed, the payer will receive the wrong diagnosis. Proofread the numbers on the computer screen or on the printed claim form.

   • The codes are complete. If the phone rang in the middle of coding a diagnosis, the last number of the code may have been omitted.

   • The highest (most specific) code is used.

should be asked to help select a more specific code, if possible.

NEC—This abbreviation means "not elsewhere classified." It is used when the ICD-9 does not provide a code specific enough for the patient's condition.

[ ] Brackets—Used around synonyms, alternative wordings, or explanations.

( ) Parentheses—Used around descriptions that do not affect the code, that is, nonessential or supplementary terms.

: Colon—Used in the Tabular List after an incomplete term that needs one of the terms that follow to make it assignable to a given category.

} Brace—Encloses a series of terms, each of which is modified by the statement that appears to the right of the brace.

Includes—This note indicates that the entries following it refine the content of a preceding entry. For example, after the three-digit diagnosis code for acute sinusitis, the word *includes* is followed by the types of conditions that the code covers.

Excludes—These notes, which are boxed and italicized, indicate that an entry is not classified as part of the preceding code. The note may also give the correct location of the excluded condition.

Use additional code—This note indicates that an additional code should be used, if available.

Code first underlying disease—This instruction appears when the category is not to be used as the primary diagnosis. These codes may not be used as the first code; they must always be preceded by another code for the primary diagnosis.

A New Revision: The ICD-10-CM

The tenth edition of the ICD was published by the World Health Organization in the mid-1990s. In the United States, the new *Clinical Modification* (ICD-10-CM) is being reviewed by health-care professionals. It is expected to be adopted as the HIPAA-required diagnosis code set before 2010. Major changes include the following:

- The ICD-10 contains more than 2000 categories of diseases, many more than the ICD-9. This creates more codes to permit more specific reporting of diseases and newly recognized conditions, such as SARS.

- Codes are alphanumeric, containing a letter followed by up to five numbers. The sixth digit is added to capture clinical details. For example, all codes that relate to pregnancy, labor, and childbirth include a digit that indicates the patient's trimester.

- Codes are added to show which side of the body is affected when a disease or condition can be involved with the right side, the left side, or bilaterally.

It is generally acknowledged that experienced ICD-9 coders will require only brief training to work effectively and efficiently with ICD-10.

Procedure Codes: The CPT

After an office visit, each procedure and service performed for a patient is reported on health-care claims using a **procedure code.** These codes represent medical procedures, such as surgery and diagnostic tests, and medical services, such as an examination to evaluate a patient's condition. Medical assistants often verify procedure codes and use them to report physicians' services.

The most commonly used system of procedure codes is found in the *Current Procedural Terminology,* a book published by the American Medical Association (AMA) that is commonly known as **CPT.** CPT is the HIPAA-required code set for physicians' procedures.

An updated edition of the CPT is published every year to reflect changes in medical practice. Newly developed procedures are added, and old ones that have become obsolete are deleted. These changes are also available in a computer file because some medical offices use a computer-based version of the CPT.

Medical offices should have the current year's CPT available for reference and keep forms up to date. Previous years' books should also be kept in case there is a question about health-care claims that were previously submitted.

Using the CPT

CPT codes are five-digit numbers, organized into six sections:

Section	Range of Codes
Evaluation and Management	99201–99499
Anesthesiology	00100–01999
Surgery	10021–69990
Radiology	70010–79999
Pathology and Laboratory	80048–89356
Medicine	90281–99602

Except for the first section, the CPT reference book is arranged in numerical order. Codes for evaluation and management are listed first, out of numerical order, because they are used most often.

Each section opens with important guidelines that apply to its procedures. This material should be checked carefully before a procedure code is chosen. The sections of the CPT are divided into categories. These in turn are further divided into headings according to the type of test, service, or body system. Code number ranges included on a particular page are found in the upper right corner. This helps to locate a code quickly after using the index. An example is shown in Figure 16-2.

Locate correct procedure codes by first looking up the term in the CPT's index. Bold-faced main terms may be followed by descriptions and groups of indented terms. The correct code is selected by reviewing each description and indented term under the main term.

Although it may seem tempting to record the procedure code directly from the index, resist the shortcut. Explanations and notes in the guidelines and main sections

Surgery

General

(10000-10020 have been deleted. To report see 10060, 10061)

10021 Fine needle aspiration; without imaging guidance
➔ *CPT Assistant* Aug 02:10; *CPT Changes: An Insider's View* 2002

10022 with imaging guidance
➔ *CPT Changes: An Insider's View* 2002

(For radiological supervision and interpretation, see 76003, 76360, 76393, 76942)

(For percutaneous needle biopsy other than fine needle aspiration, see 20206 for muscle, 32400 for pleura, 32405 for lung or mediastinum, 42400 for salivary gland, 47000, 47001 for liver, 48102 for pancreas, 49180 for abdominal or retroperitoneal mass, 60100 for thyroid, 62269 for spinal cord)

(For evaluation of fine needle aspirate, see 88172, 88173)

Integumentary System

Skin, Subcutaneous and Accessory Structures

Incision and Drainage

(For excision, see 11400, et seq)

10040 Acne surgery (eg, marsupialization, opening or removal of multiple milia, comedones, cysts, pustules)

10060 Incision and drainage of abscess (eg, carbuncle, suppurative hidradenitis, cutaneous or subcutaneous abscess, cyst, furuncle, or paronychia); simple or single

10061 complicated or multiple

10080 Incision and drainage of pilonidal cyst; simple

10081 complicated

(For excision of pilonidal cyst, see 11770-11772)

10120 Incision and removal of foreign body, subcutaneous tissues; simple

10121 complicated

(To report wound exploration due to penetrating trauma without laparotomy or thoracotomy, see 20100-20103, as appropriate)

(To report debridement associated with open fracture(s) and/or dislocation(s), use 11010-11012, as appropriate)

10140 Incision and drainage of hematoma, seroma or fluid collection
➔ *CPT Changes: An Insider's View* 2002

(If imaging guidance is performed, see 76360, 76393, 76942)

10160 Puncture aspiration of abscess, hematoma, bulla, or cyst
➔ *CPT Changes: An Insider's View* 2002

(If imaging guidance is performed, see 76360, 76393, 76942)

10180 Incision and drainage, complex, postoperative wound infection

(For secondary closure of surgical wound, see 12020, 12021, 13160)

Excision—Debridement

(For dermabrasions, see 15780-15783)

(For nail debridement, see 11720-11721)

(For burn(s), see 16000-16035)

11000 Debridement of extensive eczematous or infected skin; up to 10% of body surface

+ 11001 each additional 10% of the body surface (List separately in addition to code for primary procedure)

(Use 11001 in conjunction with code 11000)

11010 Debridement including removal of foreign material associated with open fracture(s) and/or dislocation(s); skin and subcutaneous tissues
➔ *CPT Assistant* Mar 97:1, Apr 97:10, Aug 97:6

11011 skin, subcutaneous tissue, muscle fascia, and muscle
➔ *CPT Assistant* Mar 97:1, Apr 97:10, Aug 97:6

11012 skin, subcutaneous tissue, muscle fascia, muscle, and bone
➔ *CPT Assistant* Mar 97:1, Apr 97:10, Aug 97:6

11040 Debridement; skin, partial thickness
➔ *CPT Assistant* Fall 93:21, May 96:6, Feb 97:7, Aug 97:6

11041 skin, full thickness
➔ *CPT Assistant* Fall 93:21, May 96:6, Feb 97:7, Aug 97:6

11042 skin, and subcutaneous tissue
➔ *CPT Assistant* Winter 92:10, May 96:6, Feb 97:7, Aug 97:6

11043 skin, subcutaneous tissue, and muscle
➔ *CPT Assistant* May 96:6, Feb 97:7, Apr 97:11, Aug 97:6

11044 skin, subcutaneous tissue, muscle, and bone
➔ *CPT Assistant* Fall 93:21, Mar 96:10, May 96:6, Feb 97:7, Apr 97:11, Aug 97:6

(Do not report 11040-11044 in addition to 97601, 97602)

Figure 16-2. Examples of CPT codes, surgical section.

Source: American Medical Association, *Current Procedural Terminology,* copyright 2003.

more accurately lead to finding main numbers and modifiers that reflect the services performed. That is the only way to ensure reimbursement at the highest allowed level.

Add-On Codes. A plus sign (+) is used for **add-on codes,** indicating procedures that are usually carried out in addition to another procedure. For example, code 90471 covers one immunization administration, and code 90472 covers administering an additional shot. Add-on codes are never reported alone. They are used together with the primary code.

Modifiers. One or more two-digit **modifiers** may be assigned to the five-digit main number. Modifiers are written with a hyphen after the five-digit number and before the two-digit number. The use of a modifier shows that some special circumstance applies to the service or procedure the physician performed. For example, in the surgery section, the modifier -62 indicates that two surgeons worked together, each performing part of a surgical procedure during an operation. Each physician will be paid part of the amount normally reimbursed for that procedure code. Appendix A of the CPT explains the proper use of each modifier. Some section guidelines also discuss the use of modifiers with the section's codes.

Category II Codes, Category III Codes, and Unlisted Procedure Codes. Category II codes are used to track health-care performance measures, such as programs and counseling to avoid tobacco use. Category III codes are temporary CPT codes for emerging technology, services, and procedures. When no code is available to completely describe a procedure, a code for an unlisted procedure is selected. Unlisted procedure codes are used for new services or procedures that have not yet been assigned codes in CPT. When these codes are used, which is rare, a written explanation of the procedure or service is needed.

Evaluation and Management Services

To diagnose conditions and plan treatments, physicians use a wide range of time, effort, and skill for different patients and circumstances. Evaluation and management codes **(E/M codes)** are often considered the most important of all CPT codes, because they can be used by all physicians in any medical specialty.

The E/M section guidelines explain how to code different levels of these services. Three key factors documented in the patient's medical record help determine the level of service:

1. The extent of the patient history taken
2. The extent of the examination conducted
3. The complexity of the medical decision making

Payers also want to know whether the physician treated a **new patient** or an **established patient.** Physicians often spend more time during new patients' visits than during visits from established patients, so the E/M codes for the two types of patients are separate. For reporting purposes, the CPT considers a patient "new" if that person has not received professional services from the physician within the past three years. An established patient is one who has seen the physician within the past three years. (Note that the current visit need not be for a problem treated previously.) Emergency patients are not classified as either new or established patients.

The CPT has a range of five codes each for new-patient or established-patient encounters. The lowest-level code is often called a Level I code; the highest-level code is a Level V code. For example, code 99213 is the Level III code for an established patient's office visit.

The location of the service is also important because different E/M codes apply to services performed in a physician's office, a hospital inpatient room, a hospital emergency room, a nursing facility, an extended-care facility, or a patient's home.

Surgical Procedures

Figure 16-2 illustrates a series of codes from the integumentary part of the surgical section. Codes listed in the surgery section represent all the procedures that are normally a part of that operation, including local anesthesia, the surgery itself, and routine follow-up care. This combination of services is called a surgical package. Payers assign a fee to each of these codes that pays for all the services provided under them.

The period of time that is covered for follow-up care is called the **global period.** For example, the global period for repairing a tendon might be set at 15 days. A global period for major surgery such as an appendectomy might be set at 100 days. After the global period ends, additional services can be reported separately for payment.

To make the coding process more efficient, medical offices often list frequently used CPT codes on superbills. After seeing the patient, the physician checks off the appropriate procedures or services. An example of a dermatology practice's superbill is shown in Figure 16-3. This sample superbill lists the E/M codes for new and established patient office visits as well as common procedures for the office.

Laboratory Procedures

Organ or disease-oriented **panels** listed in the pathology and laboratory section of the CPT include tests frequently ordered together. An electrolyte panel, for example, includes tests for carbon dioxide, chloride, potassium, and sodium. Each element of the panel has its own procedure code. However, when the tests are performed together, the code for the panel must be used rather than the separate procedure codes.

VALLEY ASSOCIATES, P.C.
David Rosenberg, M.D. - Dermatology
555-321-0987
FED I.D. #06-2345678

PATIENT NAME	APPT. DATE/TIME	
Scott Yeager	10/14/2003	11:00am

PATIENT NO.	DX
YEAGESCO	1. 919.7 superficial foreign body without
	2. major open wound. Infected
	3.
	4.

DESCRIPTION	✓	CPT	FEE	DESCRIPTION	✓	CPT	FEE
EXAMINATION				**PROCEDURES**			
New Patient				Acne Surgery		10040	
Problem Focused		99201		I&D Cyst/Abscess		10060	
Expanded Problem Focused	✓	99202	50	I&D Multiple		10061	
Detailed		99203		I&D Remove Foreign Body	✓	10120	60
Comprehensive		99204		Debridement		11000	
Comprehensive/Complex		99205		Paring/Curett. (Benign)		11055	
Established Patient				Paring/Curett. (2-4)		11056	
Minimum		99211		Paring/Curett. (Over 4)		11057	
Problem Focused		99212		Excision Skin Tags (1-15)		11200	
Expanded Problem Focused		99213		Cyrosurgery		17340	
Detailed		99214		Skin Biopsy		11100	
Comprehensive/Complex		99215		Skin Biopsy (EA additional)		+11101	

Figure 16-3. Superbill with procedure codes.

If each test in a panel or procedure in a surgical package is listed separately, it will unbundle the panel or package. The review performed by the insurance carrier's claims department will rebundle the services under the appropriate code, which could delay payment. Note that when unbundling is done intentionally to receive more payment than is correct, the claim is likely to be considered fraudulent.

Immunizations

Injections and infusions of immune globulins, vaccines, toxoids, and other substances require two codes, one for giving the injection and one for the particular vaccine or toxoid that is given. An E/M code is not used along with the codes for immunization unless a significant evaluation and management service is also performed by the doctor.

HCPCS

The **Health Care Common Procedure Coding System,** commonly referred to as **HCPCS,** was developed by the Centers for Medicare and Medicaid Services (CMS) for use in coding services for Medicare patients. The HCPCS (pronounced "hic-picks") coding system has two levels:

1. HCPCS Level I codes duplicate those from CPT.
2. **HCPCS Level II codes,** issued by CMS, are called national codes and cover many supplies, such as sterile trays, drugs, and DME (durable medical equipment). Level II codes also cover services and procedures not included in the CPT.

The HCPCS codes for Level II have five characters, either numbers, letters, or a combination of both. At times there are also two-character modifiers, either two letters or a letter with a number. These modifiers are different from

Locating a CPT Code

Objective: To locate correct CPT codes

Materials: Patient record, CPT

Method

1. Become familiar with the CPT.
   Read the introduction and main section guidelines and notes. For example, look at the guidelines for the evaluation and management section. They include definitions of key terms, such as *new* and *established patient, chief complaint, concurrent care,* and *counseling.* They also explain the method for selecting E/M codes.

2. Find the services listed in the patient's record.
   Check the patient's record to see which services were performed. For E/M procedures, look for clues as to the extent of history, examination, and decision making that were involved.

3. Look up the procedure code(s).
   First, pick out a specific procedure or service, organ, or condition. Find the procedure code in the CPT index. Remember, the number in the index is the five-digit code, not a page number. In some cases, the patient's medical record shows an abbreviation, an *eponym* (a person or place for which a procedure is named), or a synonym. For example, the record might state "treated for bone infection." In CPT's index, the entry for "Infection, Bone," is followed by the instruction "See Osteomyelitis."

   Example 1: To find the code for "dressing change," first look alphabetically in the index for the procedure. Then turn to the procedure code in the body of the CPT to be sure the code accurately reflects the service performed. The procedure code 15852 explains the dressing change for "other than burns" and "under anesthesia (other than local)." A dressing for a burn is listed as procedure codes 16010–16030.

   Example 2: To code the excision of a vaginal cyst, you can first look under "Excision." There is a listing for "Cyst" beneath "Excision," followed by a list of organs, regions, or structures involved. Look for "Vagina" to find the code. Another way to find the code is to look under "Vagina" and then find the listing for "Cyst Excision" beneath it.

4. Determine appropriate modifiers.
   Check section guidelines and Appendix A to choose a modifier if needed to explain a situation involving the procedure being coded, such as difficult work or a discontinued procedure.

   Example: A bilateral breast reconstruction requires the modifier -50. Find the code for "breast reconstruction with free flap": 19364. To show the insurance carrier that the procedure was performed on both breasts, attach the -50: 19364-50.

5. Record the procedure code(s) on the health-care claim.
   After the procedure code is verified, it is posted to the health-care claim. The primary procedure—performed for the condition listed as the primary diagnosis—is listed first. Match additional procedures with their corresponding diagnoses.

the CPT modifiers. For example, HCPCS modifiers may indicate social worker services or equipment rentals.

Examples of Level II codes are:

Code Number	Description
A0225-QN	Ambulance service, neonatal transport, base rate, emergency transport, one way, furnished directly by the provider of services
E0781	Ambulatory infusion pump
G0001	Routine venipuncture
G0104	Colorectal cancer screening; flexible sigmoidoscopy
Q0091	Screening Papanicolaou (Pap) smear; obtaining, preparing, and conveyance of cervical or vaginal smear to laboratory
V5299	Hearing service, miscellaneous

In medical offices where the HCPCS system is used, regulations issued by CMS are reviewed to determine the correct code and modifier for claims.

Avoiding Fraud: Coding Compliance

Physicians have the ultimate responsibility for proper documentation and correct coding as well as for compliance with regulations. Medical assistants help ensure maximum appropriate reimbursement for reported services by submitting correct health-care claims. These claims, as well as the process used to create them, must comply with the rules imposed by federal and state law and with payer requirements.

Code Linkage

On correct claims, each reported service is connected to a diagnosis that supports the procedure as necessary to investigate or treat the patient's condition. Insurance company representatives analyze this connection between the diagnostic and the procedural information, called **code linkage,** to evaluate the medical necessity of the reported charges. Correct claims also comply with many other regulations from government agencies.

The possible consequences of inaccurate coding and incorrect billing include:

- Denied claims
- Delays in processing claims and receiving payments
- Reduced payments
- Fines and other sanctions
- Loss of hospital privileges
- Exclusion from payers' programs
- Prison sentences
- Loss of the physician's license to practice medicine

To avoid errors, the codes on health-care claims are checked against the medical documentation. A code review checks these key points:

- Are the codes appropriate to the patient's profile (age, gender, condition; new or established), and is each coded service billable?
- Is there a clear and correct link between each diagnosis and procedure?
- Have the payer's rules about the diagnosis and the procedure been followed?
- Does the documentation in the patient's medical record support the reported services?
- Do the reported services comply with all regulations?

Insurance Fraud

Almost everyone involved in the delivery of health care is a trustworthy person devoted to patients' welfare. However, some people are not. For example, according to the Department of Health and Human Services (HHS), in one year alone, the federal government recovered more than $1.3 billion in judgments, settlements, and other fees in health-care fraud cases. Fraud is an act of deception used to take advantage of another person or entity. For example, it is fraudulent for people to misrepresent their credentials or to forge another person's signature on a check.

Claims fraud occurs when physicians or others falsely represent their services or charges to payers. For example,

a provider may bill for services that were not performed, overcharge for services, or fail to provide complete services under a contract. A patient may exaggerate an injury to get a settlement from an insurance company or ask a medical assistant to change a date on a chart so that a service is covered by a health plan.

A number of coding and billing practices are fraudulent. Investigators reviewing physicians' billings look for patterns like these:

- Reporting services that were not performed.
  Example: A lab bills Medicare for a general health panel (CPT 80050), but fails to perform one of the tests in the panel.
- Reporting services at a higher level than was carried out.
  Example: After a visit for a flu shot, the provider bills the encounter as an evaluation and management service plus a vaccination.
- Performing and billing for procedures that are not related to the patient's condition and therefore not medically necessary.
  Example: After reading an article about Lyme disease, a patient is worried about having worked in her garden over the summer and requests a Lyme disease diagnostic test. Although no symptoms or signs have been reported, the physician orders and bills for the Lyme disease test.
- Billing separately for services that are bundled in a single procedure code.
  Example: When a physician orders a comprehensive metabolic panel (CPT 80053), the provider bills for the panel as well as for a quantitative glucose test, which is in the panel.
- Reporting the same service twice.

Note that HIPAA calls for penalties for giving remuneration to anyone eligible for benefits under federal health-care programs. The forgiveness or waiver of co-payments may violate the policies of some payers; others may permit forgiveness or waiver if they are aware of the reasons for the forgiveness or waiver, such as the patient's inability to pay. Routine forgiveness or waiver of co-payments may constitute fraud under state and federal law. The physician practice should ensure that its policies on co-payments are consistent with applicable law and with the requirements of their agreements with payers.

Compliance Plans

To avoid the risk of fraud, medical offices have a **compliance plan** to uncover compliance problems and correct them. A compliance plan is a process for finding, correcting, and preventing illegal medical office practices. Its goals are to:

- Prevent fraud and abuse through a formal process to identify, investigate, fix, and prevent repeat violations

Medical Coder, Physician Practice

Medical coding specialists work in a number of health-care settings, including medical practices, hospitals, government agencies, and insurance companies. Coders who work in physician practices review patients' medical records and assign diagnosis and procedure codes. They are knowledgeable about the coding rules and procedures for physicians' work, which are different than those for coding hospital services. The position of medical coding specialist is growing in importance in physician practices. Accurate coding is a critical part of ensuring that claims follow the legal and ethical requirements of Medicare and other third-party payers as well as HIPAA regulations.

Medical office employees may gain required health-care work experience and then attain coding positions through coding education from seminars or college classes. Certification as a professional coder offers an excellent route to success as a medical coder in the medical practice setting. Some employers require certification for employment; others state that certification must be earned after a certain amount of time in the position, such as six months. Coding classes followed by examinations are used to obtain certification. Three physician-office coding certifications are available. All require a high school diploma or equivalent.

- The American Health Information Management Association offers the Certified Coding Associate (CCA) credential and the Certified Coding Specialist—Physician-based (CCS-P) credential. The CCA is an entry-level title; completion of either a training program or six months' job experience is recommended. The CCS-P requires at least three years of coding experience.

- The American Academy of Professional Coders offers the Certified Professional Coder (CPC) credential, also requiring coursework and on-the-job experience.

Medical assistants who hold these credentials and have coding experience may advance to coding management and coding compliance auditor positions. Becoming expert in a specialty such as surgical coding also offers advancement opportunities.

relating to reimbursement for health-care services provided

- Ensure compliance with applicable federal, state, and local laws, including employment laws and environmental laws as well as antifraud laws
- Help defend physicians if they are investigated or prosecuted for fraud by showing the desire to behave compliantly and thus reduce any fines or criminal prosecution

When a compliance plan is in place, it demonstrates to payers such as Medicare that honest, ongoing attempts have been made to find and fix weak areas of compliance with regulations. The development of this written plan is led by a compliance officer and committee with the intention to (1) audit and monitor compliance with government regulations, especially in the area of coding and billing, (2) develop written policies and procedures that are consistent, (3) provide for ongoing staff training and communication, and (4) respond to and correct errors.

Although coding and billing compliance are the plan's major focus, it covers all areas of government regulation of medical practices, such as equal employment opportunity (EEO) regulations (for example, hiring and promotion policies) and OSHA regulations (for example, fire safety and handling of hazardous materials such as blood-borne pathogens).

Summary

The ICD-9-CM is used for diagnostic coding in the United States. ICD-9 codes are required for reporting patients' conditions on health-care claims. Codes are made up of three, four, or five numbers and a description. New codes are issued annually, and current codes should be used because they can affect billing and reimbursement.

The ICD-9 has two volumes that are used in medical practices: the Tabular List (Volume 1) and the Alphabetic Index (Volume 2). To find a code, use the Alphabetic Index first. Its main terms may be followed by related terms. The codes themselves are organized into 17 chapters and are listed in numerical order in the Tabular List. Code categories consist of three-digit groupings of a single disease or a related condition. Further clinical detail is shown by four- or five-digit codes. The conventions used in the ICD-9 must be observed to correctly select codes.

V codes identify encounters for reasons other than illness or injury and are used for healthy patients receiving routine services, for therapeutic encounters, for a problem that is not currently affecting the patient's condition, and for preoperative evaluations. E codes, which are never used as primary codes, classify the injuries resulting from various environmental events.

CPT provides a standardized list of five-digit procedure codes for medical, surgical, and diagnostic services. Add-on codes and modifiers may also be selected.

CPT is divided into six sections: (1) evaluation and management, (2) anesthesiology, (3) surgery, (4) radiology, (5) pathology and laboratory, and (6) medicine. The three main factors that influence the level of service for coding purposes are the type and extent of (1) history, (2) examination, and (3) medical decision making. Surgical packages and laboratory panels should be coded as single procedures rather than broken into component parts.

The Health Care Common Procedure Coding System (HCPCS), used to code Medicare services, has codes from CPT as well as Level II national codes.

Diagnoses and procedures must be correctly linked when services are reported for reimbursement because payers analyze this connection to determine the medical necessity of the charges. Correct claims also comply with all applicable regulations and requirements. Codes should be appropriate and documented as well as compliant with each payer's rules.

A medical practice compliance plan addresses compliance concerns of government and private payers. Furthermore, having a formal process in place is a sign that the practice has made a good-faith effort to achieve compliance in coding.

CASE STUDY QUESTIONS

Now that you have completed this chapter, review the case study at the beginning of the chapter and answer the following questions:

1. How would you select the ICD-9 and CPT codes for a health-care claim for this visit?
2. What diagnosis and procedure codes will result in the correct payment for these services?
3. How should the claim show the medical necessity of the procedures?
4. Locate the ICD-9 code for the patient's asthma. How many digits are required? What code did you assign?
5. Locate the CPT code for the cardiovascular stress test. What information did you use to select it from the list of related codes?

Discussion Questions

1. What are the differences among the three code sets discussed in the chapter?
2. Are *see* cross-references in the Alphabetic Index of the ICD-9 followed by codes? Why?
3. Would you expect to locate codes for the following services or procedures in CPT? What range or series of codes would you investigate?
   a. Routine obstetric care including antepartum care, cesarean delivery, and postpartum care
   b. Echocardiography (cardiac)
   c. Radiologic examination, nasal bones, complete
   d. Home visit for evaluation and management of an established patient
   e. Drug test for amphetamines
   f. Anesthesia for cardiac catheterization
4. Why are both the ICD-9 and CPT codes updated each year?

Critical Thinking Questions

1. What is the proper order in which to select a diagnosis code?
2. Why is it necessary to report the most specific diagnosis codes available?
3. What could result if a medical assistant enters an incorrect diagnosis code on a claim?

4. How can improving physicians' documentation of diagnoses and procedures help ensure compliance?
5. A patient asked a medical assistant to help her out of a tough financial spot. Her medical insurance authorized her to receive four radiation treatments for her condition, one every 35 days. Because she was out of town, she did not schedule her appointment for the last treatment until today, which is one week beyond the approved period. The health plan will not reimburse her for this procedure. The patient asks the MA to change the date on the record to last Wednesday so that it will be covered, explaining that no one will be hurt by this change, and anyway, she pays the insurance company plenty.

    What type of action is the patient asking the MA to do? How should the request be handled?

Application Activities

1. A. A female patient is taking a medication that is known to affect the lining of the endometrium. She received an endometrial biopsy and pelvic ultrasound to monitor changes. What type of ICD-9 code is used to describe the medical need for these services?

    B. A patient fell off a ladder while on the job, spraining his left ankle and fracturing the right femur. In addition to the main code, what type of ICD-9 code is used to report his diagnosis?
2. Study Table 1 in the guidelines for the evaluation and management section of CPT. What code range is used for emergency department services? Now turn to Appendix A. Is it correct to use modifier -21 with E/M codes? Modifier -51?
3. Underline the main term in each of the following diagnoses and then determine the correct ICD-9 codes.
   a. cerebral atherosclerosis
   b. spasmodic asthma with status asthmaticus
   c. congenital night blindness
   d. recurrent inguinal hernia with obstruction
   e. incomplete bundle branch heart block
4. Find the following codes in the index of CPT. Underline the key term you used to find the code.
   a. Intracapsular lens extraction
   b. Coombs test
   c. X-ray of duodenum
   d. Unlisted procedure, maxillofacial prosthetics
   e. DTAP immunization

REVIEW

CHAPTER **16**

1. Both the American Health Information Management Association (AHIMA) and the American Academy of Professional Coders (AAPC) are national associations that certify medical coders and provide information on coding issues. Visit their Web sites and investigate the ways these associations keep their members up-to-date about changes in procedural coding. Also review the activities of these organizations in your local area.

2. Access the Web site of the National Center for Health Statistics and locate information on the current year's ICD-9-CM new codes. Also research and report on the status of ICD-10-CM.

3. Visit the American Medical Association's Web site and search on the terms *Category II* and *Category III*. Review the latest codes in these categories.

CHAPTER 17

Patient Billing and Collections

AREAS OF COMPETENCE

2003 Role Delineation Study

ADMINISTRATIVE

Practice Finances
- Apply bookkeeping principles
- Manage accounts receivable

CHAPTER OUTLINE

- Basic Accounting
- Standard Payment Procedures
- Standard Billing Procedures
- Standard Collection Procedures
- Credit Arrangements
- Common Collection Problems

OBJECTIVES

After completing Chapter 17, you will be able to:

17.1 Discuss the importance of accounts receivable to a medical practice.

17.2 Explain how to accept and account for payment from patients.

17.3 Prepare an invoice.

17.4 Manage a billing cycle efficiently.

17.5 Describe standard collection techniques.

17.6 Explain how to perform a credit check.

17.7 Identify credit arrangements.

17.8 Recognize common collection problems.

KEY TERMS

accounts payable
accounts receivable
age analysis
class action lawsuit
credit
credit bureau
cycle billing
damages
disclosure statement
legal custody
open-book account
punitive damages
single-entry account
statement
statute of limitations
superbill
written-contract account

Introduction

Medical assisting is a multifaceted career. As such, a person in that career may be required to take on many duties in the medical office that are administrative in nature. The medical office has customers who have various payment arrangements, such as third-party payers (usually insurance carriers) and payment plans, and who may also have large outstanding balances. A proper understanding and administration of billing—for both third-party payers and patients—as well as payment collection methods is therefore required.

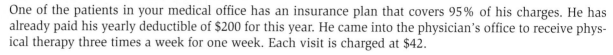
One of the patients in your medical office has an insurance plan that covers 95% of his charges. He has already paid his yearly deductible of $200 for this year. He came into the physician's office to receive physical therapy three times a week for one week. Each visit is charged at $42.

As you read this chapter, consider the following questions:
1. What is the total owed for this patient's visits?
2. How much of the total is not covered by insurance and should be billed to the patient?

Basic Accounting

In any business, basic accounting involves managing accounts receivable and accounts payable. **Accounts receivable** is the term for income, or money, owed to the business. **Accounts payable** is the term for money owed by the business. In a medical practice, accounts receivable represents the money patients owe in return for medical services. Accounts payable describes the money the medical practice must pay out to run the practice.

Billing and collections are vitally important tasks because they convert the practice's accounts receivable into readily available income, or cash flow, from which the accounts payable can be paid. Unless billing and collections are carried out effectively, a practice might have plenty of money due in accounts receivable without having enough cash flow for accounts payable.

There are methods of improving billing and collection procedures to increase income for the practice. You will need to know about standard payment, billing, and collection procedures as well as about credit arrangements and common problems in collecting payment.

Standard Payment Procedures

Most physicians prefer to collect payment from patients at each office visit. Immediate payment not only brings income into the practice faster, but it saves the cost of preparing and mailing bills and collecting on past-due accounts. For these reasons, many physicians' offices post a small sign at the reception desk that states, for example, "Payment is requested when services are rendered unless other arrangements are made in advance."

As a medical assistant, you are responsible for collecting these payments. If the patient cannot pay at the time of the visit, it is your responsibility to bill for the physician's services. A bill, the paperwork sent to patients to inform them of payment or balance due, is referred to as an invoice.

Determining Appropriate Fees

A fee schedule is a price list for the medical practice. Figure 17-1 shows an example. The fee schedule lists the services the doctor offers and the corresponding charges for those services. Fees are not randomly assigned. They reflect the cost of services, the doctor's experience, charges of other doctors in the area, and other factors. Sometimes the fee allowed by insurance policies is a determining factor. The practice may use a particular system to determine how much to charge for each service. Following are descriptions of these systems.

Usual and Customary Fees.   A usual fee is the fee a doctor charges for a service or procedure. A customary fee is either the average fee charged for a service or procedure by all comparable doctors in the same region or the ninetieth percentile of all fees charged by comparable doctors in the same region for the same procedure. There is a growing tendency, however, to determine fees by national rather than regional trends.

Relative Value Unit.   Section 121 of the Social Security Act Amendments of 1994 required CMS to develop a methodology for a resource-based system. This system was created to determine practice expense relative value units (RVUs) for all Medicare physician fee schedule services. Effective January 1, 1999, Phase 1 of resource-based practice expense was put into effect.

For each medical service, an RVU is assigned that reflects the following factors:

- The doctor's skill and time required
- The professional liability expenses related to that service, such as malpractice insurance
- The overhead costs associated with that service

The RVUs are converted to dollar amounts. These dollar amounts form the basis of the RVU fee schedule. This schedule creates uniform payments that are adjusted for geographic differences.

This methodology has reduced the growth rate of spending for doctors' professional services, related services and supplies, and other Medicare Part B services.

Processing Charge Slips

Fees must be determined in order to create a charge slip, the original record of the doctor's services and the charges for those services. Figure 17-2 shows an example of a

John Q. Davis, MD

Adult and Pediatric Urology-Infertility

SERVICE RENDERED	CPT	FEE	SERVICE RENDERED	CPT	FEE
Initial OV	99204	$100.00	Condyloma Treatment	54050	$40.00
Follow-up Visit	99214	$65.00	Cystoscopy	52000	$300.00
Fertility Consultation	99243	$140.00	Catheterization	93975	$45.00
Office Consultation	99244	$140.00	Vasectomy	55250	$775.00
Hospital Admission	99223	$150.00	Ultrasonic Guide Needle Biopsy	76942	$395.00
Hospital Consultation	99254	$150.00	Prostate Biopsy	55700	$325.00
ER Visit	99284	$75.00–$150.00	Biopsy Gun	A9270	$45.00
Hospital Visit	99232	$55.00	Uroflowmeter	51741	$80.00
Urinalysis w/ Micro	81000	$14.00	Renal Ultrasound	76775	$295.00
Culture	87086	$45.00	Scrotal Ultrasound	76870	$295.00
Stone Analysis	32360	$60.00	Acidic Acid	99070	$20.00
Venipuncture	36415	$10.00	Foley Catheter Starter Set	A4329	$35.00

Figure 17-1. The fee schedule shows the charges for services provided by the practice.

DATE	DESCRIPTION–CODE	CHARGE	PAYMENT	CURRENT BALANCE

(918) 555-9680

Tax ID No. 11-0004004

Patricia Belden, MD

111 Roosevelt Boulevard
Lawrence, OK 77527

99205 Office Visit, New Patient
99215 Office Visit, Established Patient
99213 Office Visit, Established, Brief
88155 Pap
84703 Urine Pregnancy Test

36425 Venipuncture
57454 Colposcopy with Biopsy
57511 Cryosurgery
58100 Endometrial Biopsy
56600 Vulva Biopsy

59025 NST
54150 Circumcision
58300 IUD Insertion
57170 Diaphragm Fitting

NAME_____ DX _____

No. 0005807

Figure 17-2. A charge slip shows the services performed for a patient and the charges for those services.

charge slip. Charge slips are also called fee slips or transaction slips. They are usually numbered consecutively. They may be preprinted with common services and charges for the practice. Charge slips are used in several ways.

Some doctors keep a pad of charge slips on their desk. After seeing a patient, they fill in the services and charges on the charge slip. They give the charge slip to the patient and ask the patient to give it to you on the way out of the office.

In other offices, you may write the patient's name on the charge slip and give the slip to the doctor along with the patient's medical record. The doctor then fills in the services performed and asks you to fill in the charges according to the fee schedule. If questions arise about the fee for a particular service, you can refer to the fee schedule and tell the patient how much that service will cost.

Accepting Payment

When the patient comes to you with the charge slip, you complete the charge slip and ask for payment. There are several effective yet diplomatic ways to request payment. Two examples are, "For today's visit, the total charge is $50. How would you like to pay?" and "The charge for your laboratory work today is $80. Would you like to pay for that now?" Most practices accept several forms of payment, including cash, check, credit card, and insurance. Insurance payment is discussed in detail in Chapter 15.

Cash. If the patient chooses to pay in cash, count the money carefully to be sure you have received the proper amount. Next, record the payment on the patient's ledger card, and give the patient a receipt. (Patient ledger cards are explained in Chapter 18.)

Some practices use a combination charge slip/receipt, which is discussed in Chapter 18. If your practice does not, prepare a cash receipt manually, as shown in Figure 17-3. Then place the money in the cash drawer or cash box.

Check. If the patient pays by check, be sure the check is written properly, including the current date. The amount of the check should match the total amount listed on the charge slip, unless the patient has made prior arrangements to pay only part of the amount. The name of the doctor or practice should appear in the "Pay to the Order of" section and should be properly spelled. The check should be signed by the person whose name is printed on the check. After accepting the check, endorse it immediately, and deposit it in the practice bank account.

Credit Card. Many doctors' offices accept credit cards, such as Visa or MasterCard. This payment method offers advantages for both the practice and the patient. For the practice, it provides prompt payment from the credit card company, thus increasing cash flow. It also reduces the amount of time and money spent on preparing and mailing bills, thus decreasing expenses. For the patient, it is convenient and allows a large bill to be paid in several smaller amounts, usually once a month.

Credit cards have one major disadvantage for the practice—cost. The credit card company deducts a percentage of each charge for its collection service, usually between 1% and 5%. If a patient charges $100 in services on a credit card, for example, the practice receives only $95 to $99. The credit card company keeps the difference. A disadvantage for patients is the accrued interest charges on unpaid balances.

If the practice accepts credit card payments, the American Medical Association (AMA) suggests several guidelines.

- Do not set higher fees for patients who pay by credit card.
- Do not encourage patients to use credit cards for payment.
- Do not advertise outside the office that the practice accepts credit cards.

If a patient chooses to pay by credit card, process the transaction carefully to ensure that the credit card company charges the patient correctly. To begin, inform the patient of the amount due, and ask for the credit card.

Check the expiration date on the front of the credit card. If the card has not expired, place it in the credit card machine, and place a credit card voucher on top of it. Slide the imprint arm firmly to the right and back across the machine. Remove the voucher from the machine. Write in the date, and circle the type of credit card, such as Visa or MasterCard, after it is removed from the machine.

Next, obtain the authorization code from the credit card company. Some offices have devices that read the magnetic strip on the credit card and automatically transmit the information to the credit card company by telephone line (Figure 17-4). If your office has such a device, type in the amount to be charged on its keypad. Then, the credit card company issues an authorization code, which appears on the device's screen.

No. _____	Date _____, 20_____

Received of _____

_____

_____ **Dollars**

For Professional Services	Amount Account	$_____
	This Payment	$_____
	Balance	$_____

Thank You!

Lauren Harris, MD

Medical Arts Bldg. 117 City Line Road Newtown, NJ 08944 (201) 555-0000

Figure 17-3. After writing a receipt for cash, record the payment on the patient's ledger card.

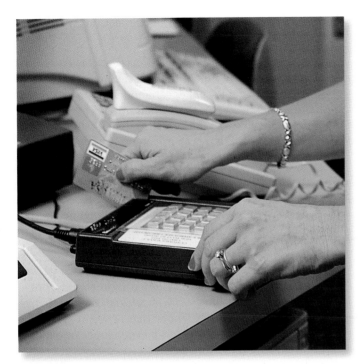

Figure 17-4. Using a device like this one, you can swipe the patient's card through the machine and obtain instant authorization from the credit card company.

If your office does not have such a device, call the credit card company for the authorization code. Give the operator the patient's credit card number and the amount of the payment. The operator then gives you the authorization code.

Write the authorization code in the box marked "Authorization" on the credit card voucher. Initial the voucher in the appropriate box. Then, fill in the services provided and the amount of the charges. Enter the total charges in the box marked "Total."

Give the voucher to the patient to sign. Compare the patient's signature on the voucher with the signature on the back of the credit card (they should, of course, be identical). Keep one copy of the voucher for the office. Give the other copy and the credit card to the patient.

Using the Pegboard System for Posting Payments

Some physicians' offices use the pegboard system to post payments and generate receipts for patients. If your office uses the pegboard system, you may use the pegboard to record the payment on the ledger card and receipt simultaneously. You handle this task in basically the same way, whether the patient pays immediately or later, in response to a bill.

Determining Payment Responsibility

Generally the patient is responsible for payments for medical services. To help promote timely payments, however, you need to know exactly who is responsible for them.

Third-Party Liability. Third-party liability refers to the responsibility of the patient's insurance company to pay for certain medical expenses, which may include doctors' services. Each practice decides how to handle its patients' health insurance claims.

Some practices do not accept any insurance, although these practices are rare. The patient must pay the doctor directly and file an insurance claim for reimbursement. If you work in such a practice, you must give the patient the necessary medical information to fill out the insurance claim. A completed superbill (discussed later in this chapter) provides the information.

Practices increasingly handle all their patients' insurance paperwork to ensure accuracy, timely submission, and prompt payment. Some practices charge a fee for handling patients' insurance claims. Some practices handle paperwork only for patients who find it particularly difficult, such as those who are frail or disabled.

If you work in an office that handles insurance paperwork, you can submit insurance claims manually or electronically. Regardless of which method you use, be sure to use the proper forms, complete them correctly, and submit them within the time limits set by insurers. (Procedures for completing insurance forms and filing claims are discussed in Chapter 15.)

TRICARE, which provides health insurance for dependents of active-duty and retired military personnel, operates differently from other insurers. TRICARE pays the doctor through a local fiscal agent. Patients pay any co-payments and deductible amounts. You must adjust for the difference between the billed fees and the amounts received from TRICARE and the patient. If a TRICARE patient fails to pay the patient's portion, you may take steps to obtain payment just as you would with any other patient.

Responsibility for Minors. When a child's parents are married, either parent may consent (agree) to treatment for the minor child (child under age 18). Both parents are responsible for payment for the minor's treatment. If you must send them a bill, you should address it to both parents to ensure payment. There is one exception to this process. Anyone under the age of 18 who is no longer living at home and is self-supporting is considered an emancipated minor and is responsible for payment. For example, a 16-year-old girl who is pregnant and leaves her parents' home to set up a household with her boyfriend is considered an emancipated minor.

Divorce or separation can create confusion about which parent can consent to the child's treatment and which of the two is responsible for payment. The parent who has **legal custody,** or the court-decreed right to make decisions about a child's upbringing, is the parent who has consent ability and payment responsibility. A divorced couple's legal and financial arrangements are considered private information, however. Therefore, you should assume that the parent who brings the child for treatment has consent ability and payment responsibility. The physician should inform the responsible parent of this assumption before providing treatment.

Professional Courtesy. As a matter of professional courtesy, a doctor may treat some patients free of charge or for just the amount covered by the patient's insurance. These patients often include other doctors and their families, the practice's staff members (including medical assistants) and their families, other health-care professionals (including pharmacists and dentists), clergy members, and hospital employees. If the patient is part of a managed care organization or has Medicare, the provider must collect any co-payment or deductible as part of the contracted agreement with the provider. It may be considered fraud to consistently not collect co-payments or deductibles.

Be sure you know the doctor's policy so that you do not bill these patients in error. If, for example, the doctor agrees to accept only the amount paid by the patient's insurance, note this professional courtesy on the patient's ledger card, and do not request co-payment.

Standard Billing Procedures

If the physician extends credit to patients, you need to know how to prepare invoices. You also have to manage related billing responsibilities, such as establishing and maintaining billing cycles.

Preparing Invoices

As a medical assistant, part of your job is to prepare an invoice to mail to the patient who does not pay when services are rendered or who makes only a partial payment. Figure 17-5 shows an invoice with an itemized list of services. You can obtain most of the information for the invoice from the patient ledger card. The invoice should include the following information:

- Physician's name, address, and telephone number
- Patient's name and address
- Balance (if any) from the previous month(s)
- Itemized list of services and charges, by date, for the current month
- Payments from the patient or insurer during the month
- Total balance due

Whatever invoicing procedure you use, enclose a self-addressed envelope with the invoice to encourage prompt payment.

Using Codes on the Invoice. Write the name of each procedure on the itemized list, or use codes for common procedures, such as OV for office visit. If you use codes, be sure that an explanation of the codes appears with the invoice. (Many practices use invoices with a key to the codes printed at the bottom.) Using an itemized list on invoices is standard procedure in most physicians' offices and is required by all health insurance plans. After completing the invoice, fold it in thirds, and mail it in a typewritten business envelope.

Using the Patient's Ledger Card as an Invoice. As an alternative to writing or typing the invoice, you may photocopy the patient's ledger card and fold the photocopy so that the patient's address shows through the window in a window envelope. If you prepare invoices this way, be sure there are no stray marks or comments written on the card. Also, be sure the photocopy is clean and easy to read.

Generating the Invoice by Computer. In computerized offices, you may print out an invoice for each patient account that has a balance due. Follow the instructions in the software manufacturer's manual. You can then fold the printouts and mail them in window envelopes.

Using an Independent Billing Service. Large practices may have invoices handled by an independent billing service. The billing service may rapidly copy ledger cards for patients with balances due. Then it mails the copies to patients, usually with an envelope for sending payment directly to the physician's office.

Sending Invoices Electronically to Insurance Companies. Invoices to insurance companies may be prepared using one of the methods just described. Physicians' offices that have a computer and modem may bill insurance companies electronically, as discussed in Chapter 15.

Using the Superbill

Some doctors' offices use a **superbill,** which includes the charges for services rendered on that day, an invoice for payment or insurance co-payment, and all the information for submitting an insurance claim. Figure 17-6 shows an example of a superbill. Having all this information on one form saves time and paperwork. These forms are often printed on NCR (no-carbon-required) paper with copies for the practice, patient, and insurance company.

Complete as much of the superbill as possible at the beginning of the patient's visit. (See Procedure 17-1 for specific instructions.) Some practices use a computerized version of the superbill, printing it out instead of completing the initial information by hand. Attach the superbill to the patient's medical record, and give them both to the doctor before he sees the patient.

Managing Billing Cycles

Many practices send out their bills just after the end of each month. You can send out bills at any regular time, however, such as once a week or twice a month. You may also send bills at a particular time of the month at the patient's request.

Cycle billing is a common billing system that bills each patient only once a month but spreads the work of billing over the month. Using this system, you send invoices to groups of patients every few days.

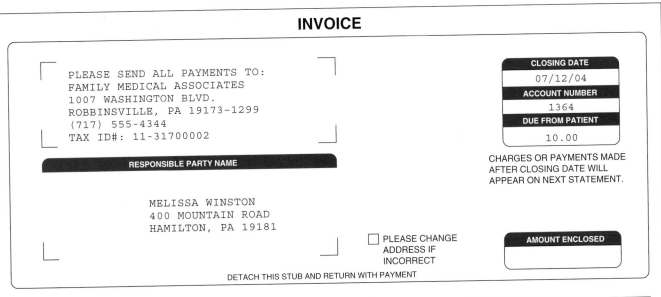

INVOICE

PLEASE SEND ALL PAYMENTS TO:
FAMILY MEDICAL ASSOCIATES
1007 WASHINGTON BLVD.
ROBBINSVILLE, PA 19173-1299
(717) 555-4344
TAX ID#: 11-31700002

CLOSING DATE
07/12/04
ACCOUNT NUMBER
1364
DUE FROM PATIENT
10.00

CHARGES OR PAYMENTS MADE
AFTER CLOSING DATE WILL
APPEAR ON NEXT STATEMENT.

RESPONSIBLE PARTY NAME

MELISSA WINSTON
400 MOUNTAIN ROAD
HAMILTON, PA 19181

☐ PLEASE CHANGE
ADDRESS IF
INCORRECT

AMOUNT ENCLOSED

DETACH THIS STUB AND RETURN WITH PAYMENT

DATE OF SERVICE	PROCEDURE CODE	DIAGNOSTIC CODE	SERVICE DESCRIPTION	ORIGINAL CHARGE	INSURANCE PAID	ADJ.	PATIENT PAID	AMOUNT DUE	DUE FROM
5/13/04	99213	473.9	EXT PAT-INTER	50.00	40.00	.00	.00	10.00	PAT
5/13/04	92567	473.9	TYMPANOGRAM	35.00	35.00	.00	.00	.00	INS
5/02/04	99203	706.2	NEW PAT-INTER	80.00	70.00	.00	10.00	.00	INS

PLEASE NOTE: ANY BALANCE NOW DUE BY THE PATIENT HAS BEEN SUBMITTED TO
THE PATIENT'S INSURANCE (IF ANY) AND PROCESSED AND IS NOW THE
RESPONSIBILITY OF THE PATIENT.

ACCOUNT NO.	SOCIAL SECURITY #	CURRENT	OVER 30 DAYS	OVER 60 DAYS	OVER 90 DAYS	OVER 120 DAYS	INSURANCE PENDING	**DUE FROM PATIENT**
1364	140-62-0000	10.00	.00	.00	.00	.00	.00	10.00

Figure 17-5. The invoice shows an itemized list of services and charges, organized by date, for the current month.

Lakeridge Medical Group
262 East Pine Street, Suite 100
Lakeridge, NJ 07500

☐ **PRIVATE** ☐ **BLUECROSS** ☐ **IND.** ☐ **MEDICARE** ☐ **MEDI-CAL** ☐ **HMO** ☐ **PPO**

PATIENT'S LAST NAME	FIRST	ACCOUNT #	BIRTHDATE / /	SEX ☐ MALE ☐ FEMALE	TODAY'S DATE / /
INSURANCE COMPANY		SUBSCRIBER	PLAN #	SUB. #	GROUP

ASSIGNMENT: I hereby assign my insurance benefits to be paid directly to the undersigned physician. I am financially responsible for non-covered services. SIGNED: (Patient, or Parent, if Minor)　　DATE: / /	RELEASE: I hereby authorize the physician to release to my insurance carrers any information required to process this claim. SIGNED: (Patient, or Parent, if Minor)　　DATE: / /

✔	DESCRIPTION	M/Care	CPT/Mod	DxRe	FEE	✔	DESCRIPTION	M/Care	CPT/Mod	DxRe	FEE	✔	DESCRIPTION	M/Care	CPT/Mod	DxRe	FEE
	OFFICE CARE						PROCEDURES						INJECTIONS/IMMUNIZATIONS				
	NEW PATIENT						Tread Mill (In Office)		93015				Tetanus		90718		
	Brief		99201				24 Hour Holter		93224				Hypertet	J1670	90782		
	Limited		99202				If Medicare (Set up Fec)		93225				Pneumococcal		90732		
	Intermediate		99203				Physician Interpret		93227				Influenza		90724		
	Extended		99204				EKG w/Interpretation		93000				TB Skin Test (PPD)		86585		
	Comprehensive		99205				EKG (Medicare)		93005				Antigen Injection-Single		95115		
							Sigmoidoscopy		45300				Multiple		95117		
	ESTABLISHED PATIENT						Sigmoidoscopy, Flexible		45330				B12 Injection	J3420	90782		
	Minimal		99211				Sigmoidos. , Flex. w/Bx.		45331				Injection, IM		90782		
	Brief		99212				Spirometry, FEV/FVC		94010				Compazine	J0780	90782		
	Limited		99213				Spirometry, Post-Dilator		94060				Demerol	J2175	90782		
	Intermediate		99214										Vistaril	J3410	90782		
	Extended		99215										Susphrine	J0170	90782		
	Comprehensive		99215				LABORATORY						Decadron	J0890	90782		
							Blood Draw Fee		36415				Estradiol	J1000	90782		
	CONSULTATION-OFFICE						Urinalysis, Chemical		81005				Testosterone	J1080	90782		
	Focused		99241				Throat Culture		87081				Lidocaine	J2000	90782		
	Expanded		99242				Occult Blood		82270				Solumedrol	J2920	90782		
	Detailed		99243				Pap Handling Charge		99000				Solucortef	J1720	90782		
	Comprehensive 1		99244				Pap Life Guard		88150-90				Hydeltra	J1690	90782		
	Comprehensive 2		99245				Gram Stain		87205				Pen Procaine	J2510	90788		
	Dr.						Hanging Drop		87210								
	Case Management		98900				Urine Drug Screen		99000				INJECTIONS - JOINT/BURSA				
													Small Joints		20600		
	Post-op Exam		99024										Intermediate		20605		
							SUPPLIES						Large Joints		20610		
													Trigger Point		20550		
													MISCELLANEOUS				

DIAGNOSIS:	ICD-9									
___ Abdominal Pain	789.0	___ Gout	274.0	___ C.V.A. - Acute	436.	___ Electrolyte Dis.	276.9	___ Herpes Simplex	054.9
___ Abscess (Site)	682.9	___ Asthma	493.90	___ Cere. Vas. Accid. (Old)	438	___ Fatigue	780.7	___ Herpes Zoster	053.9
___ Adverse Drug Rx	995.2	___ Asthmatic Bronchitis	493.90	___ Cerumen	380.4	___ Fibrocys. Br. Dis	610.1	___ Hydrocele	603.9
___ Alcohol Detox	291.8	___ Atrial Fib.	427.31	___ Chestwall Pain	786.59	___ Fracture (Site)	829.0	___ Hyperlipidemia	272.4
___ Alcoholism	303.90	___ Atrial Tachi.	427.0	___ Cholecystitis	575.0	___ Open/Close		___ Hypertension	401.9
___ Allergic Rhinitis	477	___ Bowel Obstruct.	560.9	___ Cholelithiasis	574.00	___ Fungal Infect. (Site)	110.8	___ Hyperthyroidism	242.9
___ Allergy	995.3	___ Breast Mass	611.72	___ COPD	492.8	___ Gastric Ulcer	531.90	___ Hypothyroidism	244.9
___ Alzheimer's Dis.	290.1	___ Bronchitis	490	___ Cirrhosis	571.5	___ Gastritis	535.0	___ Labyrinthitis	386.30
___ Anemia	285.9	___ Bursitis	727.3	___ Cong. Heart Fail.	428.9	___ Gastroenteritis	558.9	___ Lipoma (Site)	214.9
___ Anemia - Pernicious	281.0	___ Cancer, Breast (Site)	174.9	___ Conjunctivitis	372.30	___ G.I. Bleeding	578.9	___ Lymphoma	202.8
___ Angina	413.9	___ Metastatic (Site)	199.1	___ Contusion (Site)	924.9	___ Glomerulonephritis	583.9	___ Mit. Valve Prolapse	424.0
___ Anxiety Synd.	300.00	___ Colon	153.9	___ Costochondritis	733.99	___ Headache	784.0	___ Myocard. Infarction (Area)	410.9
___ Appendicitis	541	___ Cancer, Rectal	154.1	___ Depression	311.	___ Headache, Tension	307.81	___ M.I., Old	412
___ Arterioscl. H.D.	414.0	___ Lung (Site)	162.9	___ Dermatitis	692.9	___ Migraine (Type)	346.9	___ Myositis	729.1
___ Arthritis, Osteo.	715.90	___ Skin (Site)	173.9	___ Diabetes Mellitus	250.00	___ Hemorrhoids	455.6	___ Nausea/Vomiting	787.0
___ Rheumatoid	714.0	___ Card. Arrhythmia (Type)	427.9	___ Diabetic Ketosis	250.1	___ Hernia, Hiatal	553.3	___ Neuralgia	729.2
___ Lupus	710.0	___ Cardiomyopathy	425.4	___ Diverticulitis	562.11	___ Inguinal	550.9	___ Nevus (Site)	216.9
		___ Cellulitis (Site)	682.9	___ Diverticulosis	562.10	___ Hepatitis	573.3	___ Obesity	278.0

DIAGNOSIS: (IF NOT CHECKED ABOVE)

SERVICES PERFORMED AT: ☐ Office ☐ E.R. ☐ CLAIM CONTAINS NO ORDERED REFERRING SERVICE	REFERRING PHYSICIAN & I.D. NUMBER

RETURN APPOINTMENT INFORMATION: 5 - 10 - 15 - 20 - 30 - 40 - 60　　[DAYS] [WKS.] [MOS.] [PRN]	NEXT APPOINTMENT M - T - W - TH - F - S DATE / / TIME:	AM PM	ACCEPT ASSIGNMENT? ☐ YES ☐ NO	DOCTOR'S SIGNATURE

INSTRUCTIONS TO PATIENT FOR FILING INSURANCE CLAIMS:	☐ CASH	TOTAL TODAY'S FEE	
1. Complete upper portion of this form, sign and date.	☐ CHECK # _____	OLD BALANCE	
2. Attach this form to your own insurance company's form for direct reimbursement. **MEDICARE PATIENTS - DO NOT SEND THIS TO MEDICARE. WE WILL SUBMIT THE CLAIM FOR YOU.**	☐ VISA ☐ MC	TOTAL DUE	
	☐ CO-PAY	AMOUNT REC'D. TODAY	

Figure 17-6. A superbill is a form that can also be used as a charge slip and invoice and can be submitted with insurance claims.

PROCEDURE 17.1

How to Bill With the Superbill

Objective: To complete a superbill accurately

Materials: Superbill, patient ledger card, patient information sheet, fee schedule, insurance code list, pen

Method

1. Make sure the doctor's name and address appear on the form.
2. From the patient ledger card and information sheet, fill in the patient data, such as name, sex, date of birth, and insurance information.
3. Fill in the place and date of service.
4. Attach the superbill to the patient's medical record, and give them both to the doctor.
5. Accept the completed superbill from the patient after the patient sees the doctor. Make sure that the doctor has indicated the diagnosis and the procedures performed.
6. If the doctor has not already recorded the charges, refer to the fee schedule for procedures that are marked. Then fill in the charges next to those procedures.
7. In the appropriate blanks, list the total charges for the visit, and the previous balance (if any). Deduct any payments or adjustments received before this visit.
8. Calculate the subtotal.
9. Fill in the amount and type of payment (cash, check, money order, or credit card) made by the patient during this visit.
10. Calculate and enter the new balance.
11. Have the patient sign the authorization-and-release section of the superbill.
12. Keep a copy of the superbill for the practice records. Give the original to the patient along with one copy to file with the insurer.

For example, you may bill on the fifth of the month for patients whose last names begin with A through D. Then, on the tenth of the month, you may bill patients whose names begin with E through H, and so on. In a larger office with more patients, you may prefer to bill more frequently but to smaller groups of patients.

Standard Collection Procedures

Although most patients pay invoices within the standard 30-day period, some do not. When a patient does not pay an invoice during the standard period, you need to take steps to collect the payment. For example, you may need to call or write the patient to determine the reason for nonpayment or to set up a payment arrangement.

Whether you use telephone calls, notes, or letters, there are laws, such as statutes of limitations, and professional standards to guide your efforts to collect overdue payments from patients.

State Statute of Limitations

A **statute of limitations** is a state law that sets a time limit on when a collection suit on a past-due account can legally be filed. The time limit varies with the type of account.

Open-Book Account. An **open-book account** is one that is open to charges made occasionally as needed.

Most of a physician's long-standing patients have this type of account. An open-book account uses the last date of payment or charge for each illness as the starting date for determining the time limit on that specific debt.

Written-Contract Account. A **written-contract account** is one in which the physician and patient sign an agreement stating that the patient will pay the bill in more than four installments. Some states allow longer time limits for these accounts than for open-book accounts. Written-contract accounts are regulated by the Truth in Lending Act, discussed later in this chapter.

Single-Entry Account. A **single-entry account** is an account with only one charge, usually for a small amount. For example, someone vacationing in your area might come in for treatment of a cold. This person's account would list only one office visit. If the vacationer did not become a regular patient, the account would be considered a single-entry account. Some states impose shorter time limits on single-entry accounts than on open-book accounts.

Using Collection Techniques

Individual practices have their own ways of approaching the task of collection. Most begin the process with telephone calls, letters, or statements.

Initial Telephone Calls or Letters. When calling a patient or sending a letter about collections, be friendly and sympathetic. (Do not call a patient at work and leave a message. That type of phone call is an invasion of privacy. Call the patient at home.) Assume that the patient forgot to pay or was temporarily unable to pay. If you do not receive a response to your telephone call or initial collection letter, your next letters may need to be more urgent in tone. Standard collection letters, such as the one shown in Figure 17-7, are available for you to fill in the details, or you can create a letter to reflect the style of the practice.

Preparing Statements. You might send the patient a statement for an account that is 30 days past due. A **statement** is similar to an invoice except that it contains a courteous reminder that payment is due. This reminder can be a typewritten note on the statement, a brightly colored sticker, or a separate handwritten note attached to the statement.

If an account is 60 days past due, you could send a collection letter that says, for example, "If you are unable to pay your account in full this month, please telephone our office at [number] to make payment arrangements."

If an account is 90 days past due, your collection letter can contain stronger wording. For example, it might say, "Please let us know when you plan to pay the $250 past-due balance. We have sent you three monthly reminders. If you cannot pay in full now, please contact us at [number] to make payment arrangements. We want to be understanding but need your cooperation."

If an account is 120 days or more past due, you can send a final letter. It might state, "Every courtesy has been extended to you in arranging for payment of your long overdue account. Unless we hear from you by [date], the account will be given to [name of collection agency] for collection." Be sure to note the cutoff date on the patient's ledger card. By law, you cannot threaten to send an account to a collection agency unless it will actually be sent on that cutoff date. Therefore, you must be sure you are ready to do so before you send such a letter.

If you still cannot collect payment, the physician may indeed choose to hire an outside collection agency. Once an agency has taken over the account, there should not be any more correspondence on this matter between the physician's office and the patient.

Preparing an Age Analysis

Age analysis is the process of classifying and reviewing past-due accounts by age from the first date of billing. A quarterly or more frequent age analysis, such as that shown in Figure 17-8, helps you keep on top of past-due accounts and determine which ones need follow-up.

You can do an age analysis by computer or by hand. An age analysis should list all patient account balances, when the charges originated, the most recent payment date, and any special notes concerning the account.

In a single doctor's office or a small group practice, information for the age analysis may come from the patient ledger cards. You may place color-coded tags on the patient ledger cards to indicate the number of days past due. For example, a yellow tag might be placed on the ledger card of an account that is 60 days past due. An orange tag might be used for an account that is 90 days past due. A red tag might be used for an account that is 120 days or more past due. In a large practice, however, age analysis is typically done on the computer. The use of patient ledger cards has been phased out as more practices have become computerized.

Following Laws That Govern Debt Collection

Federal and state laws govern debt collection. Table 17-1 outlines the penalties for violating laws that regulate credit and debt.

Fair Debt Collection Practices Act of 1977. This act (also called Public Law 95-109) governs the methods that can be used to collect unpaid debts. It prevents you from threatening to take an action that is either illegal or that you do not actually intend to take. The aim of this law is to eliminate abusive, deceptive, or unfair debt collection practices. For example, the law requires that after you have said you are going to give an account to a collection agency if it is not paid within 1 month, you must actually do so. Not doing what you threaten to do can be construed as harassment, and your practice can be liable for a harassment charge. Following are guidelines for sending letters and making calls requesting payment from patients.

- Do not call the patient before 8 A.M. or after 9 P.M. Calling outside those hours can be considered harassment.
- Do not make threats or use profane language. For example, do not state that an account will be given to a collection agency in 7 days if it will not be.
- Do not discuss the patient's debt with anyone except the person responsible for payment. If the patient is represented by a lawyer, discuss the problem only with the lawyer, unless the lawyer gives you permission to talk to the patient.
- Do not use any form of deception or violence to collect a debt. For example, do not pose as a government employee or other authority figure to try to force a debtor to pay.

Telephone Consumer Protection Act (TCPA) of 1991. This act protects telephone subscribers from unwanted telephone solicitations, commonly known as telemarketing. The act prohibits autodialed calls to emergency service providers, cellular and paging numbers, and patients' hospital rooms. It prohibits prerecorded calls to homes without prior permission of the resident, and it prohibits unsolicited advertising via fax machine.

These regulations do not apply to people who have an established business relationship with the telemarketing

City Medical Group

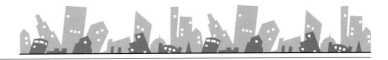

1234 Wayne Street
Smithtown, OR 93689
(503) 555-1217

Internal Medicine
Marianne Harris, MD
Karen Payne-Johnson, MD

May 5, 2004

Mr. J. J. Andrews
1414 First Avenue
Smithtown, OR 93668

Dear Mr. Andrews:

It has been brought to my attention that your account in the amount of <u>$240.00</u> is past due.

Normally at this time the account would be placed with a collection agency. However, we would prefer to hear from you regarding your preference in this matter.

(   )   Payment in full is enclosed.

(   )   Payment will be made in _____ days.

(   )   I would like to make regular weekly/monthly payments of $ _____ until this account is paid in full. My first payment is enclosed.

(   )   I would prefer that you assign this account to a collection agency for enforcement of collection. (Failure to return this letter within 30 days will result in this action.)

(   )   I don't believe I owe this amount for the following reason(s):

Signed: _____

Please indicate your preference and return this letter within 30 days. Please do not hesitate to call if you have any questions regarding this matter.

Sincerely,

Diana Sanchez
Office Manager

Figure 17-7. Standard collection letters are available for you to fill in the details.

ACCOUNTS RECEIVABLE–AGE ANALYSIS

Date: October 1, 2003

Patient	Balance	Date of Charges	Most Recent Payment	30 days	60 days	90 days	120 days	Remarks
Black, K.	120.00	5/24	5/24			75.00	45.00	3rd Notice
Brown, R.	65.00	8/30	8/30	65.00				
Green, C.	340.00	8/25						Medicare filed
Jones, T.	500.00	6/1	6/30		125.00	125.00	250.00	3rd Notice
Perry, S.	150.00	7/28	7/28	75.00	75.00			1st Notice
Smith, J.	375.00	6/15	7/1			375.00		2nd Notice
White, L.	200.00	6/24	7/5	20.00	30.00	150.00		2nd Notice

Figure 17-8. An age analysis organizes past-due accounts by age.

firm or people who have previously given the telemarketing firm permission to call. The law also does not apply to telemarketing calls placed by tax-exempt nonprofit organizations, such as charities.

Although most provisions of this federal law do not apply to medical practices, you should be aware of the law. One way to avoid an unknowing violation of this law is to limit your calls to patients to the hours between 8 A.M. and 9 P.M. (some states, however, have exceptions for the TCPA provisions). Also, place your calls yourself. Do not use an automated dialing device for calls to patients.

Observing Professional Guidelines for Finance Charges and Late Charges

According to the AMA, it is appropriate to assess finance charges or late charges on past-due accounts if the patient is notified in advance. Advance notice may be given by posting a sign at the reception desk, giving the patient a pamphlet describing the practice's billing practices, or including a note on the invoice.

The physician must adhere to federal and state guidelines that govern these charges. The physician should also use compassion and discretion when assigning charges, especially in hardship cases.

Using Outside Collection Agencies

If your collection efforts do not result in payment, the doctor may wish to select a collection agency to manage the account. Because doctors adhere to the humanitarian and ethical standards of the medical profession, they must be careful to avoid collection agencies that use harsh or harassing collection practices. The Tips for the Office section

TABLE 17-1 Laws That Govern Credit and Collections

Law	Requirements	Penalties for Breaking Law
Equal Credit Opportunity Act (ECOA)	• Creditors may not discriminate against applicants on the basis of sex, marital status, race, national origin, religion, or age. • Creditors may not discriminate because an applicant receives public assistance income or has exercised rights under the Consumer Credit Protection Act.	• If an applicant sues the practice for violating the ECOA, the practice may have to pay **damages** (money paid as compensation), penalties, lawyers' fees, and court costs. • If an applicant joins a class action lawsuit against the practice, the practice may have to pay damages of up to $500,000 or 1% of the practice's net worth, whichever is less. (A **class action lawsuit** is a lawsuit in which one or more people sue a company that wronged all of them the same way.) • If the Federal Trade Commission (FTC) receives many complaints from applicants stating that the practice violated the ECOA, the FTC may investigate and take action against the practice.
Fair Credit Reporting Act (FCRA)	• This act requires credit bureaus to supply correct and complete information to businesses to use in evaluating a person's application for credit, insurance, or a job.	• If one applicant sues the practice in federal court for violating the FCRA, the practice may have to pay damages, **punitive damages** (money paid as punishment for intentionally breaking the law), court costs, and lawyers' fees. • If the FTC receives many complaints from applicants stating that the practice violated the FCRA, the FTC may investigate and take action against the practice.
Fair Debt Collection Practices Act (FDCPA)	• This act requires debt collectors to treat debtors fairly. It also prohibits certain collection tactics, such as harassment, false statements, threats, and unfair practices.	• If one debtor sues the practice in a state or federal court for violation of the FDCPA, the practice may have to pay damages, court costs, and lawyers' fees. • If the debtor joins a class action suit against the practice, the practice may have to pay damages of up to $500,000 or 1% of the practice's net worth, whichever is less. • If the FTC receives many complaints from debtors stating that the practice violated the FDCPA, the FTC may investigate and take action against the practice.
Truth in Lending Act (TLA)	• This act requires creditors to provide applicants with accurate and complete credit costs and terms, clearly and obviously.	• If one applicant sues the practice in a federal court for violation of the TLA, the practice may have to pay damages, court costs, and lawyers' fees. • If the FTC receives many complaints from applicants stating that the practice violated the TLA, the FTC may investigate and take action against the practice.

gives information about selecting an outside collection agency.

When giving a patient's account to an agency, supply the following information about the patient:

- Full name and last known address
- Occupation and business address
- Name of spouse, if any
- Total debt
- Date of last payment or charge on the account
- Description of actions you took to collect the debt
- Responses to collection attempts

Color-coded tabs on the patient ledger cards make this information easy to gather. Note on the patient ledger card that the account has been given to a collection agency. When the agency reports progress toward a settlement, record that information on the card too.

After the account is given to the agency, do not send bills to or contact the patient in any way. If the patient

Tips for the Office

Choosing a Collection Agency

If a patient does not respond to your final collection letter or has twice broken a promise to pay, the doctor may choose to seek the help of a collection agency. This step should be taken carefully, however. Some collection agencies use illegal and unethical tactics to obtain payment. For example, some collectors have made repeated, profane phone calls to frighten debtors. Others have threatened debtors with prison for nonpayment. A good collection agency reflects the humanitarian and ethical standards of the medical profession.

To help select an effective—and ethical—collection agency, ask for a referral from the doctor's colleagues, fellow specialists, or hospital associates. You may also contact one of the following organizations:

American Collectors Association International
P.O. Box 390106
Minneapolis, MN 55439

Medical-Dental-Hospital Bureaus of America
1161 Wayzata Boulevard East
Wayzata, MN 55391

After obtaining a referral, contact the agency and request samples of its letters, reminder notices, and other print material for debtors. Be sure this material is courteous and reflects the way you would handle the collection. Also, be sure the agency uses a persuasive approach rather than simply suing debtors. Ask if the agency reports cases that deserve special consideration to the doctor's office.

Determine what methods the agency uses for out-of-town accounts. For example, it may use out-of-town services to help with those collections. Ask the agency about its collection percentage and fees for large, small, and out-of-town accounts. Be sure the percentages and fees are appropriate for the collection amounts.

After selecting a collection agency, supply all pertinent data to the agency, such as the patient's name, address, and full amount of the debt. Mark the patient's ledger card so that you do not call or write to the patient about the debt. If the patient contacts the office about the account, refer the patient to the collection agency.

If you receive any payments from the debtor, alert the collection agency immediately. (The agency takes a portion of any payments it collects.) Also, contact the agency if you learn anything new about the patient's address or employer.

---

wants to discuss payment, refer the patient to the agency. If the patient sends a payment, forward it to the agency; or, if the agency and the practice agree, keep the payment for the practice, and forward the collection fee to the agency.

The arrangement with the agency should give the doctor the final word on the uncollected account. In other words, the doctor should decide whether to write off the debt or take the matter to court.

Insuring Accounts Receivable

To protect the practice from lost income because of nonpayment, the practice may buy accounts receivable insurance. One type of accounts receivable policy pays when a large number of patients do not pay and the physician must absorb the lost income. It protects the practice's cash flow and helps ensure that the practice will have sufficient income to cover expected expenses.

Credit Arrangements

Sometimes a doctor agrees to extend credit to a patient who is unable to pay immediately. This situation is not uncommon when a patient's medical bills are high. By extending **credit,** the doctor gives the patient time to pay for

services, which are provided on trust. If the doctor knows the patient well, she may offer credit without checking the patient's credit history. Otherwise, the doctor may ask you to perform a credit check.

Performing a Credit Check

To perform a credit check, be sure you have the most current information. You will need the patient's address, telephone number, and Social Security number and the patient's employer's name, address, and telephone number. With this information you can verify employment and generate a credit bureau report.

Employment Verification. Explain to the patient that you will be calling his employer to verify employment. Many employers have someone designated to handle such calls. The patient may be able to give you that name before you call the place of employment.

After calling, record the updated information on the patient's registration card, along with any credit references you obtain from the patient.

Credit Bureau Report. A **credit bureau** is a company that provides information about the creditworthiness of a person seeking credit. If a patient's credit history is in

		File No.		
		Date 1/8/04		
		Amount Received $15.00		Payment Type
		Credit Card No.		Exp. Date

To the Consumer:
This is a copy of your current credit file. It is being furnished to you based on the information you have provided in accordance with the "Fair Credit Reporting Act." Please use the file number shown on this report on all correspondence. Refer to the reverse side for explanations of codes and abbreviations used in this disclosure.

In File Since	10/94

Consumer Name and Address	SSN	Date Rptd.
	Spouse Name SSN	
	Tel.	
	Date Rptd.	

| Former Address | |

Present Employer and Address	Position Income	Empl. Date	Date Verif.
Former Employer and Address			
Spouse's Employer and Address			

Subscriber Name	Subscriber Code	Date Opened	High Credit	Date Verif.	Balance Owed	Amount Past Due	Payment Pattern 1–12 Months / 13–24 Months	Type Account & MOP
Account Number		Terms	Credit Limit	Dated Closed	Date	Amount	MOP / Historical Status No. of Months 25–39 40–59 60+	
Collateral					Remarks	Type Loan		
MIDLANTIC	B382D021	4/92		11/98A	$325	$0	111111111111	R01
	MIN10		$850				X11111111111	
							12 0 0 0	
LINCOLN SAV B	B814M006	6/88		10/94A	$16K	$0	1111X11X1111	M01
	360M34		$30.5K				111X11111X1X	
							29 0 0 0	
BANK AMER	B196P017	11/89		10/96A	$1136	$0	111111111111	R01
	10M		$5000				11111111111X	
							48 0 0 0	
MACY D	D787D008	1/84	$475	11/97A	$0	$0*	111XXXXXXXXX	R01
	MIN20		$1000				1111111111XX	
				*CREDIT LINE CLOSED BY CUSTOMER			48 0 0 0	
UJ BK MC	33DB0002	7/91		3/96A	$310	$0	111111111111	R01
	MIN20		$3000				111X111111XX	
							47 0 0 0	

Figure 17-9. Credit reports are generated by credit bureaus.

question, you may request a report from a credit bureau. A sample credit report is shown in Figure 17-9. A credit bureau collects information about an individual's payment history on credit cards, student loans, and similar accounts. Three leading national credit bureaus are TRW Inc., Equifax Inc., and Trans Union Credit Information Company.

The physician may decide not to extend credit, based on the credit report. If so, the Fair Credit Reporting Act states that you must inform the patient in writing that credit was denied. You must also provide the name and address of the credit bureau. This information allows the patient to contest the credit report and to correct any incorrect information the credit bureau may have.

Following Laws Governing Extension of Credit

When you help the doctor decide whether to grant credit to a patient, you must comply with certain laws governing extension of credit.

Equal Credit Opportunity Act. This act states that credit arrangements may not be denied based on a patient's sex, race, religion, national origin, marital status, or age. Also, credit cannot be denied because the patient receives public assistance or has exercised rights under the Consumer Credit Protection Act, such as disputing a credit card bill or a credit bureau report.

Under the Equal Credit Opportunity Act, the patient has a right to know the specific reason that credit was denied. Some reasons might include having too little income or not being employed for a certain period of time. Vague reasons about not meeting minimum standards or not receiving enough points on a credit-scoring system are not acceptable.

Truth in Lending Act. This act is Regulation Z of the Consumer Credit Protection Act. The Truth in Lending Act covers credit agreements that involve more than four payments. It requires the physician and patient to discuss, sign, and retain copies of a **disclosure statement** (frequently called a federal Truth in Lending statement), which

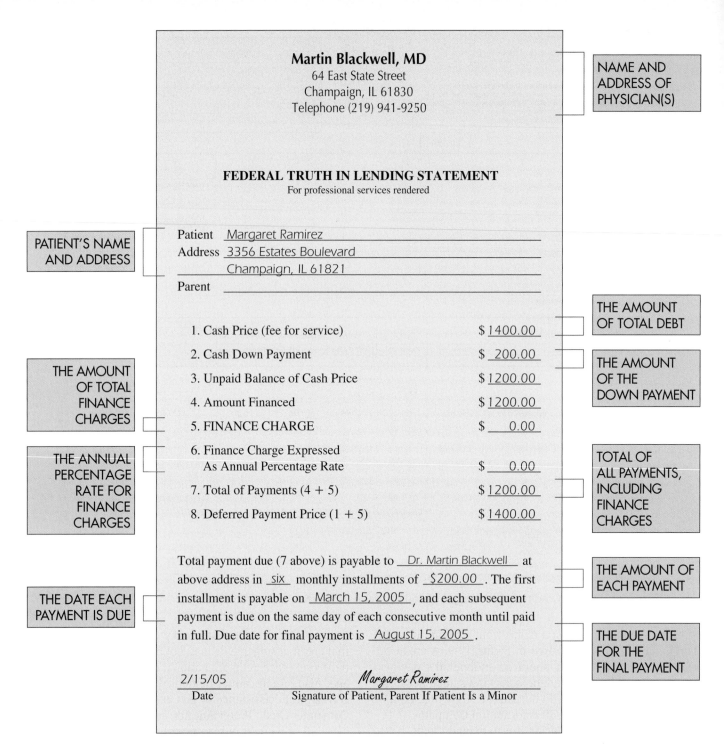

Figure 17-10. The federal Truth in Lending Act mandates that a written disclosure statement be completed and signed by the physician and patient.

is a written description of the agreed terms of payment (Figure 17-10).

According to the Truth in Lending Act, a disclosure statement must meet the following two requirements.

1. The agreement must be discussed with the patient when the terms are first determined. The physician and the patient must agree on the payment terms.

2. Both the physician and the patient must sign the document to indicate mutual agreement on the written terms.

Further, a disclosure statement must include the following six pieces of information:

1. The amount of total debt (the amount for which the patient is receiving credit).

Coding, Billing, and Insurance Specialist

To gain medical assistant credentials, you must fulfill the requirements of either the American Association of Medical Assistants (for a Certified Medical Assistant) or the American Medical Technologists (for a Registered Medical Assistant). After obtaining your medical assistant certification or registration, you may wish to acquire additional skills in specialty areas through course work or on-the-job training. Although this course work or training may not lead to an additional certification or degree, it will enable you to expand your role in the medical office and advance your career as the demand for skilled health professionals increases.

Skills and Duties

A coding, billing, and insurance specialist analyzes the data in patients' charts to provide accurate information for insurance claims. She is also responsible for processing insurance forms and obtaining fees for procedures performed, either from patients or from their insurance companies.

For the purpose of processing insurance claims, there is a code for every recognized disease, condition, problem, and diagnosis. The codes used in medical records come from the International Classification of Disease (ICD) system, issued by the World Health Organization (WHO). There is also a separate system of codes for medical procedures, known as the *Physicians' Current Procedural Terminology*, released annually by the AMA. Coders are encouraged to take a course each year to stay informed about coding changes and updates.

After coding the medical record, the specialist bills the responsible party for the charges incurred by the patient's diagnosis and treatment. She may bill the patient, Medicare or Medicaid, and/or an insurance company. If the insurance company has questions about a bill, it may request the patient's medical records to verify that a particular procedure was medically necessary.

The coding, billing, and insurance specialist may also assist patients with the claims process. She can explain what information the patient must provide to streamline the process. When patients are responsible for submitting claims to their insurance companies,

the coding, billing, and insurance specialist may tell the patient what forms to use.

The coding, billing, and insurance specialist also processes responses from the insurance companies, including the explanation of benefits (EOB) form. She checks the EOB against the claim form to make sure that the insurance company addressed all procedures that were performed. Sometimes a balance remains because the insurance company did not pay the total amount due on all procedures. In those cases the coding, billing, and insurance specialist sends a bill to the patient or responsible party. She may discover an error in the EOB. In such instances she looks for the source of the error and then contacts the insurance company to correct it.

Workplace Settings

Coding, billing, and insurance specialists work in many health-care settings, including hospitals, nursing homes, and physicians' practices. Some are employed by insurance companies.

Education

Coding specialists may receive part of their training on the job or through workshops, seminars, and courses. A high school diploma or its equivalent is required to be eligible for this training. After completing the training, a coding specialist may take certification exminations through the American Health Information Management Association (AHIMA) or the American Academy of Professional Coders (AAPC).

Where to Go for More Information

American Health Information Management
Association
233 North Michigan Avenue, Suite 2150
Chicago, IL 60611-5800
(800) 335-5535

American Academy of Professional Coders
300 West 700 South
Salt Lake City, UT 84101
(801) 236-2227

---

2. The amount of the down payment (which is sometimes greater than the weekly or monthly payments that follow).

3. The amount of each payment (which may be weekly or monthly or for another period) and the date it is

due. (Frequently the total number of payments to be made after the down payment is also included.)

4. The due date for the final payment.

5. The interest rate, if interest is to be paid, expressed as an annual percentage.

6. The total finance charges, if any. (If interest is charged, the total amount of interest accrued during the course of the debt will be entered here.)

The practice and the patient should each keep a copy of the signed disclosure agreement.

Under the Truth in Lending Act, you must send the patient a statement of account at the end of each billing cycle. This statement must include the previous balance, any payments or charges, the periodic and annual interest rates, finance charges (if any) for the billing cycle, the new balance, and a description of how the new balance was obtained.

Extending Credit

If the doctor decides to extend credit, several possible arrangements can be made. Two common arrangements are the unilateral decision and the mutual agreement.

Unilateral Decision. The doctor may decide that the patient will be billed every month for the full amount owed and should make whatever payment is possible each month. This type of arrangement is considered a unilateral decision of the doctor and is not regulated by the Truth in Lending Act.

Mutual Agreement. Another option is a mutual, or bilateral, agreement between physician and patient. They might agree that the patient will be billed for the full amount owed each month and will pay a minimum amount each month. If the physician does not assess finance charges, and if the total number of payments is four or fewer, this type of agreement is also not covered by the Truth in Lending Act. If the physician and patient make a bilateral agreement that includes more than four payments, or if the physician assesses finance charges, the agreement is subject to the requirements of the Truth in Lending Act.

Common Collection Problems

There are two common collection problems that medical practices encounter. The first is patients who cannot pay—also called hardship cases—and the second is patients who have moved and have not received an invoice.

Hardship Cases

A physician may decide to treat some patients without charge—or at a deep discount—simply because they cannot pay. These patients may be poor, uninsured or underinsured, or elderly and on a limited income. They may be patients who have suffered a severe financial loss or family tragedy. Medical ethics require physicians to provide care to individuals who need it, regardless of their ability to pay. Nevertheless, free treatment for hardship cases is at the physician's discretion.

Patient Relocation and Address Change

Sometimes an invoice remains unpaid because the patient has moved and has not received the invoice. Obviously, you will have a problem if you are trying to call such a patient about an invoice.

Remember not to discuss a debt with anyone except the person responsible for the charges. When you make a telephone call for collection, however, you may ask a third party for the patient's new address. If the third party claims not to know the new address, do not call again unless there is reason to believe that the third party has learned of the person's address since the first inquiry.

Summary

Most doctors prefer to obtain payment by cash, check, or credit card at the time medical services are provided. As a medical assistant, you may assign the fee for these services and collect payment. For various reasons, however, some patients cannot pay immediately. To accommodate these patients, the doctor may want to extend credit. If so, you may be asked to check credit references or to obtain a credit report.

When patients have made credit arrangements with the doctor, you must regularly prepare invoices from information on the patient ledger cards. To simplify this task, you may use a multipurpose superbill and send out invoices in billing cycles.

If patients do not pay their bills within 30 days, you may be asked to act as the doctor's collection agent. Through telephone calls and collection letters, you can try tactfully to collect payments. Federal and state laws govern collections and carry harsh penalties for infractions.

If your efforts to collect a payment are not effective, the doctor may ask you to help find an outside collection agency. A good collection agency should reflect the humanitarian standards of the medical profession. You will need to supply the agency with the pertinent account information.

CASE STUDY *QUESTIONS*

Now that you have completed this chapter, review the case study at the beginning of the chapter and answer the following questions:

1. What is the total owed for this patient's visits?
2. How much of the total is not covered by insurance and should be billed to the patient?

Discussion Questions

1. Discuss the responsibility of a divorced or separated patient who has the legal custody to make decisions for her or his child.
2. What information is required to prepare invoices?
3. What are some of the techniques used in the task of collections?
4. Under what conditions may a physician decide to treat patients without charge because they cannot pay?

Critical Thinking Questions

1. What are the most common collection problems? Give examples of how you would handle these problem cases. Who has the final decision on who receives discounted rates for services?
2. How is an accounts receivable age analysis prepared?

Application Activities

1. With a partner, role-play a scenario in which you, as a medical assistant, are making an initial request for payment over the phone to a patient who is late in paying a bill but has not yet been sent any collection letters. Your partner should act as the patient, offering any information or explanation she wants.
2. Give a fictional example of a "special consideration" collection case for which you might set up a payment schedule. How would you handle the case?
3. Using the guidelines described in this chapter, write a collection letter to a fictional patient. The patient owes the doctor $125, and the account is 60 days past due. Share your letter with a classmate to analyze how well you complied with federal collection guidelines.

CHAPTER 18

Accounting for the Medical Office

KEY TERMS

ABA number
asset
bookkeeping
cash flow statement
cashier's check
certified check
charge slip
check
counter check
dependent
employment contract
endorse
gross earnings
journalizing
limited check
money order
negotiable
net earnings
patient ledger card
pay schedule
payee
payer
pegboard system
petty cash fund
power of attorney
quarterly return
reconciliation
tax liability
third-party check
tracking
traveler's check
voucher check

AREAS OF COMPETENCE

2003 Role Delineation Study

ADMINISTRATIVE

Practice Finances

- Apply bookkeeping principles
- *Manage accounts payable*
- *Process payroll*
- *Document and maintain accounting and banking records*

GENERAL

Operational Functions

- Apply computer techniques to support office operations

*Denotes advanced skills.

CHAPTER OUTLINE

- The Business Side of a Medical Practice
- Bookkeeping Systems
- Banking for the Medical Office
- Managing Accounts Payable
- Managing Disbursements
- Handling Payroll
- Calculating and Filing Taxes
- Managing Contracts

OBJECTIVES

After completing Chapter 18, you will be able to:

18.1 Describe traditional bookkeeping systems, including single-entry and double-entry.
18.2 Define a pegboard system.
18.3 Explain the benefits of performing bookkeeping tasks on the computer.
18.4 List banking tasks in a medical office.
18.5 Describe the logistics of accepting, endorsing, and depositing checks from patients and insurance companies.
18.6 Reconcile the office's bank statements.
18.7 Give several examples of disbursements.
18.8 Record disbursements in a disbursement journal.
18.9 Set up and maintain a petty cash fund.
18.10 Create employee payroll information sheets.
18.11 Compute an employee's gross earnings, total deductions, and net earnings.
18.12 Prepare an employee earnings record and payroll register.

18.13 Set up the practice's tax liability accounts.

18.14 Complete federal, state, and local tax forms.

18.15 Submit employment taxes to government agencies.

18.16 Describe the basic parts of an employment contract.

Introduction

Accounting is another of the administrative competences in the medical assisting career. A person in this career may be required to take on many duties in the medical office that would typically be done by an office manager. This chapter describes the key areas of accounting and book-keeping that may be encountered.

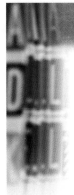

CASE STUDY

Ben is a medical assistant at a family practice clinic. A patient gave him a check for $85 for payment on her account. As you read this chapter, consider the following question:

1. What should Ben do to properly record the payment?

The Business Side of a Medical Practice

A medical practice is a business. If it is to prosper, its income must exceed its expenses. In other words, it must produce a profit. To determine whether the business is making a profit, you may be asked to do **bookkeeping,** or systematic recording of business transactions. Your records will later be analyzed by an accountant or by a more experienced medical assistant.

Bookkeeping and banking are two key responsibilities of medical assistants. To fulfill these responsibilities, you need an understanding of basic accounting systems and certain financial management skills.

Importance of Accuracy

Whenever you do bookkeeping or banking, strive for 100% accuracy. Because bookkeeping records form a chain of information, an undetected error at the first link will be carried through all other links in the chain. Undetected errors can result in billing a patient twice for the same visit, omitting bank deposits, or making improper payments to suppliers. These actions can result in lost money—and patients—for the practice.

Establishing Procedures

A set procedure not only helps you remember important aspects of bookkeeping and banking but also helps ensure

that your books are accurate. Here are some general suggestions for maintaining accuracy in bookkeeping and banking procedures for a medical practice.

- Maintain the practice's bookkeeping and banking procedures in a logical and organized way.
- Be consistent. Always handle the same kinds of transactions in exactly the same way. For example, endorse all checks with the same information, regardless of who wrote them or when you will be depositing them.
- Use check marks as you work to avoid losing your place if you are interrupted. For example, place a red check mark on each check stub as you reconcile the bank statement.
- Write clearly, and always use the same type of pen. If more than one person performs bookkeeping and banking tasks, each person might use a different color ink to identify her work. It is recommended that as few people as possible perform these tasks, however. You may use pencil for trial balances and worksheets, but you should use pen for bookkeeping entries.
- Double-check your work frequently to detect—and correct—any errors. To correct errors, draw a straight line through the incorrect figure, and write the correct figure above it. Do not erase errors or delete them with correction fluid or tape.
- Keep all columns of figures straight, so that decimal points align correctly.

Using set procedures will help you organize your work, help ensure accuracy, and make you a more valuable member of the practice staff.

Bookkeeping Systems

Three types of manual accounting systems are commonly used in a medical practice: single-entry, double-entry, and pegboard. A computerized system may also be used. All bookkeeping systems record income, charges (money owed to the practice), disbursements (money paid out by the practice), and other financial information. The choice of system is based on the size and complexity of the practice.

Traditional Bookkeeping Methods

Even practices that use computers for many other administrative and clinical functions may still perform bookkeeping methods on paper. This choice is not old-fashioned but simply the preference of the physician/owner or the office manager. Some people believe that working with numbers on paper forces you to be especially careful and to pay close attention to detail—more so than working on a computer, which has built-in mechanisms for checking arithmetic, decimal alignment, and so on.

Single-Entry System. As the name implies, the single-entry system requires only one entry for each transaction. Therefore, it is the easiest system to learn and use. Unlike the double-entry system, however, the single-entry system is not self-balancing. In addition, it does not detect errors as readily and has fewer accuracy checkpoints. This system is also more likely to produce errors because information must be posted (copied) to the bookkeeping forms.

The single-entry system uses several basic records, as well as auxiliary records:

- A daily log (also called a general ledger, day sheet, or daily journal) to record charges and payments
- Patient ledger cards or an accounts receivable ledger, which shows how much each patient owes
- A checkbook register or cash payment journal, which shows the practice expenses
- Payroll records, which show salaries, wages, and payroll deductions
- Petty cash records, which show disbursements for minor office expenses

The double-entry and pegboard systems, discussed later in this chapter, also use these records.

Daily Log. The daily log is a chronological list of the charges to patients and the payments received from patients each day, as shown in Figure 18-1. In the daily log, you write the name of each patient seen that day. Across from the name, you record the service provided, the fee charged, and the payment received (if any). This process

Dr. _____		Date _____		
Hour	**Patient**	**Service Provided**	**Charge**	**Paid**
1				
2				
3				
4				
5				
6				
7				
8				
9				
10				
11				
12				
13				
14				
15				
16				
			Totals	

Figure 18-1. A daily log is used to record charges and payments.

is called **journalizing.** You then post (copy) the charges and payments from the daily log to patient ledger cards (described in the next section). Using a daily or monthly cash control sheet, you record checks and cash received as well as deposits made each day.

Some physicians keep a daily log at their desks for entering information after they see each patient. In such cases, it may be helpful to write the name of each scheduled patient in the log to provide an appointment list. You may be responsible for this task.

In other offices, the medical assistants maintain the daily log. You can obtain the information for the log from charge slips and from checks received from patients or insurance companies. (Note: A **charge slip** is the original record of the doctor's services and the charge for those services. Some practices use a combination charge slip/receipt, which automatically creates a receipt to tear off for the patient. Typically, a charge slip/receipt includes a duplicate copy underneath to use for bookkeeping purposes. Remember, you need to track charges *and* receipts for payment, regardless of whether the practice uses separate charge slips and receipts or a combination.) There may also be records of outside visits, such as to nursing homes or hospital emergency rooms.

Be sure to record any night calls or other unscheduled visits in the daily log. Simply check with the physician each morning. If the physician has not noted the charge amount on a charge slip/receipt or record of outside visits, remember to apply the correct fee.

Record in the daily log all payments that come in the mail. If a check from an insurance company includes payment for more than one patient (which frequently is the case), post the appropriate amount to each patient ledger card.

If extra columns are available, you can record additional financial information in the daily log. For example, in addition to showing the total amount charged to the patient, you can show a breakdown of that total into the amounts generated by different physicians in a group practice or by different functions of the office, such as laboratory or x-ray.

At the end of each day, total the charges and receipts in the daily log, and post these totals to the monthly summary of charges and receipts. To double-check your totals, perform the following procedures:

- Ensure that the day's total cash and check receipts are the same as the day's total bank deposit.
- Ensure that the sum of the day's charges for each type of service is the same as the total of the day's charges.

Patient Ledger Cards. Another bookkeeping task is preparing a patient ledger card for each patient. The **patient ledger card** includes the patient's name, address, home and work telephone numbers, and the name of the person who is responsible for the charges (if different from the patient). The ledger card also lists the patient's insurance information, Social Security number, employer's name, and any special billing instructions. Figure 18-2 shows an example of a patient ledger card.

You use the patient ledger card to record charges incurred by the patient, payments received, and the resulting balance owed to the doctor. Because these cards document the financial transactions of the patient account, they are sometimes called account cards. In some practices, they are photocopied for use as monthly statements.

The information for the patient ledger cards comes from the daily log or from charge slips. It is best to complete all the cards at the end of the day. If this is not possible, you may complete them as time permits during the day. To prevent double or omitted postings, put a small check mark next to each entry in the daily log after you post it to the proper ledger card.

Take great care when posting, because errors on ledger cards will be reflected on invoices. To ensure accuracy, add up the total charges and receipts from the ledger cards, and make sure the information matches the total charges and receipts in that day's daily log.

Accounts Receivable. Every day, you must also update the accounts receivable record, which shows the total owed to the practice. Total up the items on the accounts receivable record, and then total up the outstanding balances on the patient ledger cards. The two numbers should match. If they do not, recheck your work to find the cause of the discrepancy.

Accounts Payable. Accounts payable are the amounts the practice owes to vendors. If your responsibilities include accounts payable, keep careful records of equipment and supplies ordered, and compare orders received against the invoices. In the checkbook register, keep detailed and accurate records of accounts paid.

Record of Office Disbursements. The record of office disbursements is a list of the amounts paid for such items as medical supplies, office rent, office utilities, employee wages, postage, and equipment over a certain period of time. It shows the **payee** (the person who will receive the payment), the date, the check number, the amount paid, and the type of expense. Figure 18-3 is an example of a disbursement record.

A checkbook register may be used to record office disbursements. As an alternative, a disbursement journal or the bottom section of the daily log may be used to record office disbursements. For income tax purposes, this record should include only office expenses. The doctor's personal expenses should not be listed here.

Summary of Charges, Receipts, and Disbursements. Charges, receipts, and disbursements are usually summarized at the end of each month, quarter, or year, as shown in Figure 18-4. The summary is used to compare the income and expenses of the current period with the income and expenses from any previous period.

By analyzing summaries, a physician can see which functions of the practice are profitable, the total amount charged for services, the payments received for services, the total cost of running the office, and a breakdown of

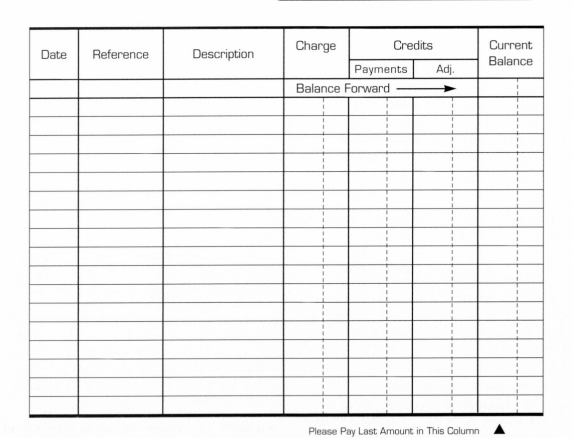

Patient's Name   Jonathan Jackson

Home Phone   (612) 555-9921   **Work Phone** (612) 555-1000

Social Security No. 111-21-4114

Employer   Ashton School District

Insurance   National Insurance Co.

Policy #   123-4-56-788

Person Responsible for Charges (if Different from Patient) _____

JONATHAN JACKSON
123 Fourth Avenue
Ashton, MN 70809-1222

Date	Reference	Description	Charge	Credits		Current Balance
				Payments	Adj.	
		Balance Forward ⟶				

Please Pay Last Amount in This Column ▲

OV—Office Visit   C—Consultation   EX—Examination
X—X-ray   NC—No Charge   INS—Insurance
ROA—Received on Account MA—Missed Appointment

Figure 18-2. Patient ledger cards are used to show how much each patient owes.

Record of Office Disbursements
April 2004

| DATE | PAYEE | CK. NO. | TOTAL AMOUNT | TYPES OF EXPENSES | | | | | | | | | | |
				RENT	UTILITIES	POSTAGE	LAB./X-RAY	MEDICAL SUPPLIES	OFFICE SUPPLIES	WAGES	INSURANCE	TAXES	TRAVEL	MISC.
01	Philips' Med. Suppl.	1778	125.00					125.00						
01	Postage	1779	16.85			16.85								
02	Medi Path	1780	32.50				32.50							
02	Quik Service Co.	1781	82.40						82.40					
02	Philips' Med. Suppl.	1782	92.00					92.00						
02	Jean Medina	1783	77.06							77.06				
05	State Dept. of Rev.	1784	189.16									189.16		
06	General Insurance	1785	165.92								165.92			
07	Postage	(Cash)	5.19			5.19								
07	Micah Smith	(Cash)	15.00										15.00	
08	IRS	1786	419.41									419.41		
12	Quik Service Co.	1787	124.00						124.00					
13	City Laundry	1788	75.00											75.00
13	National Insurance	1789	189.00								189.00			
14	Broyer Assoc.	1790	1500.00	1500.00										
14	Postage	(Cash)	12.11			12.11								
15	City Gas Co.	1791	125.00		125.00									
19	Jean Medina	1792	85.92							85.92				
19	Postage	(Cash)	8.95			8.95								
21	Philips' Med. Suppl.	1793	85.00					85.00						
23	Medi Path	1794	67.90				67.90							
24	Micah Smith	(Cash)	10.00										10.00	
24	Elena Paxson	1795	126.00							126.00				
27	Postage	1796	17.32			17.32								
28	Johnson Assoc.	1797	123.45				123.45							
	Total		3770.14	1500.00	125.00	60.42	223.85	302.00	206.40	288.98	354.92	608.57	25.00	75.00

Figure 18-3. A record of office disbursements lists the amounts paid over a certain period of time.

Quarterly Summary of Charges, Receipts, and Disbursements, 2005

					Types of Disbursements						
	1	2	3	4	5	6	7	8	9	10	11
MONTH	CHARGES	RECEIPTS	DISBURSE-MENTS	WAGES	RENT & UTILITIES	OFFICE EXPENSES	GENERAL MEDICAL	X-RAY/ LAB.	TAXES	PERSONAL	MISC.
Jan.	15400.00	14800.00	6218.14	3349.50	1625.00	129.86	93.45	241.86	589.02	100.00	89.45
Feb.	18255.00	18950.00	7050.40	3872.80	1683.08	235.00	118.72	266.00	611.20	186.60	77.00
Mar.	13850.00	13250.00	6530.14	3666.10	1702.85	43.85	243.11	187.02	577.00	88.11	22.10
Subtotal	47505.00	47000.00	19798.68	10888.40	5010.93	408.71	455.28	694.88	1777.22	374.71	188.55
Apr.											
May											
June											
Subtotal											
July											
Aug.											
Sept.											
Subtotal											
Oct.											
Nov.											
Dec.											
Subtotal											
Grand Total											

Figure 18-4. Creating a summary of charges, receipts, and disbursements is a regular bookkeeping task, performed monthly, quarterly, or yearly.

PROCEDURE 18.1

Organizing the Practice's Bookkeeping System

Objective: To maintain a bookkeeping system that promotes accurate record keeping for the practice

Materials: Daily log sheets; patient ledger cards; check register; summaries of charges, receipts, and disbursements

Method

1. Use a new daily log sheet each day. For each patient seen that day, record the patient name, the relevant charges, and any payments received.

2. Create a ledger card for each new patient, and maintain a ledger card for all existing patients. The ledger card should include the patient's name, address, home and work telephone numbers, and insurance company. It should also contain the name of the person responsible for the charges (if different from the patient) and the name of the person who referred the patient

to the office. Update the ledger card every time the patient incurs a charge or makes a payment. Be sure to adjust the account balance after every transaction.

3. Record all deposits accurately in the check register. File the deposit receipt—with a detailed listing of checks and money orders deposited—for later use in reconciling the bank statement.

4. When paying bills for the practice, enter each check in the check register accurately, including the check number, date, payee, and amount.

5. Prepare a summary of charges, receipts, and disbursements every month, quarter, or year, as directed. Be sure to double-check the calculations from the monthly summary before posting them to the quarterly summary. Also, double-check the calculations from the quarterly summary before posting them to the yearly summary.

---

expenses into various categories. Based on this information, the physician can make vital business decisions. For example, after analyzing monthly summaries, the physician may decide to budget expenses differently, collect payments more promptly, cut unprofitable services, or expand profitable services.

Although an accountant may prepare these reports, an experienced medical assistant can prepare them. If you are asked to prepare them, follow these guidelines.

- Every business day, post the total charges and receipts from the daily log to the appropriate line and column of the monthly summary.

- Every business day, also post the disbursements from the record of office disbursements to the appropriate lines and columns of the monthly summary.

- At the end of the month, total the columns on the monthly summary.

- At the end of each quarter, post the charges, receipts, and disbursements for each of the previous 3 months to the quarterly summary. Then, total each column.

- At the end of the year, post the charges, receipts, and disbursements for each of the previous 12 months (or 4 quarters) to the annual summary. Then, total each column.

Remember that the total charges and total receipts in any summary should be almost the same. They may not be identical, because some bills may not have been fully

collected. Procedure 18-1 offers a plan for setting up a medical practice bookkeeping system.

Double-Entry System. The double-entry accounting system is based on an accounting equation:

$$Assets = Liabilities + Owner\ Equity$$

Assets are goods or properties that have a dollar value, such as the medical practice building, bank accounts, office equipment, and accounts receivable. Owner equity (also called capital, net worth, or proprietorship) is the owner's right to the value of the assets. Liabilities are amounts owed by the practice to creditors, such as a mortgage on the building and accounts payable. Liabilities decrease the value of the assets. In other words, in a medical practice, the owner (the physician) has the rights to the value of the practice's assets, once the liabilities have been subtracted.

Because both sides of the accounting equation must always balance (agree), every transaction is recorded as an entry on each side of the equation. Thus, there are two entries, or a double entry. The double-entry system is accurate, detects errors easily, and provides the most complete information about the practice and its contribution to the physician's net worth. It is complex, however, and requires a great deal of time and skill to master. If it is used in a medical practice, an accountant usually establishes and maintains the system, and the medical assistant simply keeps a daily log.

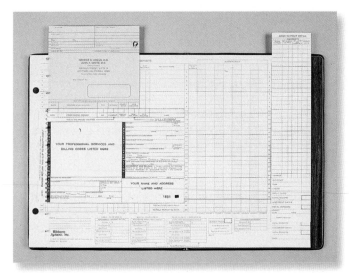

Figure 18-5. A pegboard system allows for simultaneous transfer of information while writing it only once.

Pegboard System.

The **pegboard system** lets your write each transaction once while recording it on four different bookkeeping forms. This technique can help to reduce errors and save time. The pegboard system is called the one-write system and used to be the most widely used bookkeeping system in medical practices. This system is now used less commonly in many practices.

A pegboard system usually includes a lightweight board with pegs on the left or right edges (Figure 18-5). The pegs match holes that are punched in daily log sheets, patient ledger cards, charge slips/receipts, and deposit slips. The holes allow the forms to be aligned while stacked on top of each other. Information, entered on only one form, is simultaneously transferred to the form(s) below. Generally these forms are printed on NCR (no-carbon-required) paper. If not, you must place carbon paper between the forms.

Starting the Business Day. Place a daily log sheet on the pegboard at the beginning of each day. Then, place the stack of charge slips/receipts on the pegs, aligning the top line of the first charge slip/receipt with the daily log top line. Because the charge slips/receipts are shingled, or layered one over the other from top to bottom, alignment of the first aligns all the others. The charge slips/receipts are prenumbered. This numbering promotes good cash control and theoretically prevents embezzlement.

Upon Patient Arrival. As each patient comes into the office, place the patient's ledger card under the next available charge slip/receipt. Be sure to align the card's first blank line with the carbon strip on the charge slip/receipt. Write the date, the patient's name, and the patient's previous balance on the charge slip section. The information will automatically be recorded in the daily log and on the patient ledger card.

Attaching the Charge Slip/Receipt to the Patient Chart. Next, remove the charge slip/receipt and attach it to the patient chart so that the doctor will see it. After examining the patient, the doctor fills in the appropriate charges on the charge slip/receipt, indicates when the next appointment is needed, and gives the charge slip/receipt to the patient.

Before the Patient Leaves. The patient comes to you with the completed charge slip/receipt, and you again place the ledger card between the charge slip/receipt and the daily log. Check to be sure you align it properly. On the charge slip/receipt, write the charge slip/receipt number, date, procedure (or code), charges, payments, new balance, and the date and time of the next appointment (if any). As you write this information, it should be automatically transferred onto the ledger card and daily log. Finally, tear off the receipt, and give it to the patient. You can now return the patient ledger card to the file.

Payments After the Patient Visit. If you receive payments sometime after the patient visit, either by mail or in person, record them on the patient ledger card and daily log as you normally would. Record charges for doctor visits to hospitalized patients or other out-of-office visits in the same way. If required, you can use the pegboard system to record bank deposits and petty cash disbursements in the daily log, but you will need the appropriate overlapping forms.

End of the Day. At the end of each day, total and check the arithmetic (addition and subtraction) in all columns. If you find an error, correct it immediately by drawing a line through it and making a new entry on the next available writing line. Remember to make the correction on the patient ledger card also and to issue a new receipt to the patient.

Bookkeeping on the Computer

Physicians or office managers who choose to set up the practice's bookkeeping system on the computer enjoy several important benefits over traditional bookkeeping methods. Computerized bookkeeping saves time; many repetitive tasks are done by the computer. The computer also performs mathematic calculations. Most bookkeeping software programs include built-in tax tables, which can calculate tax liabilities and so on.

As discussed in Chapter 6, many bookkeeping software programs are available on the market. Any bookkeeping software package performs the same tasks described earlier in this chapter under traditional bookkeeping systems. The practice in which you work may already have a computerized bookkeeping program in place. It is a good idea, however, to read current computer software magazines. You may learn about a new software program you might recommend to the physician or office manager, or you may read about a new or more efficient way to use the practice's current software program.

Banking for the Medical Office

Besides bookkeeping, you may be responsible for handling the banking for the practice. Because a practice may use traditional (manual) or electronic (computerized) banking methods, you should be familiar with both. Regardless of which method you use, remember to keep all banking materials secure because they represent the finances of the practice. For example, to prevent theft of checks, always put the checkbook in a securely locked place when it is not in use. Also, file deposit receipts promptly. If they are lost, you have no proof that a deposit was made. Lack of proof could cost the practice thousands of dollars.

Banking Tasks

Banking tasks for the medical practice include:

- Writing checks
- Accepting checks
- Endorsing checks
- Making deposits
- Reconciling bank statements

To perform these tasks properly, you must be familiar with several terms and concepts related to banking.

Checks. A **check** is a bank draft or order for payment. The person who writes the check is called the **payer.** By writing a check, the payer directs the bank to pay a sum of money on demand to the payee. In order to be considered **negotiable** (legally transferable from one person to another), a check must:

- Be written and signed by the payer or maker
- Include the amount of money to be paid, considered a promise to pay a specified sum
- Be made payable to the payee or bearer
- Be made payable on demand or on a specific date
- Include the name of the bank that is directed to make payment

Other Negotiable Papers. You may receive other negotiable paper in addition to standard personal and business checks.

- A **cashier's check** is a check issued on bank paper signed by a bank representative. It is usually purchased by individuals who do not have checking accounts.

- A **certified check** is a payer's check written and signed by the payer and stamped "Certified" by the bank. This certification means that the bank has already drawn money from the payer's account to guarantee that the check will be paid when submitted. (The money is set aside to cover this specific check.) Few banks offer certified checks anymore.
- A **money order** is another kind of certificate of guaranteed payment. Money orders may be purchased from banks (bank money orders) or post offices (postal money orders) or from some convenience stores.

Check Codes. The face (front) of every check contains two important items: the American Banking Association (ABA) number and the magnetic ink character recognition (MICR) code. The **ABA number** appears as a fraction, such as 60-117/310, on the upper edge of all printed checks. It identifies the geographic area and specific bank on which the check is drawn.

Found at the bottom of a check, the MICR code consists of numbers and characters printed in magnetic ink, which can be read by MICR equipment at the bank. This code enables checks to be read, sorted, and recorded by computer.

Types of Checking Accounts. A physician is likely to have three different types of checking accounts: a personal account, a business account for office expenses, and an interest-earning account. The interest-earning account will be used for paying special expenses, such as property taxes and insurance premiums. Most of your work will be with the business checking account. You may sometimes, however, make payments from, or transfer money to, the interest-earning account, as directed.

Accepting Checks. Before accepting any check, review it carefully. First be sure the check has the correct date, amount, and signature and that no corrections have been made. Figure 18-6 shows a correctly written and endorsed check. Do not accept a **third-party check** (one made out to the patient rather than to the practice) unless it is from a health insurance company. Also, do not accept a check marked "Payment in Full" unless it actually does pay the complete outstanding balance. You may accept a check signed by someone other than the payer if the person who signed the check has power of attorney. **Power of attorney** gives a person the legal right to handle financial matters for another person who is unable to do so. Frequently power of attorney is granted to a patient's spouse, son, or daughter.

Be sure to follow the policy of your practice when accepting a check. For example, if a patient is new or unfamiliar, office policy may require you to request patient identification and to compare the signature on the identification with the signature on the check. Policy may also require that you not accept a check for more than the amount due.

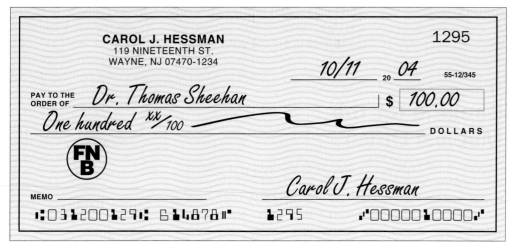

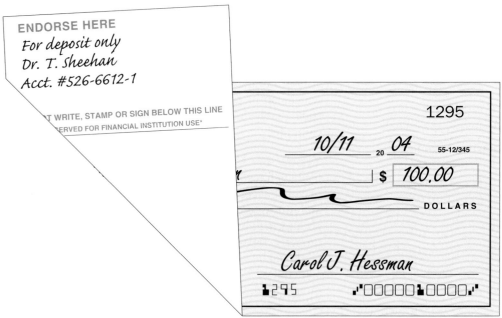

Figure 18-6. After verifying that a patient's check is correct, immediately endorse it with "For Deposit Only," the name of the practice, and the account number.

Endorsing Checks. After accepting a check, immediately **endorse** it, that is to say, write the name of the doctor or the practice on the back. Include the words "For Deposit Only" and the account number. (For convenience, this statement may be made into a rubber stamp.) This type of endorsement prevents the check from being cashed if it is lost or stolen.

Be sure to endorse the check in ink, using a pen or rubber stamp. Place the endorsement in the 1.5-inch area indicated on the back of the check. Most personal and business checks have a number of lines or a shaded area preprinted on the checks for this purpose. Leave the rest of the back of the check blank for the use of the bank.

Completing the Deposit Slip. After endorsing the check, post the payment to the patient ledger card, and put the check with others to be deposited. Then, fill out a deposit slip, as shown in Figure 18-7. The account number

is printed on deposit slips in MICR numbers that match those on the checks. As mentioned, these numbers enable checks and deposit slips to be read, sorted, and recorded by computer.

Banks will accept a list of deposited items on something other than the bank-provided deposit slip if the bank's deposit slip is attached. For example, if you are depositing 50 checks, you may create a computer printout listing the payers' names, check numbers, amount of each check, and total. You can then attach the printout to a deposit slip with the total written on the deposit slip. Another method is to attach a calculator or adding machine tape listing the individual check amounts and a total.

Making the Deposit. Plan to deposit checks and cash into the practice's bank account in person at the bank, as described in Procedure 18-2. Avoid sending cash through the mail, but if it is absolutely necessary to do so,

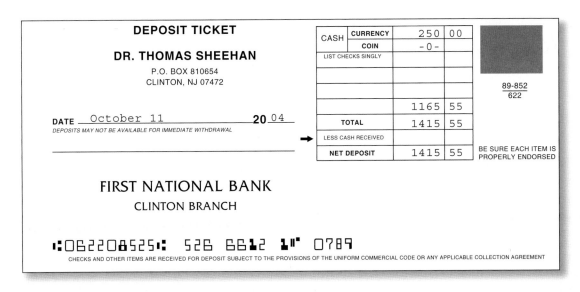

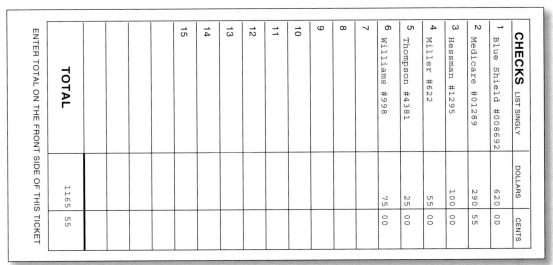

Figure 18-7. List each check on the deposit slip, including the check number and amount.

use registered mail. In any case, be sure to obtain a deposit receipt from the bank.

In a busy physician's office, you may need to make deposits every day. If the physician has a limited practice, you may make deposits less frequently. Keep in mind, however, that making deposits more frequently increases cash flow and reduces the risk of lost or bounced checks.

Reconciling Bank Statements. Another banking task is reconciling the bank statement. **Reconciliation** involves comparing the office's financial records with the bank records to ensure that they are consistent (all numbers agree) and accurate. In most practices this task is performed once a month when the practice receives the monthly checking account statement from the bank. An example of a bank statement is shown in Figure 18-8. The process of reconciliation is explained in Procedure 18-3.

Electronic Banking

Compared with traditional banking methods, electronic banking has several advantages. Electronic banking can

improve productivity, cash flow, and accuracy. The use of electronic banking can also speed up many banking tasks.

If your medical office uses electronic banking, your basic tasks will be the same as in an office that uses traditional banking methods. How these tasks are performed, however, may be quite different. When you use electronic banking, you are still responsible for recording and depositing checks, just as if you were using traditional methods, but you will see these differences.

- Rather than your recording each check in a paper checkbook and determining the new balance, the computer software calculates the new balance for you.
- Rather than your reconciling the office bank statement on paper, the computer software does it automatically.
- Rather than putting the checkbook and banking forms in a securely locked place at the end of the day, you use a computer password for security.

Many medical office software programs are available today. Each one has a different interface, uses different menus, and prompts you for information in different ways.

PROCEDURE 18.2

Making a Bank Deposit

Objective: To prepare cash and checks for deposit and to deposit them properly into a bank account

Materials: Bank deposit slip and items to be deposited, such as checks, cash, and money orders

Method

1. Divide the bills, coins, checks, and money orders into separate piles.

2. Sort the bills by denomination, from largest to smallest. Then, stack them, portrait side up, in the same direction. Total the amount of the bills, and write this amount on the deposit slip on the line marked "Currency."

3. If you have enough coins to fill coin wrappers, put them in wrappers of the proper denomination. If not, count the coins, and put them in the deposit bag. Total the amount of coins, and write this amount on the deposit slip on the line marked "Coin."

4. Review all checks and money orders to be sure they are properly endorsed with a restrictive endorsement. List each check on the deposit slip, including the check number and amount. If you do not keep a list of the check writers'

names in the office, record this information on the deposit slip also.

5. List each money order on the deposit slip. Include the notation "money order" or "MO" and the name of the writer.

6. Calculate the total deposit (total of amounts for currency, coin, checks, and money orders). Write this amount on the deposit slip on the line marked "Total." Photocopy the deposit slip for your office records.

7. Record the total amount of the deposit in the office checkbook register.

8. If you plan to make the deposit in person, place the currency, coins, checks, and money orders in a deposit bag. If you cannot make the deposit in person, put the checks and money orders in a special bank-by-mail envelope, or put all deposit items in an envelope and send it by registered mail.

9. Make the deposit in person or by mail.

10. Obtain a deposit receipt from the bank. File it in the office for later use when reconciling the bank statement.

Certain general concepts apply to all. For specific information, consult the user's manual that comes with your practice's computer software. All software will allow you to perform the following tasks:

- Record deposits
- Pay bills
- Display the checkbook
- Balance the checkbook

Record Deposits. If you select "Record Deposits," a message on the computer screen prompts you to enter information about each check to be deposited that day. This information usually includes the check writer's name and the amount of the check. The check's ABA number may also be requested. After you enter this information, the computer gives you a chance to double-check it. If all the information is correct, you continue entering and checking the other deposits, one at a time. You can then select a command to print a deposit slip that contains the information you have just entered. To make the deposit, place the cash and checks in a deposit bag along with the computerized deposit slip and the bank's deposit slip.

Pay Bills. The bill-paying function allows you to log checks that you write into a computerized checkbook register. For each check you want to write, a message on the computer screen should prompt you for information, such as the payee and the amount of the check. The computer should also give you a chance to verify and correct this information before moving on to the next check or printing the actual checks.

Some software programs automatically assign the next available check number to each new check you enter. To double-check that the computer-assigned check numbers match those on the actual checks, print a list of the checks you have entered, and compare it with the checks before mailing them.

Display the Checkbook. The checkbook display function allows you to review the electronic checkbook register. Although you cannot change information that appears in the register, you can print it out. Thus, you can be sure the checks have been recorded properly, and you can check your latest balance.

If you select "Display Checkbook" from the "Banking" menu, the computer displays a list of all checks that have

First State Bank of Englewood

1st
CN 1
Englewood WI 54534-0001

PAGE 1

ACCOUNT NO.   518-833-3

STATEMENT PERIOD
07/19/04 TO 08/20/04

CAROL J CHARLESTON
APT 49
1013 HUGHES DR
LAWRENCE SQUARE WI 54690-1226

YOUR ACCOUNT SUMMARY

DEPOSIT ACCOUNTS	BALANCE
CHECKING ACCOUNT	2,088.08
SAVINGS ACCOUNT	6.54
TOTAL	2,094.62

CHECKING ACCOUNT

CAROL J CHARLESTON

SUMMARY OF ACCOUNT   518-833-3

BEGINNING BALANCE ON 07/18/04	3,055.24
DEPOSITS AND CREDITS	+3,819.02
CHECKS & WITHDRAWALS	-4,786.18
ENDING BALANCE ON 08/20/04	2,088.08

CHECKS PAID: 38

CHECK	AMOUNT	DATE PAID	REFERENCE#	CHECK	AMOUNT	DATE PAID	REFERENCE#
CHECK	450.00	07/19/04	81569110	2226	181.00	08/12/04	05105878
2202	146.23	07/31/04	29521570	2227	24.74	08/19/04	06120827
2203	122.03	07/29/04	29141271	2228	140.00	08/12/04	05022086
2210*	43.00	07/29/04	07046380	2229	148.71	08/16/04	27248941
2211	60.09	08/01/04	04597911	2230	53.16	08/13/04	27852752
2214*	123.59	07/24/04	29470425	2231	50.00	08/14/04	01018325
2215	47.70	07/19/04	12357289	2232	50.00	08/13/04	05080148
2216	9.00	07/22/04	05479786	2233	15.00	08/16/04	04709533
2217	30.00	07/26/04	29841864	2234	13.95	08/19/04	06008593
2218	19.00	07/30/04	04330539	2235	123.59	08/14/04	27050650
2219	12.00	07/24/04	04037820	2236	50.00	08/13/04	05099115
2220	35.93	07/24/04	04068844	2237	50.00	08/15/04	03014667
2221	10.00	08/12/04	05091269	2238	20.00	08/16/04	04675854
2222	23.48	07/24/04	29465653	2239	47.70	08/14/04	06172997
2223	242.43	07/26/04	29804419	2240	24.74	08/19/04	06120925
2224	150.00	07/30/04	29405827	2243*	400.00	08/14/04	29652307
2225	830.00	08/07/04	02242873	2344	400.00	08/14/04	29652306

Figure 18-8. Each month you will receive a current bank statement, which you should reconcile with the previous statement and your checkbook register.

PROCEDURE 18.3

Reconciling a Bank Statement

Objective: To ensure that the bank record of deposits and withdrawals agrees with the practice's record of deposits and withdrawals

Materials: Previous bank statement, current bank statement, reconciliation worksheet (if not part of current bank statement), deposit receipts, red pencil, check stubs or checkbook register, returned checks

Method

1. Check the closing balance on the previous statement against the opening balance on the new statement. The balances should match. If they do not, call the bank.

2. Record the closing balance from the new statement on the reconciliation worksheet (Figure 18-9). This worksheet usually appears on the back of the bank statement.

3. Check each deposit receipt against the bank statement. Place a red check mark in the upper right corner of each receipt that is recorded on the statement. Total the amount of deposits that do *not* appear on the statement. Add this amount to the closing balance on the reconciliation worksheet.

4. Put the returned checks in numerical order.

5. Compare each returned check with the bank statement, making sure that the amount on the check agrees with the amount on the statement. Place a red check mark in the upper right corner of each returned check that is recorded on the statement. Also, place a check mark on the check stub or check register entry. Any checks that were written but that do not appear on the statement and were not returned are considered "outstanding" checks. You can find these easily on the check stubs or checkbook register because they have no red check mark.

6. List each outstanding check separately on the worksheet, including its check number and amount. Total the outstanding checks, and

---

HOW TO BALANCE YOUR CHECKING ACCOUNT

1. Subtract any service charges that appear on this statement from your checkbook balance.
2. Add any interest paid on your checking account to your checkbook balance.
3. Check off (✔) in your checkbook register all checks and pre-authorized transactions listed on your statement.
4. Use the worksheet to list checks you have written, ATM withdrawals, and Point of Sale transactions which are not listed on your statement.

5. Enter the closing balance on the statement.	$	.
6. Add any deposits not shown on the statement.	+	.
7. Subtotal	$	.
8. Subtract total transactions outstanding (from worksheet on right).	−	.
9. Account balance (should match balance in your checkbook register).	$	.

IF YOUR ACCOUNT DOES NOT BALANCE

a. Check your addition and subtraction first on this form and then in your checkbook.
b. Be sure the deposit amounts on your statement are the same as those in your checkbook.
c. Be sure all the check amounts on your statement agree with the amounts entered in your checkbook register.
d. Be sure all checks written prior to this reconcilement period but not listed on the statement are listed on the worksheet.
e. Verify that all MAC® ATM, Point of Sale, and other pre-authorized transactions have been recorded in your checkbook register.
f. Review last month's statement to be certain any corrections were entered into your checkbook.

WORKSHEET
Transactions Outstanding

Number or Date	Amount
TOTAL	

Figure 18-9. Use the reconciliation worksheet on the back of the bank statement to reconcile the statement with your checkbook register.

continued →

PROCEDURE 18.3

Reconciling a Bank Statement (continued)

subtract this total from the bank statement balance.

7. If the statement shows that the checking account earned interest, add this amount to the checkbook balance.

8. If the statement lists such items as a service charge, check printing charge, or automatic payment, subtract them from the checkbook balance.

9. Compare the new checkbook balance with the new bank statement balance. They should match. If they do not, repeat the process, rechecking all calculations. Double-check the addition and subtraction in the checkbook

register. Review the checkbook register to make sure you did not omit any items. Ensure that you carried the correct balance forward from one register page to the next. Double-check that you made the correct additions or subtractions for all interest earned and charges.

10. If your work is correct, and the balances still do not agree, call the bank to determine if a bank error has been made. Contact the bank promptly because the bank may have a time limit for corrections. The bank may consider the bank statement correct if you do not point out an error within 2 weeks (or other period, according to bank policy).

---

been entered into the register. Information includes check number, date, payee, and amount. Scrolling up and down reveals all the checks in the register. (Some banks also allow you to access this information by telephone. The Tips for the Office section gives more information about telephone banking.)

Balance Checkbook. The "Balance Checkbook" option electronically reconciles the monthly bank statement. After you enter the appropriate date or dates, the computer screen displays all the checks and deposits that were logged into the register in the order they were posted. Figure 18-10 shows an example of this function.

Tips for the Office

Telephone Banking

Telephone banking is a form of electronic banking that enables you to access your bank's computer system by phone to obtain account information and perform simple banking tasks. To use telephone banking, you should have a push-button telephone, the telephone personal identification number (TPIN) assigned to your practice by the bank, and the telephone number that accesses the telephone banking system.

The telephone banking system prompts you for information. You use the push-button pad on the telephone to provide the information. For example, an automated voice may ask you to press 1 to inquire about deposits or 2 to inquire about withdrawals. Telephone banking is especially useful for the following banking tasks:

- Checking the current balance of an account
- Determining whether deposited funds are available

- Obtaining the date and amount of the last few deposits and the last few checks paid (usually the last three)
- Finding out if a specific check has been paid
- Transferring funds between accounts (if the practice has more than one account)
- Stopping payment on checks

Although this form of electronic banking is especially useful for some services, you cannot use it to manage all banking tasks. For example, you cannot use it to make deposits or reconcile a bank statement. However, it can be quite convenient for the day-to-day banking tasks just listed. If you have a hearing impairment and have a telecommunications device for the deaf (TDD) installed on the telephone, you can bank by phone.

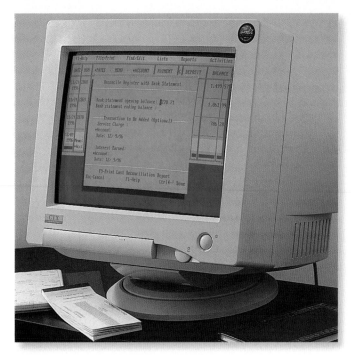

Figure 18-10. Electronic banking will allow you to see the "Balance Checkbook" menu on the screen.

The next screen highlights each check or deposit that has not been seen on a previous bank statement. You are prompted to indicate whether that item appears on the current statement, usually using Y for yes and N for no. After the computer queries these items, it may ask you to enter any items that appear on the current bank statement but are not in the checkbook, such as service charges.

Finally, a message on the screen prompts you to enter the current account balance from the bank statement. Then, the computer reconciles the bank statement. It will alert you if the system balance does not agree with the balance on the bank statement. If the balance does not agree, recheck the information you entered for possible error. If your work is correct, and the balances still do not agree, call the bank to determine if a bank error has been made.

Managing Accounts Payable

As you learned in Chapter 17, accounts payable are the practice's expenses (money leaving the business), and accounts receivable reflect a practice's income (money coming into the business). This section focuses on accounts payable, including payroll. A basic accounting principle to bear in mind is that when a practice's income exceeds its expenses, it has a profit. When a practice's expenses exceed its income, it has a loss.

Because of this relationship between income and expenses, most practices try to reduce expenses by controlling accounts payable. As a medical assistant, you play an important role in helping control accounts payable and maximize profits.

Accounts payable fall into three main groups:

1. Payments for supplies, equipment, and practice-related products and services
2. Payroll, which may be the largest of the accounts payable
3. Taxes owed to federal, state, and local agencies

A practice's accounting system usually consists of several elements. These elements include the daily log, patient ledger cards, the checkbook, the disbursements journal, the petty cash record, and the payroll register.

The daily log and patient ledger cards are used primarily for accounts receivable. The disbursements journal, petty cash record, and payroll register are used primarily in accounts payable. Procedure 18-4 tells you how to set up and use these accounting tools effectively.

Managing Disbursements

A disbursement is any payment the physician's office makes for goods or services. One of the most common disbursements is payment for office supplies. Other disbursements include payments for equipment, dues, rent, taxes, salary, and utilities. No matter what type of disbursement you make on behalf of the practice, you must keep accurate records of the purchase and the payment.

Managing Supplies

In most practices, the physician authorizes one person to handle the purchasing of supplies and other products. This person is usually the office manager or medical assistant.

Guidelines for purchasing supplies are discussed in detail in Chapter 8. When buying clinical or office supplies, keep these six principles in mind to control expenses.

1. Order only the necessary supplies, and order them only in the proper amounts. Buying too much reduces cash flow. Buying too little may cause you to run out of needed items and you may have to reorder too often.
2. Combine orders when possible. You may save money and time by placing a larger order for several items at once rather than placing a smaller order each time an item is needed.
3. Follow your practice's purchasing guidelines, if any. For example, you may have to get the physician's approval for purchases over a specific dollar amount. Employees may have to submit purchase orders (formal requests for goods or services).
4. Buy from reputable suppliers. They are more likely to provide on-time delivery and satisfactory handling of your order. If your office does not already have a list of reliable suppliers, ask for recommendations from other practices.

PROCEDURE 18.4

Setting Up the Accounts Payable System

Objective: To set up an accounts payable system

Materials: Disbursements journal, petty cash record, payroll register, pen

Method

Setting Up the Disbursements Journal

1. Write in column headings for the basic information about each check: date, payee's name, check number, and check amount.
2. Write in column headings for each type of business expense, such as rent and utilities.
3. Write in column headings (if space is available) for deposits and the account balance.
4. Record the data from completed checks under the appropriate column headings.

Setting Up the Petty Cash Record

1. Write in column headings for the date, transaction number, payee, brief description, amount of transaction, and type of expense.
2. Write in a column heading (if space is available) for the petty cash fund balance.

3. Record the data from petty cash vouchers under the appropriate column headings.

Setting Up the Payroll Register

1. Write in column headings for check number, employee name, earnings to date, hourly rate, hours worked, regular earnings, overtime hours worked, and overtime earnings.
2. Write in column headings for total gross earnings for the pay period and gross taxable earnings.
3. Write in column headings for each deduction. These may include federal income tax, Federal Insurance Contributions Act (FICA) tax, state income tax, local income tax, and various voluntary deductions.
4. Write in a column heading for net earnings.
5. Each time you write payroll checks, record earning and deduction data under the appropriate column headings on the payroll register.

---

5. Get the best-quality supplies for the best price.
6. For clinical supplies, consider the amount for which insurance companies will reimburse the practice. For example, if your office does only a few throat cultures a year, it might make more sense to send those patients elsewhere for the test than to stock the supplies required. The small reimbursement amount for a few throat cultures may not justify purchasing the supplies. Also consider shelf life. Do not buy large amounts of clinical supplies that will expire before use.

Writing Checks

Virtually all disbursements are made by check. Paying by check gives the practice complete, accurate records of all financial transactions.

Before writing a check, make sure the checking account balance is up-to-date and large enough to cover the check you want to write. Subtract the amount of each check from the previous balance, enter the new balance, and carry that balance forward to the next stub.

If you use a pegboard system, you will automatically record the date, check number, payee, and check amount

on the check register as you write out the check. You must note the reason for payment and the new balance manually, however. Record that information in the appropriate spaces on the register.

If you make an error when completing a check, write VOID in ink across the front of the check in large letters so that it cannot be used again. Then file the voided check in numerical order with the returned checks.

After filling out the check properly, detach it from the checkbook, and give it to the doctor to sign, along with the invoice to be paid. (With experience, you may be trusted to sign checks under a certain amount.) Mark the date, check number, and amount paid on the invoice. Make a copy of the invoice for your records. Keep these copies with supporting documents, such as order forms or packing slips, in a paid-invoice file. Then, mail the check and the original invoice to the payee in a neatly hand-addressed or typewritten envelope. If you use a window envelope, be sure the payee's address shows through the window.

Commonly Used Checks. Most practices use checks from a standard checkbook, or they use **voucher checks,** business checks with stubs attached. Voucher checks come in several styles. A common style is a large, ring-bound checkbook, with three checks to a page. A perforation divides each check from its matching stub, which the practice retains.

Limited checks are sometimes used for payroll. A **limited check** states that it is void after a certain time limit. Many practices use checks that are void after 90 days.

Other Types of Checks. You or the physician may sometimes need to use other types of checks. The physician may use a cashier's check to pay certain types of taxes. A cashier's check is purchased from a bank, written on the bank's own checking account, and signed by a bank official.

The physician may use a certified check to pay certain taxes or to buy property. A certified check is a standard check that the bank verifies and certifies before it is used. This certification means that funds have been set aside to guarantee payment of the check.

A **counter check** is a special bank check that allows the depositor to withdraw funds from her account only. It states, "Pay to the Order of Myself Only." The physician may use a counter check when she wants to withdraw money but has forgotten her checkbook.

A physician may use **traveler's checks** when attending an out-of-town conference or whenever using a personal check or carrying a lot of cash is not appropriate. Printed in $10, $20, $50, and $100 denominations, these checks must be signed at the location where they are purchased (usually a bank). To use traveler's checks, the physician fills in the payee's name and signs it in a second place. She must sign it in the payee's presence so the payee can ensure that the signatures match.

Recording Disbursements

You may record disbursements in a check register, in a disbursements journal, or on the bottom section of the daily log.

If you use a disbursements journal, follow these steps to record disbursements.

1. When beginning a new journal page, give each column a heading to reflect the type of expense, such as utilities or rent.
2. For each check, fill in the date, payee's name, check number, and check amount in the appropriate columns.
3. Determine the expense category of the check.
4. Record the check amount in the column for that type of business expense.
5. If you must divide a check between two or more expense columns, record the total in the check amount column. Then record the amount that applies to each type of expense in the appropriate column.

Recording disbursements in columns for each type of expense allows you to total and track expenses by category. **Tracking** (watching for changes) is important

because it helps control expenses. Before tracking, check your calculations by performing a trial balance.

1. Total the check amount column.
2. Find the total for each expense column.
3. Add together all the expense column totals. The combined expense column total should match the total in the check amount column.
4. If the amounts do not match, recheck every entry until you find the error. When you find it, draw a line through it, and record the correct information neatly above it or to the side.
5. When the two amounts match (or balance), carry forward all column totals to the disbursements journal for the next month. Remember to prepare summaries and perform balances at the end of every month, quarter, and year.

Managing Petty Cash

Occasionally, you may need to make small (petty) cash disbursements for minor expenses such as postage-due fees or holiday decorations (Figure 18-11). To avoid writing checks for such small amounts, you may pay for them from the **petty cash fund,** cash kept on hand in the office for small purchases. The doctor should determine the amount of the petty cash account (usually $50) and the minimum amount of cash to be kept on hand (such as $15).

Starting and Maintaining a Petty Cash Fund. To start the fund with $50, write a check to "Petty Cash" or "Cash" for that amount. Enter the check in the miscellaneous column of the monthly disbursement record. Then, cash the check. Because this money will be used for small disbursements, be sure to get some of it in pennies, nickels, dimes, quarters, and dollar bills. Put this money in a special petty cash box, along with a stack of petty cash vouchers.

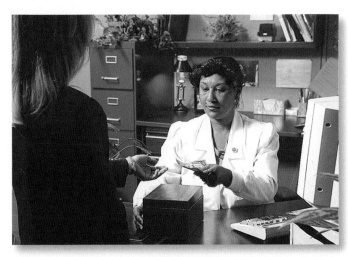

Figure 18-11. You may be in charge of maintaining the practice's petty cash fund. Count cash carefully, and keep accurate records about purchases made.

For each payment from the petty cash fund, obtain a receipt or create a petty cash voucher. The voucher should record the transaction number, date, amount paid, purpose of the expense, your signature (as the person issuing the money), and the signature of the person receiving it. Keep the receipt for any item purchased, along with the completed voucher, in the petty cash box to verify expenses later.

Also, document each petty cash withdrawal on a petty cash record form. Include the transaction number, date, payee, a brief description, amount, and type of expense (such as office expense, auto expense, or miscellaneous expense). If a space is provided, calculate and record the new balance in the petty cash fund.

Replenishing the Petty Cash Fund. At the end of the month (or whenever the fund is low), compare the latest petty cash balance to the money in the petty cash box. If you have not kept a running balance, total the receipts and vouchers, then count the cash on hand. Subtract the total amount on the receipts and vouchers (for example, $35) from the original balance (for example, $50). The difference ($15) should equal the cash on hand in the petty cash box ($15).

To replenish the account, write a check to "Cash" or "Petty Cash" for the amount spent ($35). Cash the check and add the money to the box, bringing the total back up to the original amount of $50. Record the check for $35 on the disbursement record. Also, total the receipts and vouchers by expense category. Record those totals in the appropriate columns on the disbursement record.

Understanding Financial Summaries

The physician may periodically analyze the income and expenses of the practice. Financial summaries provide an easy-to-read report on the business transactions for a given period, such as a month or a year.

An accountant usually prepares financial summaries. Although you will probably not have to create these summaries, you should understand how they are prepared.

Statement of Income and Expense. Also called a profit-and-loss statement, a statement of income and expense highlights the practice's profitability. It shows the physician the practice's total income and then lists and subtracts all expenses.

Cash Flow Statement. A **cash flow statement** shows how much cash is available to cover expenses, to invest, or to take as profits. The cash flow statement begins with the cash on hand at the beginning of the period and shows the income and disbursements made during that period. It concludes with the new amount of cash on hand at the end of the period.

Trial Balance. The doctor may review trial balances periodically to ensure that the books balance. The combined expense column total should match the total in the check amount column. If the amounts do not match, recheck every entry until you find the error.

Handling Payroll

You may be responsible for handling the office payroll (Table 18-1). If so, your duties may include:

- Obtaining tax identification numbers
- Creating employee payroll information sheets
- Calculating employees' earnings
- Subtracting taxes and other deductions
- Writing paychecks
- Creating employee earnings records
- Preparing a payroll register
- Submitting payroll taxes

Applying for Tax Identification Numbers

Every employer—whether a single physician or a corporate practice—must have an employer identification number (EIN). An EIN is required by law for federal tax accounting purposes. An EIN is obtained by completing Form SS-4 (Application for Employer Identification Number) and submitting it to the Internal Revenue Service (IRS). Some states also require employer tax reports, for which the practice must have a state identification number, obtained from the proper state agency.

Creating Employee Payroll Information Sheets

The practice must maintain up-to-date, accurate payroll information about each employee. You should prepare a payroll information sheet for each employee. Each sheet should have the following information:

- The employee's name, address, Social Security number, and marital status
- An indication that the employee has completed an Employment Eligibility Verification (Form I-9), verifying that the employee is a U.S. citizen, a legally admitted alien, or an alien authorized to work in the United States
- The employee's pay schedule, number of dependents, payroll type, and voluntary deductions

Pay Schedule. On the payroll information sheet, list the employee's **pay schedule,** showing how often the employee is paid. Common pay schedules are weekly, biweekly, and monthly.

Number of Dependents. Record the number of **dependents** (people who depend on the employee for

TABLE 18-1 Payroll Duties

Frequency	Duties
Upon assuming payroll responsibilities	• Apply for an employer identification number (EIN) with Form SS-4 if the physician does not already have an EIN.
Whenever a new employee is hired	• Have the employee complete an Employee's Withholding Allowance Certificate (Form W-4) and Employment Eligibility Verification (Form I-9). • Record the employee's name and Social Security number from the employee's Social Security card.
Every payday	• Withhold federal income tax as well as state and local income taxes (if any). • Withhold the employee's share of FICA taxes (for Social Security and Medicare). Record a matching amount for the employer's share. • Calculate how much the practice must pay for each employee's federal and state unemployment tax.
Monthly or biweekly (depending on your deposit schedule)	• Deposit withheld income taxes, withheld and employer Social Security taxes, and withheld and employer Medicare taxes.
Quarterly (by April 30, July 31, October 31, and January 31)	• File Employer's Quarterly Federal Tax Return (Form 941). With the return, pay any taxes that were not deposited earlier.
	• Deposit federal unemployment tax, if over $100.
At least once a year	• Have all employees update their W-4 forms.
On or before January 31	• Give employees their Wage and Tax Statements (Form W-2), which show total wages and various withheld taxes. • File Employer's Annual Federal Unemployment (FUTA) Tax Return (Form 940) with tax amount due.
On or before February 28	• File Transmittal of Wage and Tax Statements (Form W-3) along with the government's copies of the W-2 forms.

financial support). Dependents may include a spouse, children, and other family members.

You can find the number of dependents on the Employee's Withholding Allowance Certificate (Form W-4), which should have been completed when the employee was hired (Figure 18-12). Remember to keep the completed W-4 forms in the physician's personnel file, and update them at least annually.

Payroll Type. List the employee's payroll type—hourly wage, salary, or commission—on the payroll information sheet. An hourly wage is a set amount of money per hour of work. A salary is a set amount of money per pay period, regardless of the number of hours worked. A commission is a percentage of the amount an employee earns for the employer. Salespeople, for example, are often paid by commission.

Voluntary Deductions. Finally, document the voluntary deductions to be taken from the employee's check.

These may include additional federal withholding taxes, contributions to a 401(k) retirement plan, or payments to a company health insurance plan. Employees who want additional federal taxes taken out of their paycheck will indicate this deduction on their W-4 form.

Gross Earnings

Gross earnings refers to the total amount of income earned before deductions. Gross earnings must be calculated for each employee as a first step in the payroll process.

Calculating Gross Earnings. For every payroll period, use data from the payroll information sheet to compute each employee's gross earnings. For an hourly employee, use this equation:

Hourly Wage × Hours Worked = Gross Earnings

Form W-4 (2004)

Purpose. Complete Form W-4 so that your employer can withhold the correct Federal income tax from your pay. Because your tax situation may change, you may want to refigure your withholding each year.

Exemption from withholding. If you are exempt, complete only lines 1, 2, 3, 4, and 7 and sign the form to validate it. Your exemption for 2004 expires February 16, 2005. See **Pub. 505**, Tax Withholding and Estimated Tax.

Note: *You cannot claim exemption from withholding if: (a) your income exceeds $800 and includes more than $250 of unearned income (e.g., interest and dividends) and (b) another person can claim you as a dependent on their tax return.*

Basic instructions. If you are not exempt, complete the **Personal Allowances Worksheet** below. The worksheets on page 2 adjust your withholding allowances based on itemized deductions, certain credits, adjustments to income, or two-earner/two-job situations. Complete all worksheets that apply. **However, you may claim fewer (or zero) allowances.**

Head of household. Generally, you may claim head of household filing status on your tax return only if you are unmarried and pay more than 50% of the costs of keeping up a home for yourself and your dependent(s) or other qualifying individuals. See line **E** below.

Tax credits. You can take projected tax credits into account in figuring your allowable number of withholding allowances. Credits for child or dependent care expenses and the child tax credit may be claimed using the **Personal Allowances Worksheet** below. See **Pub. 919**, How Do I Adjust My Tax Withholding? for information on converting your other credits into withholding allowances.

Nonwage income. If you have a large amount of nonwage income, such as interest or dividends, consider making estimated tax payments using

Form 1040-ES, Estimated Tax for Individuals. Otherwise, you may owe additional tax.

Two earners/two jobs. If you have a working spouse or more than one job, figure the total number of allowances you are entitled to claim on all jobs using worksheets from only one Form W-4. Your withholding usually will be most accurate when all allowances are claimed on the Form W-4 for the highest paying job and zero allowances are claimed on the others.

Nonresident alien. If you are a nonresident alien, see the **Instructions for Form 8233** before completing this Form W-4.

Check your withholding. After your Form W-4 takes effect, use Pub. 919 to see how the dollar amount you are having withheld compares to your projected total tax for 2004. See Pub. 919, especially if your earnings exceed $125,000 (Single) or $175,000 (Married).

Recent name change? If your name on line 1 differs from that shown on your social security card, call 1-800-772-1213 to initiate a name change and obtain a social security card showing your correct name.

Personal Allowances Worksheet (Keep for your records.)

A Enter "1" for **yourself** if no one else can claim you as a dependent . . . . **A** _____

B Enter "1" if:
- You are single and have only one job; or
- You are married, have only one job, and your spouse does not work; or
- Your wages from a second job or your spouse's wages (or the total of both) are $1,000 or less.

. . **B** _____

C Enter "1" for your **spouse**. But, you may choose to enter "-0-" if you are married and have either a working spouse or more than one job. (Entering "-0-" may help you avoid having too little tax withheld.) . . . . **C** _____

D Enter number of **dependents** (other than your spouse or yourself) you will claim on your tax return . . . . . . **D** _____

E Enter "1" if you will file as **head of household** on your tax return (see conditions under **Head of household** above) . **E** _____

F Enter "1" if you have at least $1,500 of **child or dependent care expenses** for which you plan to claim a credit . . **F** _____

(**Note:** *Do not include child support payments. See **Pub. 503**, Child and Dependent Care Expenses, for details.*)

G **Child Tax Credit** (including additional child tax credit):
- If your total income will be less than $52,000 ($77,000 if married), enter "2" for each eligible child.
- If your total income will be between $52,000 and $84,000 ($77,000 and $119,000 if married), enter "1" for each eligible child plus "1" **additional** if you have four or more eligible children. . . . . **G** _____

H Add lines A through G and enter total here. Note: *This may be different from the number of exemptions you claim on your tax return.* ▶ **H** _____

For accuracy, complete all worksheets that apply.
- If you plan to **itemize or claim adjustments to income** and want to reduce your withholding, see the **Deductions and Adjustments Worksheet** on page 2.
- If you have **more than one job** or are **married and you and your spouse both work** and the combined earnings from all jobs exceed $35,000 ($25,000 if married) see the **Two-Earner/Two-Job Worksheet** on page 2 to avoid having too little tax withheld.
- If **neither** of the above situations applies, **stop here** and enter the number from line H on line 5 of Form W-4 below.

Cut here and give Form W-4 to your employer. Keep the top part for your records.

Form **W-4**

Department of the Treasury
Internal Revenue Service

Employee's Withholding Allowance Certificate

OMB No. 1545-0010

▶ Your employer must send a copy of this form to the IRS if: (a) you claim more than 10 allowances or (b) you claim "Exempt" and your wages are normally more than $200 per week.

2004

1 Type or print your first name and middle initial	Last name		2 Your social security number

Home address (number and street or rural route)	3 ☐ Single ☐ Married ☐ Married, but withhold at higher Single rate.
City or town, state, and ZIP code	Note: *If married, but legally separated, or spouse is a nonresident alien, check the "Single" box.*

4 If your last name differs from that shown on your social security card, check here. You must call 1-800-772-1213 for a new card. ▶ ☐

5 Total number of allowances you are claiming (from line **H** above **or** from the applicable worksheet on page 2) **5** _____

6 Additional amount, if any, you want withheld from each paycheck . . . . **6** $ _____

7 I claim exemption from withholding for 2004, and I certify that I meet **both** of the following conditions for exemption:
- Last year I had a right to a refund of **all** Federal income tax withheld because I had **no** tax liability **and**
- This year I expect a refund of **all** Federal income tax withheld because I expect to have **no** tax liability.

If you meet both conditions, write "Exempt" here . . . . ▶ **7** _____

Under penalties of perjury, I certify that I am entitled to the number of withholding allowances claimed on this certificate, or I am entitled to claim exempt status.

Employee's signature
(Form is not valid unless you sign it.) ▶ _____ Date ▶ _____

8 Employer's name and address (Employer: Complete lines 8 and 10 only if sending to the IRS.)	9 Office code (optional)	10 Employer identification number (EIN)

For Privacy Act and Paperwork Reduction Act Notice, see page 2.   Cat. No. 10220Q   Form **W-4** (2004)

Figure 18-12. Update all Employee's Withholding Allowance Certificates (W-4 forms) at least once a year.

An employee who earns $8 per hour and works 35 hours, for example, has gross earnings of $280 ($8 × 35 hours) per week.

For a salaried employee, use the salary amount as the gross earnings for the pay period, no matter how many hours the employee worked. An employee who earns a weekly salary of $400, for example, receives that amount whether she worked 30, 40, or 50 hours during that week.

Fair Labor Standards Act. The Fair Labor Standards Act primarily affects employees who earn hourly wages. It limits the number of hours they may work, sets their minimum wage, and regulates their overtime pay. It also requires the employer to record the number of hours they work, usually on a time card or in a time book.

For hourly employees, this act mandates payment of:

- Time and a half (1½ times the normal hourly wage) for all hours worked beyond the normal 8 in a regular workday.
- Time and a half for all hours worked on the sixth consecutive day of the work week.
- Twice the normal wage (double time) for all hours worked on the seventh consecutive workday.
- Double time, plus normal holiday pay, for all hours worked on a company-approved holiday.

The Fair Labor Standards Act also requires overtime payments for part-time hourly employees for every hour worked beyond the normal 8 in a day or 40 in a week.

Making Deductions

The law requires all employers to withhold money from employees' gross earnings to pay federal and state and local (if any) income taxes and certain other taxes. In addition, employees may wish you to make certain voluntary deductions. For example, you might be asked to deduct an amount for child care, if the practice or hospital provides on-site child care. You might also deduct employee contributions to health insurance premiums.

You must deposit all employee deductions and employer payments into separate accounts. Monies from these **tax liability** accounts are used to pay taxes to appropriate government agencies.

Income Taxes. You must withhold enough money to cover the employee's federal income tax for the pay period. You can determine this amount by finding the employee's number of exemptions (from Form W-4) and referring to the tax tables in *Circular E, Employer's Tax Guide,* published by the IRS.

Consult the state and local tax tables for other income taxes. These taxes may be simpler to calculate. For example, they may be 4% and 1% of the employee's gross earnings, respectively.

FICA Taxes. For FICA tax, withhold from the employee's check half of the tax owed for the pay period. Pay the other half from the practice's accounts. The amount of FICA tax that funds Social Security differs from the amount that funds Medicare. Report these two amounts separately. Check IRS *Circular E* for the latest FICA tax percentages and level of taxable earnings.

Unemployment Taxes. Federal unemployment tax is not a deduction from employees' paychecks, but it is based on their earnings. It is paid by the practice. The Federal Unemployment Tax Act (FUTA) requires employers to pay a percentage of each employee's income, up to a certain dollar amount. The percentage may be reduced if the employer also pays state unemployment taxes.

States calculate unemployment taxes differently. Some states tax employers and employees; others tax only employers. State unemployment tax usually varies with the employer's past employment record. Employers with few layoffs, such as physicians, have lower tax rates than those with many layoffs. To compute state unemployment tax, apply the assigned tax rate to each employee's earnings, up to a maximum for the calendar year. For details, consult your state unemployment insurance department.

Workers' Compensation. Some states require employers to insure their employees against possible loss of income resulting from work-related injury, disability, or disease. Although state laws vary, they typically require doctors to carry this insurance with a state insurance fund or state-authorized private insurer. Usually, a medical practice's insurance agent will audit the payroll books annually and then issue a bill for the workers' compensation premium due.

Calculating Net Earnings

Add each employee's required and voluntary deductions together to determine the total deductions. Then, subtract the total deductions from the gross earnings to get the employee's **net earnings,** or take-home pay. Use the following equation:

Gross Earnings − Total Deductions = Net Earnings

Preparing Paychecks

The way you prepare the practice's payroll will depend on the system the practice uses. In a small practice, you may write paychecks manually. In this case, write the check amount for the employee's net earnings, and deduct the check amount from the office checkbook. Payroll may also be handled through electronic banking; see the Tips for the Office section.

If the practice uses a payroll service, you may supply time cards or payroll data to the service by mail or electronically. The service calculates all the deductions, prepares paychecks, and mails them to the practice for distribution.

Handling Payroll Through Electronic Banking

An electronic funds transfer system (EFTS) enables you to handle the practice's payroll without writing payroll checks manually. The physician must sign up for EFTS with the bank, and employees must supply their bank account numbers to the employer. Then, the bank electronically deposits employees' paychecks into their bank accounts, as directed.

Most employees like to have their paychecks deposited automatically. The money is available on the day of deposit, and no one has to worry about losing a paycheck, getting to the bank before it closes, or carrying a paycheck around. Also, employees still receive a check stub along with a notification of deposit, so they can track their earnings and deductions.

Contact your bank for more information and specific procedures for setting up EFTS and electronic payroll.

No matter how paychecks are prepared, they should include information about how the check amount was determined. This information usually appears on the check stub. It should match the information on the employee earnings records and payroll register. Procedure 18-5 explains the process for generating payroll.

Maintaining Employee Earnings Records

You need to keep an employee earnings record for each employee (Figure 18-13). When you create the record, list the employee's name, address, phone number, Social Security number, birth date, spouse's name, number of dependents, job title, employment starting date, pay rate, and voluntary deductions.

Then, for each pay period, record the employee's gross earnings, individual deductions, net earnings, and related information. Properly completed earnings records show each employee's earning history.

Maintaining a Payroll Register

A payroll register summarizes vital information about all employees and their earnings (Figure 18-14). At the end of each pay period, record each employee's earnings to date, hourly rate, hours worked, overtime hours, overtime earnings, and total gross earnings. Also, list the gross earnings subject to unemployment taxes and FICA, all required and voluntary deductions, net earnings, and the paycheck number.

Handling Payroll Electronically

Manual payroll preparation and related tasks may take an hour per week for each employee. To save time and to provide the convenience for employees of having their paychecks automatically deposited, some practices handle payroll tasks electronically.

If you work in a relatively small practice, you may handle all payroll tasks in the office, using accounting or payroll software. If you work in a large practice, you may prepare payroll information on the computer and transmit it by modem to an outside payroll service for processing. Depending on which system and software the practice has, you may use the computer to:

- Create, update, and delete employee payroll information files
- Prepare employee paychecks, stubs, and W-2 forms
- Update and print employee earnings records
- Update all appropriate bookkeeping records, such as the payroll ledger and general ledger, with payroll data

To perform these payroll functions electronically, follow the specific instructions in the software manual or get instructions from the payroll service. Generally, you would follow these steps.

Select an option from the "Payroll" menu. Wait for the prompt, then select the appropriate employee from a list of employees.

To create an employee payroll information file for a new employee, input the same information that you would record manually on an employee payroll information sheet: name, address, Social Security number, marital status, pay schedule, number of dependents, payroll type, and voluntary deductions. Print two copies of the employee payroll information file—one for the employee and one for the physician's personnel file.

To update an employee payroll information file when an employee moves, marries, has a child, or wants to change deductions, select "Update Employee File." After making the changes, print out two copies of the file. Show one to the employee to confirm that the information is correct. Then have the employee sign and date it. Keep the signed copy for the physician's personnel file, and give the other to the employee. To ensure that payroll information is always correct and current, you should update it once a year for every employee.

Name_____ Soc. Sec. No. _____ Dependents _____ Year _____

Address_____ Birth Date _____ Deductions _____

_____ Job Title _____ Pay Rate

_____ Employed on _____

Spouse_____ Terminated on _____ Record of Changes

Phone   Reason

Pay Rate	Date	Rate

Check Number	Period Number	Earnings			Deductions					Net Pay	Cumulative FICA
		Regular	OT	Total	FICA	Fed. Tax	State	SUI	SDI		
1st Quarter Total											
2d Quarter Total											
3d Quarter Total											
4th Quarter Total											

Figure 18-13. Earnings records show the earning history of each employee at your practice.

PROCEDURE 18.5

Generating Payroll

Objective: To handle the practice's payroll as efficiently and accurately as possible for each pay period

Materials: Employees' time cards, employees' earnings records, payroll register, IRS tax tables, check register

Method

1. Calculate the total regular and overtime hours worked, based on the employee's time card. Enter those totals under the appropriate headings on the payroll register.

2. Check the pay rate on the employee earnings record. Then multiply the hours worked (including any paid vacation or paid holidays, if applicable) by the rates for regular time and overtime (time and a half or double time). This yields gross earnings.

3. Enter the gross earnings under the appropriate heading on the payroll register. Subtract any nontaxable benefits, such as health-care programs.

4. Using IRS tax tables and data on the employee earnings record, determine the amount of federal income tax to withhold based on the employee's marital status and number of exemptions. Also compute the amount of FICA tax to withhold for Social Security (6.2%) and Medicare (1.45%).

5. Following state and local procedures, determine the amount of state and local income taxes (if any) to withhold based on the employee's marital status and number of exemptions.

6. Calculate the employer's contributions to FUTA and to the state unemployment fund, if any. Post these amounts to the employer's account.

7. Enter any other required or voluntary deductions, such as health insurance or contributions to a 401(k) fund.

8. Subtract all deductions from the gross earnings to get the employee's net earnings.

9. Enter the total amount withheld from all employees for FICA under the headings for Social Security and Medicare. Remember that the employer must match these amounts. Enter other employer contributions, such as for federal and state unemployment taxes, under the appropriate headings.

10. Fill out the check stub, including the employee's name, date, pay period, gross earnings, all deductions, and net earnings. Make out the paycheck for the net earnings.

11. Deposit each deduction in a tax liability account.

Pay Period 6/1–6/14

Emp. No.	Name	Earnings to date	Hrly. Rate	Reg. Hrs.	OT Hrs.	OT Earnings	TOTAL GROSS	Earnings Subject to Unemp.	Earnings Subject to FICA	Social Security (FICA)	Medicare	Federal W/H	State W/H	Health Ins.	Net Pay	Check No.
0010	Scott, B.	9,823.14	14.00	70.00			980.00	980.00	980.00	60.50	14.10	147.92	15.10	25.00	717.38	11747
0020	Wilson, J.	14,290.38	17.00	70.00	6.50	153.00	1343.00	1343.00	1343.00	83.26	19.47	160.45	15.85	67.50	996.47	11748
0030	Diaz, J.	2,750.26	5.50	46.25			254.37	254.37	254.37	15.77	3.68	38.20	3.75		192.97	11749
0040	Ling, W.	2,240.57	6.80	30.00			204.00	204.00	204.00	12.66	2.96	26.02	3.12		159.54	11750
0050	Harris, E.	2,600.98	10.00	23.50			235.00	235.00	235.00	14.57	3.41	33.52	3.36		180.14	11751

Figure 18-14. A payroll register is designed to summarize information about all employees and their earnings.

To delete an employee payroll information file when an employee leaves the practice, select "Terminate Employee." Remember to print out and file a copy of this information before deleting it, because the physician is required to keep employees' payroll records for 4 years.

To generate paychecks and stubs, select the employee from the list of employees and choose the "Print Paycheck" option. Then, answer each prompt displayed by the computer (for example, hours worked). The computer has the employee's pay rate, payroll type, and deductions on file and automatically calculates the employee's net earnings, generates a paycheck, and prints a pay stub with the appropriate information.

To create an employee earnings record, select this option and follow the prompts for the needed information. Depending on the software used, each employee's earnings record may be updated automatically every time you generate a paycheck or make changes to other payroll files.

Calculating and Filing Taxes

In many practices, medical assistants set up tax liability accounts for money withheld from paychecks. These accounts are used to submit this money to appropriate agencies.

Setting Up Tax Liability Accounts

You must set up at least two bank accounts to hold the money deducted from paychecks until it can be sent to the appropriate government agencies. One account will hold deductions from employees' paychecks for federal, state, and local income taxes and FICA taxes. Another account will hold employer payments based on payroll, such as federal and state unemployment taxes. For these accounts, choose a bank that is authorized by the IRS to accept federal tax deposits. If the practice makes other paycheck deductions, as for workers' compensation or a 401(k) plan, set up an account for each of these also.

Each time you prepare paychecks, deposit the withheld money into the proper account. Then, record the deposited amounts as debits in the practice's checking account.

Understanding Federal Tax Deposit Schedules

You will probably deposit federal income taxes and FICA taxes (which together are known as employment taxes) on a quarterly, monthly, or biweekly (every-other-week) schedule. Every November IRS personnel decide which deposit schedule your office should use for the next year.

If the IRS does not notify you about this matter, determine your deposit schedule based on the total employment taxes your office reported on the previous year's Employer's Quarterly Federal Tax Returns (Form 941). For example, if your office reported $50,000 or less in employment taxes during the past year, you would make monthly employment tax deposits the present year. If your office reported more than $50,000 during the past year, you would make semimonthly tax deposits.

There are exceptions to the monthly or semimonthly tax deposit schedules: the $500 rule and the $100,000 rule. The $500 rule applies to employers who owe less than $500 in employment taxes during a tax period (such as a quarter). These employers do not have to make a deposit for that period. The $100,000 rule applies to employers who owe $100,000 or more in employment taxes on any one day during a tax period. These employers must deposit the tax by the next banking day after the day that ceiling is reached.

Submitting Federal Income Taxes and FICA Taxes

Some businesses must submit federal income taxes and FICA taxes to the IRS by electronic funds transfer (EFT). The EFT program, known as TAXLINK, began in 1995. Since then, more taxpayers have been required to use it each year. If your practice is not required to use EFT but wishes to do so voluntarily, contact the IRS, Cash Management Site Office, to enroll.

If your practice does not use EFT, you must submit these employment taxes with a Federal Tax Deposit (FTD) Coupon (Form 8109) (see Figure 18-15). FTD Coupons are supplied by the IRS. They are printed with the physician's name, address, and EIN. They have boxes for filling in the type of tax and the tax period for which the deposit is being made.

To make the deposit, write a single check or money order for the total amount of federal income taxes and FICA taxes withheld during the tax period. Make the check payable to the bank where you make the deposit. This must be a Federal Reserve Bank or another bank authorized to make payments to the IRS. Also, complete the FTD Coupon. Then, mail or deliver the check and FTD Coupon to the bank. The bank will give you a deposit receipt.

If you work in a practice with a large payroll, you may need to make deposits every few days. In most practices, however, you will probably make deposits once a month. Then, every 3 months, a more complete accounting is required on a **quarterly return,** called the Employer's Quarterly Federal Tax Return (Form 941).

Submitting FUTA Taxes

FUTA taxes provide money to workers who are unemployed. If the practice owes more than $100 in federal unemployment tax at the end of the quarter, deposit the tax amount with an FTD Coupon (Form 8109). At the end of the year, file an Employer's Annual Federal Unemployment (FUTA) Tax Return (Form 940) with any final taxes owed (Figure 18-16).

Generally, an employer must pay FUTA taxes if employees' wages total more than $1500 in any quarter (3-month period) and if those employees are not seasonal

AMOUNT OF DEPOSIT (Do NOT type, please print.)

DOLLARS | CENTS

MONTH TAX YEAR ENDS →

EMPLOYER IDENTIFICATION NUMBER →

BANK NAME/ DATE STAMP

Name

Address

City

State ZIP

Telephone number ( )

IRS USE ONLY

Darken only one TYPE OF TAX		and	Darken only one TAX PERIOD
941	945		1st Quarter
990-C	1120		2nd Quarter
943	990-T		3rd Quarter
720	990-PF		4th Quarter
CT-1	1042		
940			

35

FOR BANK USE IN MICR ENCODING

Federal Tax Deposit Coupon

Form 8109-B (Rev. 12-2002)

Figure 18-15. Practices that do not use TAXLINK to submit taxes electronically must submit federal income and FICA taxes with a Federal Tax Deposit (FTD) Coupon (Form 8109).

or household workers. The FUTA tax, which is 6.2%, is applied to the first $7000 of income for a year.

Filing an Employer's Quarterly Federal Tax Return

Each quarter, file an Employer's Quarterly Federal Tax Return (Form 941) with the IRS (Figure 18-17). This tax return summarizes the federal income and FICA taxes (employment taxes) withheld from employees' paychecks.

As a general rule, you should file Form 941 at the nearest IRS office by the last day of the first month after the quarter ends. If the practice has deposited all taxes on time, you have an additional 10 days after the due date to file.

Handling State and Local Income Taxes

Send withheld state and local income taxes to the proper agencies, using their forms, procedures, and schedules. If required, prepare quarterly or other tax forms for the state and local governments.

Filing Wage and Tax Statements

After the end of each year, file a Wage and Tax Statement (Form W-2) with the appropriate federal, state, and local government agencies for each employee who had federal income and FICA taxes withheld during the previous year (Figure 18-18). Also, supply copies of Form W-2 to each employee.

Form W-2 shows the employee's total taxable income for the previous year. It also shows the exact amount of federal income taxes and FICA taxes (for Social Security and Medicare) withheld, along with the amounts of state and local taxes withheld (if any).

Along with the W-2 forms, submit Form W-3, a Transmittal of Wage and Tax Statements (Figure 18-19). This form lists the employer's name, address, and EIN and summarizes the amount of all employees' earnings and the federal income taxes and FICA taxes withheld.

Managing Contracts

An **employment contract**—a written agreement of employment terms between employer and employee—may be considered a benefit because it increases employee job security. It also allows the employer to attract and keep the best employees. Although contracts are rarely offered to medical assistants, you should be aware of them because they may be used for doctors and executive management of a practice and because they may be used for medical assistants in the future.

Legal Elements of a Contract

An employment contract is a legal agreement between two or more people to perform an act in exchange for payment. To be binding, the contract must include these main elements:

- An agreement between two or more competent people to do something legal

Form 940

Department of the Treasury
Internal Revenue Service (99)

Employer's Annual Federal Unemployment (FUTA) Tax Return

► See separate Instructions for Form 940 for information on completing this form.

OMB No. 1545-0028

2003

T	
FF	
FD	
FP	
I	
T	

You must complete this section. ▶

Name (as distinguished from trade name)   Calendar year

Trade name, if any   Employer identification number (EIN)

Address (number and street)   City, state, and ZIP code

A Are you required to pay unemployment contributions to only one state? (If "No," skip questions B and C.) ☐ Yes ☐ No

B Did you pay all state unemployment contributions by February 2, 2004? ((1) If you deposited your total FUTA tax when due, check "Yes" if you paid all state unemployment contributions by February 10, 2004. (2) If a 0% experience rate is granted, check "Yes." (3) If "No," skip question C.) . . . . ☐ Yes ☐ No

C Were all wages that were taxable for FUTA tax also taxable for your state's unemployment tax? . . . . . . ☐ Yes ☐ No

If you answered "No" to any of these questions, you must file Form 940. If you answered "Yes" to all the questions, you may file Form 940-EZ, which is a simplified version of Form 940. (Successor employers, see **Special credit for successor employers** on page 3 of the separate instructions.) You can get Form 940-EZ by calling 1-800-TAX-FORM (1-800-829-3676) or from the IRS website at **www.irs.gov.**

If you will not have to file returns in the future, check here (see **Who Must File** in the separate instructions) and complete and sign the return . . . . ▶ ☐

If this is an Amended Return, check here (see **Amended Returns** in the separate instructions) . . . . . . ▶ ☐

Part I	**Computation of Taxable Wages**

1 Total payments (including payments shown on lines 2 and 3) during the calendar year for services of employees **1**

2 Exempt payments. (Explain all exempt payments, attaching additional sheets if necessary.) ▶ --

---   **2**

3 Payments of more than $7,000 for services. Enter only amounts over the first $7,000 paid to each employee (see separate instructions). Do not include any exempt payments from line 2. The $7,000 amount is the Federal wage base. Your state wage base may be different. **Do not use your state wage limitation** **3**

4 Add lines 2 and 3 . . . . **4**

5 **Total taxable wages** (subtract line 4 from line 1) . . . . ▶ **5**

Be sure to complete both sides of this form, and sign in the space provided on the back.

For Privacy Act and Paperwork Reduction Act Notice, see separate instructions.   ▼ **DETACH HERE** ▼   Cat. No. 11234O   Form **940** (2003)

Form 940-V

Department of the Treasury
Internal Revenue Service

Payment Voucher

Use this voucher only when making a payment with your return.

OMB No. 1545-0028

2003

Complete boxes 1, 2, and 3. Do not send cash, and do not staple your payment to this voucher. Make your check or money order payable to the "United States Treasury." Be sure to enter your employer identification number (EIN), "Form 940," and "2003" on your payment.

1 Enter your employer identification number (EIN).	**2** **Enter the amount of your payment.** ▶	Dollars	Cents

3 Enter your business name (individual name for sole proprietors).

Enter your address.

Enter your city, state, and ZIP code.

Figure 18-16. Tax dollars filed with FUTA tax returns (Form 940) provide money to workers who are unemployed.

Form 941
(Rev. January 2004)
Department of the Treasury
Internal Revenue Service (99)

Employer's Quarterly Federal Tax Return
▶ See separate instructions revised January 2004 for information on completing this return.
Please type or print.

OMB No. 1545-0029

Enter state code for state in which deposits were made **only** if different from state in address to the right ▶ (see page 2 of separate instructions).

Name (as distinguished from trade name)

Trade name, if any

Address (number and street)

Date quarter ended

Employer identification number

City, state, and ZIP code

T	
FF	
FD	
FP	
I	
T	

If address is different from prior return, check here ▶

IRS Use

```
1 1 1 1 1 1 1 1 1 1        2      3 3 3 3 3 3 3 3      4 4 4      5 5 5

6    7    8 8 8 8 8 8 8 8    9 9 9 9    10 10 10 10 10 10 10 10 10 10
```

A If you **do not have to file** returns in the future, check here ▶ ☐ and enter date final wages paid ▶

B If you are a seasonal employer, see **Seasonal employers** on page 1 of the instructions and check here ▶ ☐

1	Number of employees in the pay period that includes March 12th . ▶	1		
2	Total wages and tips, plus other compensation (see separate instructions)	**2**	
3	Total income tax withheld from wages, tips, and sick pay	**3**	
4	Adjustment of withheld income tax for preceding quarters of **this calendar year**	**4**	
5	Adjusted total of income tax withheld (line 3 as adjusted by line 4)	**5**	

6	Taxable social security wages	6a		× 12.4% (.124) =	**6b**	
	Taxable social security tips	6c		× 12.4% (.124) =	**6d**	
7	Taxable Medicare wages and tips . . .	7a		× 2.9% (.029) =	**7b**	

8	Total social security and Medicare taxes (add lines 6b, 6d, and 7b). **Check here if wages are not subject to social security and/or Medicare tax** . . . . ▶ ☐	**8**	
9	Adjustment of social security and Medicare taxes (see instructions for required explanation) Sick Pay $ _____ ± Fractions of Cents $ _____ ± Other $ _____ =	**9**	
10	Adjusted total of social security and Medicare taxes (line 8 as adjusted by line 9)	**10**	
11	**Total taxes** (add lines 5 and 10)	**11**	
12	Advance earned income credit (EIC) payments made to employees (see instructions) . . .	**12**	
13	Net taxes (subtract line 12 from line 11). **If $2,500 or more, this must equal line 17, column (d) below (or line D of Schedule B (Form 941))**	**13**	
14	Total deposits for quarter, including overpayment applied from a prior quarter	**14**	
15	**Balance due** (subtract line 14 from line 13). See instructions	**15**	
16	**Overpayment.** If line 14 is more than line 13, enter excess here ▶ $ _____		

and check if to be: ☐ Applied to next return **or** ☐ Refunded.

- **All filers:** If line 13 is less than $2,500, **do not** complete line 17 or Schedule B (Form 941).
- **Semiweekly schedule depositors:** Complete Schedule B (Form 941) and check here . . . . ▶ ☐
- **Monthly schedule depositors:** Complete line 17, columns (a) through (d), and check here . . . . ▶ ☐

17	**Monthly Summary of Federal Tax Liability.** (Complete **Schedule B (Form 941)** instead, if you were a semiweekly schedule depositor.)			
	(a) First month liability	**(b)** Second month liability	**(c)** Third month liability	**(d)** Total liability for quarter

Third Party Designee

Do you want to allow another person to discuss this return with the IRS (see separate instructions)? ☐ **Yes.** Complete the following. ☐ **No**

Designee's name ▶

Phone no. ▶ ( )

Personal identification number (PIN) ▶ ☐☐☐☐☐

Sign Here

Under penalties of perjury, I declare that I have examined this return, including accompanying schedules and statements, and to the best of my knowledge and belief, it is true, correct, and complete.

Signature ▶

Print Your Name and Title ▶

Date ▶

For Privacy Act and Paperwork Reduction Act Notice, see back of Payment Voucher.

Cat. No. 17001Z

Form **941** (Rev. 1-2004)

Figure 18-17. Most practices make tax deposits monthly and then make a more complete accounting once every 3 months on the Employer's Quarterly Federal Tax Return (Form 941), the first page of which is shown here.

a Control number	22222	Void ☐	For Official Use Only ▶ OMB No. 1545-0008		

b Employer identification number		1 Wages, tips, other compensation	2 Federal income tax withheld
c Employer's name, address, and ZIP code		3 Social security wages	4 Social security tax withheld
		5 Medicare wages and tips	6 Medicare tax withheld
		7 Social security tips	8 Allocated tips
d Employee's social security number		9 Advance EIC payment	10 Dependent care benefits
e Employee's first name and initial — Last name		11 Nonqualified plans	12a See instructions for box 12
		13 Statutory employee ☐ Retirement plan ☐ Third-party sick pay ☐	12b
		14 Other	12c
			12d
f Employee's address and ZIP code			

15 State Employer's state ID number	16 State wages, tips, etc.	17 State income tax	18 Local wages, tips, etc.	19 Local income tax	20 Locality name

Form **W-2** **Wage and Tax Statement** **2004** Department of the Treasury—Internal Revenue Service

For Privacy Act and Paperwork Reduction Act Notice, see back of Copy D.

Copy A For Social Security Administration — Send this entire page with Form W-3 to the Social Security Administration; photocopies are **not** acceptable.

Cat. No. 10134D

Figure 18-18. A Wage and Tax Statement (Form W-2) records the total amount of taxes withheld during the previous year for each employee.

- Names and addresses of the people involved
- Consideration (whatever is given in exchange, such as money, work, or property)
- Starting and ending dates, as well as date(s) the contract was signed
- Signatures of the employer and employee

A Medical Assistant Contract

Some medical practices use employment contracts for medical assistants. This type of contract would include these elements:

- A description of your duties and your employer's duties
- Plans for handling major changes in job responsibilities
- Salary, bonuses, and other forms of compensation
- Benefits, such as vacation time, sick days, life insurance, and participation in pension plans
- Grievance procedures
- Exceptional situations under which the contract may be terminated by either you or your employer
- Termination procedures and compensation
- Special provisions, such as job sharing, medical examinations, or liability coverage

If you are offered an employment contract, study it closely. Consider any local laws that may apply, and have a lawyer or business adviser review the contract.

Summary

The administrative and accounting duties of the medical assistant may involve several aspects of financial control through the proper understanding and management of accounts receivable and accounts payable. The use of standard bookkeeping and banking procedures is necessary in order to maintain the business of the office in proper form. The tasks involved may include the following:

- Using daily logs of charges and receipts for patient accounts
- Depositing cash and checks in bank accounts
- Summarizing patient charges and receipts
- Reconciling bank accounts to the practice records
- Disbursing funds for petty cash and office purchases
- Managing payroll for employees
- Preparing tax forms for payroll processing
- Assisting with contracts of the practice

DO NOT STAPLE OR FOLD

a Control number	33333	For Official Use Only ▶ OMB No. 1545-0008		

b Kind of Payer	☐ 941 ☐ CT-1 ☐ Military ☐ Hshld. emp. ☐ 943 ☐ Medicare govt. emp. ☐ Third-party sick pay	1 Wages, tips, other compensation	2 Federal income tax withheld

		3 Social security wages	4 Social security tax withheld
c Total number of Forms W-2	d Establishment number	5 Medicare wages and tips	6 Medicare tax withheld
e Employer identification number		7 Social security tips	8 Allocated tips
f Employer's name		9 Advance EIC payments	10 Dependent care benefits
		11 Nonqualified plans	12 Deferred compensation
		13 For third-party sick pay use only	
		14 Income tax withheld by payer of third-party sick pay	
g Employer's address and ZIP code			
h Other EIN used this year			

15 State Employer's state ID number	16 State wages, tips, etc.	17 State income tax
	18 Local wages, tips, etc.	19 Local income tax

Contact person	Telephone number ( )	For Official Use Only
Email address	Fax number ( )	

Under penalties of perjury, I declare that I have examined this return and accompanying documents, and, to the best of my knowledge and belief, they are true, correct, and complete.

Signature ▶   Title ▶   Date ▶

Form **W-3** Transmittal of Wage and Tax Statements   **2004**   Department of the Treasury
Internal Revenue Service

Send this entire page with the entire Copy A page of Form(s) W-2 to the Social Security Administration. Photocopies are not acceptable.

Do not send any payment (cash, checks, money orders, etc.) with Forms W-2 and W-3.

An Item To Note

Separate instructions. See the **2004 Instructions for Forms W-2 and W-3** for information on completing this form.

Purpose of Form

Use this form to transmit Copy A of **Form(s) W-2,** Wage and Tax Statement. Make a copy of Form W-3, and keep it with Copy D (For Employer) of Form(s) W-2 for your records. Use Form W-3 for the correct year. **File Form W-3 even if only one Form W-2 is being filed.** If you are filing Form(s) W-2 on magnetic media or electronically, **do not** file Form W-3.

When To File

File Form W-3 with Copy A of Form(s) W-2 by February 28, 2005.

Where To File

Send this entire page with the entire Copy A page of Form(s) W-2 to:

**Social Security Administration
Data Operations Center
Wilkes-Barre, PA 18769-0001**

Note: *If you use "Certified Mail" to file, change the ZIP code to "18769-0002." If you use an IRS-approved private delivery service, add "ATTN: W-2 Process, 1150 E. Mountain Dr." to the address and change the ZIP code to "18702-7997." See* **Circular E (Pub. 15),** *Employer's Tax Guide, for a list of IRS approved private delivery services.*

Do **not** send magnetic media to the address shown above.

For Privacy Act and Paperwork Reduction Act Notice, see back of Copy D of Form W-2.

Figure 18-19. Submit a Transmittal of Wage and Tax Statements (Form W-3) with the W-2 forms.

REVIEW

CHAPTER 18

CASE STUDY QUESTIONS

Now that you have completed this chapter, review the case study at the beginning of the chapter and answer the following question:

1. What should Ben do to properly record the payment?

Discussion Questions

1. Name three things that are required in a single-entry accounting system.
2. What are the three terms that are used in the double-entry accounting system?
3. Why is the reconciliation of the bank statement so important?
4. Why is a petty cash fund useful?
5. When creating a payroll information sheet, name what it should contain.

Critical Thinking Questions

1. Why is it important for an employer to have an Employer Identification Number?
2. Discuss the importance of having separate accounts for employee deductions.

3. Name some of the banking tasks of the medical practice.
4. Name some of the requirements of the Fair Labor Standards Act.

Application Activities

1. Record the following disbursements made on September 9, 2004, in a disbursements journal:
   - Check no. 1234, payee—Tom Jones (electrician), check amount—$125
   - Check no. 1235, payee—Postmaster (postage), check amount—$32
   - Check no. 1236, payee—Gateway Property Management (rent), check amount—$900
2. Simulate an office petty cash account, using your own personal expenses. Determine a starting amount, and use it for 2 weeks to buy small items. For each purchase, obtain a receipt, or write a petty cash voucher. Record each withdrawal you make from the petty cash account, using a petty cash record. At least once during the 2-week period, write a check to replenish the account.
3. Prepare your personal federal income tax return, using information from the Wage and Tax Statement (Form W-2) and the Employee's Withholding Allowance Certificate (Form W-4) provided by your employer.

APPENDIX I
Medical Assistant Role Delineation Chart

Administrative

Administrative Procedures

- Perform basic administrative medical assisting functions
- Schedule, coordinate, and monitor appointments
- Schedule inpatient/outpatient admissions and procedures
- Understand and apply third-party guidelines
- Obtain reimbursement through accurate claims submission
- Monitor third-party reimbursement
- Understand and adhere to managed care policies and procedures
- *Negotiate managed care contracts*

Practice Finances

- Perform procedural and diagnostic coding
- Apply bookkeeping principles
- Manage accounts receivable
- *Manage accounts payable*
- *Process payroll*
- *Document and maintain accounting and banking records*
- *Develop and maintain fee schedules*
- *Manage renewals of business and professional insurance policies*
- *Manage personnel benefits and maintain records*
- *Perform marketing, financial, and strategic planning*

Clinical

Fundamental Principles

- Apply principles of aseptic technique and infection control
- Comply with quality assurance practices
- Screen and follow up patient test results

Diagnostic Orders

- Collect and process specimens
- Perform diagnostic tests

Patient Care

- Adhere to established patient screening procedures
- Obtain patient history and vital signs
- Prepare and maintain examination and treatment areas
- Prepare patient for examinations, procedures, and treatments
- Assist with examinations, procedures, and treatments
- Prepare and administer medications and immunizations
- Maintain medication and immunization records
- Recognize and respond to emergencies
- Coordinate patient care information with other health-care providers
- Initiate IV and administer IV medications with appropriate training and as permitted by state law

General

Professionalism

- Display a professional manner and image
- Demonstrate initiative and responsibility
- Work as a member of the health-care team
- Prioritize and perform multiple tasks
- Adapt to change
- Promote the CMA credential
- Enhance skills through continuing education
- Treat all patients with compassion and empathy
- Promote the practice through positive public relations

Communication Skills

- Recognize and respect cultural diversity
- Adapt communications to individual's ability to understand
- Use professional telephone technique
- Recognize and respond effectively to verbal, nonverbal, and written communications
- Use medical terminology appropriately
- Utilize electronic technology to receive, organize, prioritize, and transmit information
- Serve as liaison

Legal Concepts

- Perform within legal and ethical boundaries
- Prepare and maintain medical records
- Document accurately

- Follow employer's established policies dealing with the health-care contract
- Implement and maintain federal and state health-care legislation and regulations
- Comply with established risk management and safety procedures
- Recognize professional credentialing criteria
- *Develop and maintain personnel, policy, and procedure manuals*

Instruction

- Instruct individuals according to their needs
- Explain office policies and procedures
- Teach methods of health promotion and disease prevention
- Locate community resources and disseminate information
- *Develop educational materials*
- *Conduct continuing education activities*

Operational Functions

- Perform inventory of supplies and equipment
- Perform routine maintenance of administrative and clinical equipment
- Apply computer techniques to support office operations
- *Perform personnel management functions*
- *Negotiate leases and prices for equipment and supply contracts*

* Denotes advanced skills

Source: This chart is part of the "AAMA Role Delineation Study: Occupational Analysis of the Medical Assisting Profession," released by the American Association of Medical Assistants in June 2003.

APPENDIX II
Prefixes and Suffixes Commonly Used in Medical Terms

a-, an- without, not
ab- from, away
ad-, -ad to, toward
adeno- gland, glandular
aero- air
-aesthesia sensation
-al characterized by
-algia pain
ambi-, amph-, amphi- both, on both sides, around
andr-, andro- man, male
angio- blood vessel
ano- anus
ante- before
antero- in front of
anti- against, opposing
arterio- artery
arthro- joint
-ase enzyme
-asthenia weakness
auto- self
bi- twice, double
bili- bile
bio- life
blasto-, -blast developing stage, bud
brachy- short
brady- slow
broncho- bronchial (windpipe)
cardio- heart
cata- down, lower, under
-cele swelling, tumor
-centesis puncture, tapping
centi- hundred
cephal-, cephalo- head
cerebr-, cerebro- brain
chol-, chole-, cholo- gall
chondro- cartilage
chromo- color
-cidal killing
-cide causing death
circum- around
-cise cut
co-, com-, con- together, with
-coele cavity
colo- colon
colp-, colpo- vagina
contra- against
cost-, costo- rib
crani-, cranio- skull
cryo- cold
cysto-, -cyst bladder, bag
-cyte, cyto- cell, cellular

dacry-, dacryo- tears, lacrimal apparatus
dactyl-, dactylo- finger, toe
de- down, from
deca- ten
deci- tenth
demi- half
dent-, denti-, dento- teeth
derma-, dermat-, dermato-, -derm skin
dextro- to the right
di- double, twice
dia- through, apart, between
dipla-, diplo- double, twin
dis- apart, away from
dorsi-, dorso- back
dynia- pain
dys- difficult, painful, bad, abnormal
e-, ec-, ecto- away, from, without, outside
-ectomy cutting out, surgical removal
em-, en- in, into, inside
-emesis vomiting
-emia blood
encephalo- brain
endo- within, inside
entero- intestine
ento- within, inner
epi- on, above
erythro- red
esthesio-, -esthesia sensation
eu- good, true, normal
ex-, exo- outside of, beyond, without
extra- outside of, beyond, in addition
fibro- connective tissue
fore- before, in front of
-form shape
-fuge driving away
galact-, galacto- milk
gastr-, gastro- stomach
-gene, -genic, -genetic, -genous arising from, origin, formation
glosso- tongue
gluco-, glyco- sugar, sweet
-gram recorded information
-graph instrument for recording
-graphy the process of recording
-gravida pregnant female
gyn-, gyno-, gyne-, gyneco- woman, female
haemo-, hemato-, hem-, hemo- blood
hemi- half
hepa-, hepar-, hepato- liver

herni- rupture
hetero- other, unlike
histo- tissue
homeo, homo- same, like
hydra-, hydro- water
hyper- above, over, increased, excessive
hypo- below, under, decreased
hyster-, hystero- uterus
-ia condition
-iasis condition of
-ic, -ical pertaining to
ictero- jaundice
idio- personal, self-produced
ileo- ileum
im-, in-, ir- not
in- in, into
infra- beneath
inter- between, among
intra-, intro- into, within, during
-ism condition, process, theory
-itis inflammation of
-ium membrane
-ize to cause to be, to become, to treat by special method
juxta- near, nearby
karyo- nucleus, nut
kata-, kath- down, lower, under
kera-, kerato- horn, hardness, cornea
kineto-, -kinesis, -kinetic motion
lact- milk
laparo- abdomen
latero- side
-lepsis, -lepsy seizure, convulsion
leuco-, leuko- white
levo- to the left
lipo- fat
lith-, -lith stone
-logy science of, study of
-lysis setting free, disintegration, decomposition
macro- large, long
mal- bad
-malacia abnormal softening
-mania insanity, abnormal desire
mast-, masto- breast
med-, medi- middle
mega-, megalo- large, great
meio- contraction
melan-, melano- black
meno- month
mes-, meso- middle
meta- beyond

-meter   measure
metro-, metra-   uterus
-metry   process of measuring
micro-   small
mio-   smaller, less
mono-   single, one
multi-   many
my-, myo-   muscle
myel-, myelo-   marrow
narco-   sleep
nas-, naso-   nose
necro-   dead
neo-   new
nephr-, nephro-   kidney
neu-, neuro-   nerve
niter-, nitro-   nitrogen
non-, not-   no
nucleo-   nucleus
-nuli   none
ob-   against
oculo-   eye
odont-   tooth
-odynia   pain
-oid   resembling
-ole   small, little
olig-, oligo-   few, less than normal
-oma   tumor
onco-   tumor
oo-   ovum, egg
oophor-   ovary
ophthalmo-   eye
-opia   vision
-opsy   to view
orchid-   testicle
ortho-   straight
os-   mouth, bone
-osis   disease, condition of
oste-, osteo-   bone
-ostomy   to make a mouth, opening
oto-   ear
-otomy   incision, surgical cutting
-ous   having
oxy-   sharp, acid
pachy-   thick
paedo, pedo-   child
pan-   all, every

par; para-   alongside of, with; woman who has given birth
path-, patho-, -pathy   disease, suffering
ped-, pedi-, pedo-   foot
-penia   too few, lack, decreased
per-   through, excessive
peri-   around
pes-   foot
-pexy   surgical fixation
phag-, phagia, phago-, -phage   eating, consuming, swallowing
pharyng-   throat, pharynx
phlebo-   vein
-phobia   fear, abnormal fear
-phylaxis   protection
-plasia   formation or development
-plastic   molded
-plasty   operation to reconstruct, surgical repair
-plegia   paralysis
pleuro-   side, rib
pluri-   more, several
pneo-, -pnea   breathing
pneumo-   air, lungs
-pod   foot
poly-   many, much
post-   after, behind
pre-, pro-   before, in front of
presby-, presbyo-   old age
primi-   first
procto-   rectum
proto-   first
pseudo-   false
psych-   the mind
pulmon-, pulmono-   lung
pyelo-   pelvis (renal)
pyo-   pus
pyro-   fever, heat
quadri-   four
re-   back, again
reni-, reno-   kidney
retro-   backward, behind
rhino-   nose
-rrhage, -rrhagia   abnormal or excessive discharge, hemorrhage, flow

-rrhaphy   suture of
-rrhea   flow, discharge
sacchar-   sugar
sacro-   sacrum
salpingo-   tube, fallopian tube
sarco-   flesh
sclero-   hard, sclera
-sclerosis   hardening
-scopy   examining
semi-   half
septi-, septic-, septico-   poison, infection
-spasm   cramp or twitching
-stasis   stoppage
steno-   contracted, narrow
stereo-   firm, solid, three-dimensional
stomato-   mouth
-stomy   opening
sub-   under
super-, supra-   above, upon, excess
sym-, syn-   with, together
tachy-   fast
tele-   distant, far
teno-, tenoto-   tendon
tetra-   four
-therapy   treatment
thermo-, -thermy   heat
thio-   sulfur
thoraco-   chest
thrombo-   blood clot
thyro-   thyroid gland
-tome   cutting instrument
tomo-, -tomy   incision, section
trans-   across
tri-   three
-tripsy   surgical crushing
tropho-, -trophy   nutrition, growth
-tropy   turning, tendency
ultra-   beyond, excess
uni-   one
-uria   urine
urino-, uro-   urine, urinary organs
utero-   uterus, uterine
vaso-   vessel
ventri-, ventro-   abdomen
xanth-   yellow

APPENDIX III

Latin and Greek Equivalents Commonly Used in Medical Terms

abdomen venter
adhesion adhaesio
and et
arm brachium; brachion (Gr*)
artery arteria
back dorsum
backbone spina
backward retro; opistho (Gr)
bend flexus
bile bilis; chole (Gr)
bladder vesica, cystus
blister vesicula
blood sanguis; haima (Gr)
body corpus; soma (Gr)
bone os, ossis; osteon (Gr)
brain encephalon
break ruptura
breast mamma; mastos (Gr)
buttock gloutos (Gr)
cartilage cartilago; chondros (Gr)
cavity cavum
chest pectoris, pectus; thorax (Gr)
child puer, puerilis
choke strangulo
corn clavus
cornea kerat (Gr)
cough tussis
deadly lethalis
death mors
dental dentalis
digestive pepticos
disease morbus
dislocation luxatio
doctor medicus
dose dosis (Gr)
ear auris; ous (Gr)
egg ovum
erotic erotikos (Gr)
exhalation exhalatio, expiro
external externus
extract extractum
eye oculus; ophthalmos (Gr)
eyelid palpebra
face facies
fat adeps; lipos (Gr)
female femella
fever febris
finger (or toe) digitus
flesh carnis, caro
foot pes
forehead frons
gum gingiva
hair capillus, pilus; thrix (Gr)

hand manus; cheir (Gr)
harelip labrum fissum; cheiloschisis (Gr)
head caput; kephale (Gr)
health sanitas
hear audire
heart cor; kardia (Gr)
heat calor; therme (Gr)
heel calx, talus
hysterics hysteria
infant infans
infectious contagiosus
injection injectio
intellect intellectus
internal internus
intestine intestinum; enteron (Gr)
itching pruritis
jawbone maxilla
joint vertebra; arthron (Gr)
kidney ren, renis; nephros (Gr)
knee genu
kneecap patella
lacerate lacerare
larynx guttur
lateral lateralis
limb membrum
lip labium, labrum; cheilos (Gr)
listen auscultare
liver jecur; hepar (Gr)
loin lapara
looseness laxativus
lung pulmo; pneumon (Gr)
male masculinus
malignant malignons
milk lac
moisture humiditas
month mensis
monthly menstruus
mouth oris, os; stoma, stomato (Gr)
nail unguis; onyx (Gr)
navel umbilicus; omphalos (Gr)
neck cervix; trachelos (Gr)
nerve nervus; neuron (Gr)
nipple papilla; thele (Gr)
no, none nullus
nose nasus; rhis (Gr)
nostril naris
nourishment alimentum
ointment unguentum
pain dolor; algia
patient patiens
pectoral pectoralis
pimple pustula

poison venenum
powder pulvis
pregnant praegnans, gravida
pubic bone os pubis
pupil pupilla
rash exanthema (Gr)
recover convalescere
redness rubor
rib costa
ringing tinnitus
scaly squamosus
sciatica sciaticus; ischiadikos (Gr)
seed semen
senile senilis
sheath vagina; theke (Gr)
short brevis; brachys (Gr)
shoulder omos (Gr)
shoulder blade scapula
side latus
skin cutis; derma (Gr)
skull cranium; kranion (Gr)
sleep somnus
solution solutio
spinal spinalis
stomach stomachus; gaster (Gr)
stone calculus
sugar saccharum
swallow glutio
tail cauda
taste gustatio
tear lacrima
testicle testis; orchis (Gr)
thigh femur
throat fauces; pharynx (Gr)
tongue lingua; glossa (Gr)
tooth dens; odontos (Gr)
touch tactus
tremor tremere
twin gemellus
ulcer ulcus
urine urina; ouran (Gr)
uterus hystera (Gr)
vagina vagina; kolpos (Gr)
vein vena; phlebos, phleps (Gr)
vertebra spondylos (Gr)
vessel vas
wash diluere
water aqua
wax cera
weak debilis
windpipe arteria aspera
wrist carpus; karpos (Gr)

* Parenthetical "Gr" means the preceding term is Greek. Other terms in the column are Latin.

APPENDIX IV
Abbreviations Commonly Used in Medical Notations

a before
a.c. before meals
AD right ear
ADD attention deficit disorder
ADL activities of daily living
ad lib as desired
ADT admission, discharge, transfer
AIDS acquired immunodeficiency syndrome
a.m.a. against medical advice
AMA American Medical Association
amp. ampule
amt amount
aq., AQ water; aqueous
AS left ear
ausc. auscultation
AU both ears
ax axis
Bib, bib drink
b.i.d., bid, BID twice a day
BM bowel movement
BP, B/P blood pressure
BPC blood pressure check
BPH benign prostatic hypertrophy
BSA body surface area
c., c̄ with
Ca calcium; cancer
cap, caps capsules
CBC complete blood (cell) count
cc cubic centimeter
C.C., CC chief complaint
CDC Centers for Disease Control and Prevention
CHF congestive heart failure
chr chronic
CNS central nervous system
Comp, comp compound
COPD chronic obstructive pulmonary disease
CP chest pain
CPE complete physical examination
CPR cardiopulmonary resuscitation
CSF cerebrospinal fluid
CT computed tomography
CV cardiovascular
d day
d/c, D/C discontinue, discharge
D & C dilation and curettage
DEA Drug Enforcement Administration
Dil, dil dilute
DM diabetes mellitus
DOB date of birth

DTP diptheria-tetanus-pertussis vaccine
Dr. doctor
DTs delirium tremens
D/W dextrose in water
Dx, dx diagnosis
ECG, EKG electrocardiogram
ED emergency department
EEG electroencephalogram
EENT eyes, ears, nose, and throat
EP established patient
ER emergency room
ESR erythrocyte sedimentation rate
FBS fasting blood sugar
FDA Food and Drug Administration
FH family history
Fl, fl, fld fluid
F/u follow-up
Fx fracture
GBS gallbladder series
GI gastrointestinal
Gm gram
gr grain
gt, gtt drops
GTT glucose tolerance test
GU genitourinary
GYN gynecology
HB, Hgb hemoglobin
HEENT head, ears, eyes, nose, throat
HIV human immunodeficiency virus
HO history of
h.s., hs, HS hour of sleep/at bedtime
Hx history
ICU intensive care unit
I & D incision and drainage
I & O intake and output
IM intramuscular
inf. infusion; inferior
inj injection
IT inhalation therapy
IUD intrauterine device
IV intravenous
KUB kidneys, ureters, bladder
L1, L2, etc. lumbar vertebrae
lab laboratory
liq liquid
LLL left lower lobe
LLQ left lower quadrant
LMP last menstrual period
LUQ left upper quadrant
MI myocardial infarction
MM mucous membrane
MRI magnetic resonance imaging

MS multiple sclerosis
NB newborn
NED no evidence of disease
no. number
noc, noct night
npo, NPO nothing by mouth
NPT new patient
NS normal saline
NSAID nonsteroidal anti-inflammatory drug
NTP normal temperature and pressure
N & V nausea and vomiting
NYD not yet diagnosed
OB obstetrics
OC oral contraceptive
o.d. once a day
OD overdose
O.D., OD right eye
oint ointment
OOB out of bed
OPD outpatient department
OPS outpatient services
OR operating room
O.S., OS left eye
OTC over-the-counter
O.U., OU both eyes
P & P Pap smear (Papanicolaou smear) and pelvic examination
PA posteroanterior
Pap Pap smear
Path pathology
p.c., pc after meals
PE physical examination
per by, with
PH past history
PID pelvic inflammatory disease
p/o postoperative
POMR problem-oriented medical record
PMFSH past medical, family, social history
PMS premenstrual syndrome
p.r.n., prn, PRN whenever necessary
Pt patient
PT physical therapy
PTA prior to admission
PVC premature ventricular contraction
pulv powder
q. every
q2, q2h every 2 hours
q.a.m., qam every morning

q.d., qd every day

q.h., qh every hour

qhs every night, at bedtime

q.i.d., QID four times a day

qns, QNS quantity not sufficient

qod every other day

qs, QS quantity sufficient

RA rheumatoid arthritis; right atrium

RBC red blood cells; red blood (cell) count

RDA recommended dietary allowance, recommended daily allowance

REM rapid eye movement

RF rheumatoid factor

RLL right lower lobe

RLQ right lower quadrant

R/O rule out

ROM range of motion

ROS/SR review of systems/systems review

RUQ right upper quadrant

RV right ventricle

Rx prescription, take

SAD seasonal affective disorder

s.c., SC, SQ, subq, SubQ subcutaneously

SIDS sudden infant death syndrome

Sig directions

sig sigmoidoscopy

SOAP subjective, objective, assessment, plan

SOB shortness of breath

sol solution

S/R suture removal

ss, s̄s̄ one-half

Staph staphylococcus

stat, STAT immediately

STD sexually transmitted disease

Strep streptococcus

subling, SL sublingual

surg surgery

S/W saline in water

SX symptoms

T1, T2, etc. thoracic vertebrae

T & A tonsillectomy and adenoidectomy

tab tablet

TB tuberculosis

TBS, tbs. tablespoon

TIA transient ischemic attack

t.i.d., tid, TID three times a day

tinc, tinct, tr tincture

TMJ temporomandibular joint

top topically

TPR temperature, pulse, and respiration

tsp teaspoon

TSH thyroid stimulating hormone

Tx treatment

U unit

UA urinalysis

UCHD usual childhood diseases

UGI upper gastrointestinal

ung, ungt ointment

URI upper respiratory infection

US ultrasound

UTI urinary tract infection

VA visual acuity

VD venereal disease

Vf visual field

VS vital signs

WBC white blood cells; white blood (cell) count

WNL within normal limits

wt weight

y/o year old

APPENDIX V
Symbols Commonly Used in Medical Notations

Apothecaries' Weights and Measures

℞ minim
℈ scruple
ʒ dram
fʒ fluidram
℥ ounce
f℥ fluidounce
O pint
℔ pound

Other Weights and Measures

\# pounds
° degrees
′ foot; minute
″ inch; second
μm micrometer
μ micron (former term for micrometer)
mμ millimicron; nanometer
μg microgram
mEq milliequivalent
mL milliliter
dL deciliter
mg% milligrams percent; milligrams per 100 mL

Abbreviations

a̅a̅, A̅A̅ of each
c̅ with

M mix (Latin *misce*)
m- meta-
o- ortho-
p- para-
p̅ after
s̅ without
ss, s̅s̅ one-half (Latin *semis*)

Mathematical Functions and Terms

\# number
+ plus; positive; acid reaction
− minus; negative; alkaline reaction
± plus or minus; either positive or negative; indefinite
× multiply; magnification; crossed with, hybrid
÷, / divided by
= equal to
≈ approximately equal to
> greater than; from which is derived
< less than; derived from
≮ not less than
≯ not greater than
≤ equal to or less than
≥ equal to or greater than
≠ not equal to
√ square root
³√ cube root
∞ infinity

: ratio; "is to"
∴ therefore
% percent
π pi (3.14159)—the ratio of circumference of a circle to its diameter

Chemical Notations

Δ change; heat
⇌ reversible reaction
↑ increase
↓ decrease

Warnings

Ⓒ Schedule I controlled substance
Ⓒ Schedule II controlled substance
Ⓒ Schedule III controlled substance
Ⓒ Schedule IV controlled substance
Ⓒ Schedule V controlled substance
☠ poison
☢ radiation
☣ biohazard

Others

℞ prescription; take
□, ♂ male
○, ♀ female
i̇ one
i̇i̇ two
i̇i̇i̇ three

APPENDIX VI
Professional Organizations and Agencies

American Academy of Dental Practice Administrators
1063 Whippoorwill Lane
Palatine, IL 60067
(312) 934-4404

American Academy of Medical Administrators
30555 Southfield Road, Suite 150
Southfield, MI 48076
(313) 540-4310

American Academy of Ophthalmology
655 Beach Street
San Francisco, CA 94109
(415) 561-8500

American Academy of Pediatrics
PO Box 927
Elk Grove, IL 60009-0927
(708) 228-5005

American Association for Medical Transcription
PO Box 576187
Modesto, CA 95355
(209) 527-9620

American Association for Respiratory Care
11030 Ables Lane
Dallas, TX 75229
(214) 243-2272

American Association of Medical Assistants
20 N. Wacker Drive, Suite 1575
Chicago, IL 60606
(312) 899-1500

American Cancer Society
777 Third Avenue
New York, NY 10017
(212) 586-8700

American College of Cardiology
9111 Old Georgetown Road
Bethesda, MD 20814
(301) 897-5400

American College of Physicians
2011 Pennsylvania Avenue, NW
Washington, DC 20006
(202) 261-4500

American Diabetes Association
Two Park Avenue
New York, NY 10016
(212) 683-7444

American Dietetic Association
216 West Jackson Boulevard, Suite 800
Chicago, IL 60606-6995
(800) 366-1655

American Health Information Management Association
(formerly the American Medical Record Association)
233 N. Michigan Avenue, Suite 2150
Chicago, IL 60601-5800
(312) 233-1100

American Heart Association
National Center
7272 Greenville Avenue
Dallas, TX 75231-4596
(800) 242-8721, or call your local center

American Hospital Association
One North Franklin, Suite 2706
Chicago, IL 60606
(312) 422-3000

American Lung Association
1740 Broadway
New York, NY 10019
(212) 315-8700

American Medical Association
Division of Allied Health Education and Accreditation
515 North State Street
Chicago, IL 60610
(312) 464-5000

American Medical Technologists
710 Higgins Road
Park Ridge, IL 60068
(847) 823-5169

American Occupational Therapy Association
4720 Montgomery Lane
PO Box 31220
Bethesda, MD 20824-1220
(301) 948-9626

American Pharmacists Association
2215 Constitution Avenue, NW
Washington, DC 20037-2985
(202) 628-4410

American Physical Therapy Association
1111 North Fairfax Street
Alexandria, VA 22314
(703) 684-2782

American Red Cross
17th and D Streets, NW
Washington, DC 20006
(202) 728-6400, or call your local chapter

American Red Cross
HIV/AIDS Education, Health and Safety Services
8111 Gatehouse Road, 6th Floor
Falls Church, VA 22042
(703) 206-7180

American Society for Cardiovascular Professionals
120 Falcon Drive, Unit 3
Fredericksburg, VA 22408
(540) 891-0079

American Society for Clinical Laboratory Science
7910 Woodmont Avenue, Suite 1301
Bethesda, MD 20814
(301) 657-2768

American Society of Clinical Pathologists
2100 West Harrison Street
Chicago, IL 60612
(312) 738-1336

American Society of Hand Therapists
401 North Michigan Avenue
Chicago, IL 60611
(312) 321-6866

American Society of Phlebotomy Technicians
PO Box 1831
Hickory, NC 28603
(704) 322-1334

American Society of Radiologic Technologists
15000 Central Avenue SE
Albuquerque, NM 87123
(505) 298-4500

The Arthritis Foundation
1314 Spring Street, NW
Atlanta, GA 30309
(404) 872-7100

Association of Surgical Technologists
7108-C South Alton Way
Englewood, CO 80112
(303) 694-9130

Association of Technical Personnel in Ophthalmology
50 Lee Road
Chestnut Hill, MA 02167
(617) 232-4433

Asthma and Allergy Foundation of America
1717 Massachusetts Avenue, Suite 305
Washington, DC 20036
(202) 265-0265

International Society for Clinical Laboratory Technology
818 Olive Street, Suite 918
St. Louis, MO 63101
(314) 241-1445

Joint Commission on Allied Health Personnel in Ophthalmology
2025 Woodlane Drive
St. Paul, MN 55125-2995
(800) 284-3937

Medical Group Management Association
104 Inverness Terrace East
Englewood Cliffs, CA 80112
(313) 799-1111

National Accrediting Agency for Clinical Laboratory Services
8410 West Bryn Mawr Avenue, Suite 670
Chicago, IL 60631
(312) 714-8880

National AIDS Hotline
215 Park Avenue South, Suite 714
New York, NY 10003
(800) 342-AIDS
(800) 344-SIDA (Spanish)

National Association of Medical Staff Services
PO Box 23590
Knoxville, TN 37933-1590
(615) 531-3571

National Cancer Institute
9000 Rockville Pike
Building 31, Room 10A18
Bethesda, MD 20205
(800) 4-CANCER

National Clearinghouse for Alcohol and Drug Information
PO Box 2345
Rockville, MD 20852
(301) 468-2600

National Health Council
1730 Street NW, Suite 500
Washington, DC 20036
(202) 785-3910

National Health Information Center
PO Box 1133
Washington, DC 20013-1133
(800) 336-4797

National Institute of Mental Health
Office of Communications
6001 Executive Boulevard, Room 8184,
MSC 9663
Bethesda, MD 20892-9663
(301) 443-4513

National Institute on Aging
Building 31, Room 5C27
31 Center Drive, MSC 2292
Bethesda, MD 20892
(301) 496-1752

National Kidney Foundation
30 East 33rd Street
New York, NY 10016
(212) 889-2210

National Mental Health Association
2001 N. Beauregard Street, 12th Floor
Alexandria, VA 22311
(703) 684-7722

National Organization for Rare Disorders
100 Route 37, PO Box 8923
New Fairfield, CT 06812
(800) 999-NORD

National Phlebotomy Association
5615 Landover Road
Hyattsville, MD 20784
(301) 386-4200

National Rehabilitation Association
633 South Washington Street
Alexandria, VA 22314
(703) 836-0850

National Society for Histotechnology
4201 Northview Drive, Suite 502
Bowie, MD 20716-1073
(301) 262-6221

President's Council on Physical Fitness and Sports
Department of Health and Human Services
Washington, DC 20001
(202) 272-3421

Society of Diagnostic Medical Sonographers
12770 Coit Road, Suite 508
Dallas, TX 75251
(214) 239-7367

Glossary

Note: (†) Pronunciation from Stedman's Medical Dictionary 26th edition, all others from American Heritage 4th edition, in case you need to consult.

abandonment (ə-băn′dən-mənt) A situation in which a health-care professional stops caring for a patient without arranging for care by an equally qualified substitute. (3*)

ABA number (nŭm′bər) A fraction appearing in the upper right corner of all printed checks that identifies the geographic area and specific bank on which the check is drawn. (18)

accounts payable (ə-kounts′ pā′-ă-bəl) Money owed by a business; the practice's expenses. (17)

accounts receivable (ə-kounts′ rĭ-sē′və-bəl) Income or money owed to a business. (17)

accreditation (ə-krĕd′ĭ-tā′shən) The documentation of official authorization or approval of a program. (1)

active file (ăk′tiv fīl) A file used on a consistent basis. (10)

active listening (ăk′tiv lĭs′əning) Part of two-way communication, such as offering feedback or asking questions; contrast with **passive listening.** (4)

acupuncturist (ăk′yoo-pŭngk′chər-ĭst) A practitioner of acupuncture. The acupuncturist uses hollow needles inserted into the patient's skin to treat pain, discomfort, or systemic imbalances. (2)

advance scheduling (ăd-văns skĕj′ool-ĭng) Booking an appointment several weeks or even months in advance. (12)

age analysis (āj ə-năl′ĭ-sĭs) The process of clarifying and reviewing past due accounts by age from the first date of billing. (17)

agenda (ə-jĕn′də) The list of topics discussed or presented at a meeting, in order of presentation. (12)

agent (ā′-jənt) (legal) A person who acts on a physician's behalf while performing professional tasks; (clinical) an active principle or entity that produces a certain effect, for example, an infectious agent. (3)

aggressive (ə-grĕs′ĭv) Imposing one's position on others or trying to manipulate them. (4)

allergist (ăl′ər-jĭst) A specialist who diagnoses and treats physical reactions to substances including mold, dust, fur, pollen, foods, drugs, and chemicals. (2)

allowed charge (ə-loud′ chärj) The amount that is the most the payer will pay any provider for each procedure or service. (15)

alphabetic filing system (ăl′fə-bĕt′ĭkəl fī′lĭng sĭs′təm) A filing system in which the files are arranged in alphabetic order, with the patient's last name first, followed by the first name and middle initial. (10)

Alphabetic Index (ăl′fə-bĕt′ĭk ĭn′dĕks′) One of two ways diagnoses are listed in the ICD-9-CM. They appear in alphabetic order with their corresponding diagnosis codes. (16)

American Association of Medical Assistants (AAMA)(ə-mĕr′ĭkən ə-sō′sē-ā′shən mĕd′ĭ-kəl ə-sĭs′tənts) The professional organization that certifies medical assistants and works to maintain professional standards in the medical assisting profession. (1)

Americans With Disabilities Act (ADA) (ə-mĕr′ĭ-kəns dĭs′ə-bĭl′ĭ-tēs ăkt) A U.S. civil rights act forbidding discrimination against people because of a physical or mental handicap. (13)

anesthetist (ă-nĕs′thĕ-tist)(†) A specialist who uses medications to cause patients to lose sensation or feeling during surgery. (2)

annotate (ăn′ō-tāt′) To underline or highlight key points of a document or to write reminders, make comments, and suggest actions in the margins. (7)

arbitration (är′bĭ-trā′shən) A process in which opposing sides choose a person or persons outside the court system, often someone with special knowledge in the field, to hear and decide a dispute. (3)

assault (ə-sôlt′) The open threat of bodily harm to another. (3)

assertive (ə-sûrt′tĭv) Being firm and standing up for oneself while showing respect for others. (4)

asset (ăs′ĕt′) An item owned by the practice that has a dollar value, such as the medical practice building, office equipment, or accounts receivable. (18)

assignment of benefits (ə-sīn′mənt bĕn′ə-fĭts) An authorization for an insurance carrier to pay a physician or practice directly. (15)

authorization (ô′thər-ĭ-zā′shən) A form that explains in detail the standards for the use and disclosure of patient information for purposes other than treatment, payment, or health-care operations. (3)

balance billing (băl′əns bĭl′ĭng) Billing a patient for the difference between a higher usual fee and a lower allowed charge. (15)

battery (băt′ə-rē) An action that causes bodily harm to another. (3)

benefits (bĕn′ə-fĭts) Payments for medical services. (15)

birthday rule (bûrth′dā′rool) A rule that states that the insurance policy of a policyholder whose birthday comes first in the year is the primary payer for all dependents. (15)

bioethics (bī-ō-ĕth′ĭks) Principles of right and wrong in issues that arise from medical advances. (3)

body language (bŏd′ē lăng′gwĭj) Nonverbal communication, including facial expressions, eye contact, posture, touch, and attention to personal space. (4)

bookkeeping (book′kē′pĭng) The systematic recording of business transactions. (18)

breach of contract (brēch kŏn′trăkt′) The violation of or failure to live up to a contract's terms. (3)

burnout (′bər-naut) The end result of prolonged periods of stress without relief. Burnout is an energy-depleting condition that can affect one's health and career. It can be common for those who work in health care. (4)

capitation (kăp′ĭ-tā′shən) A payment structure in which a health maintenance organization prepays an annual set fee per patient to a physician. (15)

cardiologist (kär′dē-ŏl′ə-jĭst) A specialist who diagnoses and treats diseases of the heart and blood vessels (cardiovascular diseases). (2)

* Parenthetical numbers indicate the chapter in which the entry is a key term or is first defined in context. Entries not followed by a chapter number are important terms related to material covered but not specifically defined in the text.

cash flow statement (kăsh flō stā´mənt) A statement that shows the cash on hand at the beginning of a period, the income and disbursements made during the period, and the new amount of cash on hand at the end of the period. (18)

cashier's check (kă-shîrz´ che´k) A bank check issued by a bank on bank paper and signed by a bank representative; usually purchased by individuals who do not have checking accounts. (18)

CD-ROM (sē´dē´rŏm´) A compact disc that contains software programs; an abbreviation for "compact disc—read-only memory." (6)

Centers for Medicare and Medicaid Services (CMS) (sĕn´tərs mĕd´ĭ-kâr´ mĕd´ĭ-kăd´ sûr´vĭs-əz) A congressional agency designed to handle Medicare and Medicaid insurance claims. It was formerly known as the Health Care Financing Administration. (15)

central processing unit (CPU) (sĕn´trəl prŏs´es´ĭng yoo´nĭt) A microprocessor, the primary computer chip responsible for interpreting and executing programs. (6)

certified check (sûr´tə-fīd´ chĕk) A payer's check written and signed by the payer, which is stamped "certified" by the bank. The bank has already drawn money from the payer's account to guarantee that the check will be paid. (18)

Certified Medical Assistant (CMA) (sûr´tə-fīd´ mĕd´ĭ-kəl ə-sĭs´tənt) A medical assistant whose knowledge about the skills of medical assistants, as summarized by the 2003 AAMA Role Delineation Study areas of competence, has been certified by the Certifying Board of the American Association of Medical Assistants (AAMA). (1)

CHAMPVA (Civilian Health and Medical Program of the Veterans Administration) (sī-vĭl´yən hĕlth mĕd´ĭ-kəl prō´grăm vĕt´ər-enz ăd-mĭn´ĭ-strā´shən) A type of health insurance that covers the expenses of families (dependent spouses and children) of veterans with total, permanent, and service-connected disabilities. It also covers the surviving families of veterans who die in the line of duty or as a result of service-connected disabilities. (15)

charge slip (chärj slĭp) The original record of services performed for a patient and the charges for those services. (18)

check (chĕk) A bank draft or order written by a payer that directs the bank to pay a sum of money on demand to the payee. (18)

chiropractor (kī´rə-prăk´tôr) A physician who uses a system of therapy, including manipulation of the spine, to treat illness or pain. This treatment is done without drugs or surgery. (2)

civil law (sĭv´əl lô) Involves crimes against persons. A person can sue another person, business, or the government. Judgments often require a payment of money. (3)

clarity (klăr´ĭ-tē) Clearness in writing or stating a message. (7)

class action lawsuit (klăs-ăk´shən lô´soot´) A lawsuit in which one or more people sue a company or other legal entity that allegedly wronged all of them in the same way. (17)

clearinghouse (klîr´ĭng-hous´) A group that takes nonstandard medical billing software formats and translates them into the standard EDI formats. (15)

Clinical Laboratory Improvement Amendments (CLIA '88) (klē´ə) A law enacted by Congress in 1988 that placed all laboratory facilities that conduct tests for diagnosing, preventing, or treating human disease or for assessing human health under federal regulations administered by the Health Care Financing Administration (HCFA) and the Centers for Disease Control and Prevention (CDC). (1)

closed file (klōzd fīl) A file for a patient who has died, moved away, or for some other reason no longer consults the office for medical expertise. (10)

closed posture (klōzd pŏs´chər) A position that conveys the feeling of not being totally receptive to what is being said; arms are often rigid or folded across the chest. (4)

cluster scheduling (klŭs´tər skĕj´ool-ĭng) The scheduling of similar appointments together at a certain time of the day or week. (12)

code linkage (kōd lĭng´kĭj) Analysis of the connection between diagnostic and procedural information in order to evaluate the medical necessity of the reported charges. This analysis is performed by insurance company representatives. (16)

coinsurance (kō-ĭn-shoor´əns) A fixed percentage of covered charges paid by the insured person after a deductible has been met. (15)

color family (kŭl´ər făm´ə-lē) A group of colors that share certain characteristics, such as warmth or coolness, allowing them to blend well together. (13)

compactible file (kəm-păkt´-əbəl fīl) Files kept on rolling shelves that slide along permanent tracks in the floor and are stored close together or stacked when not in use. (10)

compliance plan (kəm-plī´əns plăn) A process for finding, correcting, and preventing illegal medical office practices. (16)

conciseness (kən-sīs´nəs) Brevity; the use of no unnecessary words. (7)

conflict (kŏn´flĭkt´) An opposition of opinions or ideas. (4)

consumer education (kən-soo´mər ĕj´ə-ka´shən) The process by which the average person learns to make informed decisions about goods and services, including health care. (14)

contagious (kən-tā´jəs) Having a disease that can easily be transmitted to others. (13)

contaminated (kən-tăm´ə-nāt´ĕd) Soiled or stained, particularly through contact with potentially infectious substances; no longer clean or sterile. (1)

contract (kŏn´trăct´) A voluntary agreement between two parties in which specific promises are made. (3)

conventions (kən-vĕn´shənz) A list of abbreviations, punctuation, symbols, typefaces, and instructional notes appearing in the beginning of the ICD-9. The items provide guidelines for using the code set. (16)

coordination of benefits (kō-ôr´dn-ā´shən bĕn´ə-fĭts) A legal principle that limits payment by insurance companies to 100% of the cost of covered expenses. (15)

co-payment (kō-pā´mənt) A small fee paid by the insured at the time of a medical service rather than by the insurance company. (15)

counter check (koun´tər chĕk) A special bank check that allows a depositor to draw funds from his own account only, as when he has forgotten his checkbook. (18)

courtesy title (kûr´tĭ-sē tīt´l) A title used before a person's name, such as Dr., Mr., or Ms. (7)

cover sheet (kŭr´ər shēt) A form sent with a fax that provides details about the transmission. (5)

CPT See *Current Procedural Terminology.* (16)

credit (krĕd´ĭt) An extension of time to pay for services, which are provided on trust. (17)

credit bureau (krĕ´-dit byür´-o) A company that provides information about the credit worthiness of a person seeking credit. (17)

crime (krīm) An offense against the state committed or omitted in violation of public law. (3)

criminal law (krĭm´ə-nəl lô) Involves crimes against the state. When a state or federal law is violated, the government brings criminal charges against the alleged offender. (3)

cross-reference (krôs´rĕf´ər-əns) The notation within the ICD-9 of the word *see* after a main term in the index. The *see* reference means that the main term first checked is not correct. Another category must then be used. (16)

cross-referenced (krôs´rĕf´ər-ənsd) Filed in two or more places, with each place noted in each file; the exact contents of the file may be duplicated, or a cross-reference form can be created, listing all the places to find the file. (10)

cross-training (krós-trā´-ning) The acquisition of training in a variety of tasks and skills. (1)

Current Procedural Terminology (CPT) (kûr´ənt prə-sē´jər-əl tûr´mə-nŏl´ə-jē) A book with the most commonly used system of procedure codes. It is the HIPAA-required code set for physicians' procedures. (16)

cursor (kûr´sər) A blinking line or cube on a computer screen that shows where the next character that is keyed will appear. (6)

cycle billing (sī´kəl bĭl´ĭng) A system that sends invoices to groups of patients every few days, spreading the work of billing all patients over the month while billing each patient only once. (17)

damages (dăm´ĭjz) Money paid as compensation for violating legal rights. (17)

database (dā´tə-bās) A collection of records created and stored on a computer. (6)

dateline (dāt´līn´) The line at the top of a letter that contains the month, day, and year. (7)

deductible (dĭ-dŭk´tə-bəl) A fixed dollar amount that must be paid by the insured before additional expenses are covered by an insurer. (15)

defamation (dĕf´ə-mā´shən) Damaging a person's reputation by making public statements that are both false and malicious. (3)

dementia (dĭ-mĕn´shə) The deterioration of mental faculties from organic disease of the brain. (14)

dependent (dĭ-pĕn´dənt) A person who depends on another person for financial support. (18)

dermatologist (der-mă-tŏl´ō-jist)(†) A specialist who diagnoses and treats diseases of the skin, hair, and nails. (2)

diagnosis (Dx) (dī´əg-nō´sĭs) The primary condition for which a patient is receiving care. (16)

diagnosis code (dī´əg-nō´sĭs kōd) The way a diagnosis is communicated to the third-party payer on the health-care claim. (16)

differently abled (dĭf´ər-ənt-lē ā´bəld) Having a condition that limits or changes a person's abilities and may require special accommodations. (13)

disability insurance (dĭs´ə-bĭlĭ-tē ĭn-shōōr´əns) IInsurance that provides a monthly, prearranged payment to an individual who cannot work as the result of an injury or disability. (15)

disbursement (dĭs-bûrs´mənt) Any payment of funds made by the physician's office for goods and services. (8)

disclaimer (dĭs-klā´mər) A statement of denial of legal liability. (5)

disclosure (dĭ-sklō´zhər) The release of, the transfer of, the provision of access to, or the divulgence in any manner of patient information. (3)

disclosure statement (dĭ-sklō´zhər stāt´mənt) A written description of agreed terms of payment; also called a federal Truth in Lending statement. (17)

doctor of osteopathy (dok´tər ŏs´tē-ŏp´ə-thē) A doctor who focuses special attention on the musculoskeletal system and uses hands and eyes to identify and adjust structural problems, supporting the body's natural tendency toward health and self-healing. (2)

documentation (dŏk´yə-mən-tā´shən) The recording of information in a patient's medical record; includes detailed notes about each contact with the patient and about the treatment plan, patient progress, and treatment outcomes. (9)

dot matrix printer (dŏt mā´trĭks prĭn´tər) An impact printer that creates characters by placing a series of tiny dots next to one another. (6)

double-booking system (dŭb´əl bŏŏk´ĭng sĭs´təm) A system of scheduling in which two or more patients are booked for the same appointment slot, with the assumption that both patients will be seen by the doctor within the scheduled period. (12)

durable item (dōōr´ə-bəl ĭ´təm) A piece of equipment that is used repeatedly, such as a telephone, computer, or examination table; contrast with **expendable item.** (8)

durable power of attorney (dōōr´ə-bəl pouár ə-tûr´nē)(†) A document naming the person who will make decisions regarding medical care on behalf of another person if that person becomes unable to do so. (3)

E code (ē kōd) A type of code in the ICD-9. E-codes identify the external causes of injuries and poisoning. (16)

editing (ĕd´ĭt-ĭng) The process of ensuring that a document is accurate, clear, and complete; free of grammatical errors; organized logically; and written in the appropriate style. (7)

efficiency (ĭ-fĭsh´ən-sē) The ability to produce a desired result with the least effort, expense, and waste. (8)

electronic data interchange (EDI) (ĭ-lĕk-trŏn´ĭk dā´tə ĭn´tər-chānj´) Transmitting electronic medical insurance claims from providers to payers using the necessary information systems. (15)

electronic mail (ĭ-lĕk´trŏn´ĭks) A method of sending and receiving messages through a computer network; commonly known as e-mail. (6)

electronic transaction record (ĭ-lĕk´trŏn´ĭk trăn-săk´shən rĭ-kôrd) The standardized codes and formats used for the exchange of medical data. (3)

E/M code (ē/ĕm kōd) Evaluation and management codes that are often considered the most important of all CPT codes. The E/M section guidelines explain how to code different levels of services. (16)

empathy (ĕm´pə-thē) Identification with or sensitivity to another person's feelings and problems. (4)

employment contract (ĕm-ploi´mənt kŏn´trăkt´) A written agreement of employment terms between employer and employee that describes the employee's duties and the considerations (money, benefits, and so on) to be given by the employer in exchange. (18)

enclosure (ĕn-klō´zhərz) Materials that are included in the same envelope as the primary letter. (7)

endocrinologist (ĕn´də-kra-nŏl´ə-jĭst) A specialist who diagnoses and treats disorders of the endocrine system, which regulates many body functions by circulating hormones that are secreted by glands throughout the body. (2)

endorse (ĕn-dôrs´) To sign or stamp the back of a check with the proper identification of the person or organization to whom the check is made out, to prevent the check from being cashed if it is stolen or lost. (18)

enunciation (ĭ-nŭn´sē-ā´shən) Clear and distinct speaking. (11)

established patient (ĭ-stăb´lĭsht pā´shənt) A patient who has seen the physician within the past three years. This determination is important when using E/M codes. (16)

ethics (ĕth´ĭks) General principles of right and wrong, as opposed to requirements of law. (3)

etiquette (ĕt´ĭ-ket´) Good manners. (11)

exclusion (ĭk-sklōōzh´ən) An expense that is not covered by a particular insurance policy, such as an eye examination or dental care. (15)

expendable item (ĭk-spĕn´dəbəl ī´təm) An item that is used and must then be restocked; also known collectively as supplies. Contrast with **durable item.** (8)

expressed contract (ĭk-sprĕst´ kŏn´trăct) A contract clearly stated in written or spoken words. (3)

externship (ĭk-stûrn´shĭp) A period of practical work experience performed by a medical assisting student in a physician's office, hospital, or other health-care facility. (1)

facsimile machine (făk-sĭm´ə-lē mə-shēn´) A piece of office equipment used to send a facsimile, or fax, over telephone lines from one modem to another; more commonly called a fax machine. (11)

family practitioner (făm´ə-lē prăk-tĭsh´ə-nər)(†) A physician who does not specialize in a branch of medicine but treats all types and ages of patients; also called a general practitioner. (2)

feedback (fēd´băk´) Verbal and nonverbal evidence that a message was received and understood. (4)

fee-for-service (fē fôr sûr´vĭs) A major type of health plan. It repays policyholders for the costs of health care that are due to illness and accidents. (15)

fee schedule (fē skĕj´ōōl) A list of the costs of common services and procedures performed by a physician. (15)

felony (fĕl´ə-nē) A serious crime, such as murder or rape, that is punishable by imprisonment. In certain crimes, a felony is punishable by death. (3)

file guide (fīl´gīd) A heavy cardboard or plastic insert used to identify a group of file folders in a file drawer. (10)

formulary (fôr´myū-lā-rē)(†) An insurance plan's list of approved prescription medications. (15)

fraud (frôd) An act of deception that is used to take advantage of another person or entity. (3)

full-block letter style (fōōl blŏk lĕt´ər stīl) A letter format in which all lines begin flush left; also called block style. (7)

gastroenterologist (găs´trō-ĕn-ter-ol´ō-jist)(†) A specialist who diagnoses and treats disorders of the entire gastrointestinal tract, including the stomach, intestines, and associated digestive organs. (2)

gerontologist (jĕr´ən-tŏl´ə-jĭst) A specialist who studies the aging process. (2)

global period (glō´bəl pîr´ē-əd) The period of time that is covered for follow-up care of a procedure or surgical service. (16)

gross earnings (grōs ûr´nĭngz) The total amount an employee earns before deductions. (18)

gynecologist (gī´nĭ-kŏl´ə-jĭst) A specialist who performs routine physical care and examinations of the female reproductive system. (2)

hard copy (härd kŏp´ē) A readable paper copy or printout of information. (6)

hardware (härd´wâr´) The physical components of a computer system, including the monitor, keyboard, and printer. (6)

HCPCS Level II codes (ăch sē pē sē ĕs lĕv´əl tōō kōdz) Codes that cover many supplies such as sterile trays, drugs, and durable medical equipment; also referred to as national codes. They also cover services and procedures not included in the CPT. (16)

Health Care Common Procedure Coding System (HCPCS) (hĕlth kâr kŏm´ən prə-sē´jər kōd´ĭng sĭs´təm) A coding system developed by the Centers for Medicare and Medicaid Services that is used in coding services for Medicare patients. (16)

health maintenance organization (HMO) (hĕlth mān´tə-nəns ôr´gə-nĭ-zā´shən) A health-care organization that provides specific services to individuals and their dependents who

are enrolled in the plan. Doctors who enroll in an HMO agree to provide certain services in exchange for a prepaid fee. (15)

hierarchy (hī´ə-rär´kē) A term that pertains to Abraham Maslow's hierarchy of needs. This hierarchy states that human beings are motivated by unsatisfied needs and that certain lower needs must be satisfied before higher needs can be met. (4)

HIPAA (Health Insurance Portability and Accountability Act) (hĭp´ə) A set of regulations whose goals include the following: (1) improving the portability and continuity of health-care coverage in group and individual markets; (2) combating waste, fraud, and abuse in health-care insurance and health-care delivery; (3) promoting the use of a medical savings account; (4) improving access to long-term care services and coverage; and (5) simplifying the administration of health insurance. (1)

homeostasis (hō´mē-ō-stā´sĭs) A balanced, stable state within the body. (4)

hospice (hŏs´pĭs) Volunteers who work with terminally ill patients and their families. (4)

ICD-9 See *International Classification of Diseases, Ninth Revision, Clinical Modification.* (16)

icon (ī´kŏn´) A pictorial image; on a computer screen, a graphic symbol that identifies a menu choice. (6)

identification line (ī-dĕn´tə-fĭ-kā´shən lĭn) A line at the bottom of a letter containing the letter writer's initials and the typist's initials. (7)

implied contract (ĭm-plīd´ kŏn´trăct´) A contract that is created by the acceptance or conduct of the parties rather than the written word. (3)

inactive file (ĭn-ăk´tĭv fīl) A file used infrequently. (10)

infectious waste (ĭn-fĕk´shəs wāst) Waste that can be dangerous to those who handle it or to the environment; includes human waste, human tissue, and body fluids as well as potentially hazardous waste, such as used needles, scalpels, and dressings, and cultures of human cells. (13)

informed consent form (ĭn-fôrmd´ kən-sĕnt´ fôrm) A form that verifies that a patient understands the offered treatment and its possible outcomes or side effects. (9)

ink-jet printer (ĭngk´jĕt´ prĭn´tər) A nonimpact printer that forms characters by using a series of dots created by tiny drops of ink. (6)

interactive pager (ĭn′tər-ăk′tĭv pāj′ər) A pager designed for two-way communication. The pager screen displays a printed message and allows the physician to respond by way of a mini keyboard. (5)

interim room (ĭn′tər-ĭm rōōm) A room off the patient reception area and away from the examination rooms for occasions when patients require privacy. (13)

***International Classification of Diseases, Ninth Revision, Clinical Modification* (ICD-9)** (ĭn′tər-năsh′ə-nəl klăs′ə-fĭ-kā′shən dĭ-zēz′əz nīnth rĭ-vĭzh′ən klĭn′ĭ-kəl mŏd′ə-fĭ-kā′shən) Code set that is based on a system maintained by the World Health Organization of the United Nations. The use of the ICD-9 codes in the health-care industry is mandated by **HIPAA** for reporting patients' diseases, conditions, and signs and symptoms. (16)

Internet (ĭn′tər-nĕt′) A global network of computers. (6)

internist (ĭn-tûr′nĭst) A doctor who specializes in diagnosing and treating problems related to the internal organs. (2)

interpersonal skills (ĭn′tər-pûr′sə-nəl skĭlz) Attitudes, qualities, and abilities that influence the level of success and satisfaction achieved in interacting with other people. (4)

inventory (ĭn′vən-tôrē) A list of supplies used regularly and the quantities in stock. (8)

invoice (ĭn′vois′) A bill for materials or services received by or services performed by the practice. (8)

itinerary (ī-tĭn′ə-rĕr′ē) A detailed travel plan listing dates and times for specific transportation arrangements and events, the location of meetings and lodgings, and phone numbers. (12)

journalizing (jûr′nə-līz′ĭng) The process of logging charges and receipts in a chronological list each day; used in the single-entry system of bookkeeping. (18)

laser printer (lā′zər prĭn′tər) A high-resolution printer that uses a technology similar to that of a photocopier. It is the fastest type of computer printer and produces the highest-quality output. (6)

lateral file (lăt′ər-əl fīl) A horizontal filing cabinet that features doors that flip up and a pull-out drawer, where files are arranged with sides facing out. (10)

law (lô) A rule of conduct established and enforced by an authority or governing body, such as the federal government. (3)

law of agency (lô ā′jən-sē) A law stating that an employee is considered to be acting on the physician's behalf while performing professional duties. (3)

lease (lēs) To rent an item or piece of equipment. (5)

legal custody (lēgəl kŭs′tə-dē) The court-decreed right to have control over a child's upbringing and to take responsibility for the child's care, including health care. (17)

letterhead (lĕt′ər-hĕd′) Formal business stationery, with the doctor's (or office's) name and address printed at the top, used for correspondence with patients, colleagues, and vendors. (7)

liable (lī′ə-bəl) Legally responsible. (3)

liability insurance (lī′ə-bĭl′ĭ-tē ĭn-shōōr′əns) A type of insurance that covers injuries caused by the insured or injuries that occurred on the insured's property. (15)

lifetime maximum benefit (līf′tīm′ măk′sə-məm bĕn′ə-fĭt) The total sum that a health plan will pay out over the patient's life. (15)

limited check (lĭm′ĭ-tĭd chĕk) A check that is void after a certain time limit; commonly used for payroll. (18)

living will (lĭv′ĭng wĭl) A legal document addressed to a patient's family and health-care providers stating what type of treatment the patient wishes or does not wish to receive if he becomes terminally ill, unconscious, or permanently comatose; sometimes called an advance directive. (3)

locum tenens (lō′kum tĕn′ens) (†) A substitute physician hired to see patients while the regular physician is away from the office. (12)

maintenance contract (mān′tə-nəns kŏn′trăkt′) A contract that specifies when a piece of equipment will be cleaned, checked for worn parts, and repaired. (5)

malpractice claim (măl-prăk′tĭs klām) A lawsuit brought by a patient against a physician for errors in diagnosis or treatment. (3)

managed care organization (MCO) (măn′ijd kâr ôr′gə-nī-zā′shən) A health-care business that, through mergers and buyouts, can deliver health care more cost-effectively. (1)

massage therapist (mə-säzh′thĕr′ə-pĭst) An individual who is trained to use pressure, kneading, and stroking to promote muscle and full-body relaxation. (2)

Material Safety Data Sheet (MSDS) (mə-tîr′ē-əl sāf′tē dā′tə shĕt) A form that is required for all hazardous chemicals or other substances used in the laboratory and that contains information about the product's name, ingredients, chemical characteristics, physical and health hazards, guidelines for safe handling, and procedures to be followed in the event of exposure. (8)

matrix (mā′trĭks) The basic format of an appointment book, established by blocking off times on the schedule during which the doctor is able to see patients. (12)

Medicaid (mĕd′ĭ-kād′) A federally funded health cost assistance program for low-income, blind, and disabled patients; families receiving aid to dependent children; foster children; and children with birth defects. (15)

Medicare (mĕd′ĭ-kâr′) A national health insurance program for Americans aged 65 and older. (15)

Medicare + Choice Plan (mĕd′ĭ-kâr′ chois plăn) Medicare benefit in which beneficiaries can choose to enroll in one of three major types of plans instead of the **Original Medicare Plan.** (15)

Medigap (mĕd′ĭ-găp′) Private insurance that Medicare recipients can purchase to reduce the gap in coverage—the amount they would have to pay from their own pockets after receiving Medicare benefits. (15)

microfiche (mī′krō-fēsh′) Microfilm in rectangular sheets. (5)

microfilm (mī′krə-fĭlm′) A roll of film stored on a reel and imprinted with information on a reduced scale to minimize storage space requirements. (5)

minutes (mĭ-nōōtz′) A report of what happened and what was discussed and decided at a meeting. (12)

misdemeanor (mĭs′dĭ-mē′nər) A less serious crime such as theft under a certain dollar amount or disturbing the peace. A misdemeanor is punishable by fines or imprisonment. (3)

modeling (mŏd′l-ĭng) The process of teaching the patient a new skill by having the patient observe and imitate it. (14)

modem (mō′dəm) A device used to transfer information from one computer to another through telephone lines. (6)

modified-block letter style (mŏd´ə-fīd blŏk lĕt´ər stīl) A letter format similar to full-block style, except that the dateline, complimentary closing, signature block, and notations are aligned and begin at the center of the page or slightly to the right of center. (7)

modified-wave schedule (mŏd´ə-fīd wāv skĕj´ōōl) A scheduling system similar to the wave system, with patients arriving at planned intervals during the hour, allowing time to catch up before the next hour begins. (12)

modifier (mŏd´ə-fī´ər) One or more two-digit codes assigned to the five-digit main code to show that some special circumstance applied to the service or procedure that the physician performed. (16)

money order (mŭn´ē ôr´dər) A certificate of guaranteed payment, which may be purchased from a bank, a post office, or some convenience stores. (18)

moral values (môr´əl văl´yōōz) Values or types of behavior that serve as a basis for ethical conduct and are formed through the influence of the family, culture, or society. (3)

motherboard (mŭth´ər-bôrd´) The main circuit board of a computer that controls the other components in the system. (6)

multimedia (mŭl´tē-mē´dē-ə) More than one medium, such as in graphics, sound, and text used to convey information. (6)

multitasking (mŭl´tē-tăs´kĭng) Running two or more computer software programs simultaneously. (6)

negligence (nĕg´lĭ-jəns) A medical professional's failure to perform an essential action or performance of an improper action that directly results in the harm of a patient. (3)

negotiable (nĭ-gō´shē-ə-bəl) Legally transferable from one person to another. (18)

nephrologist (ne-frol´ō-jĭst)(†) A specialist who studies, diagnoses, and manages diseases of the kidney. (2)

net earnings (nĕt ûr´nĭngz) Take-home pay, calculated by subtracting total deductions from gross earnings. (18)

network (nĕt´wûrk´) A system that links several computers together. (6)

neurologist (nōō-rəl´ə-jē) A specialist who diagnoses and treats disorders and diseases of the nervous system, including the brain, spinal cord, and nerves. (2)

new patient (nōō pā´shənt) Patient that, for CPT reporting purposes, has not received professional services from the physician within the past three years. (16)

noncompliant (nŏn´kəm-plī´ent) The term used to describe a patient who does not follow the medical advice given. (9)

no-show (nō shō) A patient who does not call to cancel and does not come to an appointment. (12)

Notice of Privacy Practices (NPP) (nō´tĭs prī´və-sē prăk´tis-əs) A document that informs patients of their rights as outlined under **HIPAA.** (3)

numeric filing system (nōō-mĕr´ĭk fīl´ĭng sĭs´təm) A filing system that organizes files by numbers instead of names. Each patient is assigned a number in the order in which she joins the practice. (10)

objective (əb-jĕk´tĭv) Pertaining to data that is readily apparent and measurable, such as vital signs, test results, or physical examination findings. (9)

Older Americans Act of 1965 (ōl´dər ə-mĕr´i-kəns ăkt) A U.S. law that guarantees certain benefits to elderly citizens, including health care, retirement income, and protection against abuse. (13)

oncologist (ŏn-kŏl´ə-jĭst) A specialist who identifies tumors and treats patients who have cancer. (2)

open-book account (ō´pən bŏok ə-kount´) An account that is open to charges made occasionally as needed. (17)

open hours scheduling (ō´pən ourz skĕj´ōōl-ĭng) A system of scheduling in which patients arrive at the doctor's office at their convenience and are seen on a first-come, first-served basis. (12)

open posture (ō´pən pŏs´chər) A position that conveys a feeling of receptiveness and friendliness; facing another person with arms comfortably at the sides or in the lap. (4)

Original Medicare Plan (ə-rĭj´ə-nəl mĕd´i-kâr´ plăn) The Medicare fee-for-service plan that allows the beneficiary to choose any licensed physician certified by Medicare. (15)

orthopedist (ôr´thə-pēdĭst) A specialist who diagnoses and treats diseases and disorders of the muscles and bones. (2)

OSHA (Occupational Safety and Health Act) (ō´shə) A set of regulations designed to save lives, prevent injuries, and protect the health of workers in the United States. (1)

osteopathic manipulative medicine (OMM) (ŏs´tē-ō-păth´ĭk mə-nĭp´ū-lā´tĭv mĕd´ĭ-sĭn) A system of hands-on techniques that help relieve pain, restore motion, support the body's natural functions, and influence the body's structure. Osteopathic physicians study OMM in addition to medical courses. (2)

otorhinolaryngologist (ō-tō-rī´nōlar-ing-gol´ō-jist) A specialist who diagnoses and treats diseases of the ear, nose, and throat. (2)

out guide (out gīd) A marker made of stiff material and used as a placeholder when a file is taken out of a filing system. (10)

overbooking (ō´vər-bŏok´ĭng) Scheduling appointments for more patients than can reasonably be seen in the time allowed. (12)

panel (păn´əl) Tests frequently ordered together that are organ or disease oriented. (16)

participating physicians (pär-tĭs´ə-pāt´ĭng fĭ-zĭsh´ənz) Physicians who enroll in managed care plans. They have contracts with MCOs that stipulate their fees. (15)

passive listening (păs´ĭv lĭs´ən-ĭng) Hearing what a person has to say without responding in any way; contrast with **active listening.** (4)

pathologist (pă-thŏl´ə-jĭst) A medical doctor who studies the changes a disease produces in the cells, fluids, and processes of the entire body. (2)

patient ledger card (pā´shənt lĕj´ər kärd) A card containing information needed for insurance purposes, including the patient's name, address, telephone number, Social Security number, insurance information, employer's name, and any special billing instructions. It also includes the name of the person who is responsible for charges if this is anyone other than the patient. (18)

patient record/chart (pā´shənt rĕk´ərd/chärt) A compilation of important information about a patient's medical history and present condition. (9)

payee (pā-ē´) A person who receives a payment. (18)

payer (pā´ər) A person who pays a bill or writes a check. (18)

pay schedule (pā skĕj´ōōl) A list showing how often an employee is paid, such as weekly, biweekly, or monthly. (18)

pediatrician (pē′dē-ə-trĭshən) A specialist who diagnoses and treats childhood diseases and teaches parents skills for keeping their children healthy. (2)

pegboard system (pĕg′bôrd sĭs′təm) A bookkeeping system that uses a lightweight board with pegs on which forms can be stacked, allowing each transaction to be entered and recorded on four different bookkeeping forms at once; also called the one-write system. (18)

personal space (pûr′sə-nəl spās) A certain area that surrounds an individual and within which another person's physical presence is felt as an intrusion. (4)

petty cash fund (pĕt′ē kăsh fŭnd) Cash kept on hand in the office for small purchases. (18)

philosophy (fĭ-lŏs′ə-fē) The system of values and principles an office has adopted in its everyday practice. (14)

physiatrist (fiz-ī′ə-trist) (†) A physical medicine specialist, who diagnoses and treats diseases and disorders with physical therapy. (2)

physician assistant (PA) (fĭ-zĭsh′ən ə-sĭs′tənt) A health-care provider who practices medicine under the supervision of a physician. (2)

pitch (pĭch) The high or low quality in the sound of a person's speaking voice. (11)

plastic surgeon (plăs′tĭk sûr′jən) A specialist who reconstructs, corrects, or improves body structures. (2)

POMR (pē′ō-ĕm-är) The problem-oriented medical record system for keeping patients' charts. Information in a POMR includes the database of information about the patient and the patient's condition, the problem list, the diagnostic and treatment plan, and progress notes. (9)

portfolio (pôrt-fō′lē-ō′) A collection of an applicant's résumé, reference letters, and other documents of interest to a potential employer. (1)

power of attorney (pou′ər ə-tûr′nē) The legal right to act as the attorney or agent of another person, including handling that person's financial matters. (18)

practitioner (prăk-tĭsh′ə-nər) One who practices a profession. (1)

preferred provider organization (PPO) (prĭ-fûrd′ prə-vīd′ər or′gə-nĭ-zā′shən) A managed care plan that establishes

a network of providers to perform services for plan members. (15)

premium (prē′mē-əm) The basic annual cost of health-care insurance. (15)

primary care physician (prī′mĕr′ē kâr fĭ-zĭsh′ən) A physician who provides routine medical care and referrals to specialists. (2)

Privacy Rule (prī′və-sē rool) Common name for the **HIPAA** Standard for Privacy of Individually Identifiable Health Information, which provides the first comprehensive federal protection for the privacy of health information. The Privacy Rule creates national standards to protect individuals' medical records and other personal health information. (3)

procedure code (prə-sē′jər kōd) Codes that represent medical procedures, such as surgery and diagnostic tests, and medical services, such as an examination to evaluate a patient's condition. (16)

pronunciation (prə-nun′cē-ā′shən) The sounding out of words. (11)

proofreading (proof′rēd′ĭng) Checking a document for formatting, data, and mechanical errors. (7)

protected health information (PHI) (prə-tĕkt-əd hĕlth ĭn′fər-mā′shən) Individually identifiable health information that is transmitted or maintained by electronic or other media, such as computer storage devices. The core of the **HIPAA Privacy Rule** is the protection, use, and disclosure of protected health information. (3)

punitive damages (pyoo′nĭ-tĭv dăm′ĭjz) Money paid as punishment for intentionally breaking the law. (17)

purchase order (pûr′chĭs ôr′dər) A form that authorizes a purchase for the practice. (8)

purchasing groups (pur′chĭs-ĭng groops) Groups of medical offices associated with a nearby hospital that order supplies through the hospital to obtain a quantity discount. (8)

quarterly return (kwŏr′tar-lē rĭ-tûrn′) The Employer's Quarterly Federal Tax Return, a form submitted to the IRS every 3 months that summarizes the federal income and employment taxes withheld from employees' paychecks. (18)

radiologist (rā′dē-ŏl′ ə-jĭst) A physician who specializes in taking and reading x-rays. (2)

random access memory (RAM) (răn′dəm ăk′sĕs mĕm′ə-rē) The temporary, or

programmable, memory in a computer. (6)

rapport (ră-pôr′) A harmonious, positive relationship. (4)

read only memory (ROM) (rēd ōn′lē mĕm′ə-rē) A computer's permanent memory, which can be read by the computer but not changed. It provides the computer with the basic operating instructions it needs to function. (6)

reconciliation (rĕk′ən-sĭl′ē-ā′shən) A comparison of the office's financial records with bank records to ensure that they are consistent and accurate; usually done when the monthly checking account statement is received from the bank. (18)

records management system (rĭ-kôrdz măn′ij-mənt sĭs′təm) How patient records are created, filed, and maintained. (10)

referral (rĭ-fûr′əl) An authorization from a medical practice for a patient to have specialized services performed by another practice; often required for insurance purposes. (15)

Registered Medical Assistant (RMA) (rĕj′ĭ-stərd mĕd′ĭ-kəl ə-sĭs′tənt) A medical assistant who has met the educational requirements and taken and passed the certification examination for medical assisting given by the American Medical Technologists (AMT). (1)

remittance advice (RA) (rĭ-mĭt′ns ăd-vīz′) A form that the patient and the practice receive for each encounter that outlines the amount billed by the practice, the amount allowed, the amount of subscriber liability, the amount paid, and notations of any service not covered, including an explanation of why that service is not covered; also called an explanation of benefits. (15)

reputable (rĕp′yə-tə-bəl) Having a good reputation. (8)

requisition (rĕk′wĭ-zĭsh′ən) A formal request from a staff member or doctor for the purchase of equipment or supplies. (8)

resource-based relative value scale (RBRVS) (rē′sôrs′ bāst rĕl′ə-tĭv văl′yoo skāl) The payment system used by Medicare. It establishes the relative value units for services, replacing the providers' consensus on usual fees. (15)

résumé (rĕz′oo-mā′) A typewritten document summarizing one's employment and educational history. (1)

retention schedule (rĭ-těnʹshən skĕjʹōol) A schedule that details how long to keep different types of patient records in the office after they have become inactive or closed and how long the records should be stored. (10)

return demonstation (rĭ-tûrnʹ dĕmʹən-străʹshən) Participatory teaching method in which the technique is first described to the patient and then demonstrated to the patient; the patient is then asked to repeat the demonstration. (14)

salutation (sălʹyə-tāʹshən) A written greeting, such as "Dear," used at the beginning of a letter. (7)

scanner (skănʹər) An optical device that converts printed matter into a format that can be read by the computer and inputs the converted information. (6)

screening (skrēnʹĭng) Performing a diagnostic test on a person who is typically free of symptoms. (14)

screen saver (skrēn sāʹvər) A program that automatically changes the monitor display at short intervals or constantly shows moving images to prevent burn-in of images on the computer screen. (6)

Security Rule (sĭ-kyoōrʹĭ-tē roōl) The technical safeguards that protect the confidentiality, integrity, and availability of health information covered by **HIPAA**. The Security Rule specifies how patient information is protected on computer networks, the Internet, disks, and other storage media. (3)

sequential order (sĭʹkwĕnʹshəl ôrʹdər) One after another in a predictable pattern or sequence. (10)

service contract (sûrʹvĭs kŏnʹtrăktʹ) A contract that covers services for equipment that are not included in a standard maintenance contract. (5)

sign (sīn) An objective or external factor, such as blood pressure, rash, or swelling, that can be seen or felt by the physician or measured by an instrument. (9)

simplified letter style (sĭmʹplə-fīdʹ lĕtʹər stīl) A modification of the full-block style in which the salutation and complimentary closing are omitted and a subject line typed in all capital letters is placed between the address and the body of the letter. (7)

single-entry account (sĭngʹgəl-ĕnʹtrē ə-kountʹ) An account that has only one charge, usually for a small amount, for a patient who does not come in regularly. (17)

SOAP (sōp) An approach to medical records documentation that documents information in the following order: S (**subjective** data), O (**objective** data), A (assessment), P (plan of action). (9)

software (sôftʹwârʹ) A program, or set of instructions, that tells a computer what to do. (6)

statement (stātʹmənt) A form similar to an invoice; contains a courteous reminder to the patient that payment is due. (17)

statute of limitations (stăchʹoōt lĭmʹĭ-tāʹshənz) A state law that sets a time limit on when a collection suit on a past-due account can legally be filed. (17)

subjective (səb-jĕkʹtĭv) Pertaining to data that is obtained from conversation with a person or patient. (9)

subpoena (sə-pēʹnə) A written court order that is addressed to a specific person and requires that person's presence in court on a specific date at a specific time. (3)

superbill (soōʹpər-bĭlʹ) A form that combines the charges for services rendered, an invoice for payment or insurance co-payment, and all the information for submitting an insurance claim. (17)

surgeon (sûrʹjən) A physician who uses hands and medical instruments to diagnose and correct deformities and treat external and internal injuries or disease. (2)

symptom (sĭmʹtəm) A subjective, or internal, condition felt by a patient, such as pain, headache, or nausea, or another indication that generally cannot be seen or felt by the doctor or measured by instruments. (9)

tab (tăb) A tapered rectangular or rounded extension at the top of a file folder. (10)

Tabular List (tăbʹyə-lər lĭst) One of two ways that diagnoses are listed in the **ICD-9**. In the Tabular List, the diagnosis codes are listed in numerical order with additional instructions. (16)

tax liability (tăk līʹə-bĭlʹĭ-tē) Money withheld from employees' paychecks and held in a separate account that must be used to pay taxes to appropriate government agencies. (18)

telephone triage (tĕlʹə-fōnʹ trē-äzhʹ) A process of determining the level of urgency of each incoming telephone call and how it should be handled. (11)

teletype (TTY) device (tĕlʹə-tīp) A specially designed telephone that looks very much like a laptop computer with a cradle for the receiver of a traditional telephone. It is used by the hearing impaired to type communications onto a keyboard. (13)

template (tĕmʹplĭt) A guide that ensures consistency and accuracy. (7)

third-party check (thûrd pärʹtē chĕk) A check made out to one recipient and given in payment to another, as with one made out to a patient rather than the medical practice. (18)

third-party payer (thûrd pärʹtē pāʹər) A health plan that agrees to carry the risk of paying for patient services. (15)

tickler file (tĭkʹlər fīl) A reminder file for keeping track of time-sensitive obligations. (10)

time-specified scheduling (tīm spěsʹə-fīd skĕjʹoōl-ĭng) A system of scheduling where patients arrive at regular, specified intervals, assuring the practice a steady stream of patients throughout the day. (12)

tort (tôrt) In civil law, a breach of some obligation that causes harm or injury to someone. (3)

tower case (touʹər kās) A vertical housing for the system unit of a personal computer. (6)

tracking (trăkʹĭng) (financial) Watching for changes in spending so as to help control expenses. (18)

transcription (trăn-skrĭpʹshən) The transforming of spoken notes into accurate written form. (9)

transfer (trăns-fûrʹ) To give something, such as information, to another party outside the doctor's office. (9)

traveler's check (trăvʹəlz chĕk) A check purchased and signed at a bank and later signed over to a payee. (18)

treatment, payments and operations (TPO) (trētʹmənt pāʹmənts ŏpʹə-rāʹshəns) The portion of **HIPAA** that allows the provider to use and share patient health-care information for treatment, payment, and operations (such as quality improvement). (3)

triage (trē-äzhʹ) To assess the urgency and types of conditions patients present as well as their immediate medical needs. (2)

TRICARE (trīʹkâr) A program that provides health-care benefits for families of military personnel and military retirees. (15)

troubleshooting (trŭbʹəl-shoōʹtĭng) Trying to determine and correct a problem without having to call a service supplier. (5)

tutorial (tōō-tôrʹē-əl)   A small program included in a software package designed to give users an overall picture of the product and its functions. (6)

underbooking (ŭnʹdər-bŏŏkĭng)   Leaving large, unused gaps in the doctor's schedule; this approach does not make the best use of the doctor's time. (12)

uniform donor card (yōōʹnə-fôrmʹ dōʹnər kärd)   A legal document that states a person's wish to make a gift upon death of one or more organs for medical research, organ transplants, or placement in a tissue bank. (3)

unit price (yōōʹnĭt prīs)   The total price of a package divided by the number of items that comprise the package. (8)

urologist (yŏŏ-rŏlʹə-jĭst)   A specialist who diagnoses and treats diseases of the kidney, bladder, and urinary system. (2)

use (yōōz)   The sharing, employing, applying, utilizing, examining, or analyzing of individually identifiable health information by employees or other members of an organization's workforce. (3)

V code (vē kōd)   A code used to identify encounters for reasons other than illness or injury, such as annual checkups, immunizations, and normal childbirth. (16)

vertical file (vûrʹtĭ-kəl fil)   A filing cabinet featuring pull-out drawers that usually contain a metal frame or bar equipped to handle letter- or legal-sized documents in hanging file folders. (10)

voice mail (vois māl)   An advanced form of answering machine that allows a caller to leave a message when the phone line is busy. (5)

void (void)   (legal) A term used to describe something that is not legally enforceable. (3)

voucher check (vouʹchər chĕk)   A business check with an attached stub, which is kept as a receipt. (18)

walk-in (wôkʹĭn)   A patient who arrives without an appointment. (12)

warranty (wôkʹən-tē)   A contract that specifies free service and replacement of parts for a piece of equipment during a certain period, usually a year. (5)

wave scheduling (wāv skĕjʹōol-ĭng)   A system of scheduling in which the number of patients seen each hour is determined by dividing the hour by the length of the average visit and then giving that number of patients appointments with the doctor at the beginning of each hour. (12)

written-contract account (rĭtʹn kŏnʹtrăktʹ ə-kountʹ)   An agreement between the physician and patient stating that the patient will pay a bill in more than four installments. (17)

X12 837 Health Care Claim (hĕlth kâr klām)   An electronic claim transaction that is the **HIPAA** Health Care Claim or Equivalent Encounter Information ("HIPAA claim"). (15)

Photo Credits

CHAPTER 1
Fig. 1.1: Robert Mathews; Fig. 1.2, Page 13, Fig. 1.4: © David Kelly Crow.

CHAPTER 2
Fig. 2.1, 2.2: © Kathy Sloane; Fig. 2.3: © David Kelly Crow; Page 27, Fig. 2.4, Fig. 2.5, Fig. 2.6: © David Kelly Crow; Fig. 2.7: © Will and Deni McIntyre.

CHAPTER 3
Fig. 3.2: © Volker Steger/Peter Arnold, Inc.; Fig. 3.3, Fig. 3.4: © Cliff Moore.

CHAPTER 4
Fig. 4.2, Fig. 4.3, Fig. 4.4, Fig. 4.5: © Cliff Moore.

CHAPTER 5
Fig. 5.1, Fig. 5.3, Fig. 5.4, Fig. 5.5, Fig. 5.6, Fig. 5.7: © Terry Wild Studio.

CHAPTER 6
Fig. 6.1: © Terry Wild Studio; Fig. 6.3: Courtesy Total Care Programming; Fig. 6.4, Fig. 6.8, Fig. 6.9, Fig. 6.10, Page 116: © Terry Wild Studio.

CHAPTER 7
Fig. 7.1: © David Kelly Crow; Fig. 7.7, Fig. 7.8, Fig. 7.9, Fig. 7.10: © Cliff Moore.

CHAPTER 8
Fig. 8.1, Fig. 8.6: © David Kelly Crow.

CHAPTER 9
Fig. 9.1: © Hank Morgan/Photo Researchers, Inc.; Fig. 9.5: © David Kelly Crow; Fig. 9.6: Courtesy Total Care Programming; Fig. 9.8, Fig. 9.9: © David Kelly Crow; Page 170: © Kathy Sloane; Fig. 9.10: © David Kelly Crow.

CHAPTER 10
Fig. 10.1: © Terry Wild Studio; Fig. 10.2: Courtesy Bibbero Systems, Inc. Petaluma, CA (800) 242-2376, www.bibbero.com; Fig. 10.5, 10.7: © Terry Wild Studio; Fig. 10.8: © David Kelly Crow; Page 192: © Terry Wild Studio.

CHAPTER 11
Fig. 11.3: Courtesy Total Care Programming; Fig. 11.4: © Terry Wild Studio; Fig. 11.5: Shirley Zeiberg.

CHAPTER 12
Fig. 12.6, Fig. 12.7: © Terry Wild Studio.

CHAPTER 13
Fig. 13.1: Courtesy Total Care Programming; Fig. 13.2, Fig. 13.3: © Terry Wild Studio; Fig. 13.4: © Cliff Moore; Fig. 13.5, Fig. 13.6: © Terry Wild Studio; Fig. 13.7: Shirley Zeiberg; Fig. 13.8: © Terry Wild Studio.

CHAPTER 14
Fig. 14.1: © Kathy Sloane; Fig. 14.2: © Terry Wild Studio; Fig. 14.4, Fig. 14.5: © Kathy Sloane; Fig. 14.6: © Terry Wild Studio; Page 252: © Ken Lax.

CHAPTER 15
Fig. 15.3: © David Kelly Crow; Fig. 15.9: © Terry Wild Studio.

CHAPTER 17
Fig. 17.4: © Terry Wild Studio.

CHAPTER 18
Fig. 18.5: Courtesy Bibbero Systems, Inc. Petaluma, CA (800) 242-2376, www.bibbero.com; Fig. 18.10, Fig. 18.11: © Terry Wild Studio.

Text and Line Art Credits

CHAPTER 1
Context (pg 18–19) The Medical Assistant Role Delineation Chart, courtesy of the American Association of Medical Assistants.

CHAPTER 3
Fig. 3.1: *Source:* Medicolegal Forms With Legal Analysis, American Medical Association, © 1991; Fig. 3.6: The AAMA's Code of Ethics, (Reprinted with permission of the American Association of Medical Assistants.). Context (pg 40) The Four Ds of Negligence, courtesy of the American Medical Association (AMA).

CHAPTER 4
Table 4.1: From *YOUR PERFECT RIGHT: Assertiveness and Equality in Your Life and Relationships, 8th Edition* © 2001 by Robert E. Alberti and Michael L. Emmons. Reproduced for Ramutkowski et al. by permission of Impact Publishers, Inc., PO Box 6016, Atascadero, CA

93423. Further reproduction prohibited. Context (pg 76) "Preventing Burnout." Section adapted from *The Stress Solution* by Lyle H. Miller, PhD and Alma Dell Smith, PhD, American Psychological Association, 1997.

CHAPTER 6
Fig. 6.5: Windows 2000-Screen shot reprinted by permission from Microsoft Corporation; Fig. 6.6: I. Hoffmann + Associates Inc. (H + a) Image from the Epilepsy CD-ROM of the H + a Medical Series. All rights reserved; Fig. 6.7: Screen capture Corel Corporations.

CHAPTER 10
Table 10.1: Adapted from William A. Sabin, *The Gregg Reference Manual,* 8th ed. (Columbus, OH: Glencoe/McGraw-Hill, 1996), 288–295.

CHAPTER 14
Context (pg 244) Data for in-home deaths of people of all ages, provided by National Safety Council.

CHAPTER 15
Fig. 15.1: *Source:* Mercer's National Survey of Employer Sponsored Health Plans, 2003. Copyright 2003, The Managed Care Information Center; Fig. 15.4: *Source:* Blue Cross and Blue Shield Association; Fig. 15.7: *Source:* Center for Medicare and Medicaid Services.

CHAPTER 16
Fig. 16.1: *Source:* International Classification of Diseases, Ninth Revision, Clinical Modification, 2004, Volumes 1 and 2. International Classification of Diseases, Ninth Revision, Clinical Modification http://www.cdc.gov/nchs/about/otheract/icd9/abticd9.htm; Fig. 16.2: *Source:* American Medical Association, *Current Procedural Terminology,* copyright 2003.

Index

Page numbers in **boldface** indicate figures. Page numbers followed by (b) indicate box features, (p) procedures, and (t) tables, respectively.

AAMA. *See* American Association of Medical Assistants (AAMA)
AAMT. *See* American Association of Medical Transcription (AAMT)
Abandonment
    letter of withdrawal from case and, 43
    as negligence, 40
ABA number, 321
Abbreviations
    in appointment book, 212
    medical, **166**
    state, 123(t)
ABHES. *See* Accrediting Bureau of Health Education Schools (ABHES)
ABMS. *See* American Board of Medical Specialties (ABMS)
Acceptance, as stage of death, 72
Accepting assignment, 260
Account cards, 315
Accounting. *See also* Billing; Collections
    banking tasks, 321–323
    bookkeeping systems, 314–321
    calculating and filing taxes, 338–339
    disbursement management, 328–331
    employment contracts, 339, 342
    establishing procedures for, 313
    importance of accuracy, 313
    payroll, 331–338
    software for, 108
    understanding financial summaries, 331
Accounts
    open-book account, 301
    single-entry account, 301
    written-contract account, 301
Accounts payable, 294
    disbursement management, 328–331
    payroll, 331–338
    setting up system, 329(p)
    in single-entry bookkeeping system, 315
Accounts receivable, 294
    insurance for, 306
    in single-entry bookkeeping system, 315
Accreditation, 10
Accredited Record Technician (ART), 26, 28, 192(b)
Accrediting Bureau of Health Education Schools (ABHES), 9, 10
Accuracy
    bookkeeping and, 313
    of patient records, 167
ACP. *See* American College of Physicians (ACP)
Active files, 187
Active listening, 64, **65**
Activity-monitoring systems, 114
Acupuncturists, 26

ADA. *See* Americans with Disabilities Act
Adding machines, 90
Add-on codes, 285
Address
    in business letter, **122,** 123
    format of, 132–133
    inside, **122,** 123–124
    patient address change and collections, 310
    placement on envelope, 132, **133**
Address books, online address books, 110(b)
Adjustments, chiropractor, 26
Administrative duties
    daily duties of medical assistant, 14
    legal issues and, 43
    simplification of, by HIPAA, 54, 56
Administrative office supplies, 141, **142,** 143
ADN. *See* Associate degrees in nursing (ADN)
Advance Beneficiary Notice, 269, **270**
Advance directive, 44
Advance scheduling, 217
Advice, patient calling requesting, 201
Age analysis, 302, **304**
Agenda, 223
Agent, 41
Aggressive behavior
    vs. assertiveness, 67, 67(t)
    in communication, 67, 67(t)
AHA. *See* American Hospital Association (AHA)
AHIMA. *See* American Health Information Management Association (AHIMA)
AIDS/HIV infection
    communicating with patients, 72–73
    OSHA regulations and, 44–45
Airborne Express, 136
Airmail supplies, 134
Allergies, specialty, 23
Allergists, 23
Allowable charge, 268
Allowed amount, 268
Allowed fee, 268
Alphabetic filing system, **180,** 181, 181(t)
    color coding and, 182
    rules for filing personal names, 181(t)
Alphabetic Index, 279–281, **280**
Alternative therapies, right to information about, 50
Alzheimer's Association, **251**
AMA. *See* American Medical Association (AMA)
American Academy of Dental Practice Administrators, 116(b)
American Academy of Medical Administrators, 27(b)

American Academy of Pediatrics, **251**
American Academy of Professional Coders, 289(b), 309(b)
American Association of Medical Assistants (AAMA)
    certification by, 8–9
    certification examination by, 8–9
    code of ethics, 8, **50**
    creation of, 7–8
    creed of, 8
    definition of medical assisting profession, 11
    on malpractice insurance, 41
    membership requirements and advantages of, 34–35, 34(t)
    pin worn by medical assistants certified by, **7**
    professional benefits from membership, 9–10
    purpose of, 7–8
    Role Delineation Chart, 18–19
    on standard of care, 42–43
    standards for accredited programs, 10
American Association of Medical Transcription (AAMT), 170(b)
    membership requirements and advantages of, 34(t), 35
American Banking Association, 321
American Board of Medical Specialties (ABMS), 22
American Cancer Society, **251**
American Collectors Association International, 306(b)
American College of Physicians (ACP), membership requirements and advantages of, 34(t), 35
American Diabetes Association, **251**
American Dietetic Association, **251**
American Health Information Management Association (AHIMA), 289(b), 309(b)
American Heart Association, **251**
American Hospital Association (AHA), 13(b)
    membership requirements and advantages of, 34(t), 35
    Patient's Bill of Rights, 50
    on retention of patient records, 191
American Medical Association (AMA), 7
    code of ethics, 49
    on credit card payments, 296
    four Ds of negligence, 40
    on Internet, 111(t)
    membership requirements and advantages of, 34(t), 35
    reception area furniture, 229
    on retention of patient records, 191

American Medical Record Association (AMRA), 192(b)
American Medical Technologists (AMT), 7
  membership requirements and advantages of, 34(t), 35
  pin worn by registrants of, **7**
  professional benefits from membership, 10
  RMA credentials, 9
American Pharmaceutical Association (APhA), membership requirements and advantages of, 34(t), 35
American Red Cross, **251**
  volunteer opportunities, 11
American Society of Clinical Pathologists (ASCP), 29, 34(t)
American Society of Phlebotomy Technicians (ASPT), 34(t)
Americans with Disabilities Act, 236–237
  on office access, 232
AMRA. *See* American Medical Record Association (AMRA)
AMT. *See* American Medical Technologists (AMT)
Anatomical models, patient education and, 249–250
Anatomic pathologists, 25
Anesthesiology, 23
Anesthetists, 23
Anesthetist's assistant, 31
Anger, as stage of death, 72
Anger, patient, communicating with, 68
Annotate, mail, 137–138
Answering machine, 86
Answering service, 86–87
  retrieving messages from, 206(p)
Anxiety, patient
  communicating with, 68, 69(p)
  preoperative education to relieve, 250
Appearance
  of medical assistant, 16–17
  of patient records, 167
Appointment book, 211–214, **213**
  commonly used abbreviations, 212
  legal importance of, 43
  as legal record, 212, 214
  matrix, 211–212, **213**
  missed appointments and documentation of, 43
  obtaining patient information, 212
  standard procedure times, 212
Appointment card, 218, **218**
Appointment reminders, 218, **218**
Appointments, scheduling, 210–225
  appointment book for, 211–214, **213**
  arranging appointments, 218–219
  cancellations, 220, 222
  emergency appointments, 219, 219(b)
  fasting patients, 220
  information on, 246
  late arrivals and, 220
  maintaining physician's schedule, 222–224
  missed appointments, 220

new patients, 218
outside appointments, 221–222
patients with diabetes, 220
physician scheduling situations, 220–221
referrals, 219–220, 221–222
reminders for, 218, **218**
repeat visits, 220
return appointments, 218
scheduling and confirming surgery, 221(p)
scheduling systems for, 214, **215–216,** 217–218
software for, 108
walk-ins, 220
Appointment scheduling system
  advance scheduling, 217
  cluster scheduling, 217, 217(p)
  combination scheduling, 217
  computerized scheduling, **217,** 217–218
  double-booking system, 214
  modified-wave scheduling, 214, **216**
  open-hours scheduling, 214
  time-specified scheduling, 214, **215**
  wave scheduling, 214
Arbitration, 41
Areas of competence (AOC), 18
  administrative procedures, 83(b), 119(b), 156(b), 176(b), 210(b), 256(b)
  communication skills, 5(b), 59(b), 100(b), 119(b), 156(b), 196(b), 240(b), 256(b)
  fundamental principles, 37(b)
  instruction, 240(b)
  legal concepts, 21(b), 37(b), 59(b), 156(b), 226(b), 256(b)
  operational functions, 83(b), 100(b), 140(b), 312(b)
  patient care, 156(b), 256(b)
  practice finances, 293(b), 312(b)
  professionalism, 5(b), 21(b), 59(b), 196(b), 210(b)
Arthritis Foundation, **251**
ASCP. *See* American Society of Clinical Pathologists (ASCP)
Assault, 39
Assertiveness skills, 67, 67(t)
Assessment, in SOAP, 167
Assets, in double-entry bookkeeping system, 319
Assignment of benefits statement, 268
Associate degrees in nursing (ADN), 30
Associations, as patient education resource, **251,** 252
Asthma and Allergy Foundation of America, **251**
Attention
  to details, as medical assistant skill, 15
  in telephone techniques, 204
Attention line, 124
Attitude, of medical assistant, 17
Attorneys, handling calls from, 202
Authorization of disclosure form, 53, 57
Autoclave, 45

Automated menu telephone system, 86, 86(b)
Automation equipment, office
  adding machines and calculators, 90
  check writers, 93
  dictation-transcription equipment, 92–93, 92(p)
  microfilm and microfiche readers, **94,** 94–95
  paper shredders, **93,** 93–94
  photocopiers, 89–90
  postage meters, **90,** 90–91, 91(p)
  postage scales, 91–92
Awakening Phase of burnout, 76

Baccalaureate nurse, 30
Bachelor of science in nursing (BSN), 30
Backup systems, for office equipment, 97
Balance billing, 268
Balasa, Donald A., 8
Bandages, storage of, 143
Banking
  accepting checks, 321
  electronic, 323–324, 327–328
  endorsing checks, 322, **322**
  establishing procedures for, 313
  making deposits, 322–323, **323,** 324(p)
  reconciling bank statements, 323
  telephone, 327(b)
  writing checks, 321
Bank statements, reconciling, 323, 326(p)–327(p)
Bargaining, as stage of death, 72
Battery, defined, 39
Battery power backup, 97
Beepers, 87
Benefits
  explanation of, 266
  health insurance, 257
  review for allowed, 266
Bilirubin, testing urine for, **48**
Billing. *See also* Collections
  accepting payment, 296–297
  basic accounting for, 294
  coding, billing, and insurance specialist, 309(b)
  credit arrangements, 306–310
  determining appropriate fees, 294
  ethical behavior and, 49
  insurance fraud and, 288
  managing billing cycles, 298, 301
  preparing invoices, 298, **299**
  processing charge slips, 294, **295,** 296
  software for, 108
  standard payment procedures and, 294–298
  standard procedures for, 298–301
  telephone inquiries, 201
  using superbill, 298, **300,** 301(p)
Billing service, independent, 298
Binders, 180
Bioethics, 49–50
Biohazardous waste, disposal of, 45, **46**
Birthday rule, 264
Block style letter, 125, **126**

Blood-borne pathogens. *See also* AIDS/HIV infection
  exposure, 45
  Exposure Control Plan, 47
  OSHA regulations and, 44–45
Bloodborne Pathogens Standard, OSHA (1991), 44
Blood glucose, testing, 48, **48**
Blue Cross and Blue Shield (BCBS), 262, **263**
Body, of business letter, **122,** 124
Body language, 63–64
  eye contact, 64
  facial expression, 63–64
  personal space, 64
  posture, 64
  touch, 64
Bookkeeping
  on computer, 320–321
  double-entry system, 319
  establishing procedures for, 313
  organizing, 319(b)
  pegboard system, 320
  single-entry system, 314–319
Booklets, as patient education, 242–243
Books, 233, 234(b)
Breach of contract, 40, 41
Brochures, as patient education, 242–243
Brownout Phase of burnout, 76
Bulletin board, in reception area, 234–235
Burnout
  preventing, 75–76
  stages of, 76
Business letter, parts of, **122,** 122–124
Business side of medical practice. *See* Banking; Bookkeeping

CAAHEP. *See* Commission on Accreditation of Allied Health Education Programs (CAAHEP)
Calculators, 90
Cancellations
  by patient, 220
  by physicians, 222
Cancer, symptoms and warning signs of, 245
Candidate's Guide to the Certification Examination (AAMA), 9
Capitalization, rules of, 131(t)
Capitation, 258, 268
Cardiologists, 23
Cardiology, 23
Career opportunities
  dental office administrator, 116(b)
  medical coder, physician practice, 289(b)
  medical office administrator, 27(b)
  medical record technologist, 191(b)–192(b)
  medical transcriptionist, 170(b)
  multiskill training and, 11, 13
  occupational therapy assistant, 252(b)–253(b)
  specialty career options, 31–33
  unit secretary, 13(b)

Carpal tunnel syndrome, 104(b)
Carpets, in reception area, 228
Cash
  accepting payment in, 296
  petty cash fund, 330–331
Cash flow statement, 331
Cashier's check, 321, 330
Categorization scheduling, 217
Caution
  maintaining cleanliness standards in reception area, 231(b)
  multicultural attitudes about modern medicine, 70(b)
  notifying those at risk for sexually transmitted disease, 55(b)–56(b)
CDC. *See* Center for Disease Control and Prevention (CDC)
CD-ROM, 105
  care and maintenance of, 115, **115**
  changes in research and, 110, **112**
CD-R technology, 117
Cell phones, 97
Center for Disease Control and Prevention (CDC). *See also* Universal Precautions
  on Internet, 110
  OSHA regulations and, 45
Centers for Medicare and Medicaid Services (CMS), 259
Central processing unit (CPU), 105
Certification
  benefits of, 9, 10
  process of, 8–9
  tests for, 9
Certified check, 321, 330
Certified laboratory assistant, 31
Certified mail, 135, **135,** 137(b)
Certified Medical Assistant (CMA)
  examination by, 9
  professional support for, 9–10
Certified Medical Assistants: HealthCare's Most Versatile Professionals (AAMA), 9
Certified registered nurse anesthetist (CRNA), 23
Charges, summary of, 315, **318,** 319
Charge slip, 315
  in pegboard slip system, 320
  processing, 294, **295,** 296
Charting. *See also* Patient records
  Security Rule of HIPAA, 53–54
  six C's of, 164–165
Charts, 158. *See also* Patient records
Checkbook, electronic, 324, 327–328
Checking accounts, types of, 321
Checks
  accepting checks, 321
  endorsing checks, 322, **322**
  making deposits, 322–323, **323,** 324(p)
  producing/voiding on check writer, 93
  reconciling bank statements, 323, 326(p)–327(p)
  types of, 321, 329–330
  writing checks, 321
  writing for disbursements, 329–330
Check writers, 93
Chief complaint, 279

Children
  communicating with, 72
  confidentiality of patient records, 173–174
  payment responsibility and, 297–298
  reception area for, 230, 235, 236(p)
  retention of patient records, 189, 191
Chiropractors, 26
Cholesterol, tests for, 48
Chronological order, in patient records, 165
Circular E, Employer's Tax Guide, 334
Civil law, 39
  malpractice and, 40–41
Civil penalties, of HIPAA violations, 54
Civil Rights Act of 1964, Title VII of, 18
Claims. *See* Insurance claims, processing
Claim scrubber, 276
Clarity
  in patient records, 164–165
  telephone techniques and, 198
  of writing style, 125
Classes, as patient education, 243
Classification, color coding filing system and, 182
Classification of Disease system, 309(b)
Cleaning, of reception area, 230–232, 231(b)
Clearinghouse, 271
Clerical duties, unit secretary and, 13(b)
CLIA (Clinical Laboratory Improvements Act), credentialed medical assistants and, 8
Client's words, in charting, 164
Clinical duties, daily duties of medical assistant, 14
Clinical Laboratory Improvement Amendments of 1988 (CLIA '88), 48
Clinical Modification (ICD-10-CM), 283
Clinical office supplies, 141, **142,** 143–144
Clinics, recycling procedures, 15(b)
Closed files, 187
Closed posture, 64
Cluster scheduling, 217, 217(p)
CMA. *See* Certified Medical Assistant (CMA)
CMS-1500 claim, 269, 271, **272,** 273(p)–274(p)
Code linkage, 288
Code of ethics, 49, **50**
Code of Medical Ethics: Current Opinions with Annotations (AMA), 49
Coding, billing, and insurance specialist, 309(b)
Coding, filing, 185
  color coding, **182,** 182–183
Coding, medical
  avoiding fraud, 287–289
  code linkage, 288
  coding, billing, and insurance specialist, 309(b)
  compliance plans, 288–289
  diagnosis codes, 279–283
  HCPCS, 286–287
  procedure codes, 283–286

Cohesiveness, telephone techniques and, 198
Coinsurance, 257
Collection agencies, outside, 302, 304–306, 306(b)
Collections. *See also* Billing
  accounts receivable insurance, 306
  age analysis, 302, **304**
  basic accounting for, 294
  coding, billing, and insurance specialist, 309(b)
  common problems of, 310
  credit arrangements, 306–310
  finance charges and late fees, 304
  initial telephone call or letters, 301–302, **303**
  laws governing, 302, 304, 305(t)
  outside agencies for, 304–306, 306(b)
  standard payment procedures and, 294–298
  standard procedures for, 301–306
  state statute of limitations, 301
Color, in reception area, 228
Color coding filing system, **182,** 182–183
Color family, 228
Combination scheduling, 217
Commercial records centers, 188, **189**
Commission on Accreditation of Allied Health Education Programs (CAAHEP), 9, 10, 192(b)
Communication, 59–79. *See also* Patient education; Telephone techniques
  with AIDS or HIV-positive patients, 72–73
  with angry patient, 68
  with anxious patient, 68, 69(p)
  assertiveness skills, 67, 67(t)
  body language, 63–64
  channels of, 73
  with children, 72
  conflict and, 74
  with coworkers, **73,** 73–74
  customer service and, 60–61
  defense mechanisms and, 66–67
  dental office administrator, 116(b)
  with elderly patients, 71–72
  electronic, 109–110
  feeling over telephone, 205
  five C's of, 198
  hierarchy of needs and, 62–63
  humanizing process in medical office, 62
  improving your, 64–67
  interpersonal skill, 64–65
  legal issues and, 44
  listening skills, 64
  with mentally/emotionally disturbed patients, 71
  negative, 63
  office equipment for, 84–89
  with older patients, 164(b)
  with parents and families, 72
  with patients and families, 60–61, 67–73
  patients' bills, 268–269

  with patients from other cultures, 68–70, 70(b)
  patients with hearing impairment, 71, **71**
  policy and procedures manual, 76–78, **77**
  positive, 63, 73–74
  preventing lawsuits and, 41
  in special circumstances, 67–73
  stress management and, 74–75
  with superiors, 74
  for telephone use, 197–198
  with terminally ill patients, 72
  therapeutic communication skills, 65–67
  types of, 63–64
  unit secretary and, 13(b)
Communication circle, **61,** 61–62
Communication skills, of medical assistant, 18
Community-assistance directory, 243
Community resources, as patient education resource, 252
Compactible files, 178
Compensation, as defense mechanism, 66
Competitive pricing of supply vendors, 147, 149
Complaint, patient calling with, 201–202
Completeness
  in patient records, 165
  telephone techniques and, 198
Compliance plans, 288–289
Complimentary closing, of business letter, **122,** 124
Computerized scheduling, **217,** 217–218
Computers in office, using, 100–118
  activity-monitoring systems, 114
  adding a network, 113
  backup system for, 97
  bookkeeping on, 320–321
  carpal tunnel syndrome, 104(b)
  choosing a vendor, 113–114
  components of, 103–107
  converting to computerized office, 112
  in the future, 117
  hardware, 103–106
  history of computer, 102
  making and storing backup files, 114, **114**
  output devices, 106
  passwords, 114
  as patient education resource, 252
  for patient records, 169
  preventing system contamination, 114–115
  processing devices, 105
  safeguarding confidential files, 114
  security issues, 114–115
  Security Rule of HIPAA, 53–54
  selecting equipment, 112
  software, 106–112, 113
  storage devices, 105–106
  storage of files on, 188
  system care and maintenance, 115
  types of, 102–103

  upgrading office system, 112–113
  viruses, 114–115
  word processing program to create form letter, 108(p)
Conciseness
  in patient records, 165
  telephone techniques and, 198
  of writing style, 125
Conference calls, 207
Confidentiality. *See also* Privacy
  for electronic claims transmission, 276
  fax machines and, 208
  leaving messages on answering/fax machines, 85, 88
  legal obligation for, 44
  mandatory disclosure, 56–57
  notifying those at risk for sexually transmitted disease, 55(b)–56(b)
  patient confidentiality statement, 246–247
  patient records, 165, 173–174
  securing confidential files on computer, 114
  taking messages and maintaining patient, 206
  telephone calls and, 198, 202
Conflict, with coworkers and dealing with, 74
Confusion, elderly patients and, 71–72
Consideration, in communication, 65
Consumer education, 243
Contagious patients
  in reception area, 230
  reception area and, 238
Contaminated supplies, 14
Continuing education credits, 50
Contracts
  breach of, 40, 41
  defined, 39
  employment, 339, 342
  legal elements of, 39–40, 339, 342
  medical assistant contract, 342
  types of, 40
Controlled substances, legal issues, 43
Conventional records, 165
Conventions, of ICD-9-CM, 282–283
Conversion factor, 266
Coordination of benefits, 264, 264(t)
Co-payment, 257–258
Copier machines, 89–90
Correcting patient records, 171, 172(p)
Correspondence, 119–130. *See also* Letters; Mail
  basic rules of writing, 131(t)
  business letter, **122,** 122–124
  editing, 128
  effective writing for, 125
  general formatting guidelines for letters, 124–125
  letter styles, 125, **126, 127**
  in patient record, 162
  professionalism and, 120
  proofreading, 128–130
  punctuation style, 124
  reference books for, 125, 128
  signing letters, 130

style and language usage for, 128
supplies, choosing, 120–122
templates for, 122
types of, 122
written, 122–130
Cotton fiber bond paper, 121
Counter check, 330
Courier services, 137
Courtesy, telephone techniques and, 198, 204
Courtesy title, 123
Cover sheet, for faxes, 88, **88**
Coworkers, communicating with, 73–74
CPT, 283, **284,** 285
add-on codes, 285
Category II codes, Category III codes and Unlisted procedures, 285
evaluation and management codes (E/M codes), 285
laboratory procedures, 285–286
locating a code, 287(p)
modifiers, 285
surgical procedures, **284,** 285
Credentials, 8–9
Credit
arrangements for, 306–310
following laws governing extension of credit, 307–310
performing credit check, 306–307
unilateral decision, 310
Credit bureau report, 306–307, **307**
Credit cards, accepting payment in, 296–297, **297**
Credit check, performing, 306–307
Crime, 39
Criminal law, 39
Criminal penalties, of HIPAA violations, 54
Critical thinking skills, of medical assistant, 15
CRNA. *See* Certified registered nurse anesthetist (CRNA)
Cross-references, 185, 281
Cross-trained, 14
Cultural differences and considerations
communicating with patients and, 68–70, 70(b)
eye contact, 64
patient education, 248–249
view of illness, symptoms and treatment expectations, 70(b)
Current Procedural Terminology, 283, **284,** 285
Cursor, 103
Customary fees, 294
Customer service
defined, 60
importance of, 60–61
Cyberspace Hospital, 111(t)
Cycle billing, 298, 301

Daily log, in single-entry bookkeeping system, **314,** 314–315
Damages, negligence and, 40
Data, in SOAP, 167

Database, 107
in POMR, 165
Database management software, 108
Data elements, 269, 271, 275(b)
Data errors, in correspondences, 128
Dateline, **122,** 122–123
Death, stages of dying, 72
Debt collection. *See* Collections
Decontamination, OSHA regulations, 45
Decor, in reception area, 228–229
Deductible, 257
Deductions, payroll, 334
Defamation, 39
Defense Enrollment Eligibility Reporting System (DEERS), 261
Defense mechanisms, 66–67
Deficiency needs, 62
Delayed treatment, 40
Dementia, 248
Denial
as defense mechanism, 66
elderly patients and, 71–72
as stage of death, 72
Dental assistant, 31
Dental office administrator, 116(b)
Dependents, 331–332
Deposits
in electronic banking, 324
making bank, 322–323, **323,** 324(p)
Deposit slips, 322, **323**
Depression, as stage of death, 72
Derelict, negligence and, 40
Dermatologists, 23
Dermatology, 23
Desktop computer, 102
Despair, in burnout, 76
Detail persons, 223
Diabetes, scheduling appointments for patients with, 220
Diagnosis, in patient records, 159
Diagnosis codes, 279–283
defined, 279
Diagnosis (Dx), 279
Diagnostic summary, in POMR, 166
Dictation
dictation-transcription equipment, 92–93, 92(p)
direct dictation, 171
equipment for, 171
recorded dictation, 170–171
steps doctors take in, 93
Dietitians, 29
Differently abled patients, 235–237
creating accessible waiting room, 237(p)
Diplomacy, of medical assistant, 17
Diploma graduate nurse, 30
Direct cause, negligence and, 40
Direct data entry (DDE), 271
Disability insurance, 258
Disbursements, 152–153
electronic banking and, 324
petty cash, 330–331
recording, 330
record of, in single-entry bookkeeping system, 315, **317**

summary of, 315, **318,** 319
for supplies, 328–329
understanding financial summaries, 331
writing checks for, 329–330
Disbursements journal
recording in, 330
setting up, 329(p)
Discharge summary form, 159, 162
Discharging patients, ethical behavior and, 49
Disclaimer, for faxes, 88
Disclosure
confidentiality and mandatory disclosure, 56–57
in Privacy Rule of HIPAA, 52–53
Disclosure statement, 307–310, **308**
Diseases and disorders. *See also specific diseases*
carpal tunnel syndrome, 104(b)
medical coding, 279–282, **281**
patient education in about preventing, 245
Diskette drive, 105
Diskettes, care and maintenance of, 115
Dismissals, documentation of, 43
Displacement, as defense mechanism, 66
Disposable gloves, 45
Dissociation, as defense mechanism, 66
Divorce, children of
coordinating benefits of, 264(t)
payment responsibility, 297–298
DNR (do not resuscitate) orders, 44
Doctor of osteopathy, 23
Doctors. *See* Physicians
Documentation. *See also* Patient records
convention, records, 165
dismissals, 43
follow-up, 163–164
legal importance of, 43
medical history forms, 163
missed appointments, 43
OSHA regulations, 47
of patient statements, 163
problem-oriented medical records (POMR), 165–167
quality assurance programs and, 48
referrals, 43
six C's of charting, 164–165
SOAP, 167, **168**
telephone calls, 159, 167
of telephone calls, 205–206
test results, 163
DOS, 107
Dot matrix printers, 106
Double-booking system, 214
Double-entry bookkeeping system, 319
Download files, 110(b)
Dressings, storage of, 143
Drug(s)
handling drug and product samples, 138
patient education about, 244–245
storage of, 143–144
telephone inquiries about prescription renewals, 201

Durable items, 141
Durable power of attorney, 44
Duties
    coding, billing, and insurance
        specialist, 309(b)
    daily, of medical assistant, 14–15
    dental office administrator, 116(b)
    medical office administrator, 27(b)
    medical record technologist,
        191(b)–192(b)
    medical transcriptionist, 170(b)
    occupational therapy assistant,
        252(b)–253(b)
    of unit secretary, 13(b)
Duty, negligence and, 40

Ear, nose, and throat (ENT) specialist, 25
Earnings
    gross, 332, 334
    net, 334
Earnings records, 335, **336**
E codes, 282
Editing, correspondence, 128
Education. *See also* Patient education
    coding, billing, and insurance
        specialist, 309(b)
    continuing, 50
    of dental office administrator, 116(b)
    medical office administrator, 27(b)
    medical record technologist, 192(b)
    medical transcriptionist, 170(b)
    occupational therapy assistant, 253(b)
    of physicians, 22
    of unit secretary, 13(b)
Educational newsletters, 243
Educational plan, in POMR, 166
EIN. *See* Employer identification
    number (EIN)
Elderly patients
    communicating with, 71–72
    denial and confusion, 71
    growth in numbers of, 7
    patient education for, 247–248, **248**
    reception area and, 237–238
    tips for talking with older
        patients, 164(b)
    touch and, 72
Electricity, backup system for, 97
Electrocardiograph technician, 26, **26**
Electroencephalographic technologist, 26
Electronic banking, 323–324, 327–328
    displaying checkbook, 324, 327
    paying bills, 324
    payroll, 335, 335(b), 338
    recording deposits, 324
    telephone banking as, 327(b)
Electronic claims transactions, 109
Electronic claims transmission, HIPAA
    claims, 269, 271, 275(b)
Electronic data interchange (EDI), 271
Electronic funds transfer system
    (EFTS), 335(b)
Electronic mail (e-mail), 109
    sending and receiving e-mail,
        109(b)–110(b)
Electronic transactions, 54, 56, 109–110

E-mail, 109
    sending and receiving e-mail,
        109(b)–110(b)
E/M codes, 285
Emergencies. *See* Medical emergencies
Emergency calls, 202, **202,** 203(p)
Emergency medical technician (EMT),
    31–32
Emergency medicine, 23
Emotionally disturbed patients,
    communicating with, 71
Emotions, as noise in communication
    circle, 62
Empathy
    in communication, 65
    as skill of medical assistant, 16
Employee earnings records, 335, **336**
Employee's Withholding Allowance
    Certificate, 332, **333**
Employer identification number (EIN),
    applying for, 331
Employer's Annual Federal
    Unemployment (FUTA), 332(t), 334
Employer's Quarterly Federal Tax Return,
    332(t), 338, 339, **341**
Employment contracts, 339, 342
Employment Eligibility Verification,
    332(t)
Employment taxes, 338
Employment verification, 306
Enclosure notation, **122,** 123
Endocrinologists, 23
Endocrinology, 23
Endorsement of checks, 322, **322**
Entrances to medical office, 232
Enunciation, 204
Envelopes
    address format, 132–133
    address placement, 132, **133**
    for airmail, 134
    folding and inserting mail into,
        133–134
    for overnight delivery, 134
    preparing envelopes, 130–133, **133**
    types of, 121
EOB. *See* Explanation of benefits
Equal Credit Opportunity Act (ECOA),
    305(t), 307
Equipment. *See also* Office equipment,
    using and maintaining
    cleaning, 230
    filing, 177–179
    for mail, 134
    for transcription, 171
Erythrocyte sedimentation rate (ESR), **48**
ESR. *See* Erythrocyte sedimentation rate
    (ESR)
Established patient, procedure coding
    and, 285
Esteem needs, 62
Ethics. *See also* Legal issues
    AAMA Code of Ethics, 8
    code of, 49, **50**
    confidentiality and mandatory
        disclosure, 56–57
    defined, 38–39

Ethnic groups, patients of diverse. *See*
    Cultural differences and
    considerations
Etiquette, proper telephone, 202–205
Evaluation and management codes (E/M
    codes), 285
Evaluations, filing systems, 187(b)
Examination gloves, 45
Exclusions, 258
Exits to medical office, 233
Expendable items, 141
Expenses, statement of, 331
Expiration dates, storing office supplies
    and, 143
Explanation of benefits, 266
Exposure Control Plan, 47
Exposure incident
    OSHA regulations on, 45–46
    postexposure procedures, 46
Express delivery services, 136–137
Expressed contract, 40
Express mail, 134–135
Externships
    duties, 11
    obtaining references through, 11
    requirements, 10–11
    time sheets, 117
Eye, on-the-job injuries and OSHA
    regulations, 47
Eye contact, as body language, 64

Fabric, in reception area, 228
Face shields, 45
Facial expression, 63–64
Fact sheets, as patient education,
    242–243
Factual preoperative teaching, 249
Fair Credit Reporting Act (FCRA),
    305(t), 307
Fair Debt Collection Practices Act
    (FDCPA), 302, 305(t)
Fair Labor Standards Act, 334
False imprisonment, 39
Families, communicating with,
    60–61, 73
Family practitioners, 22–23
Fasting patients, scheduling
    appointments for, 220
Fax (facsimile) machines, 87–89, 208
    benefits of, 87
    confidentiality and, 208
    disclaimer for, 88
    information received by, in patient
        records, 162
    ordering office supplies by, 150(b)
    paper for, 87–88
    privacy issues and leaving
        messages, 85
    receiving faxes, 89
    Security Rule of HIPAA, 54
    sending faxes, **88,** 88–89
Fax modem, 105
Fecal occult blood, **48**
Federal Express, 136
Federal income taxes, 338
Federal Register, 266

Federal Tax Deposit (FTD) Coupon (Form 8109), 338
Federal tax deposit schedule, 338
Federal Unemployment Tax Act (FUTA), 334
Feedback, in communication circle, **61,** 61–62
Fee-for-service plans, 258
    Medicare Private Fee-for-Service Plans, 260
    Original Medicare Plan, 259–260
Feeling, communicating over telephone, 205
Fees
    allowed charges, 268
    customary, 294
    determining appropriate, 294
    resource-based relative value scale (RBRVS), 266
    usual, 294
Fee schedule, 266, 294, **295**
    contracted, 268
Fee slip, 296
Felony, 39
FICA taxes, 332(t)
    as payroll deduction, 334
    submitting, 338
File folders, 179
File guides, 180
File jackets, 180
Files
    active vs. inactive files, 187
    backup, 114, **114**
    closed, 187
    compactible, 178
    cross-referencing, 185
    labeling, 178
    lateral, 178
    locating misplaced, 185–186
    making, 114
    rotary circular, 178
    safeguarding confidential, 114
    storage of, 114, **114,** 185, 187–191
    supplemental, 183–184
    tickler, 183, 184(p)
    vertical, 178
File sorters, 180
Filing
    dental office administrator, 116(b)
    medical office administrator, 27(b)
Filing cabinets, 178
Filing equipment, 177–179
Filing process, 184–187
    active vs. inactive files, 187
    coding, 185
    filing guidelines, 186
    indexing, 184–185
    inspecting, 184
    limiting access to files, 185–186
    locating misplaced files, 186–187
    sorting, 185
    storing, 185
Filing shelves, 177–178, **178**
Filing supplies, 179–180
Filing systems, 180–184
    alphabetic, **180,** 181, 181(t)

color coding, **182,** 182–183
creating, 183(p)
evaluating, 187(b)
inventory of medical supplies, 144, 145(p)
numeric, 181–182
supplemental files, 183–184
tickler files, 183, 184(p)
Finance charges, 304
Financial responsibilities. *See* Accounts payable; Banking; Billing; Bookkeeping; Collections; Contracts; Insurance claims, processing; Payroll
Fire extinguisher, maintenance of, 97
First-class mail, 134
First impressions, of reception area, 227–230
Flexibility, of medical assistant, 16
Follow-up care, in patient records, 159
Forensic pathologists, 25
Formatting errors, 128
Form letter, word processing program to create, 108(p)
Forms
    hospital discharge summary form, 159, 162
    informed consent, 159, **162,** 249
    patient medical history, 159, **161**
    patient registration form, 159, **160**
    release-of-records form, 173
    W-4, 332, **333**
Formulary, 258
Fourth-class mail, 134
Fraud, 39
    code compliance and, 287–289
Friendliness, in communication, 65
Full-block letter style, 125, **126**
Full-Scale Burnout Phase, 76
Furniture, in reception area, 229–230

Gastroenterologists, 23
Gastroenterology, 23
General office supplies, 141, **142**
General physical examination, results of, as part of patient records, 159, **161**
General practitioners, 22
Genuineness, in communication, 65
Geographic adjustment factor, 266
Gerontologists, 23–24
Gerontology, 23–24
Global period, 285
Gloves
    disposable, 45
    examination, 45
    sterile, 45
    utility, 45
Glucose, testing urine for, **48**
Goggles, 45
Grammar
    correct usage in correspondence, 128
    manuals for, 128
Graphical user interface (GUI), 107
Grief, stages of dying and, 72
Gross earnings, 332, 334
Group buying pool, 149, **149**

GUI. *See* Graphical user interface (GUI)
Guide to Record Retention Requirements, 191
Gynecologists, 24
Gynecology, 24. *See also* Obstetrics and gynecology (OB/GYN)

Hanging files, 178
Harassment
    debt collection and, 302
    sexual, 18
Hard copy, 106, **106**
Hard disk drive, 105
Hardship cases, 310
Hardware, computer
    defined, 103
    input devices, 103–105
Hazardous materials
    Exposure Control Plan, 47
    OSHA regulations, 46–47
    OSHA training requirements, 47
HBV. *See* Hepatitis B vaccination
HCPCS. *See* Health Care Common Procedure Coding System (HCPCS)
Health-care claims. *See* Insurance claims, processing
Health Care Common Procedure Coding System (HCPCS), 56, 286–287
    Level II codes, 286
Health-care costs, reducing, and multiskilled health professionals, 11
Health-care portability, 51
Health-care workers
    cultural differences in view of, 68
    HBV vaccination for, 46
Healthful habits, 243–244
Health information
    defined, 51
    disclosure, 52–53
    Privacy Rule of HIPAA, 51–53
    protected health information (PHI), 51–52
    rules for improper release of, 56–57
    Security Rule of HIPAA, 53–54
Health insurance. *See* Insurance claims, processing
Health Insurance Portability and Accountability Act (HIPAA), 50–56
    administrative simplifications, 54, 56
    for electronic claims transmission, 276
    managing and storing patient information, 52
    Notice of Privacy Practices (NPP), 53
    patient confidentiality statement, 246–247
    patient notification of compliance, 53
    Privacy Rule, 51–53
    protected health information (PHI), 51–52
    purpose of act, 50–51
    Security Rule, 53–54
    sharing information, 52–53
    telephone calls and, 202
    telephone messages and, 85
    telephone techniques and, 198
    Title I: health-care portability, 51

Health Insurance Portability and
 Accountability Act (HIPAA)—*Cont.*
 treatment, payment and operations
  (TPO), 52–53
 violations and penalties of, 54
Health maintenance organization
 (HMO), 258, **259**
HealthWeb, 111(t)
Hearing impaired patients
 communicating with, 71, **71**
 patient education, 248, 248(b)
 in reception area, 236–237
Hemoglobin, tests for, **48**
Hepatitis B vaccination
 HBV vaccination for health-care
  workers, 46
 OSHA regulations and, 44–45
Hierarchy of needs, 62–63
High-complexity tests, 48
HIPAA. *See* Health Insurance Portability
 and Accountability Act (HIPAA)
HIPAA claim, 269, 271, 275(b)
Hippocratic oath, 49
HIV. *See* AIDS/HIV infection
Hold, putting telephone call on, 204
Home, preventing injury at, **244**
Homeostasis, 62
Honesty, of medical assistant, 17
Honeymoon Phase of burnout, 76
Horizontal files, 178
Hospice, 72, 259
Hospital discharge summary form,
 159, 162
Hospitals, recycling procedures, 15(b)
Housekeeping
 for reception area, 230
 storing office supplies, 143–144
Human immunodeficiency virus. *See*
 AIDS/HIV infection

IBM-compatible computers, 107
ICD-9-CM, 56, 279–283, 309(b)
 Alphabetic Index, 279–281, **280**
 code structure, 281
 conventions of, 282–283
 E codes, 282
 locating code, 282(p)
 new revision of, 283
 Tabular List, 279, **280**, 282–283, 282(t)
 V codes, 282
Icons, 107, **107**
Identification line, of business letter,
 122, 124
Illiteracy, communication and, 44
Illnesses. *See also* Diseases and disorders
 cultural differences in view of, 70(b)
Immunization. *See also* Vaccinations
 procedure codes, 286
Immunocompromised patients, 238
Implied contract, 40, 41
Inactive files, 187
Incidental supplies, 143
Income, statement of, 331
Income tax
 as payroll deduction, 334
 submitting federal, 338

Incoming calls
 managing, 198–200
 types of, 200–202
Indexing, in filing process, 184–185
Infectious waste, 231–232. *See also*
  Biohazardous waste
Information. *See also* Patient information
 privacy of health information, 51–53
Information packet, patient. *See* Patient
 information packets
Information storage devices, care and
 maintenance of, 115
Informed consent
 in patient records, 159, **162**
 for surgery, 249
Injuries, patient education in preventing,
 244, 244–245
Ink-jet printers, 106
Input devices, 103–105
Inside address, **122**, 123–124
Inspection, in filing process, 184
Insurance
 for accounts receivable, 306
 malpractice, 41
 portability of health insurance, 51
Insurance claims, processing, 256–292
 Blue Cross and Blue Shield, 262
 calculating patient charges, 268
 CHAMPVA, 261–262
 claims process, overview, 262–266
 CMS-1500 claim, 269, 271, **272**,
  273(p)–274(p)
 coding, billing, and insurance
  specialist, 309(b)
 communications with patients about
  charges, 268–269
 coordination of benefits, 264, 264(t)
 delivering services to patient, 264–265
 determining payment responsibility,
  297
 determining primary coverage, 264(t)
 electronic claims transmission, 269,
  271, 275(b)
 fee-for-service plans, 258
 fee schedule and charges, 266–269
 generating clean claims, 275–276
 HIPAA claim, 269, 271, 275(b)
 insurance fraud, 288
 insurer's processing and payment,
  265–266
 managed care plans, 258
 Medicaid, 260–261
 Medicare, 258–260, 266
 for members of military, 261–262
 obtaining patient information,
  262–264
 payment methods, 268
 preparing health-care claims, 265
 preparing HIPAA claims, 269, 271
 reviewing insurer's RA and
  payment, 266
 security for, 276
 terminology for, 257–258
 time limits for, 265
 TRICARE, 261–262
 workers' compensation, 262

Insurance fraud, medical coding
 and, 288
Insurance policies, information on, in
 patient information packets, 246
Integrity, of medical assistant, 17
Interactive pagers, 87
Interim room, 230
Internal medicine, 24
Internal Revenue Service (IRS), 191
*International Classification of Diseases,
 Ninth Revision, Clinical
 Modification,* 279–283. *See also*
 ICD-9-CM
International mail, 135
Internet, 110
 doing research on, 110(b)
 medical resources on, 110, 111(t)
Internists, 24
Interpersonal skill, 64–65
Introjection, as defense mechanism, 66
Invasion of privacy, 39
 phone calls and, 43
Inventory, office equipment, 97–98, **98**
Inventory card, 144, **146**
Inventory of medical supplies
 filing system for, 144, 145(p)
 inventory card, 144, **146**
 reorder reminder cards, 144, 146, **147**
 scheduling, 146–147
Inventory reminder kits, 146
Invoices. *See also* Billing
 preparing, 298, **299**
 types of, 121–122
I-pagers, 87
Itinerary, 223

Joint Commission for Accreditation
 of Health Organizations (JCAHO)
 auditing charts for quality of
  treatment, 143
 file equipment, 178
 storing office supplies, 143
Journalizing, 315
Judgment, of medical assistant, 18

Ketone bodies, testing urine for, **48**
Keyboard, 103, 104(b)
Kübler-Ross, Elisabeth, 72

Labels
 for correspondence, 121
 for file folders, 179
 for filing equipment, 178
 storing office supplies and, 143
Laboratories, recycling procedures, 15(b)
Laboratory assistants, 31
Laboratory duties, daily duties of
 medical assistant, 14
Laboratory procedures, procedure codes,
 285–286
Laboratory report, telephone request
 for, 201
Laboratory testing
 high-complexity tests, 48
 moderate-complexity tests, 48
 quality assurance programs for, 48

regulations for, 48
results of, as part of patient
  records, 159
waived tests, 48, **48**
Labor Standards Act, 189
Language. *See* Body language;
  Communication
Laptop computer, 102
Laser printers, 106
Late feed, 304
Lateral files, 178
Laundry, OSHA regulations, 46
Laws, 37–57. *See also* Ethics; Legal
  issues; OSHA regulations
  of agency, 41
  credit and collection, 302, 304, 305(t),
    307–310
  defined, 38
  types of, 39
LCME. *See* Liaison Committee on
  Medical Education (LCME)
Lease agreement, 96, **96**
Leasing, office equipment, 95–96, **96**
Legal documents
  appointment book as, 43
  living will, 44
  patient and, 44
  uniform donor card, 44
Legal issues, 38–44
  administrative duties, 43
  appointment book as legal record,
    212, 214
  communication and, 44
  confidentiality issues, 44, 56–57
  contracts, 39–40
  controlled substances, 43
  courtroom conduct, 41
  effective communication and
    preventing lawsuits, 41
  Health Insurance Portability
    and Accountability Act (HIPAA),
    50–56
  importance of studying, 38
  living will, 44
  malpractice, 40–41
  OSHA regulations and inspections,
    44–47
  patient records, guidelines for, 158
  quality control and assurance, 48
  retention of patient records, 189, 191
  standard of care, 42–43
  terminating care of patient, 41–42
  uniform donor card, 44
Legibility, of patient records, 167
Letterhead paper, 121
Letters. *See also* Correspondence
  business, **122,** 122–124
  collection, 301–302, **303**
  content for, 128
  creating, 132(p)
  folding and inserting, 133–134
  general formatting guidelines for
    letters, 124–125
  preparing envelopes for, 130–133
  signing, 130
  styles for, 125, **126, 127**

of withdrawal from case, 42, **42**
word processing program to create
  form letter, 108(p)
Leukocytes, testing urine for, **48**
Liabilities, in double-entry bookkeeping
  system, 319
Liability insurance, 258
Liable, 41
Liaison Committee on Medical Education
  (LCME), 22
Libel, 39
Libraries, as patient education
  resource, 252
Licensed practical nurses (LPNs), 30
Licensed vocational nurses (LVNs), 30
Lifetime maximum benefit, 257
Lighting, in reception area, 228
Limited checks, 330
Listening skills, 64, **65**
  active, 64, **65**
  passive, 64
Living will, 44
Locum tenens, 223
Love needs, 62

Magazines, 233, 234(b)
Magnetic ink character recognition
  (MICR) code, 321
Magnetic tapes, care and maintenance
  of, 117
Mail. *See also* Correspondence; Letters
  annotating, 137–138
  distributing, 138
  e-mail, 109, 109(b)–110(b)
  equipment and supplies for, 134
  folding and inserting mail, 133–134
  handling drug and product
    samples, 138
  other delivery services, 136–137
  postage meters, **90,** 90–91, 91(p)
  postage scales, 91–92
  posting mail, 92
  preparing envelopes, 130–133, **133**
  preparing outgoing mail, 130–134
  processing, 136(p), 137–138
  recording, 137
  signing letters, 130
  sorting and opening, 136(p), 137
  spotting urgent incoming mail, 137(b)
  tracing, 135
  U.S. Postal Service delivery, 134–136
Mail-order companies, 149
Mainframe computers, 102
Maintenance
  of computers in office, 115
  of office equipment, 96–98
Maintenance contract, office
  equipment, 97
Malfeasance, 40
Malpractice, 40–41
  civil law and, 40–41
  courtroom conduct, 41
  credentialed medical assistants
    and, 8
  defined, 39
  examples of, 40

insurance, 41
  settling suits of, 41
Managed care organizations (MCOs),
  credentialed medical assistants
  and, 8
Managed care plans, 258
  Medicare Managed Care Plans, 260
Manuals
  developing, 77–78
  grammar, 128
  office equipment, 97
  policy and procedures manual as
    communication tool, 76–78, **77**
  for software, 111
Masks, 45
Maslow, Abraham, 62
Massage therapists, 26
Material Safety Data Sheets (MSDS),
  46–47, 151–152
Matrix, 211–212, **213**
Maximum allowed fee, 268
Maximum charge, 268
Mechanical errors, in correspondences,
  128
Medicaid, 260–261
  accepting assignment, 260
  assistance provided by, 260
  Medi/Medi, 260
  patients covered by, 260
  state guidelines for, 260–261
  time limits for filing claims, 265
Medical Assistant, 95
Medical assistant clinical station,
  Security Rule of HIPAA, 54
Medical assistant profession
  growth of, 7–8
  history of, 7
  importance of credentials, 8–9
  membership in medical assisting
    association, 9–10
  multiskill training, 11, 13
  training programs and learning
    opportunities, 10
Medical assistants
  certification of, 8–9
  contracts for, 342
  daily duties of, 14–15
  on-the-job rights of, 18
  personal qualifications of, 15–18
  Medical assistant's role, preoperative
    patient education, 249–250, 250(p)
Medical bag, stocking, **222,** 222–223
Medical boards, 22
Medical brochures in reception area, 234
Medical coder, physician practice, 289(b)
Medical coding, 265
  avoiding fraud, 287–289
  code linkage, 288
  compliance plans, 288–289
  diagnosis codes, 279–283
  HCPCS, 286–287
  procedure codes, 283–286
Medical-Dental-Hospital Bureaus of
  America, 306(b)
Medical dictionary, 125, 128
Medical Economics, 95

Medical emergencies
scheduling emergency appointments, 219, 219(b)
symptoms that require immediate medical help, 202, **202**, 203(p)
telephone calls that require immediate medical help, 202, **202**, 203(p)
Medical Group Management Association, 27(b)
Medical history, patient, as part of patient records, 159, **161**
Medical laboratory technician (MLT), 28
Medical law, 38–44
Medical office. *See also* Reception area, patient
contact information cards, 228
humanizing communication process in, 62
office access, 232
recycling procedures, 15(b)
safety and security, 232–233
Medical office administrator, 27(b)
Medical records, legal importance of, 43
Medical records management. *See* Records management system
Medical records technologists, 26, 28, 191(b)–192(b)
Medical secretary, 28
Medical specialties, 22
Medical technologists, 28
Medical technology, 28
Medical transcription, 169–171, 170(b)
Medical transcriptionist, 28, 170(b)
Medicare, 258–260
Advance Beneficiary Notice, 269, **270**
CMS-1500 claim, 269, 271, **272,** 273(p)–274(p)
electronic claims transmission, 269, 271, 275(b)
fee schedule, 266
Medicare + Choice Plans, 260
Medicare Managed Care Plans, 260
Medicare Preferred Provider Organization Plan (PPO), 260
Medicare Private Fee-for-Service Plans, 260
Medigap, 260
Original Medicare Plan, 259–260
Part A, 259
Part B, 259
patients covered by, 258
relative value units (RVUs), 294
resource-based relative value scale (RBRVS), 266
time limits for filing claims, 265
Medicare + Choice Plans, 260
Medicare Managed Care Plans, 260
Medicare Preferred Provider Organization Plan (PPO), 260
Medicare Private Fee-for-Service Plans, 260
Medication. *See* Drug(s)
Medigap, 260
Medi/Medi, 260
MEDLINE, 110
Meetings, planning, 223

Memory, computer, 105
Mental health technician, 28
Mentally-impaired patients
communicating with, 71
patient education, 248
Message, in communication circle, 61, **61**
Messages, telephone
documenting calls, 205–206
ensuring correct information, 206
maintaining patient confidentiality, 206
Messengers, 137
MICR. *See* Magnetic ink character recognition (MICR) code
Microcomputers, 102
Microfiche or microfilm, **94,** 94–95
storage of files on, 188
Microprocessor, 105
Military personnel, insurance claims and, 261–262
Minicomputers, 102
Minutes, meeting, 223
Misdemeanor, 39
Misfeasance, 40
Misplaced files, locating, 185–186
Missed appointments, 220
Misspelled words, commonly, **129–130**
Mixed punctuation, 124
MLT. *See* Medical laboratory technician (MLT)
Modeling, 249
Modem, 104–105
Moderate-complexity tests, 48
Modified-block letter style, 125
Modified-wave scheduling, 214, **216**
Modifiers, 285
Money order, 321
Monitor, computer, 106
care and maintenance of, 115
Moral values, 39
Motherboard, 105
Mouse, 103, **105**
MSDS. *See* Material Safety Data Sheets (MSDS)
Multicultural concerns. *See* Cultural differences and considerations
Multimedia software, 105
Multiskilled health-care professional (MSHP), 11, 13
Multiskill training, 11, 13
Multitasking system, 107
Music, in reception area, 228
Mutual agreement extending credit, 310

Names
remembering patient's name on telephone call, 204
rules for alphabetic filing of personal names, 181(t)
Narcotics, storage of, 144
National AIDS Hotline, **251**
National Association of Medical Staff Services, 27(b)
National Board of Medical Examiners (NBME), 8, 22
National Center Institute, **251**

National Childhood Vaccine Injury Act, 189
National Clearinghouse for Alcohol and Drug Information, **251**
National Committee for Clinical Laboratory Standards (NCCLS), 78
National Health Council, 13(b)
National Health Information Center, **251**
National Institutes of Health, on Internet, 110, 111(t)
National Kidney Foundation, **251**
National Library of Medicine, on Internet, 110, 111(t)
National Organization for Rare Disorders (NORD), **251**
National Phlebotomy Association, 29
NBME. *See* National Board of Medical Examiners (NBME)
NCCLS. *See* National Committee for Clinical Laboratory Standards (NCCLS)
Neatness, of patient records, 167
Needles, disposal of, 45
Needs, hierarchy of, 62–63
Negative communication, 63
Negligence
classification of, 40
defined, 39
examples of, 40
four Ds of, 40
Negotiable, 321
Nephrologists, 24
Nephrology, 24
Net earnings, 334
Network, computer, 102, **114**
adding, 113
Neurologists, 24
Neurology, 24
New England Journal of Medicine, on Internet, 111(t)
New patient, procedure coding and, 285
Newsletters, as patient education, 243
Nitrite, testing urine for, **48**
Noise, in communication circle, **61,** 62
Nonassertive aggressive behavior, 67(t)
Nonassertive behavior, 67(t)
Noncompliance, 158
Nonfeasance, 40
Nonprescription drugs. *See* Over-the-counter drugs
Nonverbal communication
eye contact, 64
facial expression, 63–64
personal space, 64
posture, 64
touch, 64
No-shows, 218
Notations, of business letter, **122,** 124
Notebook computer, 102
Notice of Privacy Practices (NPP), 53
patient confidentiality statement, 246–247
Notification, of those at risk for sexually transmitted disease, 55(b)–56(b)
Nuclear medicine, 24
Nuclear medicine technologist, 28

Numbers, rules for writing, 131(t)
Numeric filing system, 181–182
  color coding and, 182–183
Nurse practitioner (NP), 30–31
  telephone calls that can be answered
    by, 199
Nurses, 30–31
Nursing aides, 30
Nursing assistants, 30
Nutritionists, 29

Objective data, in SOAP, 167
Obstetrics and gynecology (OB/GYN), 24
Occupational Health and Safety Act
  (1970), 46–47
Occupational Safety and Health
  Administration (OSHA). See OSHA
  regulations
Occupational therapist, 28
Occupational therapist assistant, 32
Occupational therapy assistant,
  252(b)–253(b)
OCRs. See Optical character readers
  (OCRs)
Odors, removing, 231
Office access, 232, **232**
Office equipment, using and
  maintaining, 83–98. See also
  Computers in office, using
  adding machines and calculators, 90
  backup systems, 97
  check writers, 93
  dictation-transcription equipment,
    92–93, 92(p)
  equipment inventory, 97–98, **98**
  equipment manuals, 97
  evaluating office needs, 95
  fax (facsimile) machines, 87–89
  leasing vs. buying equipment, 95–96
  mailing, 134
  maintenance of, 96–98
  maintenance/service contracts, 97
  microfilm and microfiche readers, **94,**
    94–95
  pagers (beepers), 87
  paper shredders, **93,** 93–94
  photocopiers, 89–90
  postage meters, **90,** 90–91, 91(p)
  postage scales, 91–92
  purchasing decisions, 95–96
  telephone systems, 85–87
  for transcription, 171
  troubleshooting, 97
  typewriters, 89
  warranty, 95
Office hours, 246
Office medical records. See Records
  management system
Office policies and procedures, in patient
  information packets, 245–247
Office supplies, 140–155
  administrative, 141, **142,** 143
  budget for, 147
  categorizing, 141–143
  clinical, 141, **142,** 143–144
  controlling expenses for, 328–329

disbursements for, 328–329
efficiency in, 141
inventory process, 144–147, 145(p)
list of typical, **142**
Material Safety Data Sheet (MSDS),
  151–152
ordering, **147,** 147–153, **148,** 150(b),
  152, 153
organizing, 141–144
storing, 143–144
Office tips
  choosing collection agency, 306(b)
  data elements for HIPAA electronic
    claims, 275(b)
  evaluating filing system, 187(b)
  ordering supplies by telephone, fax or
    online, 150(b)
  recycling procedures, 15(b)
  routing calls through automated
    menu, 86b
  scheduling emergency appointments,
    219, 219(b)
  spotting urgent incoming mail, 137(b)
  for talking with older patients, 164(b)
Office work. See Correspondence; Mail;
  Office equipment, using and
  maintaining; Office supplies; Patient
  records; Records management system
Older Americans Act of 1965, 237–238
Oncologists, 23, 24
Oncology, 24
One-write system, 320
Online services, 109
  choosing, 109(b)
  doing research, 110(b)
  on-line help for computer software,
    111, **113**
  ordering office supplies by, 150(b)
  sending and receiving e-mail,
    109(b)–110(b)
Open-book account, 301
Open fracture, 474(t)
Open-hours scheduling, 214
Openness, in communication, 65
Open posture, 64
Open punctuation, 124
Operating room, reserving, 222
Operating system, 106–107
Operative reports, in patient records, 159
Ophthalmic assistant, 32
Ophthalmologist, 24
Ophthalmology, 24
Optical character readers (OCRs),
  130, 132
Optometrist, 24
Order forms, 151
Ordering office supplies, 146–153
  ahead of schedule, 146
  common purchasing mistakes,
    avoiding, 153
  competitive pricing and quality, 149
  establishing ordering times, 146
  local vendors, benefits of using,
    149, 151
  locating and evaluating vendors,
    147–149

payment schedules for, 151
  procedures for, 151–153
  by telephone, fax or online, 150(b)
  unanticipated shortage of supply
    item, 147
Organizational chart, 77
Original Medicare Plan, 259–260
Orthopedics, 24–25
Orthopedist, 24–25
OSHA regulations, 44–47
  Blood-borne Pathogens Standard, 44
  cleaning medical office, 232
  decontamination, 45
  documentation, 47
  exposure incidents, 45–46
  general regulations, 47
  hazardous materials, 46–47
  HBV vaccination for health-care
    workers, 46
  importance of, 44–45
  inspections, 47
  laundry, 46
  postexposure procedures, 46
  protective gear, 45, **45**
  sharp equipment, 45
  training requirements, 47
Osteopathic manipulative medicine
  (OMM), 23
Osteopathy, doctor of, 23
Otorhinolaryngologists, 25
Otorhinolaryngology, 25
Outgoing calls, placing, 206–207
Out guide, 180
Output devices, computer, 106
Overbooking, 222
Overnight mail, 137(b)
Over-the-counter drugs, patient
  education on, 244–245
Ovulation tests, **48**
Owner equity, in double-entry
  bookkeeping system, 319

PA. See Physician Assistant (PA)
Pagers (beepers), 87
Palmtop computer, 103
Paper
  for fax machines, 87–88
  letterhead, 121
  for photocopiers, 89
Paper shredders, **93,** 93–94
Paper storage of files, 188
Paramedics, 31–32
Parcel post, 134
Parents, communicating with, 72
Parking arrangements, 232
Participating physicians, 258
Participatory preoperative teaching, 249
Pascal, Blaise, 102
Passive listening, 64
Passwords, 114
  selecting, 276
Pathogens, 44. See also Blood-borne
  pathogens
Pathologists, 25
Pathologist's assistant, 32
Pathology, 25

Patient
  appointments for new, 218
  client's words in charting, 164
  communicating with, 60–61
  communication with, 67–73
  notification of Privacy Rule of
    HIPAA, 53
  telephone calls from, 200–202
Patient confidentiality statement,
  246–247
Patient education, 240–254
  additional resources for, **251,** 252
  developing patient education plan,
    242(p)
  for elderly patients, 247–248, **248**
  for hearing impaired patients, 248,
    248(b)
  importance of, 241–242
  on injury prevention, **244,** 244–245
  for mentally impaired patients, 248
  patient information packet, 234,
    245–247
  patient records and, 158
  preoperative, 249–250, 250(p)
  printed materials for, 242–243
  promoting good health through,
    243–245
  for special needs patients, 247–249
  telephone triage and, 207–208
  for visually impaired patients, 248–249
  visual materials for, 243
Patient information
  disclosure, 52–53
  managing and storing, 52
  obtaining, to schedule
    appointments, 212
  obtaining to file insurance claim,
    262–264
  protected health information, 51–52
  rules for improper release of, 56–57
  Security Rule of HIPAA, 53–54
  treatment, payment and operations
    (TPO), 52–53
Patient information packets, 245–247
  benefits of, 245
  contents of, 245–247
  distribution of, 247
  in reception area, 234
  special concerns, 247
Patient ledger cards
  age analysis and, 302
  information on, 315, **316**
  as invoice, 298
  outside collection agencies and, 305
  in single-entry bookkeeping
    system, 315
Patient medical history. *See* Medical
  history, patient
Patient reception area. *See* Reception
  area, patient
Patient records, 156–175. *See also*
  Records management system
  accuracy of, 167
  additional use of, 158
  appearance of, 167
  chart security in HIPAA, 53–54

computer records of, 169
confidentiality of, 165, 173–174
contents of, 159–163, **160–162**
convention, records, 165
correcting, 171, 172(p)
dating and initialing, 162–163
diagnosis and treatment plans, 159
examination results, 159, **161**
importance of, 158
information received by fax, 162
informed consent, 159, **162**
initiating and maintaining, 163–164
laboratory results, 159
legal guidelines for, 158
medical history, 159, **161**
medical transcription, 169–171, 170(b)
noncompliance and, 158
from other physicians or hospitals, 159
patient registration form, 159, **160**
problem-oriented medical records
  (POMR), 165–167
professional attitude and tone in, 169
release of records, 173
six C's of charting, 164–165
SOAP, 167, **168**
standards for, 158
timeliness of, 167
tips for talking with older patients,
  164(b)
types of, 165–167
updating, 171, 172(p)–173(p)
Patient registration form, 159, **160**
Patient resource rooms, 252
Patient's Bill of Rights, 50
Paychecks, preparing, 334–335
Payer, 321
Payment, procedure
  accepting payment, 296–297, **297**
  determining appropriate fees, 294
  determining payment responsibility,
    297–298
  pegboard system for posting
    payments, 297, 320
  processing charge slips, 294, **295,** 296
Payment policies
  information on, in patient information
    packets, 246
  for office supplies, 151
Payroll, 331–338
  applying for tax identification
    number, 331
  calculating net earning, 334
  creating employee payroll information
    sheets, 331–332
  electronic handling of, 335,
    335(b), 338
  generating, 337(p)
  gross earnings, 332, 334
  maintaining employee earnings
    records, 335, **336**
  maintaining payroll register, 335, **337**
  making deductions, 334
  overview of duties for, 332(t)
  preparing paychecks, 334–335
Payroll information sheet, 331–332
Payroll register, 335, **337**

Payroll schedule, 333
Payroll type, 332
Pediatrician, 25
Pediatric medical assistant, 32
Pediatrics, 25
Pegboard system, 320
  writing checks, 329
Pegboard system for, 297
Periodic supplies, 143
Personal computers, 102–103
Personality, burnout and, 75
Personal space, 64
Petty cash fund, 330–331
pH, testing urine for, **48**
Pharmaceutical sales representatives,
  scheduling appointments
    for, 223
Pharmacist, 28–29
Pharmacy, doctor of (PharmD), 29
Pharmacy technician, 29, 32–33
Philosophy, office, 245
Phlebotomist, 29
Phoenix Phenomenon, 76
Phone calls. *See* Telephone techniques
Photocopiers, 89–90
Physiatrists, 25
Physical medicine, 25
Physical therapist (PT), 29
Physical therapy assistant (PTA), 33
Physician assistant (PA), 29
  telephone calls that can be answered
    by, 199
Physicians
  calls from other, 202
  code of ethics and, 49–50
  education and licensure of, 22
  information on qualifications
    in patient information packet,
    245–246
  maintaining physician's schedule,
    222–223, **224**
  scheduling situations of, 220–221
  substitute, 223
  telephone call's requiring attention
    from, 199
*Physicians' Current Procedural
  Terminology,* 309(b)
Physicians' Desk Reference (PDR), 128
Physician's public duty, 43
Physician's services, 264–265
Physiological needs, 62
Plan of action, in SOAP, 167
Plastic surgeon, 25
Plastic surgery, 25
Plural words, rules for writing, 131(t)
Pointing device, computer, 103–104
Poisons, storage of, 144
Policies, manuals and communicating,
  76–77, **77**
Portability, health-care, 51
Portfolio, 11
Positive communication, 63, 73–74
Possessive words, rules for
  writing, 131(t)
Postage meters, **90,** 90–91, 91(p)
Postage scales, 91–92

Postexposure procedures, OSHA regulations, 46
Post operative care, malpractice and, 40
Posture
  as body language, 64
  carpal tunnel syndrome and, 104(b)
  closed, 64
  open, 64
Power of attorney, 321
Practitioners, 7
Preferred provider organizations (PPO), 258, **259**
  Medicare Preferred Provider Organization Plan (PPO), 260
Pregnancy tests, **48**
Premium, 257
Preoperative education/instructions, 249–250, 250(p)
Prescriptions
  ethics and filling, 49
  renewals, 201
President's Council on Physical Fitness and Sports, **251**
Prevention, patient education in, 245
Prices
  comparing vendors for, 147, 149
  unit, 149
Primary care physicians, 22–23
Printers, 106, **106**
  care and maintenance of, 115
  types of, 106
Priority mail, 134
Privacy
  invasion of, 39
  leaving messages on answering/fax machines, 85, 88
  Notice of Privacy Practices (NPP), 53
  patient confidentiality statement, 246–247
  Privacy Rule of HIPAA, 51–53
  in reception area, 230
  right to, 50
  of those at risk for sexually transmitted disease, 55(b)–56(b)
Privacy Rule of HIPAA, 51–53
  disclosure, 52–53
  Notice of Privacy Practices (NPP), 53
  use, 52
Problem list, in POMR, 165–166
Problem-oriented medical records (POMR), 165–167
Procedure codes, 283–286
  CPT, 283, **284**, 285
  evaluation and management codes (E/M codes), 285
  immunizations, 286
  laboratory procedures, 285–286
  superbill, 285, **286**
  surgical procedures, **284**, 285
Procedures
  manuals and communicating, **77**, 77–78
  standard procedure times, 212
Processing devices, computer, 105
Product samples in mail, handling, 138

Profession. *See* Medical assistant profession
Professional associations, 34(t)
  membership in, 9–10, 34–35
Professional courtesy, payments and, 298
Professionalism
  in correspondence, 120
  of medical assistant, 16
  professional attitude and tone in patient records, 169
Profit-and-loss statement, 331
Progress notes, in POMR, 166–167
Progress report, telephone call from patient reporting, 201
Projection, as defense mechanism, 66
Pronunciation, 204
Proofreading, correspondence, 128–130
Protected health information (PHI), 51–52
  managing and storing, 52
  rules for improper release of, 56–57
  treatment, payment and operations (TPO), 52–53
Protective gear, OSHA regulations, 45, **45**
Protein, testing urine for, **48**
Psychiatric aide, 28
Public Law 95-109, 302, 305(t)
Punctuation style, 124
Puncture exposure incident, 45–46
Purchase order, 151, **152**
Purchase requisitions, 151
Purchasing. *See also* Ordering office supplies
  file supplies, 180
  filing equipment, 179
  office equipment, 95–96
Purchasing groups, 149

Qi, 26
Quality control and assurance programs, 48
  elements of programs for, 48
  laboratory testing, 48
Quarterly return, 338

Radiation therapy technologist, 33
Radiographer, 29
Radiologic technologists, 30
Radiologists, 25
Radiology report, telephone request for, 201
Random-access memory (RAM), 105
Rapport, 73, **73**
Rationalization, as defense mechanism, 66
Reading material in reception area, 233–235
Read-only memory (ROM), 105
Recall notices, 218–219
Receipts
  for cash, 296
  summary of, 315, **318**, 319
Receiver, in communication circle, 61, **61**

Reception
  dental office administrator, 116(b)
  medical office administrator, 27(b)
  unit secretary and, 13(b)
Reception area, patient, 226–239
  for children, 230, 235, 236(p)
  decor in, 228–229
  first impressions, 227–230
  furniture, 229–230
  importance of cleanliness, 230–232
  keeping patients occupied and informed, 233–235
  patients with special needs and, 235–238
  physical components of, 232–233
  privacy and, 230
  safety and, 229
  Security Rule of HIPAA, 54
Reception desk or window, 227, **227**
Reconciliation, of bank statements, 323, 326(p)–327(p)
Record keeping. *See* Documentation
Record of office disbursements, in single-entry bookkeeping system, 315
Record page, 144, **146**
Records. *See* Patient records; Records management system
Records and filing
  dental office administrator, 116(b)
  medical office administrator, 27(b)
Records management system, 176–194
  active vs. inactive files, 187
  filing equipment for, 177–179
  filing guidelines, 186
  filing process, 184–187
  filing supplies, 179–180
  filing systems, 180–184
  importance of, 177
  records retention program, 189–191, 190(p)–192(p)
  security, 178–179
  storing files, 187–191
Records retention program, 189–191, 190(p)–192(p)
Recycling procedures, 15(b)
References
  for correspondence, 125, 128
  for job, 11
Referrals
  customer service and, 61
  documentation of, 43
  insurance claims and, 265
  scheduling, 219–220, 221–222
Refrigerator
  OSHA regulations and, 47, **47**
  for supplies storage, 144
Registered dietitians, 29
Registered mail, 135, 137(b)
Registered Medical Assistant (RMA)
  credentials, 9
  examination by, 9
  professional support for, 9–10
Registered nurse, 30
Registered pharmacist (RPh), 29
Registered Records Administrator (RRA), 26, 28

Regression, as defense mechanism, 66
Rehabilitation, as disease prevention, 245
Relative values, 266
Relative value units (RVUs), 294
Release-of-records form, 173
Reminder calls, 218
Reminder mailings, 218
Remittance advice (RA), 266, **267**
Reorder reminder cards, 144, 146, **147**
Reporting, state reporting
    requirements, 43
Repression, as defense mechanism, 66
Requisitions, purchase, 151
Requisition slip, for file, **185**
Research
    CD-ROM technology and, 110, **112**
    medical resources for, on Internet,
        110, 111(t)
    online services and, 110(b)
    patient records and, 158
Residency, 22
Res ipsa loquitur, 40
Resolution
    monitors, 106
    printers, 106
Resource-based relative value scale
    (RBRVS), 266
Respect
    communicating with patients of other
        cultures, 68–69
    in communication, 65
Respiratory therapist, 30
Respiratory therapy technician, 33
Respite care, 259
Respondeat superior, 41
Résumé, example of, **12**
Retention schedule, 189
Return appointments, 218
Return demonstration, 249
Return receipt requested, 135
Rights, of medical assistants, 18
RMA. *See* Registered Medical Assistant
    (RMA)
Role Delineation Chart, 18–19
ROM (Read-only memory), 105
Rotary circular files, 178
Routing list, 199–200, **200**
Routing telephone calls, 198–200, **200**
RRA. *See* Registered Records
    Administrator (RRA)
Rush orders, 149

Safety
    file storage and, 189
    filing equipment, 179
    in medical office, 232–233
    patient education on injury
        prevention, **244,** 244–245
    reception area and, 229
    unit secretary's responsibilities
        for, 13(b)
Safety needs, 62
Salespeople
    handling calls from, 202
    scheduling appointment with
        physicians, 223

Salutation, **122,** 124
Samples, handling drug and product
    samples, 138
Scanner, 105
    computer storage of files using, 188
Scheduling. *See also* Appointments,
    scheduling
    dental office administrator, 116(b)
    inventory and ordering of medical
        supplies, 146–147
Screening
    as disease prevention, 245
    telephone calls, 198, 199(b)
Screen saver, 115
Second-class mail, 134
Secretarial tasks, medical office
    administrator, 27(b)
Security
    activity-monitoring systems, 114
    in computerized office, 114–115
    computerized patient records, 169
    computer viruses, 114–115
    for electronic claims transmission, 276
    for filing equipment, 178–179
    making and storing backup files,
        114, **114**
    in medical office, 232–233
    passwords, 114
    preventing system contamination,
        114–115
    selecting good password, 276
Security Rule of HIPAA, 53–54
    charts, 53–54
    computers, 53
    faxes, 54
    medical assistant clinical station, 54
    reception area, 54
Security systems, 233
Self-actualization, 62–63
Self-motivation, of medical assistant, 16
Seminars, as patient education, 243
Sensitivity, in communication, 65
Sensory preoperative teaching, 249
Sequential order, 180
Servers, online, 109
Service contract, office equipment, 97
Sexual harassment, 18
Sexually transmitted diseases (STDs).
    See also AIDS/HIV infection
    communication and, 44
    notifying those at risk for, 55(b)–56(b)
    telephone technique for notifying
        those at risk for, 55(b)–56(b)
Sharp instruments/equipment, OSHA
    regulations, 45
Signature block, of business letter,
    122, 124
Signs, 166
Simplified letter style, 125, **127**
Single-entry account, 301
Single-entry bookkeeping system, 314–319
Skills
    assertiveness skills, 67, 67(t)
    coding, billing, and insurance
        specialist, 309(b)
    communication, 18

critical thinking skills, 15
    dental office administrator, 116(b)
    interpersonal, 64–65
    listening, 64, **65**
    medical office administrator, 27(b)
    medical record technologist,
        191(b)–192(b)
    medical transcriptionist, 170(b)
    occupational therapy assistant,
        252(b)–253(b)
    therapeutic communication skills,
        65–67
Slander, 39
Smoke detectors, 233
Smoking, in reception area, 231
SOAP charting, 167, **168**
Social Security number, 332(t)
Software, computer
    accounting and billing, 108
    applications, 107
    appointment scheduling, 108
    database management, 108
    defined, 103
    electronic transactions, 109–110
    manuals for, 111
    on-line help, 111
    operating system, 106–107
    research, 110
    selecting, 113
    technical support, 111–112
    training in, 110–112
    word processing, 108, 108(p)
Sorting, filing process, 185
Source, in communication circle, 61, **61**
Source-oriented records, 165
Special delivery, 135, 137(b)
Specialization, 14–15
Special needs, patients with
    patient education, 247–249
    reception area and, 235–238
Specific gravity, urine, **48**
Speech/language pathologist, 33
Speech recognition technology, 117
Spelling
    commonly misspelled words, **129–130**
    spell checkers, 128
Sperm, testing for presence of, 48
Spun microhematocrit, **48**
Stains, cleaning, 230–231
Standardized code sets, 54, 56
Standard of care, 42–43
Standard Precautions, 45
Statements
    for account past due, 302
    financial, 331
    of income and expenses, 331
    types of, 121–122
States, abbreviation for, 123(t)
Statute of limitations, 189, 191
    collection and, 301
Sterile gloves, 45
Sterilization, sharp equipment, 45
Storage
    of files, 185, 187–191
    of office supplies, 143–144, 151
    storage space as cost factor, 151

Storage cabinets, 143
Storage devices, computer, 105–106
Storage facilities, 188–189, **189**
Stream scheduling, 214, **215**
Stress
  causes of, **75**
  management of, 74–75
  preventing burnout, 75–76
  tips for reducing, 75, **75**
Subjective data, in SOAP, 167
Subject line, **122**, 124
Subluxations, 26
Subpoena, 41
Subpoena duces tecum, 41
Subscriber liability, 266
Substitute physician, 223
Substitution, as defense mechanism, 67
Sulfite bond paper, 121
Summary of charges, receipts, and
  disbursements, 315, **318**, 319
Superbill, 285, **286**, 298, **300**, 301(p)
Supercomputers, 102
Superiors, communicating with, 74
Supervision, dental office administrator,
  116(b)
Supplemental files, 183–184
Suppliers, office equipment, and
  contacting, 95
Supplies. *See also* Office supplies
  controlling expenses for, 328–329
  for correspondence, 120–122
  disbursements for, 328–329
  filing, 179–180
  for mail, 134
Supply budget, 147
Supply list, 142–143
Surgeons, 25
Surgeon's assistant, 33
Surgery, 25
  informed consent form, 249
  medical coding, **284**, 285
  patient education before, 249–250,
    250(p)
  reserving operating room, 222
  scheduling and confirming surgery,
    221(p)
Symptoms
  of cancer, 245
  cultural differences in view of, 70(b)
  defined, 166
  telephone call from patient
    reporting, 201
  that require immediate medical help,
    202, **202**, 203(p)
System unit, care and maintenance of, 115

Tabs, file folders, 179
Tabular List, 279, **280**, 282–283, 282(t)
Tape drive, 106
Taxes, calculating and filing
  Employer's Quarterly Federal Tax
    Return, 339, **341**
  federal income and FICA taxes,
    submitting, 338
  federal tax deposit schedules, 338
  FUTA taxes, submitting, 338–339, **340**

making payroll deductions, 334
setting up tax liability accounts, 338
state and local income taxes, 339
Transmittal of Wage and Tax
  Statements (Form W-3), 342, **343**
Wage and Tax Statement (Form W-2),
  339, **342**
Tax liabilities, 334
TAXLINK, 338
Tax Return (Form 940), 338–339, **340**
Teaching, types of preoperative, 249
Technical support, for software, 111–112
Technology. *See* Computers in office,
  using
Telemedicine, 117
Telephone banking, 327(b)
Telephone calls
  automated, 304
  collection, 301–302
  information on, in patient information
    packets, 246
  ordering office supplies by, 150(b)
  in patient records, 159, 167
  telemarketers and, 302, 304
Telephone log, 205
Telephone message pad, 205
Telephone numbers, locating, 206
Telephone personal identification
  number (TPIN), 327(b)
Telephone systems, 85–87
  answering machine, 86
  answering service, 86–87
  answering systems, 206
  automated menu, 86, 86(b)
  backup system for, 97
  cell phones, 97
  I-pagers, 87
  multiple lines, 85
  patient courtesy phone, 85
  voice mail, 86
Telephone techniques, 196–209
  appointment reminder calls, 218
  calls from patients, 200–202
  communication skills for, 197–198
  conference calls, 207
  confidentiality and, 198, 202, 206
  guidelines for managing incoming
    calls, 198
  importance of effective, 197
  leaving messages on answering/fax
    machines, 85
  legal issues, 43
  making a good impression, 204–205
  notifying those at risk for sexually
    transmitted disease, 55(b)–56(b)
  paging physician, 87
  placing outgoing calls, 206–207
  proper etiquette for, 202–205
  putting on hold, 204
  retrieving messages from answering
    service, 206(p)
  routing calls, 198–200, **200**
  screening calls, 198, 199(b)
  symptoms that require immediate
    medical help, 202, **202**, 203(p)
  taking messages, 205–206

telephone voice, 203–204
types of incoming calls, 200–202
Telephone triage, 207–208
Teletype (TTY) device, 237
Television in reception area, 235
Temperature, of reception area, 228
Templates, 122
Terminal illness and patients with
  communicating with, 72
  living wills and, 44
  Medicare definition of, 259
  stages of dying, 72
Terminating care of patient, 41–42
Thermal paper, 87–88
Third-class mail, 134
Third-party check, 321
Third-party liability, 297
Third-party payer, 257
Tickler files
  computerized patient records and, 169
  in records management system, 183
  setting up, 184(p)
Time, standard procedure times, 212
Timeliness of patient records, 167
Time-specified scheduling, 214, **215**
Title I of HIPAA, 51
Title II of HIPAA, 51–56
Title VII of 1964 Civil Rights Act, 18
Tort, 39, 41
Touch
  as body language, 64
  elderly patients and, 72
Touch pad, 103–104
Tower case, 102, **103**
Trackball, 103
Tracking expenses, 330
Training
  medical assisting programs, 10
  OSHA training requirements, 47
Transaction slips, 296
Transcription, 169–171, 170(b)
  dictation-transcription equipment,
    92–93, 92(p)
  from direct dictation, 171
  equipment for, 171
  medical transcriptionist, 170(b)
  from recorded dictation, 170–171
  steps doctors take in, 93
Transmittal of Wage and Tax Statements
  (Form W-3), 332(t), 342, **343**
Travel arrangements, making, 223
Traveler's check, 330
Treatment, payment and operations
  (TPO), 52–53
Treatment plan
  cultural differences in view of, 70(b)
  in patient records, 159
  in POMR, 166
Triage, 31
  telephone, 207–208
Trial balance, 331
TRICARE, 261–262, 297
Troubleshooting, office equipment, 97
Truth in Lending Act (TLA), 305(t),
  307–310, **308**
Type A personality, 76

Type B personality, 76
Typewriters, 89

Underbooking, 222
Unemployment tax, as payroll
  deduction, 334
Uniform Anatomical Gift Act, 44
Uniform donor card, 44
Unilateral decision extending
  credit, 310
United Parcel Service (UPS), 136
Unit price, 149
Unit secretary, 13(b)
Universal Precautions, OSHA regulations
  and, 45
Updating patient records, 171,
  172(p)–173(p)
Urobilinogen, testing urine for, **48**
Urologist, 25
Urology, 25
U.S. Department of Health, Education,
  and Welfare, 7
U.S. Department of Health and Human
  Services, on Internet, 111(t)
U.S. Medical Licensing Examination
  (USMLE), 22
U.S. Postal Service, 134–136
  abbreviations for states, 133(t)
  international mail, 135
  regular mail service, 134–135
  special postal service, 135
  tracing mail, 135, **135**
Use, in Privacy Rule of HIPAA, 52
Usual fees, 294
Utility gloves, 45

Vaccinations, Hepatitis B, 44–45, 46
V codes, 282
Vendors
  benefit of local, 149, 151

disreputable tactics by, 153
locating and evaluating supply
  vendors, 147–149
Vertical file, 178
Videotapes
  as patient education, 243
  in reception area, 235
Virtual Hospital, 110, 111(t)
Viruses, computer, 114–115
Visually-impaired patients, patient
  education, 248–249
Vital supplies, 142–143
Voice
  active, 125
  in correspondence, 125
  passive, 125
  telephone technique and, 203–204
Voice mail, 86
Void, 40
Voiding check, 93
Voluntary deductions, 333
Volunteer programs, 11
Voucher checks, 329

Wage and Tax Statement (Form W-2),
  339, **342**
Waived tests, 48, **48**
Walk-ins, 220
Warmth, in communication, 65
Warranty, office equipment, 95
Waste
  infectious, 231–232
  recycling procedures, 15(b)
Weed, Lawrence L., 165
W-4 Form, 332, **333**
White-coat syndrome, 68
Williams, Maxine, 8
Willingness to learn, 16
Windows 2000, 107, **107**
Windows, Microsoft, 107

Withdrawal from a case, 41–42
  letter of, 42, **42**
Word division, rules of, 131(t)
Word processor, 108
  software to create form letter,
    108(p)
  spell checkers, 128
  vs. typewriter, 89
Work, preventing injury at, **244**
Workers' compensation, 262
  as payroll deduction, 334
Workplace settings
  coding, billing, and insurance
    specialist, 309(b)
  conflict in and communication, 73
  dental office administrator, 116(b)
  medical office administrator, 27(b)
  medical record technologist,
    192(b)
  medical transcriptionist, 170(b)
  occupational therapy assistant,
    253(b)
  of unit secretary, 13(b)
World Health Organization (WHO),
  309(b)
Written-contract account, 301
Written correspondence, 122–130
  basic rules of writing, 131(t)
  business letter, **122,** 122–124
  editing and proofing, 125–130
  effective writing for, 125
  general formatting guidelines for
    letters, 124–125
  letter styles, 125, **126, 127**
  punctuation style, 124
  reference books for, 125, 128

X12 837 Health Care Claim, 269, 271,
  275(b)
X-ray technician, 29